CONGRESSIONAL POLICIES, PRACTICES AND PROCEDURES

TOP 10 REPORTS AND TESTIMONIES IN DECEMBER 2018

Congressional Policies, Practices and Procedures

Additional books and e-books in this series can be found on Nova's website under the Series tab.

CONGRESSIONAL POLICIES, PRACTICES AND PROCEDURES

TOP 10 REPORTS AND TESTIMONIES IN DECEMBER 2018

SARAH J. NYGAARD
EDITOR

snova
New York

Library of Congress Cataloging-in-Publication Data

ISBN: 978-1-53615-507-5

Published by Nova Science Publishers, Inc. † New York

CONTENTS

Preface		**vii**
Chapter 1	2017 Disaster Contracting: Action Needed to Better Ensure More Effective Use and Management of Advance Contracts *United States Government Accountability Office*	**1**
Chapter 2	2020 Census: Additional Steps Needed to Finalize Readiness for Peak Field Operations *United States Government Accountability Office*	**49**
Chapter 3	Critical Infrastructure Protection: Actions Needed to Address Significant Weaknesses in TSA's Pipeline Security Program Management *United States Government Accountability Office*	**73**
Chapter 4	Improper Payments: Additional Guidance Needed to Improve Oversight of Agencies with Noncompliant Programs *United States Government Accountability Office*	**137**
Chapter 5	Information Security: Agencies Need to Improve Implementation of Federal Approach to Securing Systems and Protecting against Intrusions *United States Government Accountability Office*	**177**
Chapter 6	National Security: Long-Range Emerging Threats Facing the United States As Identified by Federal Agencies *United States Government Accountability Office*	**235**
Chapter 7	Navy and Marine Corps: Rebuilding Ship, Submarine, and Aviation Readiness Will Require Time and Sustained Management Attention *John H. Pendleton*	**255**
Chapter 8	State and Local Governments' Fiscal Outlook: 2018 Update *United States Government Accountability Office*	**289**
Chapter 9	VA Health Care: Improvements Needed in Suicide Prevention Media Outreach Campaign Oversight and Evaluation *United States Government Accountability Office*	**329**

Chapter 10 Working Children: Federal Injury Data and Compliance Strategies Could Be Strengthened **351**
United States Government Accountability Office

Index **423**

Related Nova Publications **433**

PREFACE

This book is a compilation of significant reports and testimonies issued in December 2018.

Chapter 1 - Following Hurricane Katrina, Congress required FEMA to establish advance contracts for goods and services to enable the government to quickly and effectively mobilize resources in the aftermath of a disaster, like those that affected the United States in 2017. GAO was asked to review the federal government's response to the three 2017 hurricanes and California wildfires. This chapter assesses, among other things, (1) FEMA and USACE's use of advance contracts, (2) FEMA's planning and reporting of selected advance contracts, and (3) challenges, if any, with FEMA's use of these contracts. GAO analyzed data from the Federal Procurement Data System-Next Generation through May 31, 2018; selected a non-generalizable sample of 14 FEMA and USACE advance contracts that were competed and obligated over $50 million, or non-competed and obligated over $10 million, in response to the 2017 disasters; and interviewed FEMA and USACE officials.

Chapter 2 - The cost of the decennial census has steadily increased over the past several decades, with self-response rates declining over the same period. The largest and costliest operation that the Bureau undertakes, NRFU is the Bureau's attempt to enumerate households not initially self-responding to the census. GAO was asked to review NRFU implementation during the 2018 Census Test as well as the Bureau's overall readiness for peak field operations, which cover the actual enumeration of residents. This chapter examines (1) how peak field operations, including NRFU, were implemented during the test; and (2) the extent to which prior test implementation issues have been addressed. GAO reviewed test planning and training documentation, as well as production and payroll data. At the test site, GAO observed and interviewed enumerators, field supervisors, and managers conducting peak operations.

Chapter 3 - More than 2.7 million miles of pipeline transport and distribute oil, natural gas, and other hazardous products throughout the United States. Interstate pipelines run through remote areas and highly populated urban areas, and are vulnerable to accidents, operating errors, and malicious physical and cyber-based attack or intrusion. The energy sector accounted for 35 percent of the 796 critical infrastructure cyber incidents reported to DHS from 2013 to 2015. Several federal and private entities have roles in pipeline security. TSA is primarily responsible for the oversight of pipeline physical security and cybersecurity. GAO was asked to review TSA's efforts to assess and enhance pipeline security and cybersecurity. This chapter examines, among other objectives: (1) the guidance pipeline operators reported using to address security risks and the extent that TSA ensures its guidelines reflect the current threat environment; (2) the extent that TSA has assessed pipeline systems' security risks; and (3) the extent TSA has assessed its effectiveness in reducing pipeline security risks. GAO analyzed TSA documents, such as its *Pipeline Security Guidelines*; evaluated TSA pipeline risk assessment efforts; and interviewed TSA officials, 10 U.S. pipeline operators—selected based on volume, geography, and material transported— and representatives from five industry associations.

Chapter 4 - Government-wide estimated improper payments totaled almost $1.4 trillion from fiscal year 2003 through fiscal year 2017. IPERA requires IGs to annually assess and report on whether executive branch agencies complied with the six criteria to (1) publish an agency financial report or performance accountability report, (2) conduct program-specific improper payment risk assessments, (3) publish improper payment estimates, (4) publish corrective action plans, (5) publish and meet annual improper payment reduction targets, and (6) report a gross improper payment rate of less than 10 percent. This chapter examines the extent to which

1. CFO Act agencies complied with IPERA criteria for fiscal years 2016 and 2017, and the trends evident since 2011, as reported by their IGs;
2. CFO Act agencies addressed requirements for programs reported as noncompliant with IPERA criteria for 3 or more consecutive years, as of fiscal year 2016, and communicated their strategies to Congress for reducing improper payments and achieving compliance; and
3. OMB made determinations regarding whether additional funding would help CFO Act agency programs reported as noncompliant with IPERA criteria for 2 consecutive years, as of fiscal years 2016 and 2017, come into compliance.

GAO analyzed the IGs' fiscal years 2016 and 2017 IPERA compliance reports; reviewed prior GAO reports on agencies' IPERA compliance; reviewed agency information submitted to Congress; and made inquiries to OMB, applicable agencies, and IGs; and assessed such information based on relevant IPERA provisions and OMB and other guidance.

Chapter 5 - Federal agencies are dependent on information systems to carry out operations. The risks to these systems are increasing as security threats evolve and become more sophisticated. To reduce the risk of a successful cyberattack, agencies can deploy intrusion detection and prevention capabilities on their networks and systems. GAO first designated federal information security as a government-wide high-risk area in 1997. In 2015, GAO expanded this area to include protecting the privacy of personally identifiable information. Most recently, in September 2018, GAO updated the area to identify 10 critical actions that the federal government and other entities need to take to address major cybersecurity challenges. The federal approach and strategy for securing information systems is grounded in the provisions of the *Federal Information Security*

Modernization Act of 2014 and Executive Order 13800. The act requires agencies to develop, document, and implement an agency-wide program to secure their information systems. The Executive Order, issued in May 2017, directs agencies to use the National Institute of Standards and Technology's cybersecurity framework to manage cybersecurity risks. The *Federal Cybersecurity Enhancement Act of 2015* contained a provision for GAO to report on the effectiveness of the government's approach and strategy for securing its systems. GAO determined (1) the reported effectiveness of agencies' implementation of the government's approach and strategy; (2) the extent to which DHS and OMB have taken steps to facilitate the use of intrusion detection and prevention capabilities to secure federal systems; and (3) the extent to which agencies reported implementing capabilities to detect and prevent intrusions. To address these objectives, GAO analyzed OMB reports related to agencies' information security practices including OMB's annual report to Congress for fiscal year 2017. GAO also analyzed and summarized agency-reported security performance metrics and IG-reported information for the 23 civilian CFO Act agencies. In addition, GAO evaluated plans, reports, and other documents related to DHS intrusion detection and prevention programs, and interviewed OMB, DHS, and agency officials.

Chapter 6 - The United States faces a complex array of threats to our national security, including our political, economic, military, and social systems. These threats will continue to evolve as new and resurgent adversaries develop politically and militarily, as weapons and technology advance, and as environmental and demographic changes occur. A House committee report accompanying a bill for the National Defense Authorization Act for Fiscal Year 2018 included a provision for GAO to identify emerging threats of high national security consequence. This chapter focuses on long-range emerging threats—those that may occur in approximately 5 or more years, or those that may occur during an unknown timeframe—as identified by various respondents at the Department of Defense (DOD), Department of State (State), Department of Homeland Security (DHS), and the Office of the Director of National Intelligence (ODNI). To identify long-range emerging threats, GAO administered a questionnaire to 45 government organizations that assess emerging threats across DOD, State, DHS, and ODNI, and had a 78-percent response rate. GAO conducted a content analysis of the responses to identify specific threats and develop broad threat categories. To supplement the data from the questionnaire, GAO reviewed national security strategies and agency documents provided by DOD, State, DHS, and ODNI, and interviewed key agency officials. This chapter is a public version of a classified report that GAO issued on September 28, 2018. Information that DOD deemed classified and sensitive has been omitted.

Chapter 7 - The 2018 National Defense Strategy emphasizes that restoring and retaining readiness is critical to success in the emerging security environment. The Navy and Marine Corps are working to rebuild the readiness of their forces while growing and modernizing their aging fleet of ships and aircraft. However, achieving readiness recovery goals will take years as both services continue to be challenged to rebuild readiness amid continued operational demands. This statement provides information on current and future readiness challenges facing (1) the Navy ship and submarine fleet and

(2) Navy and Marine Corps aviation. GAO also discusses prior recommendations on Navy and Marine Corps readiness and progress to address them. This statement is based on previously published work since 2015 related to Navy and Marine Corps readiness challenges, including shipyard workforce and capital investment, ship crewing, weapon system sustainment, the fighter pilot workforce, and modernizing force structure. GAO conducted site visits to the Pacific fleet in November 2018 and analyzed updated data, as appropriate.

Chapter 8 - Fiscal sustainability presents a national challenge shared by all levels of government. Since 2007, GAO has published simulations of long-term fiscal trends in the state and local government sector, which have consistently shown that the sector faces long-term fiscal pressures. While most states have requirements related to balancing their budgets, deficits can arise because the planned annual revenues are not generated at the expected rate, demand for services exceeds planned expenditures, or both, resulting in a near-term operating deficit. This chapter updates GAO's state and local fiscal model to simulate the fiscal outlook for the state and local government sector. This includes identifying the components of state and local expenditures likely to contribute to the sector's fiscal pressures. In addition, this chapter identifies considerations related to federal policy and other factors that could contribute to uncertainties in the state and local government sector's long-term fiscal outlook. GAO's model uses the Bureau of Economic Analysis's National Income and Product Accounts as the primary data source and presents the results in the aggregate for the state and local sector as a whole. The model shows the level of receipts and expenditures for the sector until 2067, based on current and historical spending and revenue patterns. In addition, the model assumes that the current set of policies in place across state and local government remains constant to show a simulated long-term outlook.

Chapter 9 - Veterans suffer a disproportionately higher rate of suicide than the civilian population. VA has estimated that an average of 20 veterans die by suicide per day, and in 2018, VA identified suicide prevention as its highest clinical priority. VHA's suicide prevention media outreach campaign—its collective suicide prevention outreach activities—helps raise awareness among veterans and others in the community about suicide prevention resources. VHA has contracted with an outside vendor to develop suicide prevention media outreach content. GAO was asked to examine VHA's suicide prevention media outreach campaign. This chapter examines the extent to which VHA (1) conducts activities for its suicide prevention media outreach campaign, and (2) evaluates the effectiveness of its campaign. GAO reviewed relevant VHA documents and data on the amount, type, and cost of suicide prevention outreach activities since fiscal year 2013. GAO also reviewed VHA's contract for developing suicide prevention outreach content and interviewed VA and VHA officials.

Chapter 10 - Children aged 17 and under in the United States work for various reasons: some are encouraged to work to develop independence and responsibility; others work because of financial need. At the same time, research suggests working children are at risk for work-related injuries and fatalities. GAO was asked to update its 2002 child labor report to discuss the current status of working children in the United States, including those working in agriculture. This chapter examines (1) children working in the

United States since 2003, (2) work-related fatalities and injuries to such children for the period, and (3) how DOL oversees compliance with the child labor provisions of the Fair Labor Standards Act. GAO analyzed federal data from several sources, including DOL and other agencies; reviewed relevant federal laws and regulations; and interviewed officials from DOL, including staff in six WHD district offices that were selected based on factors such as investigations with at least one child labor violation, and all five regional offices. GAO also spoke with stakeholders knowledgeable about child labor, such as employer and employee labor groups.

In: Top 10 Reports and Testimonies in December 2018 ISBN: 978-1-53615-507-5
Editor: Sarah J. Nygaard

Chapter 1

2017 Disaster Contracting: Action Needed to Better Ensure More Effective Use and Management of Advance Contracts*

United States Government Accountability Office

Abbreviations

DOD	Department of Defense
DHS	Department of Homeland Security
FAR	Federal Acquisition Regulation
FEMA	Federal Emergency Management Agency
FPDS-NG	Federal Procurement Data System-Next Generation
IASC	Individual Assistance Support Contract
IA-TAC	Individual Assistance-Technical Assistance Contract
LOGHOUSE	Logistics Housing Operations Unit Installation, Maintenance, and Deactivation Contracts
MAPS	Master Acquisition Planning Schedule
PA-TAC	Public Assistance-Technical Assistance Contract
PKEMRA	Post-Katrina Emergency Management Reform Act of 2006
USACE	U.S. Army Corps of Engineers

Why GAO Did This Study

Following Hurricane Katrina, Congress required FEMA to establish advance contracts for goods and services to enable the government to quickly and effectively mobilize resources in the aftermath of a disaster, like those that affected the United States in 2017.

* This is an edited, reformatted and augmented version of United States Government Accountability Office; Report to Congressional Requesters, Publication No. GAO-19-93, dated December 2018.

GAO was asked to review the federal government's response to the three 2017 hurricanes and California wildfires. This chapter assesses, among other things, (1) FEMA and USACE's use of advance contracts, (2) FEMA's planning and reporting of selected advance contracts, and (3) challenges, if any, with FEMA's use of these contracts.

GAO analyzed data from the Federal Procurement Data System-Next Generation through May 31, 2018; selected a non-generalizable sample of 14 FEMA and USACE advance contracts that were competed and obligated over $50 million, or non-competed and obligated over $10 million, in response to the 2017 disasters; and interviewed FEMA and USACE officials.

What GAO Recommends

GAO is making nine recommendations to FEMA, including that it update its strategy and guidance to clarify the use of advance contracts, improve the timeliness of its acquisition planning activities, revise its methodology for reporting disaster contracting actions to congressional committees, and provide more consistent guidance and information to contracting officers to coordinate with and encourage states and localities to establish advance contracts. FEMA concurred with our recommendations.

What GAO Found

In response to Hurricanes Harvey, Irma, and Maria, as well as the 2017 California wildfires, the Federal Emergency Management Agency (FEMA) and U.S. Army Corps of Engineers (USACE) relied heavily on advance contracts. As of May 31, 2018, FEMA and USACE obligated about $4.5 billion for various goods and services through these contracts, see figure below.

GAO found limitations in FEMA's use of some advance contracts that provided critical goods and services to survivors, including

- an outdated strategy and unclear guidance on how contracting officers should use advance contracts during a disaster, and
- challenges performing acquisition planning.

FEMA also did not always provide complete information in its reports to congressional committees. Specifically, GAO found 29 advance contract actions that were not included in recent reports due to shortcomings in FEMA's reporting methodology, limiting visibility into its disaster contract spending.

FEMA identified challenges with advance contracts in 2017, including federal coordination with states and localities on their use. FEMA is required to coordinate with states and localities and encourage them to establish their own advance contracts with vendors. However, GAO found inconsistencies in that coordination and the information FEMA uses to coordinate with states and localities on advance contracts. Without consistent information and coordination with FEMA, states and localities may not have the tools needed to establish their own advance contracts for critical goods and services and quickly respond to future disasters.

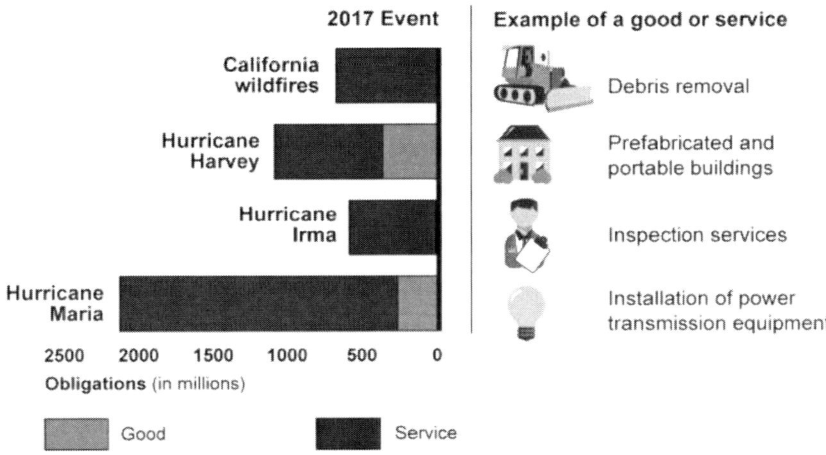

Source: GAO analysis of Federal Procurement Data System-Next Generation data. | GAO-19-93.
Note: Obligations are nominal 2017 and 2018 dollars.

Advance Contract Obligations and Examples of Goods and Services the Federal Emergency Management Agency and U.S. Army Corps of Engineers Used to Respond to the 2017 Disasters.

December 6, 2018
Congressional Requesters

The Post-Katrina Emergency Management Reform Act of 2006 (PKEMRA) required the Federal Emergency Management Agency (FEMA) to establish advance contracts—those that are established prior to disasters and that are typically needed to quickly provide life-sustaining goods and services in the immediate aftermath of disasters.[1] FEMA and the U.S. Army Corps of Engineers (USACE)—components of the Department of Homeland Security (DHS) and the Department of Defense (DOD), respectively—used advance contracts to procure goods and services provided in response to the catastrophic disasters the United States experienced in 2017: Hurricanes Harvey, Irma, and Maria; and the California wildfires.[2]

Contracts play a key role in immediate disaster response and longer-term community recovery. In February 2018, we found that early estimates for Hurricanes Harvey, Irma, and Maria placed them among the costliest hurricanes in terms of federal contract obligations since 2005, when tracking this information by hurricane began.[3] We also found that DHS and DOD accounted for about 97 percent of those obligations. In September 2015, we found

[1] Pub. L. No. 109-295, § 691 (codified at 6 U.S.C. § 791).

[2] Although PKEMRA does not apply to USACE, the agency awards advance contracts as a preparedness measure as part of its Advance Contracting Initiative, a program developed and implemented specifically for emergency and disaster scenarios. For the purposes of this report, we rely on how FEMA and USACE define advance contracts. For FEMA, this includes indefinite delivery contracts and blanket purchase agreements, including those under the Federal Supply Schedule, as well as interagency agreements, and interagency reimbursable work agreements. For USACE this includes indefinite delivery contracts. Obligations against interagency agreements are not included in this report.

[3] GAO, *2017 Disaster Contracting: Observations on Federal Contracting for Response and Recovery Efforts*, GAO-18-335 (Washington D.C.: Feb. 28, 2018).

issues related to the use of advance contracts, specifically that FEMA's contracting officers had limited awareness about advance contract requirements and how to coordinate advance contracting efforts with state and local governments.[4] We made several recommendations, including that FEMA provide guidance to contracting officers to make them aware of current information on the availability and use of advance contracts and the need to conduct outreach to state and local governments to support their use of advance contracts. FEMA agreed with our recommendations and has taken action to address them.

You asked us to review the federal government's contracting efforts for preparedness, response, and recovery efforts related to the three 2017 hurricanes and California wildfires. This chapter specifically addresses the use of advance contracts, assessing the extent to which (1) FEMA and USACE used advance contracts, (2) the planning, management, and reporting of selected FEMA and USACE advance contracts met certain contracting requirements, and (3) FEMA and USACE identified any lessons learned and challenges with their use of these contracts. We also have an ongoing review on post-disaster contracting that is expected to be completed in early 2019.

To identify the extent to which FEMA and USACE used advance contracts, we reviewed data on contract obligations for the 2017 disasters from the Federal Procurement Data System-Next Generation (FPDS-NG) through May 31, 2018.[5] Data on obligations for the California wildfires are limited to contracts that FEMA and USACE identified as being used to respond to the events because some of this information was not able to be identified in FPDS-NG. To determine which obligations were made through the use of advance contracts, we reviewed documentation provided by FEMA and USACE identifying the advance contracts they have in place and that were used in support of the 2017 disasters.[6] We assessed the reliability of FPDS-NG data by reviewing existing information about the FPDS-NG system and the data it collects— specifically, the data dictionary and data validation rules— and performing electronic testing. We determined the FPDS-NG data were sufficiently reliable for the purposes of this chapter. We also reviewed FEMA contracting policies and guidance, to identify available guidance on the use and intent of advance contracts, and federal internal control standards. We identified examples of goods that FEMA had advance contracts in place for but experienced challenges using in response to the 2017 disasters, reviewed advance and post-disaster contract documentation and FPDS-NG data related to these examples, and interviewed contracting officials involved in the award and use of the contracts in 2017.

---

[4] GAO, *Disaster Contracting: FEMA Needs to Cohesively Manage Its Workforce and Fully Address Post-Katrina Reforms*, GAO-15-783 (Washington, D.C.: Sept. 29, 2015).

[5] For the purposes of this report, contract obligations include obligations against what the General Services Administration's Federal Procurement Data System-Next Generation (FPDS-NG) categorizes as definitive vehicles (definitive contracts and purchase orders that have a defined scope of work that do not allow for individual orders under them), and against what FPDS-NG categorizes as indefinite delivery vehicles (orders under the Federal Supply Schedule, orders/calls under blanket purchase agreements, orders under basic ordering agreements, orders under government-wide acquisition contracts, and orders under other indefinite delivery vehicles, such as indefinite delivery, indefinite quantity contracts).

[6] DHS and DOD exercised the use of the special emergency procurement authorities within 41 U.S.C § 1903, as amended by § 816 of the National Defense Authorization Act for Fiscal Year 2017, Pub. L. No. 114-328 (and as implemented by DHS FAR Class Deviation 17-02 and DOD FAR Class Deviation 2017-O0007, respectively) to increase the micro-purchase threshold to $20,000 for procurements in support of these major disaster responses. As a result, contract obligations for hurricanes reported in FPDS-NG may only include obligations over that amount.

To assess the extent to which the planning, management, and reporting of advance contracts used in response to the three hurricanes and California wildfires in 2017 met selected applicable contracting requirements, we reviewed relevant documentation, including PKEMRA, the Federal Acquisition Regulation (FAR), DHS, FEMA, and USACE contracting policies. We identified a non-generalizable sample of advance contracts to serve as case studies based on obligation data from FPDSNG as of March 31, 2018. We analyzed the data to identify 10 competed and 4 non-competed contracts—valued at above $50 million and above $10 million, respectively—including 10 contracts from FEMA and 4 from USACE.[7] For additional details on the contracts we selected, see appendix I. Findings based on information collected from the 14 contracts cannot be generalized to all advance contracts. To review our selected FEMA and USACE advance contracts, we developed a data collection instrument to gather selected contract information, such as period of performance, contract type, estimated contract value, and the presence of key contract documents, among others. To assess planning we reviewed our selected advance contracts, and determined that six of FEMA's contracts met GAO's definition of a bridge contract. We interviewed FEMA officials associated with these contracts on acquisition planning efforts and factors that affected their ability to award new contracts. To assess FEMA and USACE's management of selected advance contracts, we reviewed information gathered from our data collection instrument to confirm the contract files contained required acquisition documents, such as acquisition strategies and contract modifications, which typically provide the history of a contract file, and interviewed officials at FEMA and USACE headquarters on their record keeping policies, practices, and challenges. To assess the reporting of selected advance contracts, we compared advance contract action data identified in FPDS-NG in the fourth quarter of fiscal year 2017 and first quarter of fiscal year 2018 to data reported for the same time period in FEMA's mandated reports to congressional committees on disaster contracting to identify any unreported actions. We interviewed FEMA officials to discuss the methodology and data sources for the congressional committee reports and any limitations to the accuracy of the data reported.

To assess what lessons learned and challenges FEMA and USACE identified with the use of advance contracts in 2017, we interviewed FEMA and USACE officials on what they identified as lessons learned and challenges specific to advance contracts, and any recommendations or actions planned by the agencies to address them. We reviewed PKEMRA advance contract requirements, including requirements that FEMA coordinate with state and local governments on the use of advance contracts, FEMA and USACE documentation on the use of advance contracts, after-action reports from 2017 and prior years, and federal internal control standards for information and communications. To identify challenges related to coordination with state and local officials on the use of advance contracts, we reviewed after action reports from 2017, and interviewed FEMA and USACE regional staff and state and local government officials on advance contracting efforts. We also analyzed information on available advance contracts from FEMA's June 2018 Prepositioned Contract List and FEMA's May 2018 training documentation identifying advance contracts to

[7] For the purposes of selecting our case studies, competitive contracts included contracts and orders coded in FPDS-NG as "full and open competition," "full and open after exclusion of sources," and "competed under simplified acquisition procedures." Noncompetitive contracts included contracts and orders coded in FPDS-NG as "not competed," "not available for competition," and "not competed under simplified acquisition procedures."

identify any differences in the information available to FEMA contracting officers, and their state and local contracting counterparts.[8] Appendix I provides more information about our overall scope and methodology.

We conducted this performance audit from March 2018 to December 2018 in accordance with generally accepted government auditing standards. Those standards require that we plan and perform the audit to obtain sufficient, appropriate evidence to provide a reasonable basis for our findings and conclusions based on our audit objectives. We believe that the evidence obtained provides a reasonable basis for our findings and conclusions based on our audit objectives.

BACKGROUND

The 2017 Hurricanes and California Wildfires

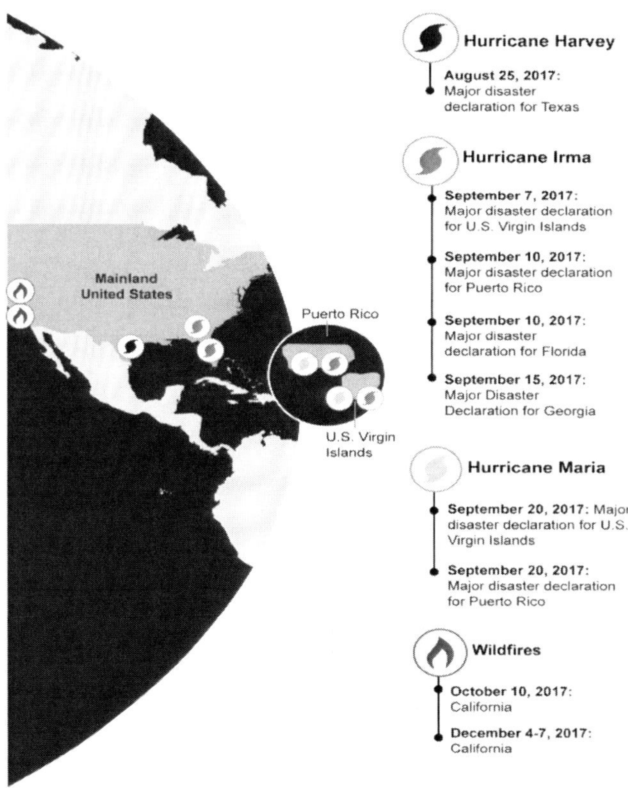

Source: GAO analysis of Federal Emergency Management Agency data. | GAO-19-93.

Figure 1. Timeline of Major 2017 Hurricanes and California Wildfires.

In 2017, three major hurricanes made landfall in the United States and historic wildfires struck California. According to FEMA, the 2017 hurricanes and wildfires collectively

[8] Prepositioned contracts are the same as advance contracts. For the purposes of this report, we use the term advance contracts and refer to FEMA's Prepositioned Contract List as the advance contract list.

affected 47 million people—nearly 15 percent of the nation's population. See Figure 1 for a timeline of these major disasters.[9]

Overview of Federal Disaster Response and Recovery

When disasters hit, state and local entities are typically responsible for disaster response efforts. The Robert T. Stafford Disaster Relief and Emergency Assistance Act established a process by which a state may request a presidential disaster declaration to obtain federal assistance.[10] According to the DHS National Response Framework—a guide to how the federal government, states and localities, and other public and private sector institutions should respond to disasters and emergencies—the Secretary of Homeland Security is responsible for ensuring that federal preparedness actions are coordinated to prevent gaps in the federal government's efforts to respond to all major disasters, among other emergencies.[11] The framework also designates FEMA to lead the coordination of the federal disaster response efforts across federal agencies.

The National Response Framework identifies 14 emergency support functions that serve as the federal government's primary coordinating structure for building, sustaining, and delivering disaster response efforts across more than 30 federal agencies. Each function addresses a specific need—such as communication, transportation, and energy—and designates a federal department or agency as the coordinating agency. For example, the emergency support function for public works and engineering assists DHS by coordinating engineering and construction services, such as temporary roofing or power, and USACE is the primary agency responsible for these functions during disaster response activities.

FEMA coordinates disaster response efforts through mission assignments—work orders that FEMA issues to direct other federal agencies to utilize the authorities and the resources granted to it under federal law. Mission assignments are authorized by the Robert T. Stafford Disaster Relief and Emergency Assistance Act and can consist of federal operations support or direct federal assistance, which includes federal contracts.

FEMA's contracting efforts are supported by its Office of the Chief Procurement Officer and its contracting workforce. While the majority of FEMA's contracting workforce is located in headquarters, contracting officers are also located in each of FEMA's 10 regional offices. See appendix II for the location of FEMA's 10 regional offices as well as the states each one is responsible for coordinating with to address National Response Framework responsibilities.

---

[9] A major disaster is any natural catastrophe (including any hurricane, tornado, storm, high water, wind driven water, tidal wave, tsunami, earthquake, volcanic eruption, landslide, mudslide, snowstorm, or drought), or, regardless of cause, any fire, flood, or explosion, in any part of the United States, which the President determines causes damage of sufficient severity and magnitude to warrant major disaster assistance to supplement the efforts and available resources of states, local governments, and disaster relief organizations in alleviating damage, loss, hardship, or suffering. See 42 U.S.C. § 5122(2).

[10] 42 U.S.C. § 5170. The Robert T. Stafford Disaster Relief and Emergency Assistance Act, as amended, permits the President to declare a major disaster after a state's governor or chief executive of an affected Indian tribal government—a governing body of an Indian or Alaska Native tribe, band, nation, pueblo, village, or community that is federally recognized—finds that the disaster is of such severity and magnitude that effective response is beyond his or her own local capacities.

[11] Department of Homeland Security, *National Response Framework* (June 2016).

PKEMRA Requirements and the Use of Advance Contracts

Congress enacted PKEMRA in 2006, which addressed various shortcomings identified in preparation for and response to Hurricane Katrina, which hit the Gulf Coast in 2005 and was one of the largest, most destructive natural disasters in U.S. history. Among the provisions included were requirements for FEMA to identify and establish advance contracts to ensure that goods and services are in place to help FEMA rapidly mobilize resources in immediate response to disasters. Examples of these goods and services are:

- Goods: construction supplies and tarps; food and water; cleaning and hygiene supplies; and power equipment and generators.
- Services: engineering; information technology and communication support; transportation of goods; and housing and lodging assistance.

As of June 2018, FEMA reported having advance contracts in place for 56 different types of goods and services.

Among other contracting requirements, PKEMRA requires FEMA to

- develop a contracting strategy that maximizes the use of advance contracts to the extent practical and cost effective;
- coordinate advance contracts with state and local governments;
- encourage state and local governments to engage in similar preplanning and contracting; and
- submit quarterly reports to the appropriate committees of Congress on each disaster contract entered into by the agency using noncompetitive procedures.[12]

According to FEMA's advance contracting strategy, the agency will maximize the use of advance contracts to the extent they are practical and cost-effective, which will help preclude the need to procure goods and services under unusual and compelling urgency. When disasters strike, contracting officers may use the unusual and compelling urgency exception to full and open competition to support non-competitive contract awards.[13] FEMA's strategy also states that advance contracts will help to ensure that goods and services are in place to help FEMA rapidly mobilize resources in immediate response to disasters.

USACE also has its own advance contracts in place as a preparedness measure. According to USACE officials, they established advance contract initiatives in 2003, two years prior to Hurricane Katrina, to help facilitate their emergency support function under the National Response Framework—public works and engineering. As of September 2018, USACE reported having advance contracts in place for three services— debris removal,

[12] While PKEMRA only requires FEMA to report on noncompetitive disaster contract actions, the Joint Explanatory Statement that accompanied PKEMRA recommends that FEMA report quarterly on all contracts issued during a disaster.

[13] Department of Homeland Security, Federal Emergency Management Agency, *Advance Contracting of Goods and Services Report to Congress* (December 2007).

temporary roofing, and temporary power. Appendix III provides details on specific advance contracts established by FEMA and USACE.

According to FEMA documentation, most of its advance contracts are indefinite delivery contracts, which can facilitate the goal of having contracts available if there is a disaster.[14] One type of indefinite delivery contract—an indefinite delivery, indefinite quantity contract—can be awarded to single or multiple vendors and provides for an indefinite quantity, within stated limits, of supplies or services during a fixed period. Under these contracts, the government places orders for individual requirements. These contracts also require the government to order and the contractor to provide at least a stated minimum quantity of supplies and services. Additionally, the contracting officer should also establish a reasonable maximum quantity for the contract based on market research, trends in similar recent contracts, or any other rational basis.[15] Minimum and maximum quantity limits can be stated as the number of units or as dollar values, and may also be referred to by contracting officers as minimum guarantees or contract ceilings, respectively.

As part of its overall acquisition strategy, FEMA officials identified other vehicles aside from its own advance contracts through which they obtain goods and services.

- DHS strategic sourcing vehicles: When a disaster occurs, FEMA contracting officers are first required to use any available DHS strategic sourcing vehicles—a broader, aggregate approach for procuring goods and services—with limited exceptions.
- Blanket purchase agreements: FEMA also relies on blanket purchase agreements, such as those established through the General Service Administration Federal Supply Schedule program, to provide some commercial goods and services needed for disaster response.[16]
- Interagency Agreements: FEMA may also leverage interagency agreements, by which it obtains needed supplies or services from another agency by an assisted or direct acquisition.

FEMA and other agencies may also award new contracts to support disaster response efforts following a disaster declaration. According to FEMA officials, these post-disaster contract awards may be required, for example, if advance contracts reach their ceilings, or if goods and services that are not suitable for advance contracts are needed.[17]

---

[14] Indefinite delivery contracts (definite-quantity contracts, requirements contracts, and indefinite quantity contracts) may be used when the exact times or quantities, or both, of future deliveries are not known at the time of contract award. FAR § 16.501-2.

[15] FAR § 16.504.

[16] The General Services Administration Federal Supply Schedule program provides agencies with a simplified way to purchase commercial goods and services. State and local governments are eligible to use these contracts for certain purchases, including those supporting disaster recovery efforts. Blanket purchase agreements are simplified methods of filling anticipated repetitive needs for supplies or services by establishing "charge accounts" with qualified sources of supply. FAR § 13.303-1. Agencies may establish blanket purchase agreements under the General Services Administration's Schedule program contracts. A blanket purchase agreement is not a contract, therefore the government is not obligated to purchase a minimum quantity or dollar amount, and the contractor is not obligated to perform until it accepts an order under a blanket purchase agreement.

[17] We plan to report on post-disaster contracts in a separate, ongoing review.

FAR Requirements

The FAR requires agencies to perform acquisition planning activities for all acquisitions to ensure that the government meets its needs in the most effective, economical, and timely manner possible.[18] Generally, program and contracting officials share responsibility for the majority of acquisition planning activities, which include the following:

- Pre-Solicitation: The program office identifies a need, and develops key acquisition documents to summarize that need, such as market research, a statement of work defining requirements, cost estimates, and a written acquisition plan.[19] The pre-solicitation process ends when the program office submits these documents, typically referred to as an acquisition package, to the contracting officer to determine what type of contract is appropriate to fulfill the requirements.
- Solicitation: The contracting officer develops a solicitation, in consultation with other agency stakeholders, to request bids or proposals from contractors. The acquisition planning process ends once a solicitation is issued.

Contracting for disaster relief and recovery efforts can also present unique circumstances in which to solicit, award, and administer contracts. Under the FAR, agencies are generally required to use full and open competition when soliciting offers and awarding contracts. However, an agency may award contracts noncompetitively when the need for goods or services is of such unusual and compelling urgency that the federal government faces the risk of serious financial or other type of injury.[20]

When it becomes evident that a base contract period and any option periods will expire before a subsequent contract to meet the same need can be awarded, contracting officers may, for example,

- extend the existing contract, or
- award a short-term stand-alone contract to the incumbent contractor on a non-competitive basis to avoid a lapse in services, along with sufficient justification and approval.

---

[18] FAR § 7.102.

[19] According to the FAR, contracting agencies should establish criteria and thresholds at which increasingly greater detail and formality in the acquisition planning process is required as the acquisition becomes more complex and costly. Additionally, the FAR states that a written acquisition plan is required for cost reimbursement and other high risk contracts other than firm-fixed-price contracts, although written plans may be required for firm-fixed-price contracts as appropriate. FAR § 7.103(e).

[20] The FAR does not require agencies to seek full and open competition for contracts awarded using the simplified acquisition procedures (used for contracts that do not exceed the simplified acquisition threshold—generally $150,000 or $7 million when acquiring commercial items), though agencies are required to compete them to the maximum extent practicable. The National Defense Authorization Act for Fiscal Year 2017 raised the simplified acquisition threshold to $250,000. Pub. L. No. 115-91, § 805. In accordance with special emergency procurement authorities, DHS and DOD increased the simplified acquisition threshold for the three 2017 hurricanes to $750,000. DHS and DOD exercised the use of the special emergency procurement authorities within 41 U.S.C. §1903, as amended by §816 of the National Defense Authorization Act for Fiscal Year 2017, Pub. L. No. 114-328 (and as implemented by DHS FAR Class Deviation 17-02 and DOD Class Deviation 2017-O0007, respectively) to increase the simplified acquisition threshold for procurements in support of the three 2017 hurricanes to $750,000.

These extensions and new sole source contracts are informally referred to as bridge contracts by some in the acquisition community, and we use that terminology in this chapter. In October 2015, we established the following definitions related to bridge contracts:

- Bridge contract: An extension to an existing contract beyond the period of performance (including base and option years), and a new, short-term contract awarded on a sole-source basis to an incumbent contractor to avoid a lapse in service caused by a delay in awarding a follow-on contract.[21]
- Predecessor contract: The contract that was in place prior to the award of a bridge contract.
- Follow-on contract: A longer-term contract that follows a bridge contract for the same or similar services. This contract can be competitively awarded or awarded on a sole-source basis.

Contracts, orders, and extensions (both competitive and non-competitive) are included in our definition of a "bridge contract" because the focus of the definition is on the intent of the contract, order, or extension.[22]

However, the FAR does not formally define bridge contracts or require that they be tracked. We recommended that the Office of Federal Procurement Policy amend the FAR to incorporate a definition of bridge contracts. The Office of Federal Procurement Policy agreed with our recommendation to provide guidance to agencies on bridge contracts and has taken steps to develop that guidance, but has not yet implemented our recommendations.[23]

If a contracting officer opts to extend the existing contract in place—often referred to as a predecessor contract—the contracting officer may use a number of different mechanisms to do this. One of these is the "option to extend services" clause. If the contract includes this clause, the contracting officer may use it to extend the contract for up to six months.[24] While this option may be exercised more than once, the total extension of performance shall not exceed 6 months.

---

[21] GAO, *Sole Source Contracting: Defining and Tracking Bridge Contracts Would Help Agencies Manage Their Use*, GAO-16-15 (Washington, D.C.: Oct. 14, 2015).

[22] GAO's definition includes all types of extensions, both those extensions of contracts that may be considered "competitive," e.g., the use of FAR 52.217-8 when it was evaluated at award, and those that are "noncompetitive," e.g., those extensions of requirements that are used to extend the period of performance beyond that of the original contract (and all the options) and require a justification and approval, when the intention is to bridge a gap in services.

[23] The Office of Federal Procurement Policy has not yet taken action on our recommendations. In the National Defense Authorization Act for Fiscal Year 2018 (Pub. L. No. 115-91), Congress established a definition of bridge contracts that is applicable to DOD requirements owners, meaning members of the armed forces (excluding Coast Guard) or a civilian employee of the Department of Defense responsible for a requirement for a service to be performed through a services contract. Specifically, Section 851 defined a bridge contract as (1) an extension to an existing contract beyond the period of performance to avoid a lapse in service caused by a delay in awarding a subsequent contract; or (2) a new short-term contract awarded on a sole-source basis to avoid a lapse in service caused by a delay in awarding a subsequent contract. Section 851 requires that by October 1, 2018, the Secretary of Defense is to ensure that a requirements owner must to the extent practicable, plan appropriately before the date a service is needed to avoid the use of a bridge contract for services. DOD issued a bridge contracts memorandum in January 2018, which defined bridge contracts as modifications to existing contracts to extend the period of performance, increase the contract ceiling or value or both, or a new interim sole-source contract awarded to the same or a new contractor to cover the timeframe between the end of the existing contract and the award of a follow-on contract.

[24] FAR § 17.208(f) provides for the use of the clause cited at FAR § 52.217-8, "Option to Extend Services" in solicitations and contracts for services when the inclusion of an option is appropriate.

FEMA and USACE Relied on Advance Contracts to Respond to the 2017 Disasters, but FEMA Lacks an Updated Advance Contracting Strategy and Guidance

FEMA and USACE obligations on advance contracts—as of May 31, 2018—accounted for about half of total federal contract obligations for the three hurricanes, and more than three quarters of the contract obligations identified by those agencies for the California wildfires. However, an outdated strategy and lack of guidance to contracting officers resulted in confusion about whether and how to prioritize and use advance contracts to quickly mobilize resources in response to the three 2017 hurricanes and the California wildfires.

Advance Contracts Accounted for about Half of Government-Wide Contract Obligations for the 2017 Hurricanes, and over Three-Quarters of FEMA and USACE's Obligations for the California Wildfires

Government-wide contract obligations for the three hurricanes were about $8.2 billion as of May 31, 2018.[25] FEMA and USACE obligated 46 percent, or about $3.8 billion, of the $8.2 billion spent government-wide on the three hurricanes through advance contracts. Data on government-wide contract obligations for the California wildfires were not able to be identified because national interest action codes were not established for them in FPDS-NG.[26] However, FEMA and USACE provided information on their contracting activities related to the wildfires. Their use of advance contracts accounted for 86 percent, or about $667 million, of the contract obligations they identified. FEMA and USACE advance contract obligations for the three hurricanes and California wildfires totaled about $4.5 billion, about 56 percent of the total contract obligations made by these agencies for these disasters. See Figure 2 for details on FEMA and USACE's advance and post-disaster contract obligations by event.

The greatest proportion of FEMA and USACE's obligations on advance contracts supported Hurricane Maria disaster relief efforts—41 percent and 59 percent, respectively. About 39 percent of USACE's obligations on advance contracts were used in support of the California wildfires, compared to less than 1 percent of FEMA's obligations. FEMA awarded orders against 72 base advance contracts in response to the three 2017 hurricanes and California wildfires, and USACE awarded orders against 15 of its advance contracts. See Figure 3 for FEMA and USACE's obligations on advance contracts by event.

---

[25] Federal agencies may continue to contract for goods and services well after a disaster has occurred. For example, federal agencies are still making contract obligations as part of recovery efforts as far back as Hurricanes Sandy and Katrina, which occurred in 2012 and 2005, respectively. In addition to DOD and DHS, the following departments had contract obligations in support of hurricanes Harvey, Irma, and Maria response efforts: the departments of Agriculture, Commerce, Energy, Health and Human Services, Housing and Urban Development, Interior, Justice, Labor, State, Transportation, Treasury, and Veterans Affairs; the Agency for International Development; the Broadcasting Board of Governors; the Corporation for National and Community Service; the Environmental Protection Agency; the Federal Communications Commission; the General Services Administration; the National Aeronautics and Space Administration; the National Archives and Records Administration; the Small Business Administration; and the Social Security Administration.

[26] National interest action codes are used to track certain contracts in support for disaster response and recovery efforts in FPDS-NG. No national interest action code was established for the 2017 California wildfires.

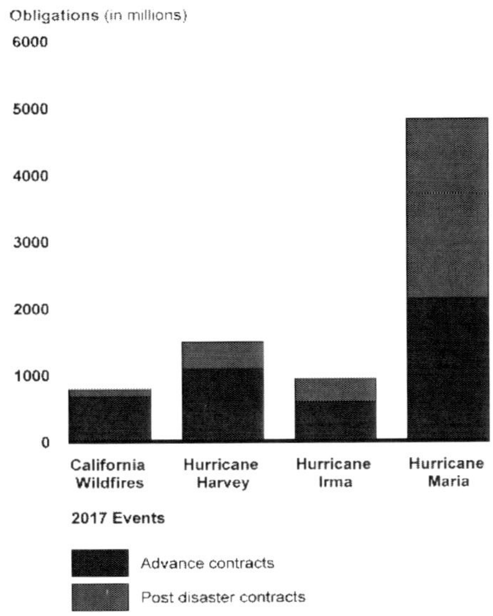

Source: GAO analysis of Federal Procurement Data System-Next Generation data. | GAO-19-93.
Notes: Obligations are nominal 2017 and 2018 dollars.
FEMA officials told us that contracts awarded in support of the U.S. Virgin Islands after Hurricane Maria impacted the islands may all be coded under Hurricane Maria, regardless of whether the contract responds to needs from Hurricane Irma or Hurricane Maria.

Figure 2. Federal Emergency Management Agency (FEMA) and U.S. Army Corps of Engineers Contract Obligations in Response to the Three 2017 Hurricanes and California Wildfires, as of May 31, 2018.

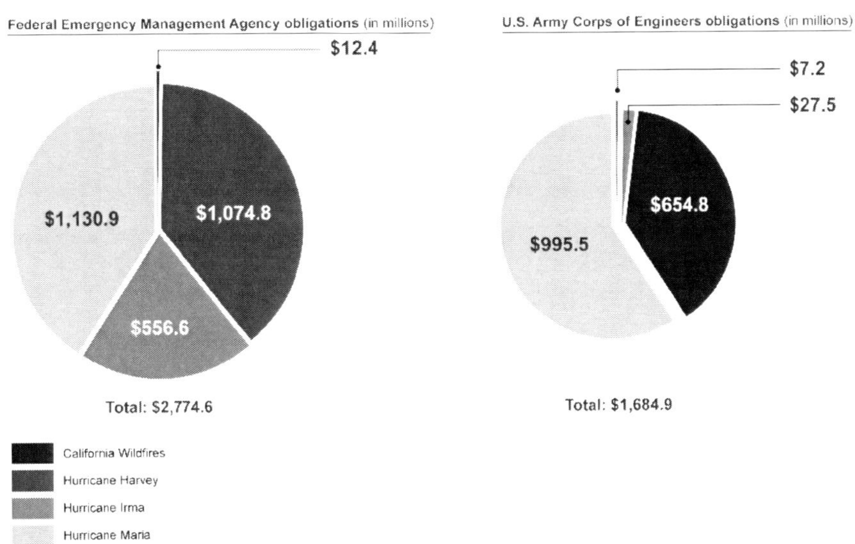

Source: GAO analysis of Federal Procurement Data System-Next Generation data. | GAO-19-93.
Note: Obligations are nominal 2017 and 2018 dollars. Numbers may not add due to rounding.

Figure 3. Federal Emergency Management Agency and U.S. Army Corps of Engineers Advance Contract Obligations in Response to the Three Hurricanes and California Wildfires in 2017, as of May 31, 2018.

Advance Contracts Were Used Primarily for Services

FEMA and USACE procured a variety of goods and services through advance contracts in response to the three hurricanes and wildfires, but about 86 percent of obligations, or $3.8 billion, were used to procure services. For example, all of USACE's $1.7 billion in advance contract obligations were for services, such as debris removal. FEMA obligated about $2.2 billion on services, such as architect and engineering services to rebuild roads and bridges. FEMA's obligations on goods totaled $624 million and included prefabricated buildings, such as manufactured housing units to provide lodging, and food and water. See Figure 4 for examples of obligations on goods or services by event.

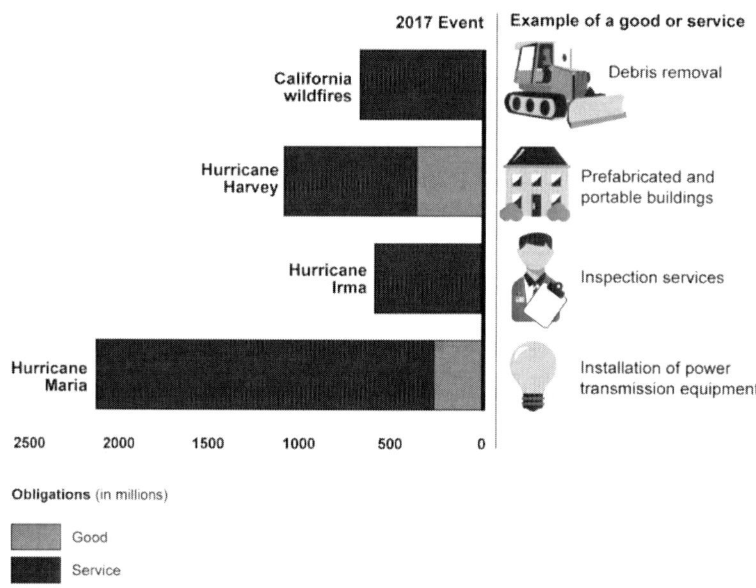

Source: GAO analysis of Federal Procurement Data System-Next Generation data. | GAO-19-93.

Notes: Obligations are nominal 2017 and 2018 dollars.

FEMA officials told us that contracts awarded in support of the U.S. Virgin Islands after Hurricane Maria impacted the islands may all be coded under Hurricane Maria, regardless of whether the contract responds to needs from Hurricane Irma or Hurricane Maria.

Figure 4. Federal Emergency Management Agency (FEMA) and U.S. Army Corps of Engineers Advance Contract Obligations and Examples of Goods and Services Used to Respond to the 2017 Hurricanes and Wildfires, as of May 31, 2018.

FEMA Lacks an Updated Strategy and Guidance on the Use of Advance Contracts

FEMA lacks an updated strategy and guidance on advance contract use, despite the PKEMRA requirement to develop a contracting strategy that maximizes their use to the extent practical and cost effective. As we found in May 2006 following Hurricane Katrina, and reiterated in our September 2015 report, agencies need to have competitively awarded contracts in place before a disaster to be effective in their response. Our current review found that FEMA has established advance contracts for goods and services to enable it to respond following a disaster. However, FEMA's lack of an updated strategy and guidance on advance contract use resulted in confusion about whether and how to maximize their use to the extent cost-effective and practical to facilitate a faster response when providing goods and services to survivors.

PKEMRA required the FEMA Administrator to identify specific goods and services that the agency could contract for in advance of a natural disaster in a cost-effective manner.[27] PKEMRA also required the FEMA Administrator to develop a contracting strategy that maximizes the use of advance contracts to the extent practical and cost-effective. Following the enactment of PKEMRA, in 2007 FEMA issued the *Advance Contracting of Goods and Services Report to Congress*, in part to address the requirement for an advance contracting strategy.[28] In addition to the strategy, FEMA provides information on advance contracts in its *Disaster Contracting Officer Desk Guide*.

The 2007 strategy notes that advance contracts will help to preclude the need to procure goods and services for disaster response under the unusual and compelling urgency exception to full and open competition, and allow FEMA to rapidly mobilize resources in immediate response to disasters. Several contracting officials we spoke with said that it is a requirement to use advance contracts before awarding new contracts. Moreover, a senior FEMA contracting official told us that advance contracts are intended to be used before awarding post-disaster contracts, even if the advance contract is not capable of fulfilling all of the requirements for a needed good or service. However, our review of the strategy found that it does not provide any specific direction on how contracting officers should award or use advance contracts to meet PKEMRA's objectives, or how they should be prioritized in relation to post-disaster contracts.[29] Further, there is no mention in FEMA's 2017 *Disaster Contracting Officer Desk Guide* that advance contracts should be considered prior to the award of post-disaster contracts.

In September 2015, we found shortfalls with the information available to contracting officers about advance contracts and recommended that FEMA provide new or updated guidance with information on how advance contracts should be used.[30] FEMA agreed with this recommendation and stated that in 2015 it included information on advance contracts and their use in training documentation. However, our review of semi-annual training documentation provided in May 2018 found that it only lists some of the advance contracts that are available, and not guidance on their use.

A report by the Senate Committee on Homeland Security and Governmental Affairs identified concerns about FEMA's use of advance contracts for self-help tarps in response to the 2017 hurricanes. Specifically, the report found that while FEMA ordered some tarps through one of its existing advance contracts, that order was placed after a post-disaster contract for tarps was signed, raising questions about whether FEMA's actions were informed by an overall strategy for using its advance contracts, in this case, for tarps. Our current review identified similar concerns, and found that the lack of an updated strategy and

---

[27] Pub. L. No. 109-295, § 691 (codified at 6 U.S.C. § 791).

[28] Department of Homeland Security, Federal Emergency Management Agency, *Advance Contracting of Goods and Services Report to Congress*.

[29] The 2007 strategy states that FEMA developed an acquisition tracker to prioritize contracts across four tiers, based on their internal and external visibility and risk. However, the strategy states the tracker only identifies contracts used in 2007 and 2008, and FEMA contracting officials we spoke with were not familiar with the acquisition tracker, and said it had been replaced by FEMA's advance contract list, which has no prioritization.

[30] GAO-15-783.

guidance on the use of advance contracts contributed to challenges in using these contracts to respond to the 2017 disasters.

In our review of advance contracts for meals and tarps, we found the following:

- Meals: Prior to the 2017 disasters, FEMA had advance contracts in place to provide meals with specific nutritional requirements. According to FEMA contracting officials, the advance contract vendors were at capacity for these specific meals following the response to Hurricane Harvey, requiring FEMA to issue a new post-disaster competitive solicitation and award new contracts with less specific nutritional requirements following Hurricane Maria. Based on our review of contract documentation, two of the existing advance contract vendors were awarded these new post-disaster contracts, but at different prices than those negotiated through their advance contracts. FEMA officials told us that contracting officers will negotiate to ensure the price of the contract is fair and reasonable and may utilize historical information or current contract prices to inform this determination. Normally, adequate price competition establishes a fair and reasonable price. According to a contracting officer involved with the award, FEMA relied on competition and historical prices, but not the existing advance contract prices, to determine that the new post-disaster contract meal prices were fair and reasonable. Guidance on the extent to which advance contract prices should be considered when comparing proposed prices to historical prices paid could help to further inform contracting officers' decision-making during a disaster.
- Tarps: Our review of FEMA's use of contracts for tarps is another example of how FEMA lacked an updated advance contracting strategy and guidance to provide goods and services to facilitate a faster response to the 2017 disasters. For example, in September 2014, FEMA awarded multiple award indefinite delivery, indefinite quantity advance contracts to three small businesses for self-help tarps, which are used to cover small areas of roof damage. In November 2014, these contracts were modified by the contracting officer to include delivery requirements for providing tarps to replenish FEMA's stock during steady state operations or during emergency response operations, such as a natural disaster. The contract modification added that during an emergency response, vendors would be expected to deliver up to 150,000 tarps within 96 hours of being issued a task order. However, these small businesses were not required to meet the emergency response delivery time frames and amounts since they would not be expected to store tarps on FEMA's behalf, limiting the use of FEMA's advance tarp contracts for immediate disaster response needs. According to a contracting officer involved with these contracts, the tarp advance contracts are typically used only to replenish tarp stockpiles in FEMA's distribution centers. However, the contracting officer also noted that not being able to fully use the existing advance contracts for tarps to respond to the three 2017 hurricanes was a challenge and required FEMA to award post-disaster contracts to meet tarp requirements.

  Furthermore, we found that FEMA awarded post-disaster contracts for tarps before utilizing its advance contracts with the small businesses. Contract file documentation for the post-disaster contracts stated that FEMA's advance contract holders for tarps had reached their capacity, and that market research had confirmed that it would be difficult for small businesses to meet the urgent delivery timeframes for tarps. Yet, after the award of the post-disaster tarp contracts, FEMA awarded task orders to one of the advance contractors to provide tarps in response to Hurricane Maria. Another small business advance contractor, which according to FEMA's post-disaster contract documentation had reached its capacity, also submitted a proposal as part of the post-disaster contract solicitation. According to FEMA, neither of the post-disaster contract holders ultimately provided the required tarps.[31] The timing and use of the existing tarp advance contracts raises questions about their ability to provide tarps immediately following a disaster, and whether an updated advance contracting strategy would have enabled FEMA to more quickly provide the needed tarps to survivors, considering the additional time and staff resources needed to award new post-disaster contracts.

FEMA established advance contracts to provide critical goods, like meals and tarps, following a disaster; however FEMA's 2007 contracting strategy does not provide direction on the objectives of advance contracts or how to maximize their use to the extent practical and cost-effective, as required by PKEMRA. According to FEMA officials, they had not considered updating the 2007 advance contracting strategy because they believed the use of advance contracts following PKEMRA had been incorporated into their disaster contracting practices. FEMA has also not communicated specific guidance to program and contracting officials on whether and how advance contracts should be prioritized before issuing new post-disaster solicitations and awarding contracts for the same or similar requirements, or how to maximize their use to the extent practical and cost-effective following a disaster, as required by PKEMRA. FEMA officials also acknowledged that additional guidance regarding advance contracts, including their availability and use during a disaster, could be useful. Without an updated strategy—and clear guidance that is incorporated into training—on the use of advance contracts and how they should be prioritized and used in relation to new post-disaster contract awards, FEMA lacks reasonable assurance that it is maximizing the use of advance contracts to quickly and cost-effectively provide goods and services following a disaster. This places FEMA at risk of continued challenges in quickly responding to subsequent disasters.

IMPROVEMENTS NEEDED IN FEMA'S PLANNING, MANAGEMENT, AND REPORTING OF ADVANCE CONTRACTS

While FEMA used a variety of advance contracts to respond to the 2017 disasters, we found weaknesses in the process of awarding and overseeing selected advance contracts in our review. These weaknesses were: (1) challenges in FEMA's acquisition planning; (2) limited record keeping or management of certain FEMA contracts; and (3) incomplete reporting on FEMA's advance contract actions to certain congressional committees. Related to USACE, we did not identify any planning or management challenges based on our review

[31] The first post-disaster contract was terminated for convenience citing shortages in available tarps following the 2017 hurricane season. A stop work order was issued for the second post-disaster contract following concerns over whether the tarps received met FEMA's specifications.

of its four selected contracts, and USACE is not required to report on its advance contract actions to the congressional committees.

Challenges in FEMA's Acquisition Planning Resulted in Bridge Contracts

FEMA has taken some steps since 2016 to improve competition and develop processes and guidance on the acquisition process for advance contracts, but shortfalls in acquisition planning have resulted in a number of bridge contracts. Bridge contracts can be a useful tool in certain circumstances to avoid a gap in providing products and services. We have previously reported that when non-competitive bridge contracts are used frequently or for prolonged periods, the government is at risk of paying more than it should for products and services.[32]

Based on our analysis, 63 of FEMA's 72 advance contracts used in response to the 2017 disasters were initially competed. All 15 of USACE's advance contracts used in responding to the three hurricanes and California wildfires in 2017 were initially competed. We found that at least 10 of FEMA's advance contracts used in 2017 were bridge contracts.[33] Within the 10 FEMA advance contracts we identified as bridge contracts, 6 were part of our selected case studies. The six advance contracts with subsequent bridges in our review obligated roughly $778 million in response to the three hurricanes and California wildfires in 2017.[34] These bridge contracts included five that are associated with two of FEMA's largest programs used in 2017—the Individual Assistance Program and Public Assistance Program—and one that is associated with a telecommunications program.

Three of the six bridge advance contracts we reviewed were awarded to support FEMA's Individual Assistance Program, which provides mass care services such as food and water as well as financial and direct assistance, among other services, to survivors whose property has been damaged or destroyed and whose losses are not covered by insurance. In 2017, this assistance was supported through the Individual Assistance-Technical Assistance Contract (IA-TAC), known as IA-TAC III. The IATAC III predecessor contracts had an original period of performance from a base year starting in May 2009 with four 1-year options that ended in May 2014. However, FEMA program and contracting officials were unable to implement changes to the requirements—recommended by FEMA senior leadership in 2010—prior to expiration. According to FEMA officials, staffing shortfalls, operational tempo, and unrealistic contract requirements led to acquisition planning delays. These challenges, in turn, led to a series of extensions from May 2014 to November 2016 and a new non-competitive bridge contract (base with options) from November 2016 to May 2018. At that point new, competitive follow-on indefinite delivery indefinite quantity contracts—the Individual Assistance Support Contract (IASC) and Logistics Housing Operations Unit Installation, Maintenance, and Deactivation (LOGHOUSE)—were awarded. See Figure 5.

---

[32] GAO-16-15.

[33] As previously noted, bridge contracts occur when an agency realizes that it will not be able to award a competed or non-competed follow-on contract before the current contract expires and can be done either by extending the current contract's period of performance or by awarding a new short term contract to the incumbent vendor(s) to avoid a lapse in service.

[34] These six contracts all had additional bridges related to the same requirement, though not all bridge contracts we identified were non-competitive.

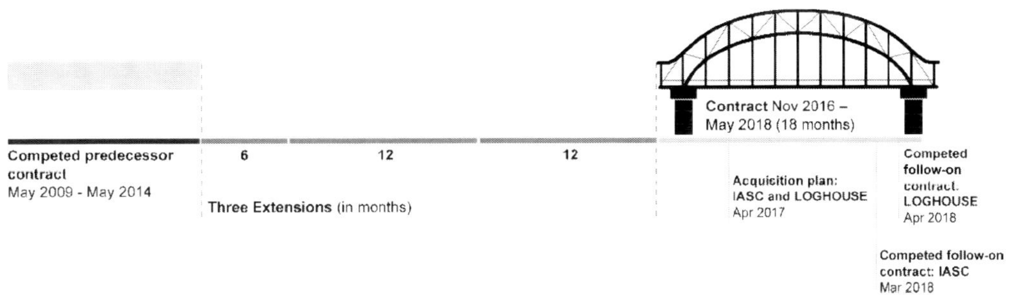

LOGHOUSE – Logistics Housing Operations Unit Installation, Maintenance, and Deactivation Contracts

IASC – Individual Assistance Support Contract

Source: GAO graphic based on information from contract file reviews and interviews with contracting officials. | GAO-19-93.

Note: The Individual Assistance Support Contract (IASC) provides the mass care and temporary housing portion of the Individual Assistance program. The Logistics Housing Operations Unit Installation, Maintenance, and Deactivation (LOGHOUSE), provides manufactured housing units to support the Logistics Manufactured Housing Unit program.

Figure 5. Timeline of the Individual Assistance-Technical Assistance Contract III Bridge.

Two of our six selected advance contracts that were bridge contracts were awarded to support FEMA's Public Assistance Program, which provides supplemental federal assistance to state, tribal, territorial, and local governments for debris removal, life-saving emergency protective measures, and the repair, replacement, or restoration of damaged facilities. The predecessor Public Assistance-Technical Assistance Contract (PA-TAC) used in 2017, known as PA-TAC III, was awarded with an original period of performance from a base year in February 2012 with four 1-year options that ended in February 2017. FEMA officials noted that changes to the PA-TAC III contract requirements and acquisition strategy were identified in 2015. Yet due to the time needed to incorporate these changes, FEMA was unable to complete required acquisition planning activities, such as finalizing the acquisition plan, prior to the expiration of PA-TAC III. Following 11 months of extensions to complete these activities, FEMA competitively awarded new contracts in December 2017. These awards were protested to the GAO and the protests were denied and are currently under review at the Court of Federal Claims. According to FEMA officials, these events required PATAC III to be extended until January 2019, as shown in Figure 6.

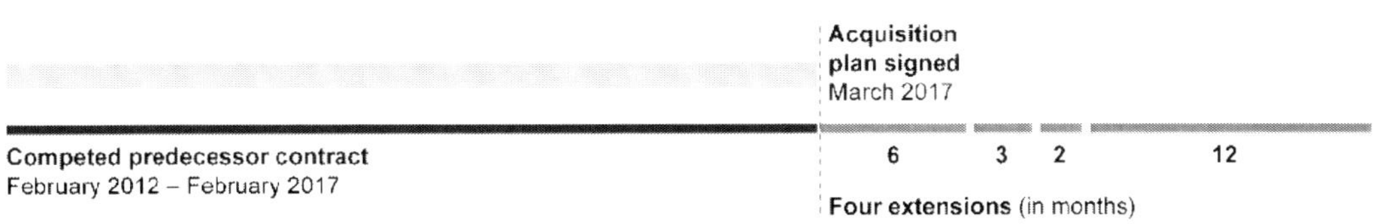

Source: GAO graphic based on information from contract file reviews and interviews with contracting officials. | GAO-19-93.

Figure 6. Timeline of Public Assistance-Technical Assistance Contract III Bridge.

The remaining bridge contract in our sample is associated with the Wireline Services Program, a telecommunication program that provides FEMA employees deployed to respond to a disaster with local and long-distance telephone, high-speed data, and cable television services. The 5 year wireline predecessor contract was awarded in 2003 and again in 2008, but FEMA was unable to award a competed contract when the 2008 contract expired in December 2013 due to the time it took to update program requirements. FEMA contracting officials extended the contract for 6 months before letting it expire altogether. Due to high staff turnover and inconsistent record keeping, at the time of our review FEMA officials were unable to determine the cause for this lapse of service, which occurred after the contract's expiration in June 2014. Starting in January 2015, FEMA contracting officials used a series of bridge contracts over more than three years to address changing contract requirements and delays in completing acquisition planning documentation, as shown in Figure 7. FEMA contracting officials anticipated awarding a competitive contract by the end of fiscal year 2018, but the award has been delayed and the existing contract extended through January 2019.

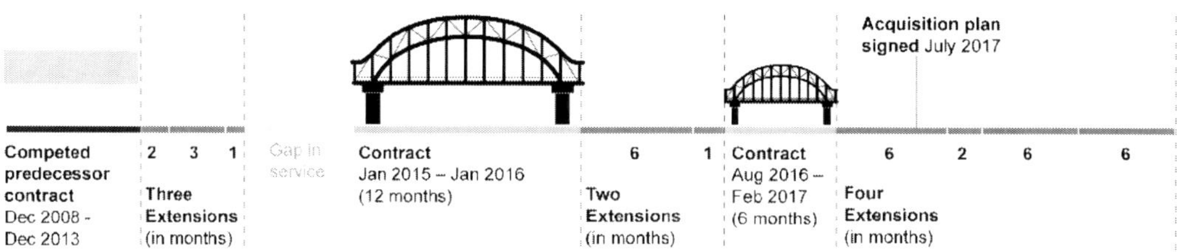

Source: GAO graphic based on information from contract file reviews and interviews with contracting officials. | GAO-19-93.

Figure 7. Timeline of Wireline Bridge.

In one of the bridge contracts included in our review, FEMA improperly used FAR clause 52.217-8. According to that clause, an agency may extend a contract's period of performance for up to 6 months and is generally used in the event of circumstances outside of the contracting officer's control that prevent the new contract award, such as a bid protest. This clause may be used multiple times to extend the contract so long as the total extension of performance does not exceed 6 months. Our analysis found that FEMA used the clause for a total of 14 months to justify two 6-month extensions and one 2-month extension to the second bridge contract. The FEMA contracting official associated with the advance contract reported uncertainty over the proper use of this clause and what other authorities should have been used instead to extend the contract. FEMA's Office of Chief Counsel and contracting officials acknowledged this error.

While not all bridge contracts that we identified during our review were non-competitive, FEMA officials acknowledged that the use of noncompetitive bridge contracts is not an ideal practice as they cannot ensure the government is paying what it should for products and services. In October 2015 we identified delays in the completion of acquisition planning documentation as one of the leading causes of awarding bridge contracts.[35] In an effort to decrease the need for non-competitive bridge contracts and provide ample time for acquisition planning, FEMA began implementing a 5-Year Master Acquisition Planning Schedule (MAPS) in 2016. MAPS is a tracking tool that monitors the status of and provides acquisition planning timeframes for certain FEMA acquisitions over $5 million, as well as for all advance

[35] GAO-16-15. Acquisition planning documentation can include an independent government cost estimate, the statement of work, acquisition plan, market research, and evaluation criteria depending on contract value.

contracts and any acquisition deemed by the agency to be mission critical, regardless of dollar value.

As we previously noted, acquisition planning includes both the pre-solicitation and solicitation phases. Based on our review of MAPS documentation, the tool generates a timeline of discretionary acquisition milestones across these two phases, based on certain considerations like the type of acquisition and whether it will be competed. Using this timeline, MAPS sends email alerts to program and contracting staff when certain acquisition milestones should occur.

Specific to the solicitation phase, FEMA's Office of the Chief Procurement Officer has developed annual lead time guidance for how long contracting officers should be given to award new contracts following the completion of the acquisition package, which is then conveyed through MAPS. For example, for acquisitions $150,000 and under, FEMA's 2018 lead time guidance states contracting officers should be given 60 days to award the contract following completion of the acquisition package. FEMA officials we spoke with acknowledged that these discretionary timeframes are frequently shortened when program office officials are delayed in completing acquisition packages. While FEMA has lead time guidance to establish timeframes for completing the solicitation phase, FEMA currently has no guidance establishing timeframes for the pre-solicitation phase, when program offices complete the acquisition packages. Figure 8 provides an example timeline of the major milestones tracked in MAPS.

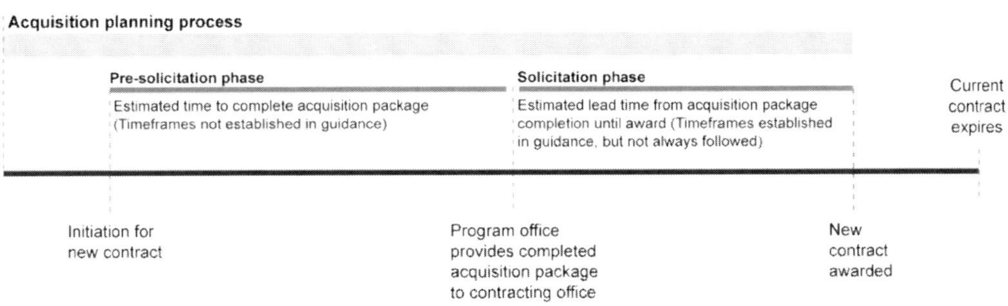

Source: GAO depiction of milestones identified in FEMA's 5 Year Master Acquisition Planning Schedule. | GAO-19-93.

Figure 8. Notional Depiction of Acquisition Planning Timeline Depicted in FEMA's 5 Year Master Acquisition Planning Schedule (MAPS).

In its analysis of 12 fiscal year 2017 contracts tracked in MAPS that were awarded late, FEMA found that half were late because contracting officials were not given enough lead time to award a new contract following the program office's completion of the acquisition package. Not adhering to suggested timeframes can place a burden on contracting officers and increase the likelihood of not awarding the contract on schedule, requiring FEMA to non-competitively extend the existing contract. According to FEMA's lead time guidance, based on the contract values for the bridge contracts in our review contracting officers should have been given between 240 and 300 days to award a new contract once the acquisition package was completed. However, as we mention earlier, due to delays from changing program requirements and acquisition strategies we found that the acquisition plans for the follow-on contracts related to these bridge contracts were not completed until after the predecessor contract had already expired, as shown in Figure 9 below.

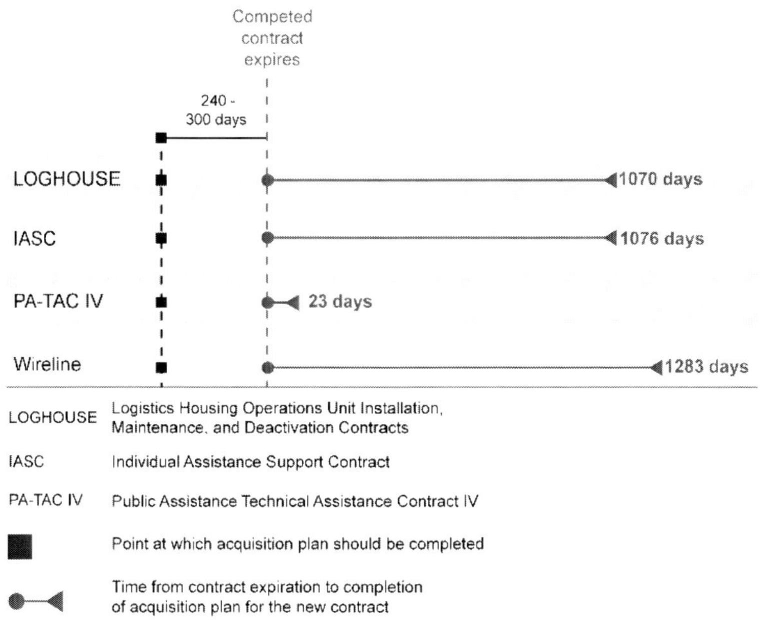

Source: GAO analysis of signed acquisition plans for identified bridge contracts. | GAO-19-93.

Note: The acquisition package can consist of documents such as an independent government cost estimate, statement of work, acquisition plan, and market research among others. The applicable documents are determined by dollar value.

Figure 9. Acquisition Plan Completion Compared to Competed Contract Expiration.

Timely completion of the acquisition package was a key challenge identified in the contracts we reviewed. However, according to officials from the Office of the Chief Procurement Officer, they do not have the authority to establish guidance for FEMA program officials on completing pre-solicitation phase activities. In August 2011, we identified challenges with acquisition planning across DHS. Specifically, we found that DHS and other agencies did not measure or incorporate into guidance the amount of time it takes to develop and obtain approvals of the acquisition planning documents required during the pre-solicitation phase.[36] We recommended that DHS procurement offices collect information about the timeframes needed for the acquisition planning process to establish timeframes for when program officials should begin acquisition planning. DHS did not concur with this recommendation, stating that its acquisition manual already encourages early planning, and has not implemented the recommendation. At the time, we maintained that program officials needed more guidance to have a better understanding of how much time to allow for completing acquisition planning steps, and that the component procurement offices are best positioned to provide guidance on how long these planning processes may take. Given the current challenges we identified with FEMA's ability to complete acquisition planning activities in a timely manner and the resulting delays in awarding new contracts for critical

[36] GAO, *Acquisition Planning: Opportunities to Build Strong Foundations for Better Services Contracts*, GAO-11-672 (Washington D.C.: Aug. 9, 2011).

advance contract goods and services, additional information and guidance on acquisition planning timeframes remains important.

Additionally, while MAPS has been in place since 2016 and FEMA officials have instituted training to communicate the system's intent, program and contracting officials we spoke with varied in their familiarity with it. For example, officials responsible for MAPS stated that by March 2016, 90 percent of FEMA's contracting staff had attended an hour long training session and additional training sessions were held for all program office staff at various points in 2016 and 2017. However, most of the program office and contracting officials responsible for the bridge contracts in our review reported limited familiarity with MAPS.

While FEMA has taken some positive steps to institute training and has guidance on timeframes for part of the acquisition planning process, program and contracting staff we spoke with were still uncertain how best to utilize MAPS to identify the time needed to effectively complete acquisition planning activities. According to federal internal control standards, agency management should internally communicate the necessary quality information to achieve their objectives.[37] Given FEMA's emphasis on planning before a disaster and using advance contracts to help reduce the need to award non-competitive contracts during a disaster, establishing clear guidance on the factors that can affect acquisition planning activities, and requiring officials to follow the timeframes needed to complete them to meet the goal of awarding competitive contracts, is essential. Until FEMA provides detailed guidance about timeframes and considerations that affect the entire acquisition planning process—both the pre-solicitation and solicitation phases—to all officials responsible for acquisition planning, and clearly communicates the intent of MAPS, it cannot ensure that MAPS will be effective at reducing the number of non-competitively awarded bridge contracts, as is FEMA's intent.

Current Record-Keeping Practices Limit Visibility into Advance Contract Management

While FEMA has procedures regarding the documentation required for its contract files, current practices limited visibility into the advance contracts in our review. Specifically we found that acquisition plans and some other contract documents were unable to be located in certain cases. Acquisition plans provide the program and contract history as well as other information on which acquisition decisions, such as the type of contract required, are based.

FEMA contracting officials were unable to locate acquisition plans for 4 of our 10 FEMA selected advance contracts despite FAR and DHS acquisition guidance requiring plans for these particular contracts to be completed and stored in the contract file.[38] Three of these acquisition plans are associated with the IA-TAC bridge contract which, as previously noted, was associated with one of FEMA's largest programs used in 2017. FEMA contracting officials were also unable to locate the acquisition plans completed for the prior iteration of IA-TAC because they were not in the hard copy contract file or contract writing system,

---

[37] GAO, *Standards for Internal Control in the Federal Government*, GAO-14-704G (Washington, D.C.: September 2014).

[38] FAR § 7.103(e) and Department of Homeland Security, *Department of Homeland Security Acquisition Manual* § 3007.103(e) (Oct. 2009).

meaning that no acquisition plan guiding the IA-TACs since before its 2009 award could be found. In 2011, the DHS Office of the Inspector General conducted a review of FEMA's IA-TAC and identified, among other things, incomplete contract files as a problem.[39] Not being able to locate acquisition plans can result in the loss of contract knowledge and lessons learned from prior awards.

Additionally, we found instances of contract documentation for advance contracts related to our case studies that contract officials could not locate. For instance, FEMA was unable to confirm whether or not an option year for the last competed Wireline contract included in the contract was exercised due to a lack of documentation. In order to obtain this answer, FEMA officials had to reach out to the vendor for their records. Moreover, the modification exercising the first option year for one of the IA-TAC III predecessor contracts was missing, as were the determination and findings documents exercising the first option year for all three of the predecessor IA-TAC III contracts that were associated with the advance contracts in our review. After we made FEMA officials aware of the missing documentation, they subsequently added clarifying memos to the contract files.

FEMA standard operating procedures state that the acquisition documents in the official contract file will be sufficient to constitute a complete history of the entire transaction for the purpose of providing a complete background, and as a basis for informed decisions at each step in the acquisition process. Additionally, these procedures require headquarters staff to place modifications to contracts and orders and associated supporting documentation in the contract file within 5 business days of awarding a contract or issuing an order. FEMA officials stated they are required to follow these procedures until DHS has fully transitioned to an electronic filing system. According to DHS officials, that system is currently in the testing phase and a timeframe for implementation has not yet been finalized. Furthermore, according to these officials, DHS has not yet decided which, if any, existing contracts will be required to be retroactively entered into the system. Until this decision has been made and implementation occurs, FEMA's official file of record for its advance contracts consists of a hardcopy file, which contracting officers at FEMA headquarters are required to add completed contract documentation to, per the standard operating procedures.[40] A FEMA official told us that some documentation, including some of the missing documentation we identified, has been lost due to staff turnover and an office move in 2016.

FEMA officials anticipate some of the challenges associated with managing the hard copy advance contract files will be alleviated after implementation of the Electronic Contract File System. However, DHS officials have not decided whether components will be required to retroactively enter contract information for any contract awarded prior to the implementation date. This would require FEMA and other DHS components to continue to maintain hardcopy files for some contracts— including large strategic sourcing vehicles and advance contracts—for the foreseeable future. For example, FEMA's $2.7 billion LOGHOUSE, and $14 million IASC advance contracts were awarded in 2018 and have a

---

[39] Department of Homeland Security Office of the Inspector General, *Improving FEMA's Individual Assistance, Technical Assistance Contracts* (Washington D.C.: Sept. 27, 2011).This report found, among others, that pricing memorandums—which help contracting officers determine if a vendor's proposed price is fair and reasonable—for two of the IA-TACs were missing from the contract files and unable to be located.

[40] While the official file of record remains hardcopy, FEMA officials said they highly encourage the use of its current contract writing system as an unofficial means of electronically storing necessary documentation. Although this is highly encouraged, FEMA officials noted they cannot require contracting officials to use this system for electronic contract file storage.

period of performance lasting until 2023. Until FEMA adheres to existing contract file management requirements, whether the contract files will be transferred into the electronic system or remain in hard copy format, it is at continued risk of having incomplete contract files and a loss of institutional knowledge regarding these advance contracts.

Information on Advance Contracts in FEMA's Disaster Contract Quarterly Reports to Congressional Committees Is Incomplete

Since December 2007, FEMA has submitted quarterly reports to congressional committees that list all disaster contracting actions in the preceding three months.[41] These quarterly reports also include details on contracts awarded by non-competitive means, as required by PKEMRA.[42] However, our analysis shows that some reports from fiscal year 2017 and 2018 have been incomplete. In September 2015, we found that FEMA's quarterly reports to congressional committees in fiscal years 2013 and 2014 did not capture all of FEMA's noncompetitive orders.[43] At that time, FEMA attributed this to an error in data compilation prior to mid-2013 and explained that it had updated its process for collecting these data and strengthened the review process, resulting in accurate reports starting in the fourth quarter of fiscal year 2013. Despite this change in the data collection process, our current analysis found that 29 contract actions associated with the 10 selected advance contracts in our review were not reported across FEMA's fourth quarter fiscal year 2017 and first quarter fiscal year 2018 reports. For example, FEMA's fourth quarter fiscal year 2017 report did not include 13 contract actions equaling about $83 million, or 15 percent, of the $558 million in total obligations associated with the 10 selected advance contracts in our review. Similarly, FEMA's first quarter fiscal year 2018 report did not include 16 contract actions equaling about $122 million, or 23 percent, of the $532 million in total obligations associated with the 10 selected advance contracts in our review. Figure 10 provides a breakdown of the total contract action obligations by extent of competition.

To compile the quarterly reports, FEMA officials told us that their methodology is to pull contract action data that is documented in their contract writing system and FPDS-NG roughly one week after the end of each fiscal quarter. Once the data are pulled from these two sources, officials said they compare the data to ensure all reported actions are captured. However, according to officials, the data may not include all contract actions. Specifically, during disaster response efforts like those in 2017, FEMA policy allows contracting officers to execute what it refers to as "notice to proceed," which is a notice to a construction contractor to begin work under certain circumstances. FEMA officials responsible for the quarterly reports stated that if notice to proceed documentation is used, information on some contract actions that were issued during the fiscal quarter, but not entered into the systems until after the quarter ended, may be missed during the data compilation process.

[41] DHS officials stated that in addition to its quarterly reports there are other methods, such as the congressional notification tool, that provide information on contract actions to the appropriations committees. However, these other methods are not in direct response to the PKEMRA requirement that FEMA report on all contracts awarded by non-competitive means.

[42] For the purpose of its congressional committee reports, FEMA considers a contract action to be an action that uses appropriated funds designated for disaster situations, excluding any that deobligate funds or constitute no-cost modifications.

[43] GAO-15-783.

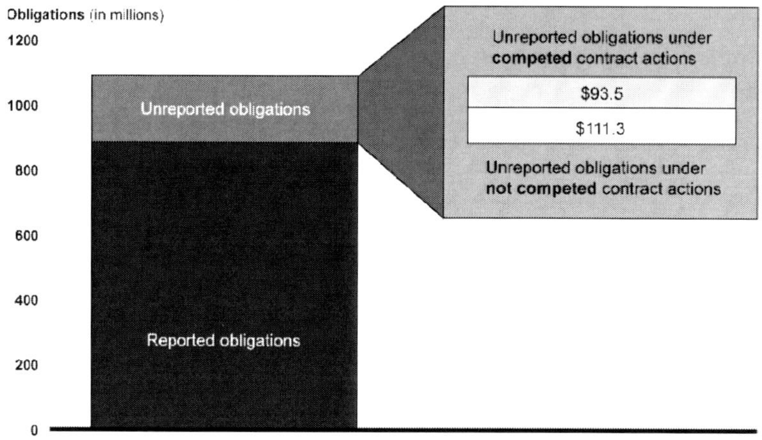

Source: GAO analysis of FEMA Fourth Quarter Fiscal Year 2017 and First Quarter Fiscal Year 2018 Quarterly Reports to Congress. | GAO-19-93.

Note: For the purpose of its congressional committee reports, FEMA considers a contract action to be an action that uses appropriated funds designated for disaster situations, excluding any that deobligate funds or constitute no-cost modifications.

Figure 10. Total Value of Contract Action Obligations from Selected Advance Contracts in Fourth Quarter Fiscal Year 2017 and First Quarter Fiscal Year 2018 Federal Emergency Management Agency (FEMA) Congressional Committee Reports.

FEMA policy requires that contracting officers who execute the notice to proceed documentation complete the contract award documentation in the contract writing system within three days of when the contracting officer receivers the contractor's acceptance of the notice. However, a FEMA policy official acknowledged that during disaster response, this does not always occur. Further, FEMA officials responsible for compiling the reports stated that it is not part of their methodology to review data from prior fiscal quarters to see whether any contract actions have been entered that were not previously reported. By not adhering to FEMA policy that establishes timeframes for entering data in a disaster response scenario, FEMA risks reporting incomplete information. Moreover, without taking steps to ensure its reporting methodology provides complete information on all competed and not competed disaster contract actions, FEMA cannot be certain it is providing the congressional committees with visibility into all of its overall disaster contract awards or the extent of non-competitive contract obligations over time.

No Challenges Identified with the Planning and Management of Selected USACE Advance Contracts

The four selected USACE advance contracts in our review—one supporting USACE's temporary power mission and three supporting its debris removal mission—were awarded in 2014 with a period of performance lasting until 2019. Since these contracts have not reached the end of their period of performance, we were unable to assess the effectiveness of USACE planning activities. According to contracting officials, USACE is performing acquisition planning activities for both the temporary power and debris removal advance contracts and anticipates awarding the new contracts prior to the current contracts' expiration.

Additionally, USACE was able to provide the acquisition plans for each of the four advance contracts in our review. Unlike FEMA, which retains hard copy files of its contract documentation, USACE uses three official systems of record to store contract file documentation electronically. Officials acknowledged that while moving between the three official systems to find documents may be time consuming, contract documents are typically able to be located.

FEMA and USACE Identified Lessons Learned from the Use of Advance Contracts in 2017, but Reported Challenges with State and Local Coordination Remain

Both FEMA and USACE have processes for identifying and assessing lessons learned following a disaster. Contracting officials from these agencies identified several lessons learned from the 2017 major hurricanes and the California wildfires that directly affected their use of advance contracts. These include the need for: (1) additional advance contracts for certain goods and services; (2) flexibility to increase contract ceilings; (3) use of USACE's debris removal advance contracts to respond to the California wildfires; and (4) federal coordination and information sharing with state and local governments on advance contracts. While officials identified some lessons learned, they also identified challenges related to FEMA's outreach with state and local governments on advance contracting efforts.

FEMA and USACE Have Identified Lessons Learned and Actions to Address Them

FEMA and USACE have processes for identifying and assessing lessons learned through after-action reviews and reports following major disasters. According to FEMA and USACE officials, they routinely perform these reviews and then compile after-action reports to identify lessons learned and proposed actions to address them. Due to the concurrent nature of hurricanes Harvey, Irma, and Maria, FEMA headquarters completed one combined after-action review for all three hurricanes in July 2018.[44] The resulting report identified 18 strategic-level key findings across five focus areas, and recommendations for improvement.[45] These recommendations included some that were specific to advance contracts, such as the need for additional advance contracts to support future disaster response efforts, and improved state and local coordination to support state and local contracting and logistics operations. In addition, USACE officials performed after-action reviews following disasters, and have a process in place to discuss challenges and recommendations for improvement on their use of advance contracts for temporary power, temporary roofing, and debris removal.

---

[44] FEMA, *2017 Hurricane Season FEMA After-Action Report* (July 12, 2018).

[45] The five focus areas are: scaling a response for concurrent, complex incidents; staffing for concurrent, complex incidents; sustained whole community logistics operations; responding during long-term infrastructure outages; mass care to initial housing operations.

Table 1. Lessons Learned and Proposed Actions Regarding Advance Contracts Identified by the Federal Emergency Management Agency (FEMA) and the U.S. Army Corps of Engineers (USACE) Following the 2017 Hurricanes and California Wildfires

Issue	Lessons Learned	Proposed Actions
Additional advance contract requirements	Both FEMA and USACE reported a need for additional advance contracts in certain areas following their response to the 2017 disasters. For example, FEMA officials explained that following the disaster response efforts for Hurricane Maria, they realized there was a need for additional advance transportation contracts, specifically for freight and barge transportation, to carry goods to areas outside the continental United States, like Puerto Rico and the U.S. Virgin Islands. USACE also reported a shortage of advance contracts for quality assurance services—inspection of the services by contractors— which officials said required them to spend extra time and resources awarding post-disaster contracts for these services.	FEMA officials confirmed that they awarded an additional advance contract for freight and barge transportation in August 2018, but stated that the contract award was being protested. USACE officials told us they are considering whether to pursue additional advance contracts for quality assurance services.
Contract ceilings	FEMA and USACE officials noted that as a result of the magnitude and timeframes of the 2017 disasters, ceilings on a number of indefinite delivery, indefinite quantity advance contracts were too low to support response and recovery efforts and were increased through modification. For example, FEMA had modified its bottled water and telecommunications advance contracts to increase the dollar value ceilings. USACE officials reported increasing ceilings for their debris removal and temporary power contracts.	FEMA and USACE officials said they have taken steps to update contract ceiling language to provide greater flexibility. For example, in August 2018, FEMA issued an alert to contracting officers to insert language into solicitations and contracts when issuing multiple award indefinite delivery, indefinite quantity contracts that allows the contracting officer to incrementally increase the contract's dollar value ceiling during a presidentially declared disaster so long as the total amount of supplies and services ordered does not exceed the total capacity of all vendors under the contract able to provide the needed goods and services. USACE officials said they have revised language in solicitations for their indefinite delivery, indefinite quantity temporary power and debris removal contracts to include higher estimated cost ceilings than those in prior advance contracts.
Debris removal pricing	USACE officials identified challenges using their debris removal advance contracts to respond to the 2017 California wildfires. According to USACE officials, the debris removal contract requirements are written broadly enough to include all kinds of debris removal, but they have primarily been used to manage hurricane debris removal. As a result, the advance contracts did not address some of the issues related to the 2017 wildfire debris removal. For example, according to USACE officials, while hurricane debris is often priced by volume, officials stated that the wildfire debris had to be priced by tonnage, and wrapped to prevent contamination.	As of August 2018, USACE officials stated that they are in the process of developing ordering instructions at the task order level based on the prices and experiences from the 2017 wildfires. Specifically, officials stated that because the unique circumstances of a disaster vary, they are developing ordering instructions that will reflect historical prices from using their debris removal contracts to respond to the wildfires that can be leveraged at the task order level in the newly awarded debris removal contracts in April 2019.

Source: GAO summary of FEMA and USACE information. I GAO-19-93.

While the scope of FEMA's and USACE's after-action reports are broader than just advance contracts, we identified, based on our review of reports and interviews with FEMA and USACE officials, several lessons learned related to advance contracts following the 2017 hurricanes and California wildfires, as shown in Table 1.

Challenges in Coordinating with and Providing Information to State and Local Governments on the Use of Advance Contracts Continued

We also found that while FEMA has updated its guidance to reflect some requirements for state and local coordination over the use of advance contracts, inconsistencies in FEMA's outreach and information on the use of advance contracts remains a challenge. PKEMRA required that FEMA encourage state and local governments to establish their own advance contracts with vendors for goods and services in advance of natural disasters.[46] In September 2015, we found that FEMA's outreach with state and local governments to encourage the establishment of advance contracts can result in more efficient contracting after a disaster.[47] PKEMRA also required that FEMA establish a process to ensure that federal advance contracts are coordinated with state and local governments, as appropriate. In our September 2015 report, we also found that these efforts can ensure that states are aware of and can access certain federal advance contracts, such as General Services Administration schedule contracts.

However, in the same report, we found that inconsistencies in whether and how the regions perform state and local outreach limited FEMA's ability to support advance contracting efforts.[48] We recommended that FEMA provide new or updated guidance to ensure that all contracting officers are aware of requirements concerning the need to conduct outreach to state and local governments to support their use of advance contracts. DHS concurred with this recommendation and in 2017 FEMA updated its *Disaster Contracting Desk Guide* to state that contracting officers should inform their state and local counterparts of the availability and use of federal advance contracts established by FEMA.[49] Our review of the guide found that it does remind contracting officers to coordinate with states and localities over the use of federal advance contracts, but does not provide any details on how often or what types of advance contract information should be shared with states and localities, or provide any instructions to contracting officers on PKEMRA's requirement to encourage states and localities to establish their own advance contracts for the types of goods and services needed during a disaster.

Our current review also found inconsistencies with FEMA's efforts to encourage states and localities to establish their own advance contracts with vendors and ensure coordination with them on their use of federal advance contracts. For example, some regional FEMA officials explained that they regularly perform outreach, which can assist states and localities with establishing advance contracts for goods and services commonly needed during a disaster, like security, transportation, and office supplies. Regional officials we spoke with said more frequent coordination allows them to avoid overlap across state and federal

[46] Pub. L. No.109-295, § 691 (codified at 6 U.S.C. § 791).
[47] GAO-15-783.
[48] GAO-15-783.
[49] FEMA Office of the Chief Procurement Officer, *Disaster Contracting Desk Guide 2017*.

contracting efforts, and know what resources the states have in place and how long states are capable of providing these resources following a disaster. However, other regional officials reported having less frequent coordination with state and local governments. For example, a FEMA official stated that one of the regions has less frequent meetings with state and local governments because the region is geographically dispersed and has fewer disasters. According to another regional official, coordination between some regional offices and state and local officials over advance contracting was minimal prior to Hurricane Harvey, and in some cases only occurred when FEMA and state and local officials were co-located during a disaster.

Officials from some state and local governments and USACE reported examples where increased coordination between FEMA, states, and localities could have improved the use of advance contracts in 2017. For example, in September 2018 we found that some localities were relying on the same contractors to perform debris removal activities following Hurricanes Harvey in Texas and Irma in Florida.[50] As a result, we reported that some contractors that were removing debris in Texas did not honor existing contracts in Florida, leading to delays in debris removal. Additional communication and coordination between FEMA and contracting officials in these states and localities about which contractors they had established advance contracts with could have helped to prevent this overlap and subsequent delay in removing debris. During our current review, USACE and California officials also reported miscommunications about state and local expectations for USACE's debris removal contracts following the wildfires. Specifically, USACE and state and local officials reported differing expectations about the work to be performed under USACE's debris removal contracts, such as what structures would be removed from private property and acceptable soil contamination levels. According to USACE officials, they relied on FEMA, as the lead for coordinating federal disaster response, to manage communication with states and localities and to identify and manage expectations about the scope of work to be performed using their advance debris removal contracts. While state and local officials we met with in California reported working closely with some FEMA officials not responsible for regional contracting during the response to the wildfires, FEMA regional contracting officials said that they had no direct coordination with California officials.

We also identified inconsistencies in the information available to FEMA's contracting officials on existing advance contracts, which can be used to facilitate coordination with states and localities on the establishment and use of advance contracts. Our review of FEMA's advance contract list found that it does not include all of the advance contracts that FEMA has in place, and contracting officers we spoke with cited other resources they also use to identify advance contracts, like biannual training documentation provided to contracting staff. For example, while FEMA officials told us the advance contract list is updated on a monthly basis, our analysis found that 58 advance contracts identified on the June 2018 advance contract list were not included in the May 2018 biannual training documentation, including contracts for telecommunications services, generators, and manufactured housing units. Further, 26 of the contracts included in the May training documentation were not included on the June advance contract list, including contracts for foreign language interpretation services, hygiene items, and short-shelf life meals. Some contracting officers

---

[50] GAO-18-472, *2017 Hurricanes and Wildfires: Initial Observations on the Federal Response and Key Recovery Challenges*, (Washington, D.C.: Sept. 4, 2018).

we spoke with said they referred to the advance contract list as the primary resource for identifying advance contracts, while others referenced the biannual training as their primary resource.

FEMA has recognized some shortcomings in how it coordinated and communicated with state and local governments over the use of advance contracts following the 2017 disasters, and identified some action to address these issues moving forward. In the *2017 Hurricane Season FEMA After-Action Report*, FEMA identified the need to expand its capabilities to support state, local, tribal, and territorial governments in improving their capabilities for advance contracting, among other issues.[51] The report recommends that FEMA should continue efforts to develop a toolkit that will provide state and local governments with recommendations for advance contracts, emergency acquisition guidance, and solicitation templates.

According to FEMA contracting officials, the development of the toolkit has been prioritized by FEMA's Administrator to help better prepare the states and localities and decrease their reliance on FEMA for assistance following a disaster. However, as of August 2018 the specific contents of the toolkit were still being decided. For example, officials familiar with the development of the toolkit originally said they intended for it to include FEMA's advance contract list, to provide states with recommendations on the types of advance contracts that may be useful. But in subsequent discussions these officials told us they did not plan to provide states and localities with a full list of advance contracts to avoid being overly prescriptive, and because not all of the contracts on the list are relevant for the types of disasters some states experience. Officials further stated that since it is the responsibility of the federal coordinator in each region to communicate available federal advance contracts to states and localities, providing a full list of advance contracts is unnecessary.

Federal internal control standards state that agency management should use quality information to achieve their objectives.[52] Agency management should also internally and externally communicate that information to achieve their objective. However, FEMA's guidance does not clearly communicate its objectives and requirements for contracting officers to encourage states and localities to enter into their own advance contracts, nor is there a consolidated resource listing available advance contracts that states and localities can use to inform their advance contracting efforts. According to FEMA officials, information on advance contracts is fluid, as new contracts are established or old contracts expire. Officials also told us that the advance contract list is updated monthly, yet as mentioned earlier, contracts identified in the May training documentation were not reflected in the list that was updated as of June. Ensuring that advance contract information is complete and updated regularly is important, because differences across FEMA's resources listing advance contracts could result in FEMA's contracting officers not being aware of the availability of certain contracts during a disaster, and states not receiving recommendations on what advance contracts may be helpful for them to establish. Without clear guidance on FEMA's expectations for coordination with states and localities on advance contracting efforts, and a centralized resource listing up to date information on FEMA's advance contracts, FEMA contracting officers and their state and local counterparts lack reasonable assurance they will

---

[51] FEMA, *2017 Hurricane Season FEMA After-Action Report* (July 12, 2018).

[52] GAO-14-704G.

have the tools needed to effectively communicate about advance contracts, and use them to respond to future disasters. Moreover, given FEMA's recent emphasis on the importance of states and localities having the capability to provide their own life-saving goods and services in the immediate aftermath of a disaster, clearly communicating consistent and up to date information on the availability and limitations of federal advance contracts through the toolkit, or other means, is critical to informing state and local disaster response efforts.

CONCLUSION

Contracting during a disaster can pose a unique set of challenges as officials face a significant amount of pressure to provide life-sustaining goods and services to survivors as quickly as possible. Advance contracts are a tool that FEMA and others within the federal government can leverage to rapidly and cost-effectively mobilize resources, while also helping to preclude the need to procure critical goods and services noncompetitively after a disaster. Given the circumstances surrounding the 2017 disasters and the importance of preparedness for future disasters, it is critical to ensure that the federal government is positioned to maximize its advance contracts to the extent practical and cost-effective to provide immediate disaster response.

Although FEMA has identified advance contracts for use during a disaster, without an updated strategy—and guidance that is incorporated into training—on how to maximize their use during a disaster, as well as the development of clear guidance on acquisition planning timeframes, FEMA is at risk of these contracts not being effectively planned and used. Furthermore, FEMA officials have not always maintained complete information on the advance contracts available for them to quickly respond to disasters, or completely reported competitively and non-competitively awarded advance contract information to better help congressional committees evaluate spending over time. Finally, without continued efforts to improve outreach with states and localities and centralize information on available advance contracts, FEMA's contracting officers and their state and local counterparts may not have the information needed to efficiently respond to a disaster.

RECOMMENDATIONS FOR EXECUTIVE ACTION

We are making nine recommendations to FEMA.

FEMA's Administrator should update the strategy identified in its 2007 *Advance Contracting of Goods and Services Report to Congress* to clearly define the objectives of advance contracts, how they contribute to FEMA's disaster response operations, and whether and how they should be prioritized in relation to new post-disaster contract awards. (Recommendation 1)

FEMA's Administrator should ensure the Head of the Contracting Activity updates the *Disaster Contracting Desk Guide* to include guidance for whether and under what circumstances contracting officers should consider using existing advance contracts prior to making new post-disaster contract awards, and include this guidance in existing semiannual training given to contracting officers. (Recommendation 2)

FEMA's Administrator should update and implement existing guidance for program office and contracting officer personnel to identify acquisition planning timeframes and considerations across the entire acquisition planning process, and clearly communicate the purpose and use of MAPS. (Recommendation 3)

FEMA's Administrator should ensure the Head of the Contracting Activity adheres to current hard copy contract file management requirements to ensure advance contract files are complete and up to date, whether they will be transferred into the new Electronic Contract Filing System or remain in hard copy format. (Recommendation 4)

FEMA's Administrator should ensure the Head of the Contracting Activity reminds contracting officers of the three day timeframe for entering completed award documentation into the contract writing system when executing notice to proceed documentation. (Recommendation 5)

FEMA's Administrator should ensure the Head of the Contracting Activity revises its reporting methodology to ensure that all disaster contracts are included in its quarterly reports to congressional committees on disaster contract actions. (Recommendation 6)

FEMA's Administrator should ensure the Head of the Contracting Activity revises the *Disaster Contracting Officer Desk* guide to provide specific guidance for contracting officers to perform outreach to state and local governments on the use and establishment of advance contracts. (Recommendation 7)

FEMA's Administrator should ensure the Head of the Contracting Activity identifies a single centralized resource listing its advance contracts and ensure that source is updated regularly to include all available advance contracts. (Recommendation 8)

FEMA's Administrator should ensure the Head of the Contracting Activity communicates information on available advance contracts through the centralized resource to states and localities to inform their advance contracting efforts. (Recommendation 9)

Agency Comments and Our Evaluation

We provided a draft of this chapter to DOD, DHS, and FEMA for review and comment. DOD did not provide any comments on the draft report. In its comments, reprinted in appendix IV, DHS and FEMA concurred with our nine recommendations. DHS and FEMA also provided technical comments, which we incorporated as appropriate.

In its written comments, FEMA agreed to take actions to address our recommendations, such as updating guidance on advance contract use and management, adding an addendum to its quarterly report that captures the contract actions that were previously unreported, and better communicating information on advance contracts to states and localities. In its concurrence with two of our recommendations, FEMA requested that we consider these recommendations resolved and close as implemented based on our actions it had previously taken.

For example, in its response to our third recommendation, FEMA agreed to update and implement existing guidance to identify acquisition timeframes and the purpose and use of its 5-Year MAPS program. In its response, FEMA reiterated that it has conducted training sessions for its contracting and program staff on the 5-Year MAPS program and provides notice to program managers when acquisition planning is set to begin, which the agency believes satisfies this recommendation. We acknowledge FEMA's training in this chapter; however, we noted that not all program and contracting staff we spoke with were familiar with 5-Year MAPS, and there is no formal guidance on timeframes for the entire acquisition planning process. We continue to believe this recommendation remains open and encourage FEMA to formalize guidance on the timeframes and considerations for planning various types of acquisitions across the entire acquisition planning process, and to document the purpose and use of the 5-Year MAPS program to ensure a uniform understanding of the program.

Further, in its concurrence with our eighth recommendation, FEMA stated that it believes its current advance contract list satisfies our recommendation for internally communicating available advance contracts. We acknowledge in this chapter that the advance contract list is updated monthly; however, we found inconsistencies in the advance contract list and other documentation identifying advance contracts, which could result in FEMA's contracting officers not having full visibility into available advance contracts. We continue to believe the recommendation remains open and encourage FEMA to identify a centralized resource with all available advance contracts and ensure that it is regularly updated for contracting staff.

We are sending copies of this chapter to the appropriate congressional committees, the Secretary of Defense, the U.S. Army Corps of Engineers Director of Contracting, the Secretary of Homeland Security, the Administrator of the Federal Emergency Management Agency, and the Federal Emergency Management Agency's Chief Procurement Officer.

Marie A. Mak
Director, Contracting and National Security Acquisitions

List of Requesters

The Honorable Michael B. Enzi
Chairman
Committee on the Budget
United States Senate

The Honorable Ron Johnson
Chairman

The Honorable Claire McCaskill
Ranking Member
Committee on Homeland Security and Governmental Affairs
United States Senate

The Honorable Rand Paul, MD
Chairman

The Honorable Gary Peters
Ranking Member
Subcommittee on Federal Spending Oversight and Emergency Management
Committee on Homeland Security and Governmental Affairs
United States Senate

The Honorable Jeb Hensarling
Chairman

The Honorable Maxine Waters
Ranking Member
Committee on Financial Services
House of Representatives

The Honorable Michael T. McCaul
Chairman

The Honorable Bennie G. Thompson
Ranking Member
Committee on Homeland Security
House of Representatives

The Honorable Trey Gowdy
Chairman

The Honorable Elijah E. Cummings
Ranking Member
Committee on Oversight and Government Reform
House of Representatives

The Honorable Bill Shuster
Chairman

The Honorable Peter DeFazio
Ranking Member
Committee on Transportation and Infrastructure
House of Representatives

The Honorable Daniel M. Donovan, Jr.
Chairman
Subcommittee on Emergency Preparedness, Response, and Communications
Committee on Homeland Security
House of Representatives

The Honorable Sean Duffy
Chairman

The Honorable Emanuel Cleaver, II
Ranking Member
Subcommittee on Housing and Insurance
Committee on Financial Services
House of Representatives

The Honorable Gary J. Palmer
Chairman
Subcommittee on Intergovernmental Affairs
Committee on Oversight and Government Reform
House of Representatives

The Honorable Ann Wagner
Chairman

The Honorable Al Green
Ranking Member
Subcommittee on Oversight and Investigations
Committee on Financial Services
House of Representatives

The Honorable Nydia M. Velazquez
House of Representatives

APPENDIX I: OBJECTIVES, SCOPE, AND METHODOLOGY

This chapter reviews the federal government's contracting efforts for preparedness, response, and recovery efforts related to the three 2017 hurricanes and California wildfires. This chapter specifically addresses the use of advance contracts, assessing the extent to which (1) the Federal Emergency Management Agency (FEMA) and the U.S. Army Corps of Engineers (USACE) used advance contracts, (2) the planning, management, and reporting of selected FEMA and USACE advance contracts met certain contracting requirements, and (3) FEMA and USACE identified any lessons learned and challenges with their use of these contracts. We also have an ongoing review on post-disaster contracting that is expected to be completed in early 2019.

To identify the extent to which FEMA and USACE used advance contracts, we reviewed data on contract obligations for the 2017 disasters from the Federal Procurement Data System-Next Generation (FPDS-NG) through May 31, 2018.[53] We identified hurricane

[53] For the purposes of this report, contract obligations include obligations against what the General Services Administration's FPDS-NG categorizes as definitive vehicles (definitive contracts and purchase orders that have a defined scope of work that do not allow for individual orders under them), and against what FPDS-NG

obligations using the national interest code, as well as the contract description. Data on obligations for the California wildfires is limited to those contracts that FEMA and USACE identified as being used to respond to those events because no national interest code was established in FPDS-NG.[54] To determine which obligations were made through the use of advance contracts, we reviewed documentation provided by FEMA and USACE identifying the advance contracts they have in place and that were used in support of the 2017 disasters.[55] We analyzed the FPDS-NG data to identify FEMA and USACE advance contract obligations compared to overall contract obligations by disaster, competition procedures used, and the types of goods and services procured. We assessed the reliability of FPDS-NG data by reviewing existing information about the FPDS-NG system and the data it collects—specifically, the data dictionary and data validation rules—and performing electronic testing. We determined the FPDS-NG data were sufficiently reliable for the purposes of this chapter.

To assess the extent to which FEMA used its advance contracts, we reviewed FEMA contracting policies and guidance, such as FEMA's 2017 *Disaster Contracting Desk Guide* and FEMA's *Advance Contracting of Goods and Services Report to Congress* to identify available guidance on the use and intent of advance contracts. Based on our review of documentation, we identified examples of goods—tarps and meals—that FEMA had advance contracts in place for, but experienced challenges using in response the 2017 disasters. We reviewed FPDS-NG data to determine whether these goods were procured through post-disaster contracts rather than advance contracts, and selected advance and post-disaster contracts for further review. To identify limitations that affected the use of tarp and meal advance contracts, we gathered and reviewed advance and post-disaster contract documentation and interviewed contracting officials involved in the award and use of the contracts in 2017.

To assess the extent to which the planning, management, and reporting of advance contracts used in response to the three hurricanes and California wildfires in 2017 met selected applicable contracting requirements, we reviewed relevant documentation, including the Post-Katrina Emergency Management Reform Act (PKEMRA), the Federal Acquisition Regulation (FAR), and Department of Homeland Security (DHS, FEMA, and USACE contracting policies. We identified a non-generalizable sample of advance contracts based on advance contract obligation data from FPDS-NG as of March 31, 2018. We analyzed the data to identify 10 competed and four h non-competed contracts.[56] To obtain a range of competed

categorizes as indefinite delivery vehicles (orders under the Federal Supply Schedule, orders/calls under blanket purchase agreements, orders under basic ordering agreements, orders under government-wide acquisition contracts, and orders under other indefinite delivery vehicles, such as indefinite delivery, indefinite quantity contracts).

[54] National interest action codes are used to track relief contracts in FPDS-NG. No national interest action code was requested for the 2017 California wildfires.

[55] DHS and DOD exercised the use of the special emergency procurement authorities within 41 U.S.C. §1903, as amended by section 816 of the National Defense Authorization Act for Fiscal Year 2017, Pub. L. No. 114-328 (and as implemented by DHS FAR Class Deviation 17-02 and DOD Class Deviation 2017-O0007, respectively) to increase the micro-purchase threshold to $20,000 for procurements in support of these major disaster responses so contract obligations for hurricanes reported in FPDS-NG may only include obligations over that amount.

[56] For the purposes of selecting our case studies, competitive contracts included contracts and orders coded in FPDS-NG as "full and open competition," "full and open after exclusion of sources," and "competed under simplified acquisition procedures." Noncompetitive contracts included contracts and orders coded in FPDS-NG as "not competed," "not available for competition," and "not competed under simplified acquisition procedures."

contracts, we identified contracts used for goods and services with obligations above $50 million. All of the non-competed contracts used were for FEMA services; to obtain a range of non-competed contracts we identified contracts with obligations above $10 million. Our selected advance contracts included 10 from FEMA and four from USACE. Findings based on information collected from the 14 contracts cannot be generalized to all advance contracts. Additional details on our selected contracts can be found in Table 2.

Table 2. Selected Federal Emergency Management Agency (FEMA) and U.S. Army Corps of Engineers (USACE) Advance Contracts

	Contract Number	Description	Obligations as of May 31, 2018
FEMA	HSFE7017D0001 HSFE7017D0003 HSFE7017D0004	Non-competed service contract supporting FEMA's individual assistance program which provides financial assistance to those with property damaged by a disaster.	$100,525,716 $39,082,653 $249,035,558
	HSFE3016D0203	Non-competed service contract which provides FEMA employees with local and long-distance telephone service, high speed data services, and cable television that can be used during disaster response.	$13,963,151
	HSFE7014D0152 HSFE7014D0150	Competed goods contract for manufactured housing units to shelter those displaced by a disaster.	$74,332,500 $70,294,193
	HSFEHQ12D0881 HSFEHQ12D0882	Competed service contract supporting FEMA's public assistance program which provides supplemental federal assistance to state, tribal, territorial, and local governments for disaster response.	$197,464,836 $177,798,052
	HSFE7017D0019	Competed goods contract for bottled water to distribute to those affected by a disaster.	$154,627,988
	HSFE8013D0070	Competed services contract which provides housing inspection services for those with property damaged by a disaster.	$321,518,435
USACE	W911WN15D0001	Competed services contract which provides temporary power for households affected by a disaster.	$718,436,308
	W912P814D0016 W912P814D0028 W912P814D0033	Competed services contract which provides debris removal for households affected by a disaster.	$166,540,852 $321,687,964 $320,351,681

Source: GAO review of Federal Procurement System Database- Next Generation and contract information I GAO-19-93.

To review our selected FEMA and USACE advance contracts, we developed a data collection instrument to gather selected contract information, such as period of performance, contract type, estimated contract value, and the presence of key contract documents, among others. To assess FEMA and USACE's planning of selected advance contracts, we reviewed information from our data collection instrument on advance contract award date and period of performance, and determined that six of FEMA's contracts met GAO's definition of a bridge contract. To identify any planning challenges that contributed to these extensions, we reviewed FEMA acquisition planning policies, timeframes and relevant contract file documentation, such as written acquisition strategies and justification and approval documents, to determine whether acquisition planning activities for the selected advance contracts were completed according to guidance. We interviewed FEMA officials associated with these contracts on acquisition planning efforts, and factors that affected their ability to award new contracts. We also reviewed documentation and interviewed officials on FEMA's acquisition planning system—the 5 Year Master Acquisition Planning Schedule (MAPS).

To assess FEMA and USACE's management of selected advance contracts, we reviewed information gathered from our data collection instrument on the presence of selected acquisition documents, such as acquisition strategies and contract modifications in the contract file, that typically provide the history of a contract. We reviewed relevant procurement regulations, the DHS Acquisition Manual, and other FEMA and USACE policies, to identify acquisition documentation requirements and record keeping processes. For contracts where documentation was not found in the contract file or system of record, we requested the missing documentation from FEMA and USACE officials to determine whether it had been completed. We also interviewed FEMA and USACE headquarters officials to supplement our understanding of FEMA and USACE's record keeping policies, practices, and challenges.

To assess the reporting of selected advance contracts, we compared advance contract action data identified in FPDS-NG to data reported in *FEMA's Disaster Contracts Quarterly Report Fourth Quarter, Fiscal Year 2017* and *Disaster Contracts Quarterly Report First Quarter, Fiscal Year 2018* to congressional committees on disaster contracting to identify any unreported actions. We interviewed FEMA officials to discuss the methodology and data sources for the congressional committee reports, and any limitations to the accuracy of the data reported.

To assess what challenges and lessons learned FEMA and USACE identified with the use of advance contracts in 2017, we reviewed PKEMRA advance contract requirements, FEMA and USACE documentation on the use of advance contracts, and after-action reports from 2017 and prior years, including the *Hurricane Sandy FEMA After-Action Report,* and *the 2017 Hurricane Season FEMA After-Action Report*, and federal internal control standards for information and communications. As part of our review, we identified FEMA and USACE's processes for documenting lessons learned following a disaster, lessons learned specific to advance contracts, and any recommendations or actions planned by the agencies to address them. We interviewed FEMA and USACE headquarters officials on reported lessons learned, any other challenges related to the use of advance contracts, and ongoing or completed actions to address them. To describe challenges related to coordination with state and local officials on the use of advance contracts, we interviewed FEMA and USACE regional staff. To obtain perspectives and examples from state and local government officials involved in disaster response efforts we interviewed officials in California on advance contracting efforts. The information gathered from these officials is not generalizable to all officials. We also analyzed information on available advance contracts from FEMA's June 2018 advance contract list and FEMA's May 2018 training documentation identifying advance contracts to identify any differences in the information available to FEMA regional contracting officers, and their state and local contracting counterparts.

We conducted this performance audit from March 2018 to December 2018 in accordance with generally accepted government auditing standards. Those standards require that we plan and perform the audit to obtain sufficient, appropriate evidence to provide a reasonable basis for our findings and conclusions based on our audit objectives. We believe that the evidence obtained provides a reasonable basis for our findings and conclusions based on our audit objectives.

APPENDIX II: FEDERAL EMERGENCY MANAGEMENT AGENCY (FEMA) REGIONAL OFFICES

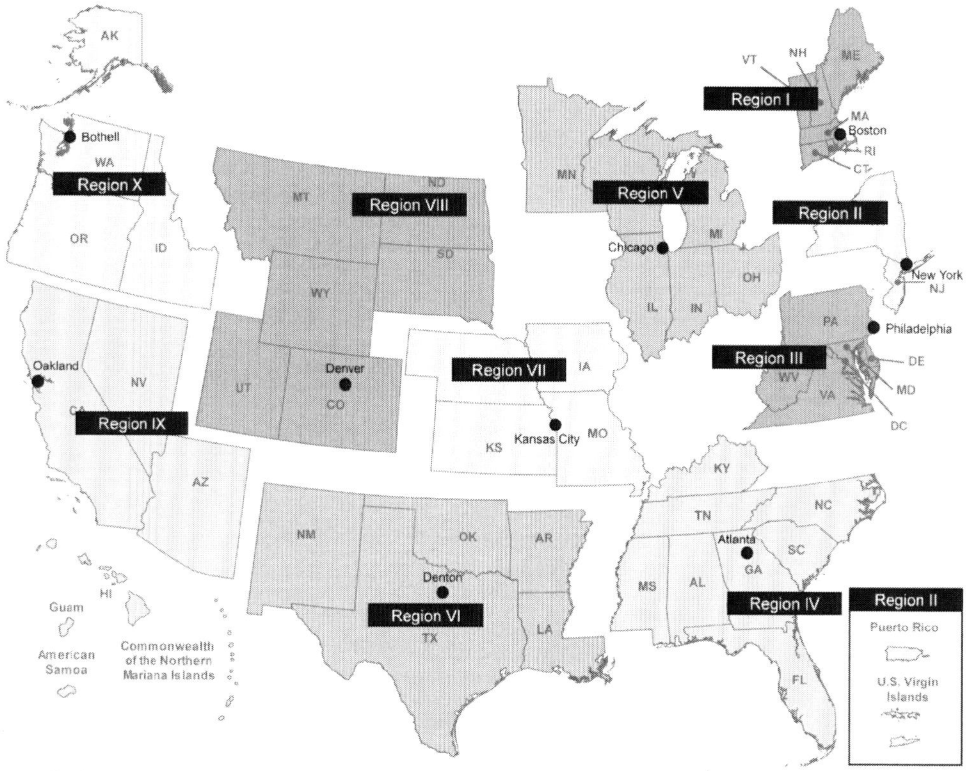

Source: Federal Emergency Management Agency; Map Resources (map). | GAO-19-93.

Figure 11. Map of Federal Emergency Management Agency (FEMA) Regions and Their Member States and Territories.

APPENDIX III: FEDERAL EMERGENCY MANAGEMENT AGENCY (FEMA) AND U.S. ARMY CORPS OF ENGINEERS (USACE)-IDENTIFIED ADVANCE CONTRACTS

Table 3. Federal Emergency Management Agency (FEMA) Identified Advance Contracts, as of June 2018

Acquisition Name	Description	Number of Contracts	Procurement Vehicle	Base Award Date
Short-term Lodging Assistance Program	Allows FEMA to use Corporate Lodging Consultant services to place disaster victims in hotels during mass evacuations.	1	GSA Schedule task order/Blanket purchase agreement	May 15, 2016

Acquisition Name	Description	Number of Contracts	Procurement Vehicle	Base Award Date
Public Assistance Technical Assistance Contract III (PA-TAC)	Supports FEMA's objectives of providing public assistance in a timely, effective, and consistent manner.	4	Indefinite delivery contract	February 17, 2012
Individual Assistance Support Contract (IASC)	Supports individual assistance and mass care in zone 2—FEMA regions 6 through 10.	2	Indefinite delivery contract	March 8, 2018
Housing Inspection Services	Provides damage inspection services in affected disaster areas in support of claims for damaged homes.	2	Indefinite delivery contract	September 30, 2013
Mail Operations	Processes incoming and outgoing mail communication and claims from disaster victims.	2	Indefinite delivery contract	September 12, 2015
Crisis Counseling Program	Provides crisis counseling assistance and training.	1	Interagency reimbursable work agreement	October 1, 2017
Disaster Readiness Account – Disaster Unemployment Assistance	Provides unemployment assistance in times of disaster.	1	Interagency agreement	December 24, 2014
Missing and Exploited Child Alert Services	Provides alert services for missing children during response and recovery of federally declared disasters.	1	Indefinite delivery contract	March 22, 2018
Individual Identity Verification Service	Verifies and authenticates the identity of personnel applying for disaster assistance to prevent duplicate or fraudulent applications for assistance.	1	Indefinite delivery contract	September 30, 2013
National and Regional Commercial Ambulance Gulf/East Coast States	Provides air and ground ambulance support services in Atlantic and Gulf Coast states. Pacific and Central Coast states are non-priced optional line items.	1	Indefinite delivery contract	July 17, 2017
Aviation and Ground Support Services for Large Scale Disasters	Provides aviation and ground support evacuation at airports in Southeastern and Gulf Coast states.	1	Indefinite delivery contract	September 21, 2016
Executive Aircraft Transport	Agreement with the Federal Aviation Administration to use executive air travel during response and recovery efforts for federally declared disasters.	1	Interagency agreement	August 11, 2016

Table 3. (Continued)

Acquisition Name	Description	Number of Contracts	Procurement Vehicle	Base Award Date
Air Transportation Support Services	Provides air transportation support services.	2	Indefinite delivery contract	April 12, 2017
Motor Coach Evacuation – Mass Transportation Services	Provides preparedness planning and operation support for large-scale motor coach evacuation of general population within the continental U.S.	1	Indefinite delivery contract	May 15, 2014
Telephone Interpretation Services	Provides telephone interpretation services at National Processing Service Center in Denton, TX during a federally declared disaster.	2	Indefinite delivery contract	February 23, 2012
RadResponder Support Services	Provides standardized radiation data collection, management, and monitoring of environmental data during a radiological or nuclear event.	1	GSA Schedule task order	August 8, 2016
Public Service Advertising Ad Council	Provides public alerts and campaigns to the general public prior to, during, and post-disaster.	1	Indefinite delivery contract	September 9, 2014
Mobile Disaster Recovery Center Satellite Airtime Service	Provides Mobile Disaster Recovery Center with satellite airtime communication and access to FEMA networks and communications for disaster operations.	1	Interagency agreement	December 21, 2014
National Responder Support Camp IT Services	Provides on-site IT support technicians, managed services, and satellite equipment.	1	GSA Schedule task order / Blanket purchase agreement	May 31, 2016
GPS Managed Services	Deploys contractors to the field to provide hands on GPS oversight.	2	Indefinite delivery contract	September 30, 2014
Deployment Tracking Systems	Tracks and deploys the national disaster workforce during response to federally declared disasters.	1	GSA Schedule task order	September 30, 2013 and September 30, 2015
Mobile Emergency Response Support Mobile Satellite Services	Provides mobile satellite services.	1	GSA Schedule task order	January 14, 2016
FEMA-Wide Wireless Telecommunications	Provides wireless telecommunications services to emergency responders.	2	Indefinite delivery contract	October 6, 2016

Acquisition Name	Description	Number of Contracts	Procurement Vehicle	Base Award Date
FEMA Wireline Telephone Services	Provides wireline and other telephone services for continental U.S. and outside continental U.S. operations.	1	Indefinite delivery contract	February 1, 2017
Centralized Operations, Maintenance and Management Information Technology	Provides operation and maintenance support for FEMA-wide systems.	4	Indefinite delivery contract	October 17, 2014
Logistics Supply Chain Management System	Provides contractor services to support operation and maintenance of Logistics Supply Chain Management System.	2	Contract(s)	August 2, 2017 and March 8, 2017
National Log House Program	Supports survivors during federally declared disasters.	6	Indefinite delivery contract	April 3, 2018
National Responder Support Camp Operation Services	Provides support services for responders, including mobilization and demobilization, site preparation, installation, and management of responder base camp.	6	Indefinite delivery contract	September 26, 2017
Consumable Medical Supply Shelter Support Items	Provides medical supply kit items for purchase on an as needed basis.	1	Indefinite delivery contract	September 26, 2017
Infant and Toddler Shelter Supply Items	Provides shelter supplies for children under the age of three.	1	Indefinite delivery contract	September 26, 2016
Logistics Support Commodities – Supplies and Services	Provides commodities and services such as tarps, cots, joint field office kits, pet supplies, and hygiene kits.	1	Interagency agreement	July 26, 2017
Caribbean Deep Sea Freight	Provides deep see freight services to be activated by FEMA Region II when a storm is about to hit the U.S. Virgin Islands or Puerto Rico.	1	Indefinite delivery contract	August 31, 2016
Shelter Leased Generators and Equipment	Provides leased generators in support of shelter operations during federally declared disasters.	2	Indefinite delivery contract	March 14, 2015
Generator Maintenance – Continental U.S.	Provides maintenance to repair non- performing generator assets for distribution centers.	1	Contract	August 25, 2017
Generator Maintenance – Caribbean Distribution Center	Provides on-site generator maintenance for Caribbean distribution center.	1	Contract	September 30, 2017

Table 3. (Continued)

Acquisition Name	Description	Number of Contracts	Procurement Vehicle	Base Award Date
Generator Maintenance – Hawaii and Guam Distribution Centers	Provides on-site generator maintenance for Hawaii and Guam distribution centers.	1	Contract	July 29, 2015
Durable Medical Equipment Cache	Provides durable medical equipment for purchase on an as needed basis.	1	Indefinite delivery contract	September 28, 2017
Commercial Cots	Provides commercial cots for continental U.S. and outside continental U.S. distribution centers.	1	Indefinite delivery contract	July 11, 2016
Supplies and Services with Defense Logistics Agency	Provides disaster commodities and services such as meals ready to eat, aviation, maritime, and land weapon systems, clothing, construction equipment, fuel, and medical supplies.	1	Interagency agreement	March 12, 2017
Commercial and Reduced Sodium Meals	Provides commercial and reduced sodium meals for survivors.	3	Indefinite delivery contract	September 28, 2017
Manufactured Housing Units	Provides 1, 2, and 3 bedroom manufactured homes in support of disaster survivors.	7	Indefinite delivery contract	September 29, 2014
National Vehicle Maintenance Service Contract	Provides maintenance of disaster response tactical vehicles.	1	Indefinite delivery contract	May 29, 2018
Self-Help Tarps	Provides 20 by 25 foot self-help tarps for small areas of roof damage.	3	Indefinite delivery contract	September 12, 2014
Boxed and Bottled Water	Provides boxed and bottled water for disaster survivors.	4	Indefinite delivery contract	September 5, 2017
Blankets	Provides blankets for disaster survivors.	2	Indefinite delivery contract	September 27, 2013
Cleaning Supplies	Provides cleaning supplies to support survivors in shelters during federally declared disasters.	3	Indefinite delivery contract	September 27, 2013
Cross Docking Operations	Provides a network of transportation and emergency cross dock and freight forwarding service operation centers to support large scale trailer operations in the continental U.S.	1	Indefinite delivery contract	September 30, 2016
Miscellaneous Shelter Items	Provides miscellaneous shelter items to disaster survivors.	3	Indefinite delivery contract	September 26, 2013

Acquisition Name	Description	Number of Contracts	Procurement Vehicle	Base Award Date
Shelter Clothing	Provides clothing for disaster survivors in shelters.	1	Indefinite delivery contract	August 2, 2016
Portable Facilities	Provides portable toilet facilities and fresh water delivery and removal services.	1	Indefinite delivery contract	September 16, 2016
Laundry Services	Provides laundry services for disaster survivors.	4	Indefinite delivery contract	May 30, 2017
Hazard Mitigation Technical Assistance Program Non-Architecture and Engineering	Provide non-architect and engineering technical assistance, research and analysis, and document development.	3	Indefinite delivery contract	March 20, 2015
Hazard Mitigation Technical Assistance Program Architect and Engineering	Provides production and technical services for architect and engineering contracts.	2	Indefinite delivery contract	November 24, 2014
Shipping and Receiving of Mail Equipment, Storage Services	Provides storage, shipping, and maintenance of mail equipment in support of disaster operations.	1	Purchase order	November 27, 2013
Warehouse Support Services	Provides warehouse support services.	1	Contract	May 4, 2015
Health and Human Services/ Federal Occupational Health Awareness Services	Provides environmental support, industrial hygiene and occupational safety support, hazardous waste, disaster safety, bio hazard safety support, and fire program development and support.	1	Interagency agreement	September 28, 2015

Source: Fiscal Year 2018 FEMA Prepositioned Contract List, June 1, 2018. I GAO-19-93.

Note: Contracts listed represent all available FEMA advance contracts, as identified by their June fiscal year 2018 prepositioned contract list, and not just contracts used in response to the three 2017 hurricanes and California wildfires.

Table 4. U.S. Army Corps of Engineers (USACE) Identified Advance Contracts, as of September 2018

Advance Contract Initiative	Description	Number of Contracts	Procurement Vehicle	Base Award Year
Temporary Power	Provides emergency power to critical public facilities	4	Indefinite Delivery Contract	2013/2014
Temporary Roofing	Provides installation of blue plastic sheeting onto roofs of damaged homes or public structures	12	Indefinite Delivery Contract	2014/2015
Debris Removal	Provides emergency debris clearance and removal	17	Indefinite Delivery Contract	2014

Source: GAO review of USACE information. I GAO 19-93.

Note: Contracts listed represent all available USACE advance contracts, and not just advance contracts used in response to the three 2017 hurricanes and California wildfires.

APPENDIX IV: COMMENTS FROM THE DEPARTMENT OF HOMELAND SECURITY

U.S. Department of Homeland Security
Washington, DC 20528

Homeland Security

November 20, 2018

Marie A. Mak
Director, Contracting and National Security Acquisition
U.S. Government Accountability Office
441 G Street, NW
Washington, DC 20548

Re: Management Response to Draft Report GAO-19-93, "2017 DISASTER CONTRACTING: Action Needed to Better Ensure More Effective Use and Management of Advance Contracts" (Job Code 102660)

Dear Ms. Mak,

Thank you for the opportunity to review and comment on the subject draft report. The U.S. Department of Homeland Security (DHS) appreciates the U.S. Government Accountability Office's (GAO) work in planning and conducting its review and issuing this report.

The Department is pleased to note GAO's recognition of the positive steps FEMA has taken to institute training and develop guidance on timeframes related to the acquisition planning process for advance contracts. Contracting during disasters can pose a unique set of challenges and significant amount of pressure to provide life-sustaining goods and services to survivors as quickly as possible. Advance contracts significantly contribute to FEMA's ability to rapidly leverage cost-effective method for mobilizing resources, while also helping to preclude the need to procure critical goods and services non-competitively. FEMA remains committed to (1) contracting in full compliance with the Post-Katrina Emergency Management Reform Act (PKEMRA), Robert T. Stafford Disaster Relief and Emergency Assistance Act, Federal Acquisition Regulation (FAR), Homeland Security Acquisition Regulation, and Homeland Security Acquisition Manual, and (2) continuously communicating to state and local governments on the availability and proper establishment and use of the advance contracts.

The draft report contained nine recommendations with which the Department concurs. Attached for our detailed responses to each recommendation. Technical comments were previously provided under separate cover.

Again, thank you for the opportunity to review and comment on this draft report. Please feel free to contact me if you have any questions. We look forward to working with you again in the future.

Sincerely,

JIM H. CRUMPACKER, CIA, CFE
Director
Departmental GAO-OIG Liaison Office

Attachment: Management Response to Recommendations Contained in GAO-19-93

GAO recommended that FEMA's Administrator:

Recommendation 1: Update the strategy identified in its 2007 *Advance Contracting of Goods and Services Report to Congress* to clearly define the objectives of advanced contracts, how they contribute to FEMA's disaster response operations, and whether and how they should be prioritized in relation to new post-disaster contract awards.

Response: Concur. FEMA's Office of the Chief Component Procurement Officer (OCPO) will update the strategy identified in the 2007 Advance Contracting of Goods and Services Report to Congress in the *Disaster Contracting Desk Guide*, outlining clear objectives and use of advance contracts in disaster operations. FEMA will memorialize a structure that prioritizes utilizing existing advance contracts related to new-post disaster contract awards. Requirements for goods and services determined to meet the requirement of advance contracts, in accordance with PKEMRA and Robert T. Stafford Disaster Relief and Emergency Assistance Act, are identified in the 5-year Master Acquisition Planning Schedule (MAPS) for accountability and advance acquisition planning purposes. Estimated Completion Date (ECD): June 30, 2019.

Recommendation 2: Ensure the Chief Procurement Officer updates the *Disaster Contracting Desk Guide* to include guidance for whether and under what circumstances contracting officers should consider using existing advance contracts prior to making new post-disaster contract awards, and include this guidance in existing semi-annual training given to the contracting officers.

Response: Concur. FEMA OCPO will update the current *Disaster Contracting Desk Guide* to establish clear guidance prioritizing the use of existing advance contracts prior to issuing any new post-disaster contract awards. The updated guidance will be communicated to contracting personnel during the next disaster webinar. ECD: June 30, 2019

Recommendation 3: Update and implement existing guidance for program office and contracting officer personnel to identify acquisition planning timeframes and considerations across the entire acquisition process and clearly communicate the purpose and use of MAPS.

Response: Concur. FEMA's OCPO conducted outreach with all of the program offices during June 2016 on the purpose and use of the 5-year MAPS program. This ensured all stakeholders have complete understanding of the tool. As a result, the program offices have full visibility into future procurement actions, and work with OCPO to conduct acquisition planning within established timelines. As a part of these efforts, all program offices receive communication from FEMA's OCPO 18 months before the expiration of their contract. This communication requests a program manager to work with OCPO Portfolio Managers to ensure solicitations are prepared in a timely manner, ensuring timely award. We request that GAO consider this recommendation resolved and closed as implemented.

Recommendation 4: Ensure the Chief Procurement Officer adheres to current hard copy contract file management requirement to ensure advance contract files are complete and up to date, whether they will be transferred into the new Electronic Contract Filing System [ECFS] or remain in hard copy format.

Response: Concur. FEMA OCPO will update the current Labeling and Organizing Official Contract File Folders Standard Operating Procedure (SOP), dated August 31, 2009, to clearly institute and enforce the policy of maintaining the official record of contract file as a hard copy unless rescinded with the implementation of a Department-wide ECFS. ECD: June 30, 2019.

Recommendation 5: Ensure the Chief Procurement Officer reminds contracting officers of the three day timeframe for entering completed award documentation into contracting writing system when executing notice to proceed documentation.

Response: Concur. FEMA OCPO will update the current Notice To Proceed SOP, dated April 23, 2013, to ensure that contracting officers know all awards must be entered into contracting writing system and Federal Procurement Data System (FPDS) within three days of award. ECD: July 31, 2019.

Recommendation 6: Ensure the Chief Procurement Officer revises its reporting methodology to ensure that all disaster contracts are included in its quarterly reports to congressional committees on disaster contract actions.

Response: Concur. To ensure accurate reporting of all disaster contracts to congressional committees, FEMA OCPO will incorporate an addendum in its quarterly report. The addendum will capture the contract actions that were not previously reported based on the exemption of FAR 4.604(b)(3), which allows any action awarded in accordance with FAR 6.302-2 or pursuant to any of the authorities listed at FAR Subpart 18.2 to be submitted in FPDS within 30 days after contract award. ECD: July 31, 2019.

Recommendation 7: Ensure the Chief Procurement Officer revises the *Disaster Contracting Officer Desk Guide* to provide specific guidance for contracting officer to perform outreach to state and local governments on the use and establishment of advance contracts.

Response: Concur. FEMA OCPO has taken the initiative to create an external acquisition toolbox website for the state, local, territorial and tribal (SLTT) governments to access templates and tools needed to establish SLTT governments' own advance contracts. Additionally, a procurement hotline was established August 23, 2018 to answer any questions or provide additional assistance when needed/requested by the SLTT governments. Finally, FEMA OCPO will update the current *Disaster Contracting Desk Guide* to provide clear and specific guidance on coordination and outreach to governments. ECD: October 31, 2019.

Recommendation 8: Ensure the Chief Procurement Officer identifies a single centralized resource listing its advance contracts and ensure that source is updated regularly to include all available advance contracts.

Response: Concur. A list of all advance contracts is provided to contracting personnel and external customers through the OCPO Reporting Dashboard SharePoint site. The list is also updated monthly and distributed to all OCPO supervisors on a monthly basis, and is available on FEMA's intranet website. We request that GAO consider this recommendation resolved and closed as implemented.

Recommendation 9: Ensure the Chief Procurement Officer communicates information on available advance contracts through the centralized resource to states and localities to inform their advance contracting efforts.

Response: Concur. FEMA's OCPO, in coordination with the Office of External Affairs and Procurement Disaster Assistance Team (PDAT) within FEMA Office of Chief Counsel, will conduct outreach with SLTT governments to communicate establishing the acquisition toolbox website. The toolbox will provide SLTTs access to the list of advance contracts, templates, and tools needed to establish their own advance contracts. In addition, PDAT will continue to engage SLTT governments and communicate guidance on procurement under grants through in-person and virtual trainings, deployments, technical assistance, and its resources and tools on the PDAT website. ECD: October 31, 2019.

In: Top 10 Reports and Testimonies in December 2018 ISBN: 978-1-53615-507-5
Editor: Sarah J. Nygaard

Chapter 2

2020 CENSUS: ADDITIONAL STEPS NEEDED TO FINALIZE READINESS FOR PEAK FIELD OPERATIONS*

United States Government Accountability Office

ABBREVIATIONS

Bureau	Census Bureau
IT	Information Technology
NRFU	Non-Response Follow-Up

WHY GAO DID THIS STUDY

The cost of the decennial census has steadily increased over the past several decades, with self-response rates declining over the same period. The largest and costliest operation that the Bureau undertakes, NRFU is the Bureau's attempt to enumerate households not initially self-responding to the census.

GAO was asked to review NRFU implementation during the 2018 Census Test as well as the Bureau's overall readiness for peak field operations, which cover the actual enumeration of residents. This chapter examines (1) how peak field operations, including NRFU, were implemented during the test; and (2) the extent to which prior test implementation issues have been addressed. GAO reviewed test planning and training documentation, as well as production and payroll data. At the test site, GAO observed and interviewed enumerators, field supervisors, and managers conducting peak operations.

* This is an edited, reformatted and augmented version of the United States Government Accountability Office Report to Congressional Requesters, Publication No. GAO-19-140, dated December 2018.

What GAO Recommends

GAO recommends that the Bureau (1) determine procedures for late-NRFU data collection; (2) align census field supervisor screening, authorities, and information flows; (3) prepare for targeted mid-operation training or guidance as needed; and (4) improve training on reporting cases that need supervisory attention and alternative ways to communicate these cases.

The Department of Commerce agreed with GAO's findings and recommendations, and the Bureau provided technical comments that were incorporated as appropriate.

What GAO Found

In preparation for the 2020 census, the Census Bureau (Bureau) set out to enumerate over 140,000 housing units during the 2018 Census Test at a site in Providence County, Rhode Island. The 2018 Census Test marked the Bureau's last chance to test enumeration procedures for peak field operations under census-like conditions before 2020. Implementation of this test identified the following concerns:

- The Bureau experienced operational issues during implementation of the Non-Response Follow-Up (NRFU) as part of the 2018 Census Test. For example, the Bureau had not finalized procedures for data collection during late phases of NRFU (e.g., after multiple attempts to interview had been made) until after the work had already started. As a result, enumerators and their supervisors did not have standardized procedures during the test, which made it difficult to evaluate the effectiveness of the test procedures. GAO also observed a range of other NRFU implementation issues during the test, such as the Bureau's use of progress reporting that overstates the number of NRFU cases not needing any additional fieldwork and the Bureau having fewer of its enumerators work Saturdays, which can be among the most productive interview days. The Bureau is taking steps to assess and mitigate these and other issues that GAO identified.
- The Bureau's field workforce was not fully prepared to face all of the enumeration challenges that arose during the test. For instance, the Bureau expects census field supervisors to provide front-line coaching to enumerators but did not screen these employees to ensure they had the needed skills. Moreover, it did not provide them with the authorities and information that would have helped them serve that role. As a result, we believe that supervisors did not have the casework expertise, information, or authority to help enumerators with procedural questions, and higher-level census field managers ended up providing direct support to enumerators.
- While the Bureau provided extensive online and in-person training to enumerators prior to NRFU fieldwork for the 2018 Census Test, the Bureau lacked any standardized form of mid-operation training or guidance as new procedures were implemented. GAO observed that during the test some enumerators continued to have questions and were uncertain about procedures. Developing targeted, location-specific training could help ensure that, in 2020, enumerators receive the guidance

they need to collect census data consistently and in accordance with NRFU procedures.

The Bureau has made progress addressing prior test implementation issues but still faces challenges. For example, the Bureau improved its collection of enumerator case notes, which reflect real-time knowledge gained during enumeration. However, enumerators did not always report cases using flags built in to their interviewing device that would benefit from supervisory review, such as for language barriers. Moreover, supervisors were not systematically analyzing case notes to identify cases not flagged properly. As a result, critical data on fieldwork challenges were not being communicated effectively to those who could analyze and use them.

December 10, 2018
Congressional Requesters

The cost of the decennial census has steadily increased over the past several decades, with enumeration costs rising from about $16 per household in 1970 to around $92 in 2010 (all in constant 2020 dollars). The Census Bureau (Bureau) estimates that overall decennial costs will increase by over $3 billion from the 2010 Census to $15.6 billion in 2020 (in current decennial time frame costs).[1] During this period of increasing costs, the percentage of households self-responding to mailed census questionnaires has declined from 78 percent in 1970 to 63 percent in 2010. The Bureau anticipates that the self-response rate will further decline to roughly 60 percent in 2020, in part because, as the Bureau has noted, the population is overloaded with requests for information and has become increasingly concerned about sharing information.

When a household does not initially respond to the census, the Bureau attempts to enumerate the residents through Non-Response Follow-Up (NRFU), an operation where enumerators personally visit to count the household. NRFU is labor intensive and is the largest and costliest operation that the Bureau undertakes. Another enumeration operation happening at about the same time is Group Quarters, when the Bureau counts residents of group facilities (such as skilled nursing facilities and correctional facilities).

The Bureau planned its 2018 Census Test in Providence County, Rhode Island, to rehearse most of the operations, systems, and procedures that it will implement during the 2020 Census.[2] Previously, the Bureau conducted operational tests from 2013 through 2017, as well as multiple small-scale tests designed to demonstrate specific functionalities (such as submitting census data over the Internet). The 2018 test is the last opportunity for the Bureau to demonstrate readiness for its major operations in 2020 and to apply lessons learned from prior tests.[3]

---

[1] According to October 2017 Commerce documents, the reported figures are "inflated to the current 2020 Census time frame (fiscal years 2012 to 2023);" the Bureau had cited constant 2020 dollars for prior figures.

[2] Address canvassing, another decennial field operation, was also tested in Pierce County, Washington, and the Bluefield-Beckley-Oak Hill area of West Virginia earlier during the test.

[3] In November 2018 Bureau officials told us they plan to conduct a randomized control test for the 2020 Census using the American Community Survey infrastructure in the summer of 2019 for the purposes of informing NRFU and the Integrated Partnership and Communications Campaign for the 2020 Census. The test will ask the 2020 questions, including a question on citizenship in one panel of the test and excluding it from the test's second panel.

You asked us to review implementation of NRFU testing during the 2018 Census Test as well as the Bureau's overall readiness for peak operations, which cover the actual enumeration of residents. This chapter examines (1) the implementation of peak operations during the 2018 Census Test at the Providence County, Rhode Island, site; and (2) the extent to which implementation issues raised in prior 2020 Census tests have been addressed and what actions the Bureau could take to address these issues.[4]

To address both of these research objectives, we visited the test site in Rhode Island to observe implementation of the peak operations being tested between May and August 2018. These visits included nongeneralizable observations of door-to-door field enumeration and office clerical work, as well as interviews with local managers. We also observed debrief sessions held with multiple levels of the census field workforce after the operations. From each of these visits, we documented observations and provided feedback to Bureau managers in near real time so that the Bureau could mitigate and adapt to issues raised by the test's implementation in a timely manner. Implementation issues are a natural part of the testing environment and are what testing is intended to uncover. We also discussed any mitigation or evaluation strategies developed in response to our observations with the cognizant Bureau headquarters officials.

In addition to our fieldwork, we collected real-time production data on the tested operations. These data included tallies of case outcomes, transactional case activity by enumerators, and hours worked by Bureau employees. After testing the case tallies and distributions and interviewing cognizant officials, we determined that these data were sufficiently reliable for our reporting purposes. We also received daily progress reports from the Bureau throughout the test, and we reviewed Bureau test-planning documentation and our work from prior tests to examine how, if at all, the Bureau planned to address prior implementation issues.

We conducted this performance audit from April 2018 to December 2018 in accordance with generally accepted government auditing standards. Those standards require that we plan and perform the audit to obtain sufficient, appropriate evidence to provide a reasonable basis for our findings and conclusions based on our audit objectives. We believe that the evidence obtained provides a reasonable basis for our findings and conclusions based on our audit objectives.

BACKGROUND

NRFU is a field-based operation that the Bureau administers following the self-response period so that it can (1) determine the occupancy status of individual non-responsive housing units and (2) enumerate them. In most instances, the Bureau typically allows up to six enumeration attempts for each nonresponsive housing unit, or case. If the Bureau is unable to enumerate the housing unit in the field, it may have to impute attributes of the household based on the demographic characteristics of surrounding housing units as well as administrative records.

[4] Peak operations include self-response and other enumeration activity. Due to the timing of our work and the schedule of the 2018 Census Test, we specifically reviewed the NRFU and Group Quarters operations.

Within the test site in Providence County, Rhode Island, the Bureau set up an area census office to administer field operations. Figure 1 provides an overview of the managerial hierarchy of the area census office. The *area census office manager* oversees day-to-day operations within the office and acts as a liaison with the Bureau's New York Regional Census Center, which is a Bureau regional office with jurisdiction over the Providence area census office. *Census field managers* are to monitor operational progress and performance indicators to understand any areas of concern and shift resources as needed within the test site. *Census field supervisors* are to act as front-line supervisors for individual performance and payroll processes and receive procedural questions from *enumerators*, who conduct the count.

The Bureau has another operation—Group Quarters—to enumerate those living or staying in a group facility that provides housing or services. Such facilities can include skilled nursing facilities, college and university student housing, and correctional facilities. Within the Group Quarters enumeration, the Bureau also enumerates places such as soup kitchens, homeless shelters, and other service-based enumeration facilities.

Prior to Group Quarters enumeration in the field, the Bureau attempts to establish the facilities' approximate population count and preferred enumeration method through the Advance Contact operation. These facilities can choose among methods including paper listing, where the facility provides a roster of residents as of census day to the Bureau, and in-person enumeration, where a team of enumerators count residents. For the 2020 cycle, the Bureau is also adding an "eResponse" option, tested on a small scale in 2016, whereby facility administrators can electronically submit enumeration data at a date of their choosing within operational time frames.

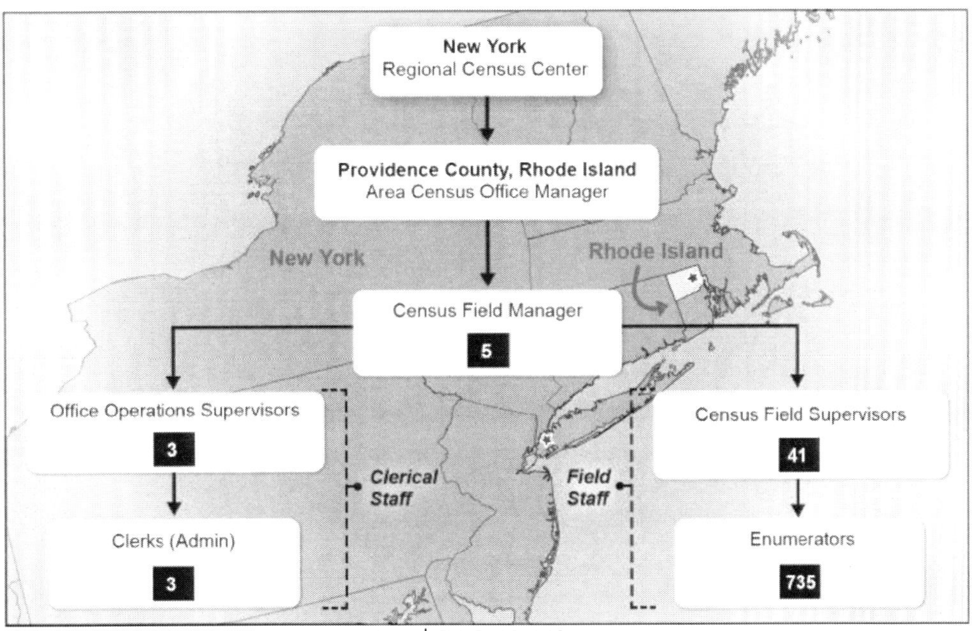

Source: GAO analysis of Census report data. | GAO-19-140.

Figure 1. Non-Response Follow-Up Was Implemented in a Multi-Tiered Structure at the Test Site.

Table 1. Time Frames for Operational Activities Observed during 2018 Census Test

Operation	Testing period
Non-Response Follow-Up	May 9 through July 31, 2018
Group Quarters Advance Contact	June 18 through July 10, 2018
Group Quarters	July 25 through August 24, 2018
Service-based Enumeration	July 25through July 27, 2018

Source: Census Bureau planning documentation. | GAO-19-140.

The Bureau's testing of the peak operations that we observed during the 2018 Census Test was intended to test collection of census data from those either not responding themselves via paper, telephone, or over the Internet or those living in group quarters. Prior to the start of NRFU during the 2018 test, roughly 45 percent of anticipated housing units in the test area of Providence County, Rhode Island, self-responded, leaving more than 140,000 remaining housing units to be attempted by NRFU itself, which took place between May 9 and July 31, 2018. The Bureau conducted a test of its Group Quarters enumeration from July 25 through August 24, 2018, including service-based enumeration. Both portions of Group Quarters fieldwork were preceded by the Advance Contact activity. Dates for the peak operations we observed during the 2018 test are listed in table 1.

The Bureau's operational plans for this phase of the fieldwork for the 2018 test incorporated two innovation areas that the Bureau hopes will produce savings for 2020.

- Reengineered field operations. For most of NRFU during the 2018 test, the Bureau relied on automated data collection methods, including a system-based, automated process for assigning work to enumerators, a smartphone-based application for collecting enumeration data in the field, and system-generated supervisory alerts.[5]
- Use of administrative records. To help reduce costly NRFU visits during the 2018 test, the Bureau reviewed and, where appropriate, applied administrative records—information already provided to the government as it administers other programs, such as Social Security, the Selective Service, or the Special Supplemental Nutrition Program for Women, Infants, and Children—to determine the occupancy status of housing units and thus remove vacant housing units from the NRFU workload, as well as to provide population counts of households not responding.[6]

The Bureau also tested multiple operational features for the first time this decennial cycle under full census-like production conditions in 2018:

- NRFU Closeout. During the 2018 test, the Bureau tested how best to relax certain business rules and enumeration procedures late in the NRFU operation so that it can

[5] Consistent with the 2016 Census Test, the Bureau had designed traditional NRFU, which began in May 2018, to involve a maximum of six enumeration attempts per non-responding housing unit. In most cases during this phase, the Bureau used its automated process for case assignments, whereby the system was to assign and route cases by geographic clusters based on multiple factors including: enumerator work availability; the likeliest time of day to successfully make contact with a resident; and spatial relationship with other open cases.

[6] For more information on the Bureau's use of Administrative Records, see: GAO, *2020 Census: Bureau Is Taking Steps to Address Limitations of Administrative Records,* GAO-17-664 (Washington, D.C.: July 26, 2017).

enumerate persistently non-responsive housing units. Examples of procedural modifications include increasing the maximum allowable number of enumeration attempts for each housing unit and manually assigning cases to the highest-performing enumerators.

- Office-Based Group Quarters Advance Contact. In the 2010 Census, the Bureau sent enumerator crews in person to each facility in advance of enumeration to establish the facility's preferred method of enumeration and to obtain an approximate population count. In the 2018 Census Test, the Bureau implemented a new method for 2020 that instead involved clerical staff contacting facilities by telephone and updating the group quarters address list and enumeration information remotely to reduce expenses associated with field visits for its enumerator crews.

The Bureau Experienced Operational Planning, Workforce Management, and Other Issues during Its 2018 Test of Peak Operations

The Bureau Did Not Determine Procedures for Late-NRFU Data Collection until after It Started the Work

The Bureau began the last phase of NRFU data collection in the 2018 test without having yet determined the procedures it would use for that critical phase.[7] Bureau planning documentation from February 2018 described a late-operation "closeout" phase of NRFU that would attempt to resolve cases that had not yet responded. However, we found that the Bureau had not determined the procedural modifications this phase would involve, either in terms of rules enumerators followed or business rules for how cases were to be assigned. By late May, nearly 3 weeks into the operation, the Bureau issued a set of closeout procedures to census areas where most cases had either been completed or where at least four of the six allowable enumeration attempt day assignments had been made. The Bureau also placed a priority on having high-performing enumerators—in terms of their ability to complete cases—available to work these cases during this phase of the NRFU testing.

Table 2 summarizes the chronology for when the Bureau implemented and documented procedural changes governing the transition from early to late-NRFU data collection, as well as the nature of those changes.

In late June 2018, the Bureau began testing the third phase of NRFU data collection, what it referred to as the "final attempt" phase, with officials citing a high incidence of non-interviews during prior phases as the reason. However, the Bureau had also begun this phase's data collection before it had established the procedural modifications it would be using. The modifications were intended to further increase the chances of enumerators completing cases in the field, such as by removing the limit on the number of attempts enumerators could make at each remaining case before NRFU ended.

---

[7] Every decennial, some housing units do not respond to the Bureau's multiple attempts to count them. In the 2018 test, NRFU included separately what it referred to as "closeout" and "final attempt" phases to maximize the participation rate of these housing units.

Table 2. Census Bureau Established Procedures for Late Non-Response Follow-Up (NRFU) after Test Implementation Had Begun

Operational Phase	Initial data collection	Final attempt
Initial scope of workload for the phase of data collection	Entire NRFU workload	NRFU areas with >3% of cases visited maximum number of times without getting a population count
Date that test data collection began for the phase	May 9, 2018	June 23, 2018
Datethat test data collection procedures were documented for the phase	January 4, 2018	July 13, 2018
Method of assigning cases	Automated assignment	Experimented with mix of manual and automated assignments
Notable changes to enumerator procedures relative to initial data collection	—	Unlimited number of attempts per day during time remaining; enumerators could sequence cases on their own

Source: GAO analysis of Bureau documentation. | GAO-19-140.
Legend: — refers to not applicable.

Standards for Internal Control in the Federal Government states that agencies should implement control activities by, for example, documenting policies.[8] However, the Bureau did not determine procedures for the final attempt phase until after testing for this phase of NRFU had begun. Enumerators and census field supervisors thus began working closeout and final attempt cases without a standardized set of test procedures.

Without determining the procedural changes the Bureau would be testing—or the business rules guiding when to make those changes—the Bureau was not well positioned to collect data to assess the alternatives it used during the test to inform planning for 2020. Bureau officials shared with us that they believed their automated case assignment approach is most effective during initial data collection but that it is less effective at targeting the toughest cases to resolve late in NRFU data collection. Yet, in part because the Bureau had not established when the transition from automated to manual case management would occur—or the business rules for determining when—some of the highest-performing enumerators were unavailable to receive assignments when the Bureau needed to begin the final attempt phase, according to the area census office manager. By not establishing the scope and timing of procedural changes for late-NRFU data collection in 2020, the Bureau may not be in a position to efficiently shift from its automated assignment approach to a manual one at the right time and position its most effective enumerators to receive assignments when needed.

In November 2018, the Bureau provided a draft contact strategy for NRFU in 2020 that included an outline of a multi-phase strategy for lateNRFU data collection. By including multiple phases of (1) shifting away from a fully-automated case assignment process and (2) relaxing management controls to complete as much casework as possible in areas with continued high non-response rates, this strategy appears to follow what the Bureau ultimately implemented during the 2018 test. It will be important, however, for the Bureau to determine

[8] GAO, *Standards for Internal Control in the Federal Government*, GAO-14-704G (Washington, D.C.: Sept. 10, 2014).

the business rules for procedural changes and their timing in advance so that it can maximize the value of NRFU in reducing the number of housing units that have to be imputed for the 2020 Census.

The Bureau Did Not Fully Ready Its Field Workforce for Enumeration Challenges

Census Field Supervisors Were Not Integrated Into Casework Management

As described in the Bureau's training and operational planning documents, census field supervisors were to be the primary points of contact in fielding and addressing enumerator questions. Census field managers—the next step above census field supervisors— were to focus their efforts on monitoring progress in completing the caseload, reviewing cases flagged by enumerators as problematic in one of a small number of pre-defined ways (e.g., dangerous addresses), and resolving significant performance issues. Among field supervisors' key responsibilities, according to the Bureau's plan for NRFU, were providing guidance to help enumerators understand procedural matters and to offer coaching and problem-solving support to enumerators who may need it. They also led enumerator training prior to the beginning of NRFU and generally were to train their specific team of enumerators.

However, census field managers and enumerators indicated that census field supervisors were often not the primary actors involved in fielding and addressing enumerator questions. Instead, enumerators and census field managers reported having direct contact with each other over procedural questions. Moreover, seven of the nine enumerators participating in the Bureau's operational debrief focus group who responded said they thought finding someone who could answer their questions was either difficult or very difficult.

We found that census field supervisors went underutilized in part because the Bureau did not recruit and position them to assume front-line supervising and coaching responsibilities. As outlined in training documentation, the Bureau vested supervisory review authority (for special cases, such as resident refusals and language barrier issues) within census field managers, the area census office manager, clerks, and office operations supervisors instead of census field supervisors. Additionally, as part of the Bureau's reengineered field operations for 2020, census field supervisors are given automated tools to monitor enumerators, and enumerators we observed told us that they generally did not interact in person with their supervisors apart from training. We believe that the combination of these factors resulted in census field supervisors having limited exposure to NRFU casework and any problematic situations enumerators might encounter. Officials also told us that the Bureau did not screen census field supervisors for their supervisory or coaching skillsets, though officials noted that this has been the practice in prior censuses, too. Rather, they hired census field supervisors based on their scores on the online enumerator training and because they reported an interest in supervising.

Additionally, census field supervisors lacked access to certain data streams from the test that could have helped them answer or troubleshoot enumerator questions. According to two census field managers, the Bureau did not regularly share consolidated records of procedural changes with census field supervisors. Information technology (IT) and census field managers also noted that the Bureau did not share or compare observations between the census field supervisor hotline and the decennial IT hotline, even though enumerators could potentially call either or both with technical or procedural questions. As a result, without sharing how best to respond to similar questions across support lines, enumerators could receive different answers for related questions depending on which hotline they contacted.

Standards for Internal Control in the Federal Government states that agency management should demonstrate a commitment to recruit, develop, and retain competent individuals.[9] Management should establish expectations for competence in key roles and should consider the level of assigned responsibility and delegated authority when establishing expectations. Yet, the role the Bureau envisioned census field supervisors having was not aligned with the authority supervisors were given, the skills for which the Bureau hired them, or the access to information that they had for the 2018 test.

When we raised this issue related to using census field supervisors, Bureau officials agreed and cited feedback they had received that census field managers felt inundated with the combination of the volume of supervisory review cases that flowed to them and with troubleshooting day-to-day enumerator questions. In October 2018, the Bureau provided documentation to us proposing a set of questions that they could use in screening applicants for the census field supervisor position to identify supervisory skills. Officials also said they were still evaluating options for granting census field supervisors more supervisory review authority. As the Bureau continues to learn from the 2018 test as part of its planning for 2020, it will be important to align census field supervisor roles with their authorities, skills, and information flows so that the Bureau does not underutilize a key portion of its field management chain. Doing so could also lessen the operational burden on higher-level census field managers.

Enumerators Did Not Receive Training To Address Mid-Operation Issues

Prior to the start of 2018 NRFU testing, the Bureau trained enumerators with a series of online training modules and assessments and one full day of in-person training facilitated by census field supervisors. The training included modules on data stewardship requirements, payroll responsibilities, and procedural directions for conducting respondent interviews. However, officials acknowledged that when the Bureau implemented its closeout and final attempt phases of NRFU, it did not provide standardized training to enumerators on the rollout of procedural changes. Five enumerators we observed during these stages said they relied on informal communications from their census field supervisors or census field managers for guidance. The initial practice had been for enumerators to receive daily assignments and follow pre-specified case sequencing and routing based on the Bureau's automated system. During the final attempt phase, enumerators were given discretion over the sequencing, routing, and number of attempts to make for cases that could be manually assigned, yet they were not given standardized training on how to handle this shift.

During our field observations, some enumerators we spoke with said they were uncertain about core procedures. For example, enumerators were not consistently aware that they had some discretion in large multi-unit settings to deviate from the assigned sequence of their cases provided by the automated system. Enumerators we observed and spoke to were also not always clear on how to flag within their field enumeration application the commonly occurring cases with confusing address markings and numberings. For example, enumerators had the

[9] GAO-14-704G.

option of selecting a case outcome of "missing unit designation," but they were not always sure whether this selection would capture the nuances of what they were seeing on the ground or how it differed from other selection options.[10]

Standards for Control in the Federal Government states that agencies should demonstrate a commitment to competence by, for example, tailoring training based on employee needs and helping personnel adapt to an evolving environment.[11] Targeted informational training would help the Bureau ensure that staff understand mid-operation procedural changes, and the training could be an opportunity for the Bureau to address commonly-observed and persistent implementation issues that may be arising. By developing brief, targeted mid-operation training, either as formal modules, guidance, or other standardized job aids, such as "frequently asked questions" worksheets, the Bureau could better position itself to react nimbly to enumerator feedback.

We have previously reported challenges the Bureau faces with its field work in other locations, such as connecting to the Internet during testing of address canvassing in rural West Virginia in 2017 and dealing with language barriers and other circumstances in unincorporated communities in southern Texas or with migrant and seasonal farmworkers in southern California during the 2000 Census.[12],[13] All challenges are not universal to all locations. Given that some of the enumeration challenges enumerators encountered in 2018 NRFU testing might not occur everywhere, and that some other areas of the country will have their own types of challenges, locally- or regionally-specific training or guidance may better address some needs. By relying solely on pre-NRFU training, the Bureau risks having little opportunity to course-correct with enumerators who may not have absorbed all of the training and are experiencing difficulty completing interviews or not collecting quality data.

The Bureau Is Assessing Other Implementation Issues That Arose during the 2018 Test

We observed and discussed with Bureau officials in real time several other implementation issues that occurred during the 2018 test. Bureau officials acknowledged these issues and, as of September 2018, were assessing them and developing mitigation strategies as part of their test evaluation process. These issues include:

- *Training certification.* Census field managers estimated that roughly 100 enumerators were unable to transmit their final test scores because the Bureau's online learning management system had an erroneous setting. According to Bureau officials, this problem delayed the start of unsupervised work for these otherwise-qualified enumerators by an average of 2 days per enumerator and resulted in the

[10] "Missing unit designation" is one of several case outcomes that refer to multi-unit address frame discrepancies. Other examples include "does not exist," "uninhabitable," and "nonresidential." Bureau officials indicated that they are reviewing the categorization of these outcomes in preparation for 2020.

[11] GAO-14-704G.

[12] GAO, *2020 Census: Actions Needed to Improve In-Field Address Canvassing*, GAO-18-414 (Washington, D.C.: June 14, 2018).

[13] GAO, *Decennial Census: Lessons Learned for Locating and Counting Migrant and Seasonal Farm Workers*, GAO-03-605 (Washington, D.C.: July 3, 2003).

attrition of some who were able to quickly find other work. Bureau officials told us they have fixed the system setting and are considering an alternative means to certify training, such as by having the option of trainees taking and verifying their final assessment as part of their final capstone day of classroom training. According to Bureau officials, development of this backup strategy will begin in December 2018.

- *Assigning cases manually in batches.* During the 2018 test, the Bureau's automated case management system was not configured for non-Headquarters staff to manually assign multiple cases to an enumerator at once. Rather, according to officials, census field managers were faced with having to manually assign thousands of cases individually during latter stages of NRFU. According to field management, this problem presented an unexpected burden on them, delayed assignments of the hardest-to-count cases, and contributed to high-performing enumerators not receiving work timely and in some cases for days in a row. Officials told us that, as a work-around, the Bureau shifted responsibility for assigning cases to a headquarters official with access rights in the system to assign large numbers of cases at once. Bureau officials acknowledge the unsustainability of this work-around if needed at a national level and the importance of resolving this before the 2020 Census. As of October 2018, Bureau officials showed us system screenshots of how census field managers would be able to manually assign batches of cases and indicated that this functionality would be ready for the 2020 Census.
- *Monitoring operational progress.* The Bureau's reporting on its progress in completing the NRFU casework for the 2018 test emphasized a process-oriented measure that overstated the extent to which the NRFU efforts were resulting in completed workload. In planning documentation, the Bureau listed the outcomes of interview attempts that it considered complete and thus not in need of further enumeration assignments. These outcomes—such as a full interview of the household or confirmation of a housing unit being vacant or nonexistent—would also result directly in reduction in the number of incomplete cases needing to have some of their missing data imputed by the Bureau later.

Yet the daily Bureau progress report and "dashboard" the Bureau provided us for the 2018 test, which decennial leadership also identified as their primary monitoring report, did not reflect these pre-planned definitions of completed workload. Rather, as officials acknowledged, it included cases that the Bureau had unsuccessfully attempted to enumerate the maximum number of allowable times for the initial phase of NRFU being tested, even though those cases could still—and did— receive additional attempts during later phases of NRFU. Officials noted that the measure reported could be helpful during early stages of the operation in determining whether enough employees had been hired, or whether case assignments were being worked quickly enough.

Figure 2 demonstrates the gap that arose during 2018 NRFU test implementation between the reported progress measure and the number of cases actually being completed. The totals reflected in the Bureau's reported measure include those that either have to be re-worked in the field during the final attempt phase as discussed or have their data imputed after fieldwork had ended. By contrast, an outcome-based measure of operational progress, like the one the Bureau designed, would capture only those cases where the Bureau had completed enumeration of the nonresponding housing units and thus be a more accurate representation of the operation's status.[14]

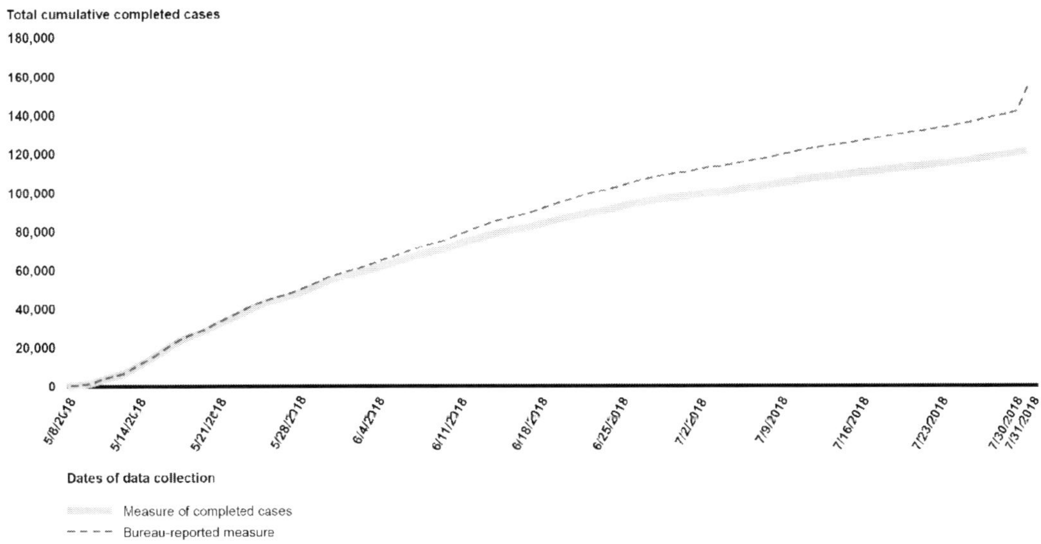

Source: GAO analysis of Census report data. | GAO-19-140.

Figure 2. The Bureau's Regular Reporting on Non-Response Follow-up Progress during the 2018 Census Test Overstated the Number of Cases Not Needing Additional Fieldwork.

Bureau officials acknowledged the need to maintain measures that focus on process as well as outcomes—such as avoiding having to impute data for cases after field work—when measuring progress completing NRFU. They said that managers in the field and in Bureau headquarters had access to alternative measures and reports that more closely identified outcomes. The officials noted that the reporting mechanism expected to be used in 2020 was not fully available in time for the beginning of NRFU testing in 2018, so the reporting format and measures will likely differ. In addition, in October 2018, the Bureau provided a draft dashboard for 2020 that included greater detail on the number of cases that could still require work to enumerate. Such detail could help assist with determining when to transition to the final-attempt phase of the operation to address cases without sufficient information yet collected.

Integrating Key Systems Settings

At the beginning of NRFU test implementation, the Bureau's case assignment and case sequencing systems were operating as if they were on time zones 4 hours apart. Bureau officials said that this resulted in enumerators receiving mismatched case assignment times, which hampered early NRFU production, and census field supervisors having to process erroneous "work not started" supervisory alerts. Bureau officials said they addressed the

[14] The Bureau-designed, outcome-oriented measure that we report also includes cases that, while not enumerated in the field, were successfully enumerated using the Bureau's sources of administrative records.

problem within the first week of the operation and that they would ensure that future updates and key settings would be coordinated across systems.

Tracking Employees and Equipment

The Bureau used two different sets of employee identification numbers to track their payroll status and use of Bureau-issued equipment (e.g., smart phones), respectively, without cross-walking them. According to census field managers, this resulted in extra work when trying to monitor changes in enumerators' employment statuses and whether enumerators had returned their equipment to the Bureau. The managers noted that office staff had to spend extra time comparing different lists of staff, while one manager developed a spreadsheet listing all staff by their two different identification numbers. Bureau officials said they considered this a priority issue to be resolved during final systems development for 2020 and had already developed a fix within their case management system so that the crosswalk between the two systems would be integrated within their management system. This would eliminate the need for manually reconciling the differing identification numbers.

Having More Enumerators Work Weekends

Until the latter stages of 2018 NRFU testing, the Bureau assigned cases to enumerators based on the alignment of the Bureau's estimated probability of finding respondents at home at certain times and enumerator-reported work availability. Bureau officials told us that Saturdays are generally one of the best days to find a household member home to respond to the census. However, during the test, our analysis showed that Saturdays had the second-fewest number of enumerators assigned to cases of any day of the week. Bureau officials said that they would review whether the incentive structure for working on Saturdays should be altered and that they would examine ways to ensure that more enumerators are working on those days. This includes exploring the feasibility of hiring and assigning work to applicants who may only want to work weekends and being clearer with enumerators about what the expected peak enumeration hours are.

Increasing Electronic Completion Rates For Group Quarters

The Bureau hopes to reduce field costs for Group Quarters (such as skilled nursing homes, college and university student housing, and correctional facilities) by, for the first time, encouraging facilities to self-enumerate electronically, when possible. As previously discussed, clerical staff first establish facility enumeration preferences during Group Quarters Advance Contact, and enumeration (either in person or otherwise) takes place afterward. During the 2018 test, the Bureau reported that only 25 of the 75 facilities that selected the "eResponse" enumeration option during Advance Contact submitted responses by the enumeration deadline. As of September 2018, Bureau officials said they were still evaluating potential causes of the low response rate by Group Quarters facilities but noted that issues with the required format for the submission of response files may have prevented some submissions. Bureau officials also acknowledged the need to conduct more active follow-up with these facilities during the eResponse period to ensure a full and accurate count of Group Quarters facilities.

THE BUREAU HAS MADE PROGRESS BUT CONTINUES TO FACE CHALLENGES ADDRESSING IMPLEMENTATION ISSUES IDENTIFIED IN PRIOR TESTS

The Bureau Has Improved Its Collection of Case Notes, but Enumerators Remain Unclear on How to Report Fieldwork Issues

We reported to the Bureau during the 2015 Census Test that information enumerators were typing into their case notes did not appear to be systematically used by their managers.[15] We also reported that, during the 2016 Census Test, the Bureau was not reviewing case notes written by enumerators providing respondent information on better times-of-day for future NRFU visits to their housing unit, and enumerators did not always have this note-taking feature available.[16] During the 2018 test, enumerators were trained to take notes and, when appropriate, identify special cases that would later require supervisory review. We also observed that enumerators appeared to be consulting case notes from prior enumerator visits when planning NRFU visits to the same housing unit. Enumerators can use markings within their automated interview instrument to describe certain types of cases (e.g., hearing barriers and dangerous situations), which the automated system would then route to receive supervisory review. Enumerators could select other case outcomes that the automated system would apply predetermined business rules to either reassign the cases (e.g., refusal, no one home) or treat them as completed (verified vacant or not a housing unit).

However, we identified multiple scenarios in which enumerators had described cases in their case notes but for which the enumerators had not selected the corresponding case flag for the situation that would have resulted automatically in a supervisory review. One census field manager described discovering several dozen cases that had been inactive where enumerators had written case notes describing language barriers encountered but had not specifically marked the flag within the device for "language barrier." Because these cases thus were not triggered for supervisory review, they were eligible to be reassigned by the Bureau's standard automated system. As a result, the Bureau was not controlling for the requisite language skills in assigning the cases for subsequent enumeration attempts.

The Bureau's use of automated systems to apply business rules to efficiently manage field casework for 2020—including identifying which cases receive supervisory review—relies critically on field staff understanding how to reflect what they are seeing on the ground within the choices provided to them with which to flag cases in their interview device. The Bureau's use of remote management as part of reengineered field operations also relies on enumerators knowing when and how to report issues to their supervisors.

We observed multiple field scenarios that called these conditions into question, however. For example, enumerators we observed during NRFU told us that they indicated address listing issues in their case notes, such as if the unit designation was missing or incorrectly marked. Yet, these enumerators did not know how to flag such cases in their interview instrument to trigger supervisory review. According to Bureau officials, this type of address listing issue

---

[15] GAO, *2020 Census: Additional Actions Would Help the Bureau Realize Potential Administrative Records Cost Savings*, GAO-16-48 (Washington, D.C.: Oct. 20, 2015).

[16] GAO, *2020 Census: Additional Actions Could Strengthen Field Data Collection Efforts*, GAO-17-191 (Washington, D.C.: Jan. 26, 2017).

turned out to be a broadly experienced challenge within the test area. Additionally, during Group Quarters, an enumerator we observed received supplemental information about the number of residents at a neighboring facility after that facility had been enumerated. The enumerator made note of this discrepancy and included the original facility's identifying information but was uncertain about how, if at all, to alert the supervisor about the discrepancy.

Moreover, we saw little evidence that census field supervisors or managers were systematically reviewing case notes for the purpose of identifying either cases not being marked properly or for which the selected flags may not have been fully describing the case characteristics. For example, a census field manager confirmed that case notes recorded at Group Quarters facilities that were enumerated would not be reviewed during clerical processing, leaving the possibility—such as we observed—that if enumerators relied on case notes to communicate information about the accuracy of data collected, it would not be acted on. Bureau officials told us that reviewing all case notes could require more staff time than budgeted for, and changing the automation process to selectively present unflagged cases for supervisory review could necessitate requirements changes to systems whose development is already pressed for time.

Standards for Internal Control in the Federal Government states that agencies should use quality information by, for example, processing reliable information to help it make informed decisions.[17] Bureau enumerators can record useful local knowledge about their cases with their choice of case type flags and within their descriptive case notes. While the Bureau has anticipated a broad range of types of cases for enumerators to select from when documenting their casework, enumerators we observed did not uniformly understand those options, and the descriptors did not fully anticipate what enumerators were encountering. Improving training and guidance to field staff on the intended use of case notes and on alternative ways to communicate their concerns about cases, such as flags for different types of cases, can help ensure the Bureau has reliable data on the cases during its field operations relying on automated interviewing instruments.

Leveraging Information on Enumerator-Reported Technical Procedural Issues Remains a Challenge

During the 2015 Census Test, we reported that certain technical and procedural problems that enumerators were encountering in the field were going unreported and that enumerators did not always know who to contact for assistance. We further noted that the Bureau was not systematically assessing or tracking the extent of these issues during testing, and we recommended that it enable such capture of information by training enumerators on where to record issues and whom to contact.[18] The Bureau agreed with our recommendation.

During the 2018 test, the Bureau had both an information technology (IT) hotline and a census-field-supervisor hotline established for technical and procedural questions, respectively. Yet, enumerators we observed told us they did not always report to their support lines the technical issues that they were easily able to resolve by, for example, turning their

[17] GAO-14-704G.
[18] GAO-16-48.

devices on and off to reset. This lack of reporting kept the Bureau from getting information on commonly-occurring challenges that might be useful real-time feedback in the testing environment. Moreover, a Bureau IT manager noted that the Bureau does not formally review and share observations and troubleshooting notes from IT hotline and census field supervisor hotline calls. Because enumerators may call either or both hotlines when having difficulty operating their Bureau-issued smart phone, operators of these hotlines could be unaware of the prevalence of or solutions to a given problem if the Bureau does not monitor troubleshooting information across the two operational silos. For the Bureau to be informed on any additional training needs or other operational decisions for 2020, it will need to continue to expand its efforts in collecting information on enumerator-reported problems per our 2015 recommendation.

The Bureau Continues to Assess How to Ensure Efficient Staffing Levels for Group Quarters

Depending on the size of a Group Quarters facility (e.g., skilled nursing facility, college and university student housing), the Bureau can use varying sizes of enumerator crews to conduct an onsite count. During the 2010 Census, we observed overstaffing during the service-based enumeration (e.g., homeless shelters and soup kitchens) portion of Group Quarters. While determining staffing levels at these facilities can be challenging, such overstaffing can lead to poor productivity and unnecessarily high labor costs. We recommended that the Bureau determine and address the factors that led to this overstaffing prior to 2020.[19] The Bureau agreed with our recommendation.

However, the Bureau has faced challenges determining the right staffing ratios in light of complications with the Advance Contact phase of Group Quarters. As previously noted, the Bureau used this phase to establish facilities' enumeration method preferences. For the 2018 test, most Group Quarters facilities selected the facility-provided paper listing and the eResponse enumeration options. Therefore, the Bureau allocated a large share of its enumerator and census field supervisor workforce in the test area to the 44 known service-based enumeration facilities, which were restricted in terms of the enumeration options they could select and tended to select in-person enumeration. However, only 11 of these facilities responded to initial inquiries, so the Bureau had less work than anticipated for its enumerator crews. At multiple sites we observed in the test area, enumerators appeared either idle or underutilized. Moreover, several of the Group Quarters facilities we observed had changed their initial choice of enumeration method on the day of enumeration.

Enumerator crews thus ran the risk of either being overstaffed (in the case of switching to a facility-provided paper listing) or understaffed (in the case of switching to an in-person enumeration).

The Bureau's Advance Contact activities have a potential benefit—if the Bureau can get accurate information on the method of enumeration and approximate population within a facility ahead of time, Bureau managers and enumerator crews can more proactively allocate

[19] GAO, *2010 Census: Key Efforts to Include Hard-to-Count Populations Went Generally As Planned; Improvements Could Make the Efforts More Effective for Next Census*, GAO-11-45 (Washington, D.C.: Dec. 14, 2010).

resources and prepare for the count. Bureau officials said they are still assessing outcomes of Advance Contact to see if these gains were realized and may have completed the assessment by as early as January 2019. Doing so will help the Bureau determine appropriate staffing sizes and thus address our prior recommendation.

The Bureau Is Working to Determine the Causes of Elevated Non-Interview Rates

According to preliminary data from the 2018 Census Test, the Bureau experienced similarly high rates of cases coded as non-interviews as it did during its last major field test of NRFU in 2016. Non-interviews are cases where enumerators collect no data or insufficient data from households either because enumerators made the maximum number of visits without a successful interview, or because of special circumstances like language barriers or dangerous situations.[20] When this happens, the Bureau may have to impute the census data for the case, such as whether the housing unit is vacant or not, the population counts of the households, or demographic characteristics of their residents. In January 2017, we reported that, during the 2016 Census Test, the Bureau incurred what it considered high non-interview rates (31 and 22 percent across the two test sites, respectively, as the Bureau preliminarily reported at the time), and we recommended that the Bureau determine the causes of these rates.[21]

Using the same method to calculate the rate of non-interviews for the test as in 2016, the 2018 Census Test had similarly high non-interview rates— 33 percent of all NRFU cases. Bureau officials said they are still examining causes of these elevated non-interview rates and whether final attempts helped to mitigate the non-interview rate and will report out on what they learn as part of their comprehensive assessment of the test, planned for December 2018. A draft of the Bureau's revised contact strategy for NRFU, provided in November 2018, indicates that as part of enumerator training in 2020 the Bureau will need to incorporate messaging that emphasizes the importance of obtaining sufficient data from interview attempts. Officials noted that any interim lessons learned from this assessment process would inform updates to the field enumeration contact strategies for 2020.

The Bureau Experienced a Programming Error While Implementing Procedures for Proxy Interviews

Enumerators are directed to try and complete a NRFU case by interviewing a proxy for a household respondent, like a neighbor, after multiple failed attempts have been made to contact someone in the household for that case. We previously observed in the 2016 Census Test that enumerators did not seem to understand the procedures for conducting these interviews and, as a result, underutilized the interviewing method. In our January 2017 report, we therefore recommended that, as part of determining the causes of its non-interview rate,

[20] According to the Bureau, it needs to collect a combination of data fields during field interviews in order to consider the interview complete.

[21] GAO-17-191.

the Bureau revise and test any needed changes to proxy procedures and associated training.[22] The Bureau agreed with our recommendation and subsequently developed automated supervisory performance alerts for census field supervisors and census field managers that would inform them when an enumerator was not following prompts to conduct proxy interviews for eligible cases.

However, in implementing proxy interview procedures for the 2018 Census Test, the Bureau experienced a technical glitch resulting in some confusion among some enumerators and their supervisors about related procedures. Early in NRFU data collection for the test, a programming error within the field enumeration application was prompting enumerators to make more than the allowable three attempts to interview a proxy respondent.[23] The Bureau reported promptly implementing a technical fix to this issue; yet, enumerators we observed reported receiving varying guidance from their supervisors on whether to abide by the erroneous prompts. While some of these enumerators appeared to understand the importance of attempting proxy interviews, some did not appear to understand Bureau guidance that enumerators should make no more than three attempts to interview a proxy respondent, and some appeared conditioned to follow the erroneous prompts.

Proxy interviews can be a substantial portion of completed interviews during the census. In 2018 NRFU testing, interviews of proxy respondents accounted for 27 percent of all successful interview-based enumerations of occupied housing units—compared to 24 percent during the 2010 Census and 9 percent during the 2016 Census Test. Given the role that proxy interviews play in completing census data collection, it will be important for the Bureau to fully implement our recommendation so that enumerators are properly pursuing and conducting these interviews.

Enumerators We Observed Were Uncertain of How to Proceed When Property Managers Were Unavailable

Initial visits to property managers of multi-unit residences can help the Bureau identify vacant and occupied housing units before sending enumerators to individual units within the facilities. We have previously reported that property managers can also be a helpful source of information on respondents who are not at home, thereby making subsequent follow-up visits to individual units more productive.[24] During the 2016 Census Test, we observed that enumerators were uncertain of how to handle individual cases within a multi-unit once they were unsuccessful in contacting a property manager initially. As a result, we recommended in January 2017 that the Bureau revise and test procedural and training modifications as needed to aid enumerators and their supervisors in these cases.[25] The Bureau agreed with this recommendation and indicated that the evaluations of the 2018 test would inform its strategies for 2020.

---

[22] GAO-17-191.

[23] The 2020 NRFU operational plan indicates that enumerators should, in most cases, only attempt three proxy interviews per visit. These interviews can be conducted with neighbors, relatives, landlords, or other sources with connections to the respondent or housing unit.

[24] GAO-17-191.

[25] GAO-17-191.

However, we observed a similar issue during the 2018 Census Test in that enumerators were unclear on what, if any, proxies to attempt if they were unsuccessful in finding the listed property manager. Additionally, we observed multiple enumerators leave voicemails with their contact information—not a central number—for the listed property manager, but it was unclear how these voicemails would produce a successful interview because, later, the automated system could reassign other enumerators to visit the manager. When we raised this concern with Bureau officials, they acknowledged that they need to continue to refine procedures for handling initial property manager visits for 2020.

The Bureau Provided Enumerators Access to Incomplete Closed Cases, but Enumerators Were Not Consistently Aware They Had Access

Previously, during the 2016 Census Test, we observed that enumerators were unable to re-open closed non-interview cases even if they happened upon the respondent in question soon after and nearby. We noted this inefficiency, since these cases would get re-assigned later, and in January 2017, we recommended that the Bureau revise and test procedures that would grant flexibility to enumerators to access cases in these circumstances.[26] The Bureau agreed with our recommendation.

For the 2018 Census Test, the Bureau provided a list in the field enumeration application of the cases that had been worked by the enumerator that day but that had not been submitted for processing or reassignment. Training for enumerators described this enumeration option, and enumerators were authorized to access these cases when needed, but not all enumerators we observed were consistently aware of how to do so. Enumerators we spoke with cited uncertainty over how to access these cases and whether enumerators were allowed to do so as considerations. Continuing to review the procedures and guidance to enumerators on this flexibility for completing interviews, consistent with our prior recommendation, will help the Bureau make better use of it in 2020.

The Bureau May Add an Extra Check on NRFU Addresses Identified by Administrative Records as Vacant or Nonexistent

As we reported in 2017, the Bureau previously modified how it would treat some of the households that did not respond to the 2020 Census and that the Bureau's use of administrative records had determined to be not occupied. The Bureau's earlier testing had determined that the Bureau should require two—instead of just one—notices from the United States Postal Service that mail could not be delivered to these households before removing their addresses from the NRFU workload.[27] After we provided a draft of this chapter to the Department of Commerce to obtain agency comments, Bureau officials provided us with findings from an evaluation of the 2018 Census Test. In the evaluation, Bureau officials observed that there were households for which they had received multiple notices from the United States Postal Service that mail was undeliverable but that Bureau enumerators

[26] GAO-17-191.
[27] GAO-17-664.

recorded as occupied. While Bureau officials believe, based on their follow-up research, that these addresses may likely be vacant or not housing units, they are concerned about possible undercounting from not enumerating people who may be at these addresses. As of November 2018, the Bureau was considering adding one physical visit for each of these cases. Bureau officials said they are continuing to analyze these evaluation results and expect to document and include changes within its final operational plan for the 2020 Census due in January 2019.

Conclusion

The 2018 Census Test offered the Bureau its last opportunity to test key procedures, management approaches, and systems under decennial-like conditions prior to the 2020 Census. As the Bureau studies the results of its NRFU and Group Quarters testing to inform 2020, it will be important that it address key program management issues that arose during implementation of the test. Namely, by not establishing the intended procedural changes for late-NRFU data collection ahead of time, the Bureau risked not getting the most out of NRFU to minimize the number of housing units having to have their information imputed by the Bureau later. Additionally, by not aligning the skills, responsibilities, and information flows for census field supervisors, the Bureau limited their role in support of enumerators within the reengineered field operation. The Bureau also lacks mid-operation training or guidance, which, if implemented in a targeted, localized manner, could further help enumerators navigate procedural modifications and any commonly-encountered problems when enumerating. Finally, without enumerators understanding how to use case notes and flags for various types of cases in their enumeration device and to report enumeration challenges to supervisors and managers, the Bureau may be unaware of field work issues that could affect the efficiency of its operations and the quality of its data.

We provided near real-time feedback to the Bureau across a range of test implementation issues. Some, such as those related to staffing ratios for the Group Quarters operation, build on long-standing implementation issues that, if addressed, can contribute to the efficiency and effectiveness of 2020 field operations. Others, like not having NRFU progress measures that provide true indications of completed workload, are issues specific to this test that the Bureau is assessing as part of its 2018 Census Test evaluations. It will be important for the Bureau to prioritize its mitigation strategies for these implementation issues so that it can maximize readiness for the 2020 Census.

Recommendations for Executive Action

We are making four recommendations to the Department of Commerce and the Census Bureau:

The Secretary of Commerce should ensure that the Director of the Census Bureau determines in advance of Non-Response Follow-Up what the procedural changes will be for the last phases of its data collection and what the business rules will be for determining when to begin those phases, which cases to assign, and how to assign them. (Recommendation 1)

The Secretary of Commerce should ensure that the Director of the Census Bureau identifies and implements changes to align census field supervisor screening, authorities, and information flows to allow greater use of the census field supervisor position to provide supervisory support to enumerators. (Recommendation 2)

The Secretary of Commerce should ensure that the Director of the Census Bureau enables area census offices to prepare targeted, mid-operation training or guidance as needed to address procedural changes or implementation issues encountered locally during Non-Response Follow-Up. (Recommendation 3)

The Secretary of Commerce should ensure that the Director of the Census Bureau improves training and guidance to field staff on the intended use of case notes and flags, as well as on alternative ways to alert supervisors and managers when case characteristics are not readily captured by those flags. (Recommendation 4)

AGENCY COMMENTS AND OUR EVALUATION

We provided a draft of this chapter to the Secretary of Commerce. In its written comments, reproduced in appendix II, the Department of Commerce agreed with our findings and recommendations and said it would develop an action plan to address them. The Census Bureau also provided technical comments and an update on their evaluation of the test, which we incorporated as appropriate.

We are sending copies of this chapter to the Secretary of Commerce, the Undersecretary of Economic Affairs, the Acting Director of the U.S. Census Bureau, and the appropriate congressional committees.

Robert Goldenkoff

Robert Goldenkoff
Director
Strategic Issues

List of Congressional Requesters

The Honorable Trey Gowdy
Chairman

The Honorable Elijah E. Cummings
Ranking Member
Committee on Oversight and Government Reform
House of Representatives

The Honorable Mark Meadows
Chairman

The Honorable Gerald E. Connolly
Ranking Member
Subcommittee on Government Operations
Committee on Oversight and Government Reform
House of Representatives

APPENDIX I: OBJECTIVES SCOPE & METHODOLOGY

This chapter examines (1) how peak field operations were implemented during the 2018 Census Test; and (2) the extent to which implementation issues raised in prior 2020 Census tests have been addressed, and what actions the Census Bureau (Bureau) is taking to address them.

To address these objectives, we reviewed 2018 Census Test and 2020 Census operational planning and training documentation. We also reviewed our prior reports and documentation on prior census testing operations. Non-Response Follow-Up (NRFU) operations took place from May 8 through July 31, 2018, while Group Quarters took place from July 25, 2018 through August 24, 2018, with the service-based enumeration portion taking place July 25, 2018 through July 27, 2018.

To review the Bureau's test implementation and mitigation strategies for previously-identified implementation issues for peak operations, we visited Providence, Rhode Island, multiple times between May and August 2018 to observe enumerators, census field supervisors, and management operations. NRFU visits took place between mid-May and late-July 2018, while we also conducted two iterations of visits of Group Quarters in late July and early-August 2018. These multiple iterations both across and within operations enabled us to see how, if at all, implementation of procedures varied over time. It also enabled us to get direct feedback from Bureau field managers on how various phases of test operations were proceeding. These visits consisted of non-generalizable observations of field enumeration and office clerical work, as well as interviews with local managers. For each of these visits, we developed data collection instruments to structure our interviews and to cover topics that were pertinent to the given phase of the operation we were observing. We also observed debrief sessions with multiple levels of the Bureau's field workforce following the field work.

To translate our observations into actionable feedback for the Bureau, we shared high-level observations in near real-time to Bureau headquarters management overseeing the operations so that the Bureau could mitigate and adapt to known issues in a timely manner. We also discussed any mitigation or evaluation strategies developed in response to our observations with the cognizant Bureau headquarters officials. For objective two specifically, we reviewed Bureau test planning documentation and our work from prior tests to examine how, if at all, the Bureau planned to address known implementation issues.

To gain insight into how implementation was proceeding when we were not directly observing test implementation, we received daily management progress reports from the Bureau throughout the NRFU operation testing that included information on the total number of NRFU cases, the final outcomes of each case, and the number of cases that the Bureau reported as completed for each day of the NRFU operation. We also received Periodic

Management Reports that summarized high level outcomes of both the NRFU and Group Quarters workload.

To fully understand the source of the Bureau's daily progress reports, we requested and received all transactional data collected during NRFU production. We reconciled case totals and outcomes with the final numbers in the NRFU progress reports and then used these data to analyze the Bureau's progress during NRFU production. We also received and analyzed Bureau payroll data on enumerator hours worked during NRFU operations. Specifically, we assessed the number of enumerators working each day, the number of enumerator' hours paid each day, and the days of the week that were worked the most by enumerators. We found the Bureau's transactional and payroll data sources to be sufficiently reliable for our reporting purposes.

We conducted this performance audit from April to December of 2018 in accordance with generally accepted government auditing standards. Those standards require that we plan and perform the audit to obtain sufficient, appropriate evidence to provide a reasonable basis for our findings and conclusions based on our audit objectives. We believe that the evidence obtained provides a reasonable basis for our findings and conclusions based on our audit objectives.

APPENDIX II: COMMENTS FROM THE DEPARTMENT OF COMMERCE

UNITED STATES DEPARTMENT OF COMMERCE
The Secretary of Commerce
Washington, D.C. 20230

December 3, 2018

Mr. Robert Goldenkoff
Director, Strategic Issues
U.S. Government Accountability Office
441 G Street, NW
Washington, DC 20548

Dear Mr. Goldenkoff:

The U.S. Department of Commerce appreciates the opportunity to comment on the U.S. Government Accountability Office's (GAO) draft report titled *2020 Census: Additional Steps Needed to Finalize Readiness for Peak Field Operations* (GAO-19-140).

The Department agrees with the findings and recommendations in this draft report. Once the GAO issues the final version of this report, the Department will prepare an action plan to document the steps we will take regarding the final recommendations.

Sincerely,

Wilbur Ross

Wilbur Ross

In: Top 10 Reports and Testimonies in December 2018
Editor: Sarah J. Nygaard

ISBN: 978-1-53615-507-5

Chapter 3

Critical Infrastructure Protection: Actions Needed to Address Significant Weaknesses in TSA's Pipeline Security Program Management*

United States Government Accountability Office

Abbreviations

AGA	American Gas Association
API	American Petroleum Institute
CFSR	Critical Facility Security Reviews
CRISP	Cybersecurity Risk Information Sharing Program
CSR	Corporate Security Reviews
DHS	Department of Homeland Security
DOE	Department of Energy
DOT	Department of Transportation
FERC	Federal Energy Regulatory Commission
ICS	Industrial Control Systems
INGAA	Interstate Natural Gas Association of America
ISAC	Information Sharing and Analysis Center
NCCIC	National Cybersecurity and Communications Integration Center
NIPP	National Infrastructure Protection Plan
NIST	National Institute of Standards and Technology
NSTS	National Strategy for Transportation Security
NTAS	National Terrorism Advisory System
OEIS	Office of Energy Infrastructure Security
PHMSA	Pipeline and Hazardous Materials Safety Administration

* This is an edited, reformatted and augmented version of United States Government Accountability Office; Report to Congressional Requesters, Publication No. GAO-19-48, dated December 2018.

SCADA	Supervisory Control and Data Acquisition
SCC	Sector Coordinating Council
TSA	Transportation Security Administration
TSOC	Transportation Security Operations Center

Why GAO Did This Study

More than 2.7 million miles of pipeline transport and distribute oil, natural gas, and other hazardous products throughout the United States.

Interstate pipelines run through remote areas and highly populated urban areas, and are vulnerable to accidents, operating errors, and malicious physical and cyber-based attack or intrusion. The energy sector accounted for 35 percent of the 796 critical infrastructure cyber incidents reported to DHS from 2013 to 2015. Several federal and private entities have roles in pipeline security. TSA is primarily responsible for the oversight of pipeline physical security and cybersecurity.

GAO was asked to review TSA's efforts to assess and enhance pipeline security and cybersecurity. This chapter examines, among other objectives: (1) the guidance pipeline operators reported using to address security risks and the extent that TSA ensures its guidelines reflect the current threat environment; (2) the extent that TSA has assessed pipeline systems' security risks; and (3) the extent TSA has assessed its effectiveness in reducing pipeline security risks.

GAO analyzed TSA documents, such as its *Pipeline Security Guidelines*; evaluated TSA pipeline risk assessment efforts; and interviewed TSA officials, 10 U.S. pipeline operators—selected based on volume, geography, and material transported— and representatives from five industry associations.

What GAO Recommends

GAO makes 10 recommendations to TSA to improve its pipeline security program management and DHS concurred.

GAO recommends, among other things, that the TSA Administrator take the following actions:

- implement a documented process for reviewing, and if deemed necessary, for revising TSA's *Pipeline Security Guidelines* at defined intervals;
- clarify TSA's *Pipeline Security Guidelines* by defining key terms within its criteria for determining critical facilities;
- develop a strategic workforce plan for TSA's Security Policy and Industry Engagement's Surface Division;
- update TSA's pipeline risk assessment methodology to include current data to ensure it reflects industry conditions and threats;
- fully document the data sources, underlying assumptions and judgments that form the basis of TSA's pipeline risk assessment methodology;

- take steps to coordinate an independent, external peer review of TSA's pipeline risk assessment methodology;
- ensure the Security Policy and Industry Engagement's Surface Division has a suite of performance measures which exhibit key attributes of successful performance measures; and
- enter information on Corporate Security Review recommendations and monitor and record their status.

WHAT GAO FOUND

Pipeline operators reported using a range of guidelines and standards to address physical and cybersecurity risks, including the Department of Homeland Security's (DHS) Transportation Security Administration's (TSA) *Pipeline Security Guidelines*, initially issued in 2011. TSA issued revised guidelines in March 2018 to reflect changes in the threat environment and incorporate most of the principles and practices from the National Institute of Standards and Technology's *Framework for Improving Critical Infrastructure Cybersecurity*. However, TSA's revisions do not include all elements of the current framework and TSA does not have a documented process for reviewing and revising its guidelines on a regular basis. Without such a documented process, TSA cannot ensure that its guidelines reflect the latest known standards and best practices for physical security and cybersecurity, or address the dynamic security threat environment that pipelines face.

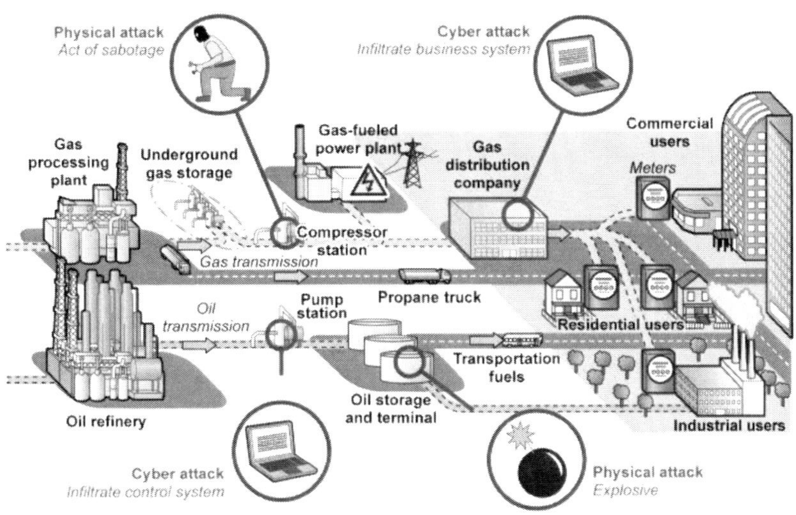

Source: GAO analysis of Transportation Security Administration information. | GAO-19-48.

U.S. Pipeline Systems' Basic Components and Vulnerabilities.

Further, GAO found that the guidelines lack clear definitions to ensure that pipeline operators identify their critical facilities. GAO's analysis showed that operators of at least 34 of the nation's top 100 critical pipeline systems (determined by volume of product transported) deemed highest risk had identified no critical facilities. This may be due, in part, to the guidelines not clearly defining the criteria to determine facilities' criticality. To assess pipeline security risks, TSA conducts pipeline security reviews— Corporate Security Reviews and Critical Facility Security Reviews—to assess pipeline systems' vulnerabilities. However, GAO found that the number of TSA security reviews has varied considerably over the last several years, as shown in the table on the following page.

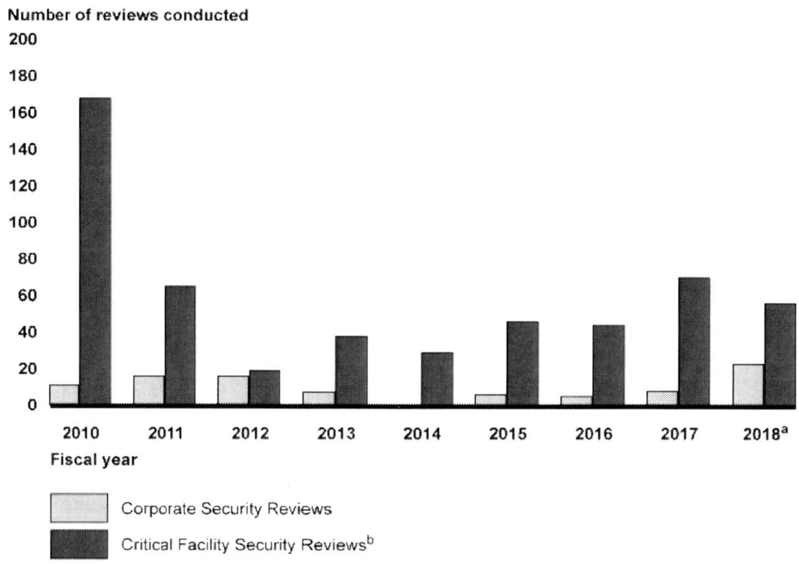

Source: GAO analysis of Transportation Security Administration-reported figures. | GAO-19-48.

[a]Fiscal year 2018 data are through July 31, 2018.
[b]Fiscal years 2010 and 2011 represent Critical Facility Inspections—the predecessor of the Critical Facility Security Review.

Pipeline Security Reviews Conducted, Fiscal Year 2010 through July 2018.

TSA officials stated that staffing limitations have prevented TSA from conducting more reviews. Staffing levels for TSA's Pipeline Security Branch have varied significantly since fiscal year 2010 with the number of staff ranging from 14 full-time equivalents in fiscal years 2012 and 2013 to 1 in 2014. Further, TSA does not have a strategic workforce plan to help ensure it identifies the skills and competencies—such as the required level of cybersecurity expertise—necessary to carry out its pipeline security responsibilities. By establishing a strategic workforce plan, TSA can help ensure that it has identified the necessary skills, competencies, and staffing.

GAO also identified factors that likely limit the usefulness of TSA's risk assessment methodology for prioritizing pipeline system reviews. Specifically, TSA has not updated its risk assessment methodology since 2014 to reflect current threats to the pipeline industry. Further, its sources of data and underlying assumptions and judgments regarding certain threat and vulnerability inputs are not fully documented. In addition, the risk assessment has not been peer reviewed since its inception in 2007. Taking steps to strengthen its risk assessment, and initiating an independent, external peer review would provide greater assurance that TSA ranks relative risk among pipeline systems using comprehensive and accurate data and methods.

TSA has established performance measures to monitor pipeline security review recommendations, analyze their results, and assess effectiveness in reducing risks. However, these measures do not possess key attributes—such as clarity, and having measurable targets—that GAO has found are key to successful performance measures. By taking steps to ensure that its pipeline security program performance measures exhibit these key attributes, TSA could better assess its effectiveness at reducing pipeline systems' security risks. Pipeline Security Branch officials also reported conducting security reviews as the primary means for assessing the effectiveness of TSA's efforts to reduce pipeline security risks. However, TSA has not tracked the status of Corporate Security Review recommendations for the past 5 years. Until TSA monitors and records the status of these reviews' recommendations, it will be hindered in its efforts to determine whether its recommendations are leading to significant reduction in risk.

December 18, 2018
Congressional Requesters

The security of the nation's pipeline systems is vital to public confidence and the nation's safety, prosperity, and well-being. More than 2.7 million miles of pipeline transport and distribute the oil, natural gas, and other hazardous liquids that U.S. citizens and businesses depend on to operate vehicles and machinery, heat homes, generate electricity, and manufacture products. The interstate pipeline system runs through remote, as well as highly populated urban areas, and is vulnerable to accidents, operating errors, and malicious attacks. In addition, pipelines increasingly rely on sophisticated networked computerized systems and electronic data, which are vulnerable to cyber attack or intrusion.

Given that many pipelines transport volatile, flammable, or toxic oil and liquids, and given the potential consequences of a successful physical or cyber attack on life, property, the economy, and the environment, pipeline systems are attractive targets for terrorists, hackers, foreign nations, criminal groups, and others with malicious intent. For example, according to the Transportation Security Administration (TSA)—the federal agency with responsibility for security in all modes of transportation, which includes the oversight of pipeline physical security and cybersecurity—a minor pipeline system disruption could result in commodity price increases while prolonged pipeline disruptions could lead to widespread energy shortages.[1] Further, disruption of any magnitude may affect other domestic critical infrastructure and industries that are dependent on pipeline system commodities.

Since the September 11, 2001, terrorist attacks, new threats to the nation's pipeline systems have evolved to include sabotage by environmental activists and cyber attack or intrusion by nations.[2] In October 2016, environmental activists forced the shutdown of five crude oil pipelines in four states.[3] In addition, the U.S. energy sector has experienced cyber intrusions by nation-state actors into their networks. For example, in March 2018, the Federal Bureau of Investigation and the National Cybersecurity and Communications Integration

---

[1] Transportation Security Administration, *Biennial National Strategy for Transportation Security: Report to Congress* (Washington, D.C.: Apr. 4, 2018).

[2] Nations, including nation-state, state-sponsored, and state-sanctioned programs, use cyber tools as part of their information-gathering and espionage activities. In addition, several nations are aggressively working to develop information warfare doctrine, programs, and capabilities.

[3] Congressional Research Service, *Pipeline Security: Recent Attacks*, IN106103 (Washington, D.C.: Apr. 11, 2017).

Center (NCCIC) reported that a nation-state had targeted organizations within multiple U.S. critical infrastructure sectors, including the energy sector, and collected information pertaining to Industrial Control Systems (ICS).[4] Also, in April 2012, the Industrial Control Systems Cyber Emergency Response Team reported that an unidentified cyber attacker had conducted a series of cyber intrusions into U.S. natural gas pipeline systems beginning in December 2011.[5]

The security of federal cyber assets has been on our High Risk list since 1997 and was expanded to include the protection of critical cyber infrastructure in 2003.[6] In September 2018, we issued an update to the information security high-risk area that identified actions needed to address cybersecurity challenges facing the nation.[7] We last reported on pipeline security in 2010 and made eight recommendations to TSA to develop outcome-based performance measures for assessing TSA's pipeline security efforts, and to track its corporate security reviews and critical facility inspections' recommendations,[8] among others.[9] We discuss some of these recommendations in more detail later in this chapter. In 2012, we reviewed information provided by TSA and closed the recommendations as implemented.

You requested that we review TSA's efforts to enhance pipeline physical security and cybersecurity. This chapter examines the following objectives:

1) how do pipeline sector stakeholders share security-related information;
2) what guidance do pipeline operators report using to address security risks and to what extent does TSA ensure its guidelines reflect the current threat environment;
3) to what extent has TSA assessed security risks to pipeline systems; and
4) to what extent has TSA assessed its effectiveness in reducing pipeline security risks.

For each objective, we interviewed representatives of the five major associations with ties to the pipeline industry: the American Petroleum Institute (API), the Association of Oil Pipe Lines, the American Gas Association (AGA), the Interstate Natural Gas Association of America (INGAA), and the American Public Gas Association. We also interviewed a

[4] Federal Bureau of Investigation and National Cybersecurity and Communications Integration Center, *Russian Government Cyber Activity Targeting Energy and Other Critical Infrastructure Sectors*, TA18-074A (Washington, D.C.: Mar., 16, 2018 (revised)). Industrial control systems include software-based systems used to monitor and control many aspects of network operation for pipeline networks.

[5] Industrial Control Systems Cyber Emergency Response Team (ICS-CERT), *ICS-CERT Monthly Monitor* (Washington, D.C.: Apr. 2012).

[6] Our biennial High Risk List identifies government programs that have greater vulnerability to fraud, waste, abuse, and mismanagement or need to address challenges to economy, efficiency, or effectiveness. We have designated federal information security as a High Risk area since 1997; in 2003, we expanded this high risk area to include protecting systems supporting our nation's critical infrastructure; and, in 2015, we further expanded this area to include protecting the privacy of personally identifiable information that is collected, maintained, and shared by both federal and nonfederal entities. See GAO, *High Risk Series: Progress on Many High Risk Areas, While Substantial Efforts Needed on Others*, GAO-17-317 (Washington, D.C.: Feb. 15, 2017).

[7] GAO, *High Risk Series: Urgent Actions Are Needed to Address Cybersecurity Challenges Facing the Nation*, GAO-18-622 (Washington, D.C.: Sept. 6, 2018).

[8] TSA conducts two types of pipeline security reviews: Corporate Security Reviews and Critical Facility Security Reviews. Corporate Security Reviews are voluntary on-site reviews of a pipeline owner's corporate policies and procedures. Critical Facility Security Reviews are voluntary on-site inspections of critical pipeline facilities, as well as other select pipeline facilities, throughout the nation. Critical Facility Inspections were the predecessor to Critical Facility Security Reviews.

[9] GAO, *Pipeline Security: TSA Has Taken Actions to Help Strengthen Security, but Could Improve Priority-Setting and Assessment Processes*, GAO-10-867 (Washington, D.C.: Aug. 2010).

nonprobability sample of security personnel from 10 pipeline operators. We selected the 10 pipeline operators from TSA's list of the top 100 critical pipeline systems.[10] We chose operators to ensure a mixture of the following characteristics: (a) type of pipeline commodity transported (i.e., natural gas or hazardous oil and liquids); (b) volume of product transported; and (c) whether or not the pipeline operators' critical facilities had been the subject of a TSA security review. We also considered the location of selected operators' pipeline systems to ensure that a single state or region was not overrepresented in our sample. We then conducted semistructured interviews to obtain operators' perspectives on pipeline security and the role of federal agencies in assisting operators with security activities. While the information gathered during operator interviews cannot be generalized to all pipeline operators, it provides a range of perspectives on a variety of topics relevant to pipeline security.

To identify how pipeline sector stakeholders share security-related information, we reviewed documents describing federal agencies' processes for sharing security-related information with federal partners and private industry. In addition, we reviewed relevant documents from TSA and other federal entities, including the Department of Transportation (DOT), DOT's Pipeline and Hazardous Materials Safety Administration (PHMSA), the Department of Energy (DOE), and the Federal Energy Regulatory Commission (FERC). We also interviewed agency and industry officials to gather their perspectives on how security information is shared among pipeline sector stakeholders.

To identify the guidance pipeline operators report using to address security risks and the extent to which TSA ensures its guidelines reflect the current threat environment, we reviewed TSA's 2018 *Pipeline Security Guidelines*[11] and compared the cybersecurity-related sections to applicable standards of the National Institute of Standards and Technology's (NIST) *Framework for Improving Critical Infrastructure Cybersecurity*.[12] We also interviewed federal officials to identify security-related standards and guidance issued. In addition, we obtained from industry officials the security-related standards and guidance they use and asked them about any challenges they experienced in implementing TSA's *Pipeline Security Guidelines*. Based on the results of our operator interviews, we analyzed TSA data on critical facility identification. Further, to assess TSA's process for updating the guidelines, we compared the process with TSA's *Pipeline Security Smart Practice Observations* for pipeline operators and our *Standards for Internal Control in the Federal Government*.[13]

To determine the extent TSA has assessed security risks to pipelines, we reviewed key threat assessments from TSA, such as its Pipeline Modal and Cyber Modal Threat Assessments and Transportation Sector Security Risk Assessments that it issued during

---

[10] According to TSA, a system is considered critical if it is so vital to the United States that its incapacitation or destruction would have a debilitating effect on security, national economic security, public health or safety, or any combination thereof. TSA determines the top 100 most critical pipeline systems based on the amount of hazardous liquid or natural gas product transported through a pipeline in 1 year.

[11] Transportation Security Administration, *Pipeline Security Guidelines* (March 2018).

[12] National Institute of Standards and Technology, *Framework for Improving Critical Infrastructure Cybersecurity, Version 1.0* (Gaithersburg, Md.: Feb. 12, 2014). In response to Executive Order 13636, NIST issued the *Framework for Critical Infrastructure Cybersecurity*, which is intended to help organizations apply the principles and best practices of risk management to improving the security and resilience of critical infrastructure. The framework consists of five concurrent and continuous functions: identify, protect, detect, respond, and recover. When considered together, these functions provide a high-level, strategic view of the life cycle of an organization's management of cybersecurity risk.

[13] GAO, *Standards for Internal Control in the Federal Government*, GAO-14-704G (Washington, D.C.: Sept. 10, 2014).

calendar years 2011 through 2017. We also evaluated TSA's identification of the 100 most critical pipeline systems, its methods for assessing relative risk among those systems, and its prioritization of its pipeline reviews. As part of that evaluation, we assessed the reliability of the data within TSA's pipeline relative risk ranking tool by performing electronic and manual checks for such things as logic errors and missing data.[14] Additionally, we interviewed TSA officials about how the risk tool is updated and maintained to ensure data reliability. We determined the data were sufficiently reliable for the purpose of our review. We also interviewed TSA officials about the methods they used to rank relative risk among pipeline systems and the extent to which those methods aligned with the *National Infrastructure Protection Plan 2013: Partnering for Critical Infrastructure Security and Resilience* (NIPP),[15] other Department of Homeland Security (DHS) priorities, and previously identified best practices for program management and risk assessment. We also analyzed information on the number of pipeline security reviews— Corporate Security Reviews (CSR) and Critical Facility Security Reviews (CFSR)—that TSA conducted by fiscal year, as well as TSA staffing levels and contractor support. Further, we interviewed TSA officials about their staffing allocation and workforce planning process and compared TSA's process to our previous work which identified principles that a strategic workforce planning process should follow.[16]

To further our understanding of TSA's pipeline security review processes, we observed TSA officials and contractors conduct one CSR of one pipeline system, and three CFSRs at three critical facilities in the Houston and Beaumont, Texas, areas. While the results of our observations cannot be generalized to all CSRs and CFSRs or all pipeline systems and critical facilities, they provided us with an understanding of how TSA conducts these reviews and inspections. We also interviewed representatives of Secure Solutions International—a security and risk management consulting firm that assists TSA in conducting CSRs and CFSRs—about critical facilities and the inspection process.

To determine the extent TSA has assessed its effectiveness in reducing pipeline security risks, we assessed key strategic documents, such as TSA's performance report, against our key characteristics of effective performance measures.[17] We also reviewed TSA guidance, such as the standard operating procedures outlining how TSA staff are to conduct pipeline security reviews and monitor operators' implementation of their recommendations. We then compared TSA's assessment efforts to our Standards for Internal Control in the Federal Government. In addition, we evaluated the databases TSA officials reported using to analyze and record the results and recommendations of pipeline security reviews. We reviewed each database to determine what information was stored in them, such as the number of observations, what fields were present, and typical entries within each field. We then reviewed and conducted electronic testing on the universe of fields and observations.

---

[14] To assess the security risks of the top 100 critical pipeline systems, TSA's Pipeline Security Branch developed its Pipeline Relative Risk Ranking Tool (risk assessment) in 2007. The risk assessment calculates threat, vulnerability, and consequence on variables such as the amount of throughput in the pipeline system.

[15] Department of Homeland Security, *2013 National Infrastructure Protection Plan, Partnering for Critical Infrastructure Security and Resilience* (Washington, D.C.: December 2013).

[16] GAO, *Human Capital: Key Principles for Effective Strategic Workforce Planning*, GAO-04-39 (Washington, D.C.: Dec. 11, 2003).

[17] GAO, *Tax Administration: IRS Needs to Further Refine Its Tax Filing Season Performance Measures*, GAO-03-143 (Washington, D.C.: Nov. 22, 2002); GAO, *Military Personnel: DOD Needs to Establish Performance Measures for the Armed Forces Sports Program*, GAO-17-542 (Washington, D.C.: June 8, 2017).

Although we identified limitations, which we discuss later in the report, we found that the data was sufficiently reliable to provide general information such as summary figures describing pipeline security reviews completed. We also interviewed TSA officials to understand TSA's efforts to assess its overall effectiveness in reducing pipeline security risks and related data collection efforts.

We conducted this performance audit from June 2017 to December 2018 in accordance with generally accepted government auditing standards. Those standards require that we plan and perform the audit to obtain sufficient, appropriate evidence to provide a reasonable basis for our findings and conclusions based on our audit objectives. We believe that the evidence obtained provides a reasonable basis for our findings and conclusions based on our audit objectives.

BACKGROUND

Overview of the U.S. Pipeline System

The national pipeline system consists of more than 2.7 million miles of networked pipelines transporting oil, natural gas, and other hazardous liquids. Hazardous liquid and natural gas pipelines—primarily buried underground in the continental United States—run under remote and open terrain, as well as densely populated areas. These pipelines are of three main types:

- Hazardous liquid: About 216,000 miles of hazardous liquid pipeline transport crude oil, diesel fuel, gasoline, jet fuel, anhydrous ammonia, and carbon dioxide.
- Natural gas transmission and storage: About 319,000 miles of pipeline—mostly interstate—transport natural gas from sources to communities.
- Natural gas distribution: About 2.2 million miles of pipeline—mostly intrastate—transport natural gas from transmission sites to consumers.

Figure 1 depicts the network of hazardous liquid and natural gas transmission pipelines in the United States.

More than 3,000 pipeline companies operate the nation's pipeline systems, which can traverse multiple states and the U.S. borders with Canada and Mexico. Many pipeline systems are comprised of the pipelines themselves, as well as a variety of facilities, such as storage tanks, compressor stations, and control centers. Most pipeline systems are monitored and moderated through automated ICS or Supervisory Control and Data Acquisition (SCADA) systems using remote sensors, signals, and preprogramed parameters to activate and deactivate valves and pumps to maintain flows within tolerances.[18]

[18] SCADA is one type of control system, which is a computer-based system used within many infrastructures and industries to monitor and control sensitive processes and physical functions. Control systems perform functions that range from simple to complex. They can be used to simply monitor processes--for example, the environmental conditions in a small office building--or to manage the complex activities of a municipal water system or a nuclear power plant. Control systems are vulnerable to cyber-attack from inside and outside the control system network.

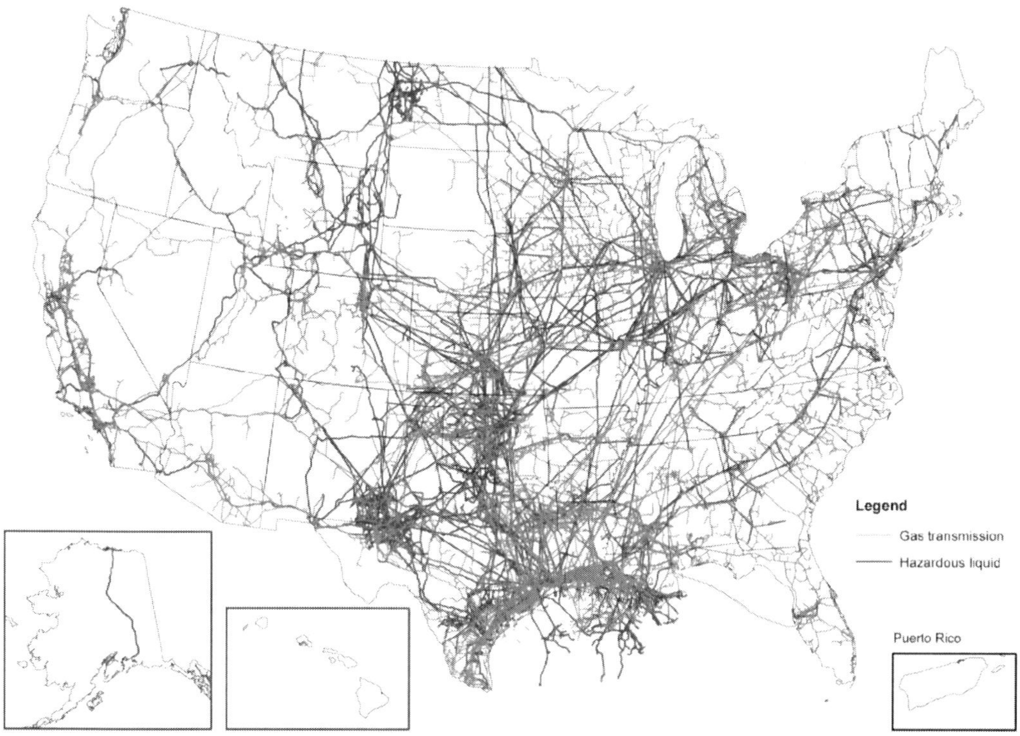

Source: U.S. Department of Transportation. | GAO-19-48.

Figure 1. Map of Hazardous Liquid and Natural Gas Transmission Pipelines in the United States, September 2018.

Federal agencies and pipeline operators determine the criticality of pipeline systems and their facilities based on their importance to the nation's energy infrastructure; service to installations critical to national defense; or, if attacked, have the potential to cause mass casualties and significant impact on public drinking water affecting major population centers. Accordingly, those determined to be critical merit increased attention to security. However, as we previously reported, the inherent design and operation of U.S. pipeline systems may reduce some potential impacts of lost service.[19] The pipeline sector is generally considered to be resilient and versatile. Historically, pipeline operators have been able to quickly respond to the adverse consequences of an incident—whether it is damage from a major hurricane or a backhoe—and quickly restore pipeline service. Pipeline infrastructure also includes redundancies such as parallel pipelines or interconnections that enable operators to reroute material through the network. Figure 2 depicts the U.S. pipeline system, its basic components, examples of vulnerabilities, and the entities to which it supplies energy and raw materials. These entities include utility companies, airports, military sites, and industrial and manufacturing facilities.

[19] GAO-10-867.

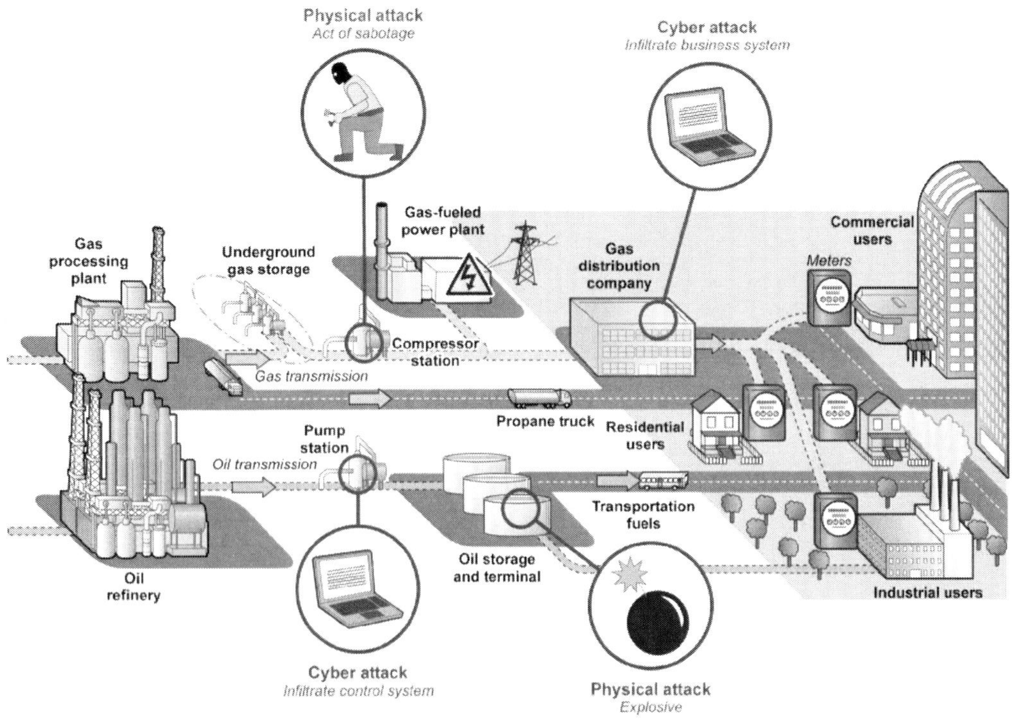

Source: GAO analysis of Transportation Security Administration information. | GAO-19-48.

Figure 2. U.S. Natural Gas and Oil Pipeline Systems' Basic Components and Examples of Vulnerabilities.

Physical and Cyber Threats to Pipeline Systems

According to TSA, pipelines are vulnerable to physical attacks—including the use of firearms or explosives—largely due to their stationary nature, the volatility of transported products, and the dispersed nature of pipeline networks spanning urban and outlying areas. The nature of the transported commodity and the potential effect of an attack on national security, commerce, and public health make some pipelines and their assets more attractive targets for attack.[20] Oil and gas pipelines have been and continue to be targeted by terrorists and other malicious groups globally.[21] Terrorists have also targeted U.S. pipelines, but have not succeeded in attacking them.[22] Further, environmental activists and lone actors seeking to

[20] Transportation Security Administration, *Biennial National Strategy for Transportation Security: Report to Congress* (Washington, D.C.: Apr. 4, 2018).

[21] For example, rebels bombed the Caño Limón oil pipeline and other pipelines in Colombia more than 600 times since 1993, with the most recent attack occurring on April 27, 2017. Militants in Nigeria have repeatedly attacked oil pipelines, including coordinated bombings of three pipelines in 2007 and the bombing of an underwater pipeline in 2016. Assailants bombed natural gas pipelines in British Columbia, Canada six times between October 2008 and July 2009, which authorities later classified as environmentally-motivated. See GAO-10-867 and Congressional Research Service, *Pipelines: Securing the Veins of the American Economy*, TE10009 (Washington, D.C.: Apr. 19, 2016).

[22] In 2006, federal authorities acknowledged the discovery of a detailed posting on a website purportedly linked to al Qaeda that reportedly encouraged attacks on U.S. pipelines, especially Trans Alaska Pipeline System, using weapons or hidden explosives. In 2007, the U.S. Department of Justice arrested members of a terrorist group planning to attack jet fuel pipelines and storage tanks at the John F. Kennedy International Airport. In 2011, a

halt the construction of new pipelines through sabotage have recently emerged as a new threat to pipelines.[23] For example, in March 2017, activists used blowtorches to cut holes in empty portions of the Dakota Access Pipeline in two states. In February 2017, local law enforcement officers fatally shot a man who used an assault rifle to damage the Sabal Trail Pipeline, a natural gas pipeline under construction in Florida.

The sophisticated computer systems that pipeline operations rely on are also vulnerable to various cyber threats.[24] According to DOE, the frequency, scale, and sophistication of cyber threats have increased, and attacks have become easier to launch. NCCIC reported that the energy sector, which includes pipelines, experienced more cyber incidents than any sector from 2013 to 2015, accounting for 35 percent of the 796 incidents reported by all critical infrastructure sectors. In 2016, NCCIC reported that the energy sector was the third most frequently attacked sector.[25] Further, according to DOE, the cost of preventing and responding to cyber incidents in the energy sector is straining the ability of companies to adequately protect their critical cyber systems.[26] For example, a 2015 study by the Ponemon Institute estimated the annualized cost of cyber crime for an average energy company to be about $28 million.[27]

Ineffective protection of cyber assets from these threats can increase the likelihood of security incidents and cyber attacks that disrupt critical operations; lead to inappropriate access to and disclosure, modification, or destruction of sensitive information; and threaten national security, economic well-being, and public health and safety. Unintentional or nonadversarial threat sources may include failures in equipment or software due to aging, resource depletion, and errors made by end users. They also include natural disasters and failures of critical infrastructure on which the organization depends, but that are outside of the control of the organization.

Intentional or adversarial threats may include corrupt employees, criminal groups, terrorists, and nations that seek to leverage the organization's dependence on cyber resources (i.e., information in electronic form, information and communications technologies, and the communications and information-handling capabilities provided by those technologies). These threat adversaries vary in terms of their capabilities, their willingness to act, and their

---

man planted a bomb, which did not detonate, along a natural gas pipeline in Oklahoma. In 2012, a man unsuccessfully attempted to bomb a natural gas pipeline in Plano, Texas. See GAO-10-867 and Congressional Research Service, Testimony TE10009, *Pipelines: Securing the Veins of the American Economy*, by Paul W. Parfomak, Apr. 19, 2016.

[23] Congressional Research Service, *Pipeline Security: Recent Attacks*, IN106103 (Washington, D.C.: Apr. 11, 2017).

[24] Once accessible to an attacker, a SCADA system can be exploited in a number of specific ways to carry out a cyber attack: issuing unauthorized commands to control equipment; sending false information to a control-system operator that initiates inappropriate actions; disrupting control system operation by delaying or blocking the flow of information through the control network; making unauthorized changes to control system software to modify alarm thresholds or other configuration settings; and rendering resources unavailable by propagating malicious software (e.g., a virus, worm, Trojan horse) through the control network. Congressional Research Service, *Cybersecurity for Energy Delivery Systems*, R44939 (Washington, D.C.: Aug. 28, 2017).

[25] NCCIC collects data on cyber incidents that attempt to gain access to both business and control systems infrastructure. These incidents, reported on a voluntary basis by critical infrastructure owners and operators, include, for example, unauthorized access to SCADA devices or exploitation of software vulnerabilities. NCCIC reports data on critical infrastructure sectors, such as energy, but does not report data on subsectors, such as pipelines.

[26] Department of Energy, Office of Electricity Delivery and Reliability, *Multiyear Plan for Energy Sector Cybersecurity, 2018* (Washington, D.C.: Mar. 2018).

[27] Ponemon Institute, *2015 Cost of Cyber Crime Study: United States*, 2016.

motives, which can include seeking monetary gain or seeking an economic, political, or military advantage.

Cyber threat adversaries make use of various techniques, tactics, practices, and exploits to adversely affect an organization's computers, software, or networks, or to intercept or steal valuable or sensitive information. For example, an attacker could infiltrate a pipeline's operational systems via the internet or other communication pathways to potentially disrupt its service and cause spills, releases, explosions, or fires.[28] Moreover, ICS, which were once largely isolated from the Internet and the company's information technology systems, are increasingly connected in modern energy systems, allowing cyber attacks to originate in business systems and migrate to operational systems. For example, malicious nation-state actors used spear-phishing[29] and other similar approaches in 2018 against energy sector organizations to gain access to their business systems, conduct reconnaissance, and collect information about their ICS.[30] Similarly, in April 2012, the Industrial Control Systems Cyber Emergency Response Team reported that an unidentified cyber attacker had conducted a series of cyber intrusions into U.S. natural gas pipeline systems beginning in December 2011.[31]

Key Critical Infrastructure Protection Guidance and Presidential Directives

Federal policy and public-private plans establish roles and responsibilities for the protection of critical infrastructure, including pipelines. These include Presidential Policy Directive 21 (PPD-21), the NIPP, and Executive Order 13636. PPD-21, issued in February 2013, reflects an all-hazards approach to protecting critical infrastructure, including natural disasters, terrorism, and cyber incidents.[32] The directive also identifies the 16 critical

[28] In 2007, researchers working with DHS conducted an experiment to prove such an attack is possible by sending two sets of commands to a diesel-fueled electric generator, which caused the generator to destroy itself without the operators knowing. In addition, according to DOE, in 2015, unidentified attackers used spear phishing emails to gain access to three Ukrainian utilities' information technology networks resulting in power loss for 225,000 customers for several hours. Once inside, among other things, they stole credentials and hijacked the distribution management system to systematically open breakers and cause a power outage. The attackers then accessed the industrial control system network and disabled the uninterruptible power supply, operational control systems, and computers and prevented infected computers from rebooting.

[29] "Spear-phishing" involves sending official-looking emails to specific individuals to insert harmful software programs (malware) into protected computer systems; to gain unauthorized access to proprietary business information; or to access confidential data such as passwords, social security numbers, and private account numbers.

[30] NCCIC and the Federal Bureau of Investigation characterized the intrusions as a multistage intrusion campaign by an identified nation state's actors on U.S. Government entities and organizations within the energy, nuclear, commercial facilities, water, aviation, and critical manufacturing sectors. According to the agencies, the campaign targeted small commercial facilities' networks where they staged malware, conducted spear phishing, and gained remote access into energy sector networks. After obtaining access, the actors conducted network reconnaissance, moved laterally, and collected information pertaining to industrial control systems. Federal Bureau of Investigation and National Cybersecurity and Communications Integration Center, Russian Government Cyber Activity Targeting Energy and Other Critical Infrastructure Sectors TA18-074A (Washington, D.C.: Mar., 16 2018 (revised)).

[31] Industrial Control Systems Cyber Emergency Response Team (ICS-CERT), *ICS-CERT Monthly Monitor* (Washington, D.C.: Apr. 2012).

[32] White House, *Presidential Policy Directive/PPD-21: Critical Infrastructure Security and Resilience* (Washington, D.C.: Feb. 12, 2013). The term "all-hazards" is defined by the directive as a threat or an incident, natural or manmade, which warrants action to protect life, property, the environment, and public health or safety, and to minimize disruptions of government, social, or economic activities. "All-hazards," as further defined in the

infrastructure sectors[33] and assigns roles and responsibilities for each critical infrastructure sector among nine designated federal sector-specific agencies.[34]

While PPD-21 identified the critical infrastructure sectors and assigned responsibility for each sector's sector-specific agency, the NIPP outlines critical infrastructure stakeholder roles and responsibilities regarding critical security and resilience. It describes a voluntary partnership model as the primary means of coordinating government and private sector efforts to protect critical infrastructure. As part of the partnership structure, the designated sector-specific agencies serve as the lead coordinators for security programs of their respective sector. As sector-specific agencies, federal departments or agencies lead, facilitate, or support the security and resilience programs and associated activities of their designated critical infrastructure sector. For example, DHS and DOT are both designated as sector-specific agencies for the transportation systems sector, which includes pipelines. Each sector also has a government coordinating council,[35] consisting of representatives from various levels of government, and many have a sector coordinating council (SCC) consisting of owner-operators of these critical assets or members of their respective trade associations.[36] For example, the Transportation Government Coordinating Council has been established, and the Pipeline Modal SCC has been established to represent pipeline operators.[37]

The NIPP also outlines a risk management framework for critical infrastructure protection. As shown in Figure 3, the NIPP uses a risk management framework as a planning methodology intended to inform how decision makers take actions to manage risk. The risk management framework calls for public and private critical infrastructure partners to conduct risk assessments to understand the most likely and severe incidents that could affect their operations and communities, and use this information to support planning and resource allocation.

---

directive, includes natural disasters, cyber incidents, industrial accidents, pandemics, acts of terrorism, sabotage, and destructive criminal activity targeting critical infrastructure.

[33] The 16 critical infrastructure sectors are Chemical; Commercial Facilities; Communications; Critical Manufacturing; Dams; Defense Industrial Base; Emergency Services; Energy; Financial Services; Food and Agriculture; Government Facilities; Health Care and Public Health; Information Technology; Nuclear Reactors, Materials, and Waste; Transportation Systems; and Water and Wastewater Systems.

[34] PPD-21 was developed to advance a national unity of effort to strengthen and maintain secure, functioning, and resilient critical infrastructure. It defines resilience as the ability to prepare for and adapt to changing conditions and withstand and recover rapidly from disruptions, and includes the ability to withstand and recover from deliberate attacks, accidents, or naturally occurring threats or incidents. Stated another way, resilience can reduce the consequences associated with an incident, event, or occurrence. Resilience is an area that may be included in vulnerability assessments to determine the extent to which critical infrastructure is prepared to withstand and recover from disruptions. Such disruptions could include exposure to a given hazard or incidents arising from the deliberate exploitation of vulnerabilities of sector-specific strategies, policies, activities, and issues.

[35] Government coordinating councils coordinate strategies, activities, policy, and communications across government entities within each sector and consist of representatives across various levels of government (i.e., federal, state, local, and tribal) as appropriate. For example, DHS and DOE are designated as the co-chairs of the Energy Government Coordinating Council.

[36] SCCs are self-organized, self-run, and self-governed private sector councils that interact on a wide range of sector-specific strategies, policies, and activities. SCC membership can vary from sector to sector, but is meant to be representative of a broad base of owners, operators, associations, and other entities—both large and small—within the sector.

[37] Pipeline operators may also participate in the Oil and Natural Gas Subsector Coordinating Council of the Energy SCC.

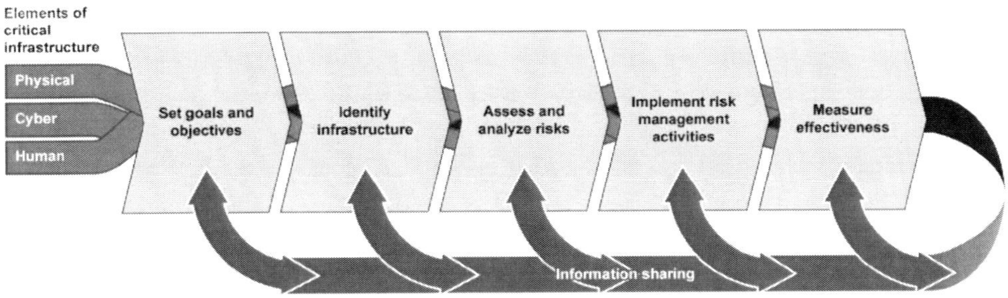

Source: Department of Homeland Security National Infrastructure Protection Plan 2013. | GAO-19-48.

Figure 3. The National Infrastructure Protection Plan's Critical Infrastructure Risk Management Framework.

According to DHS, the risk management framework is influenced by the nature and magnitude of a threat, the vulnerabilities to that threat, and the consequences that could result, as shown in Figure 4.

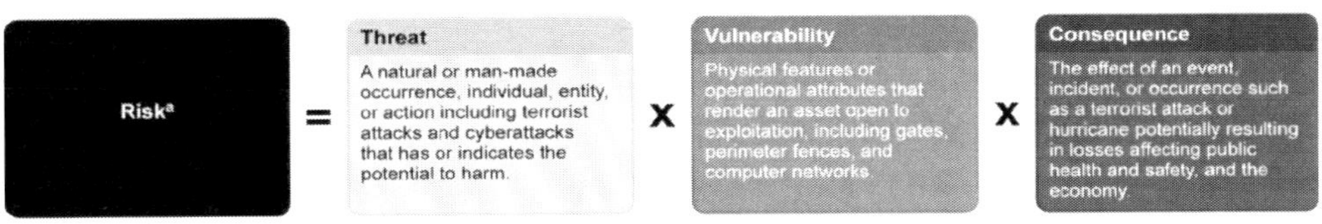

Source: GAO analysis of the Department of Homeland Security's National Infrastructure Protection Plans (2009 and 2013). | GAO-19-48.

[a]As noted in DHS's Risk Management Fundamentals Doctrine, risk is generally recognized as a function of threats, vulnerabilities, and consequences—elements that may explicitly be considered for many homeland security risks, such as those related to infrastructure protection. Risk Management Fundamentals, Homeland Security Risk Management Doctrine (Washington, D.C.: April 2011).

Figure 4. Determination of Risks Related to Infrastructure Protection.

Federal policy has encouraged voluntary information-sharing mechanisms between the federal government and critical infrastructure owners and operators.[38] For example, Information Sharing and Analysis Centers (ISAC) are formed by critical infrastructure owners and operators to gather, analyze, appropriately sanitize, and disseminate intelligence and information related to critical infrastructure. They typically collect, analyze and disseminate actionable threat information to their members and provide members with tools to mitigate risks and enhance resiliency. ISACs in which pipeline operators may participate have been formed including the Oil and Natural Gas ISAC, Downstream Natural Gas ISAC, and Electricity ISAC.

Finally, in February 2013, the president issued Executive Order 13636, *Improving Critical Infrastructure Cybersecurity*, which cited repeated cyber intrusions into critical

[38] Among other things, Presidential Decision Directive 63, for example, encouraged the development of ISACs to serve as mechanisms for gathering, analyzing, and disseminating information on cyber infrastructure threats and vulnerabilities to and from owners and operators of the sectors and the federal government. White House, *Presidential Decision Directive 63: Critical Infrastructure Protection: Sector Coordinators*, (Washington, D.C.: May 22, 1998). Presidential Decision Directive 63 has been superseded by Homeland Security Policy Directive 7, which was revoked by PPD-21.

infrastructure as demonstrating the need for improved cybersecurity.[39] Executive Order 13636 outlined actions for improving critical infrastructure cybersecurity, including direction for the National Institute of Standards and Technology (NIST) to lead the development of a voluntary risk-based cybersecurity framework that would comprise a set of industry standards and best practices to help organizations manage cybersecurity risks.[40] NIST issued the framework in 2014 and updated it in April 2018.[41] The order also addressed the need to improve cybersecurity information sharing and collaboratively develop risk-based standards and stated that U.S. policy was to increase the volume, timeliness, and quality of cyber threat information shared with private sector entities so that these entities may better protect and defend themselves against cyber threats.

Pipeline Stakeholders' Security Roles and Responsibilities

Protecting the nation's pipeline systems is a responsibility shared by both the federal government and private industry. As a result, several federal departments, agencies, and the private sector have significant roles in pipeline physical and cyber-related security. These entities include the following:

Transportation Security Administration (TSA)

TSA, within DHS, has primary oversight responsibility for the physical security and cybersecurity of transmission and distribution pipeline systems.[42] Within TSA, the Security Policy and Industry Engagement's Pipeline Security Branch is charged with overseeing its pipeline security program. Pursuant to its authority, TSA's Pipeline Security Branch first issued its voluntary *Pipeline Security Guidelines* in 2011, and released revised guidelines in March 2018.[43] In accordance with the 9/11 Commission Act, TSA's Pipeline Security Branch

---

[39] Exec. Order No. 13636 (Feb. 12, 2013), 78 Fed. Reg. 11,737 (Feb. 19, 2013). Executive Order 13800, *Strengthening the Cybersecurity of Federal Networks and Critical Infrastructure,* issued in May 2017, directs the Secretary of Homeland Security, in coordination with the heads of other appropriate departments and agencies, to among other things, identify authorities and capabilities that agencies could use to support the cybersecurity efforts of critical infrastructure entities identified pursuant to section 9 of Executive Order 13636 to be at greatest risk of attack that could result in catastrophic results on public health or safety, economic security, or national security. See Exec. Order No. 13800 (May 11, 2017), 82 Fed. Reg. 22,391 (May 16, 2017).

[40] Exec. Order No. 13636, 78 Fed. Reg. at 11,740-41. The National Institute of Standards and Technology (NIST) is a standards-setting agency under the U.S. Department of Commerce.

[41] National Institute of Standards and Technology, *Framework for Improving Critical Infrastructure Cybersecurity* (Feb. 12, 2014); *Framework for Improving Critical Infrastructure Cybersecurity* Version 1.1 (Apr. 16, 2018).

[42] Pursuant to the Aviation and Transportation Security Act, TSA is the federal entity with responsibility for security in all modes of transportation, which includes the nation's interstate pipeline systems. See Pub. L. No. 107-71, 115 Stat.597 (2001); 49 U.S.C. § 114(d).

[43] The Implementing Recommendations of the 9/11 Commission Act of 2007 (9/11 Commission Act) directs the Secretary of Homeland Security, in conjunction with the Secretary of Transportation, to develop and transmit to pipeline operators security recommendations for natural gas and hazardous liquid pipelines and pipeline facilities and, if deemed appropriate, shall promulgate regulations and carry out necessary inspection and enforcement actions. See Pub. L. No. 110-53, § 1557(d), 121 Stat. 266, 475-76; 6 U.S.C. § 1207(d). TSA has not issued regulations for the pipeline sector under this authority but instead relies on voluntary compliance with the agency's security guidelines and best practice recommendations.

identifies the top 100 critical pipeline systems in the nation.[44] To do so, it uses system annual throughput, which is based on the amount of hazardous liquid or natural gas product transported through a pipeline in 1 year (i.e., annual throughput). TSA also ranks the relative risk among the top 100 critical pipeline systems, discussed later in the report. Additionally, TSA's Pipeline Security Branch is responsible for conducting voluntary Corporate Security Reviews (CSR) and Critical Facility Security Reviews (CFSR), which assess the extent to which the 100 most critical pipeline systems are following the intent of TSA's *Pipeline Security Guidelines*.[45] See Figure 5 below for an overview of the CSR and CFSR processes.

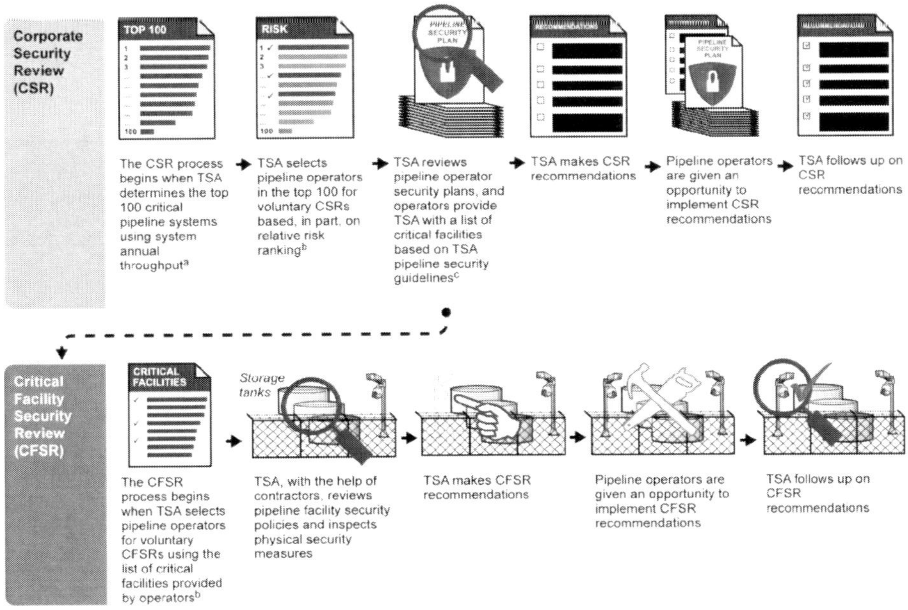

Source: GAO analysis of TSA information. | GAO-19-48.

[a]TSA uses system annual throughput in determining the top 100 critical pipeline system, which is based on the amount of hazardous liquid or natural gas product transported through a pipeline in 1 year (i.e., annual throughput measured in therms). Also, some pipeline operators own or operate more than one of the 100 most critical systems.

[b]Because of the voluntary nature of TSA's pipeline security program, TSA requests selected operators to participate in its pipeline security reviews—the CSR and CFSR. An operator may choose not to participate in these reviews. However, according to TSA officials, no operator has declined to participate in a CSR or CFSR to date.

[c]Under TSA's Pipeline Security Guidelines, pipeline operators are to self-identify the critical facilities within their pipeline system and report their critical facilities to TSA. However, operators may identify no critical facilities in their systems.

Figure 5. Overview of the Transportation Security Administration's (TSA) Voluntary Security Review Processes with Pipeline Operators.

---

[44] See 6 U.S.C. § 1207(b). According to Pipeline Security Branch officials, even though there are over 3,000 pipeline operators in the U.S., the top 100 critical pipeline systems in the country represent approximately 85 percent of the energy in the nation.

[45] CSRs are voluntary on-site reviews of a pipeline owner's corporate policies and procedures. CFSRs are voluntary onsite reviews of critical pipeline facilities, as well as other selected pipeline facilities throughout the nation. TSA requests selected operators to participate in these reviews, but operators can decline to participate. However, according to TSA officials, no operator has declined to participate in a CSR or CFSR to date.

In addition, TSA Intelligence and Analysis is responsible for collecting and analyzing threat information related to the transportation network, and sharing relevant threat information to pipeline stakeholders.

National Cybersecurity and Communications Integration Center (NCCIC)

Within DHS, NCCIC assists critical infrastructure owners in addressing cyber incidents and attacks, including those targeting industrial control systems.[46] The NCCIC's mission is to reduce the likelihood and severity of incidents that may significantly compromise the security and resilience of the nation's critical information technology and communications networks.[47] NCCIC's role is to serve as the federal civilian interface for sharing information related to cybersecurity risks, incidents, analysis, and warnings with federal and nonfederal entities, and to provide shared situational awareness to enable real-time actions to address cybersecurity risks and incidents to federal and nonfederal entities.

Pipeline and Hazardous Materials Safety Administration (PHMSA)

PHMSA, within DOT, is responsible for regulating the safety of hazardous materials transportation and the safety of pipeline systems, some aspects of which can be related to pipeline security.[48] In 2004, PHMSA and TSA entered into a memorandum of understanding regarding their respective roles in all modes of transportation. In 2006, they signed an annex to the memorandum of understanding that further delineates lines of authority and responsibility between TSA and PHMSA on pipeline and hazardous materials transportation security. The annex identifies TSA as the lead federal entity for transportation security, including hazardous materials and pipeline security, and PHMSA as responsible for administering a national program of safety in natural gas and hazardous liquid pipeline transportation, including identifying pipeline safety concerns and developing uniform safety standards.

Department of Energy (DOE)

DOE is responsible for protecting electric power, oil, and natural gas delivery infrastructure and, in December 2015, was identified in statute as the sector-specific agency for cybersecurity for the energy sector.[49] The Office of Cybersecurity, Energy Security, and Emergency Response is the lead for DOE's cybersecurity efforts.[50] In addition, DOE operates the National SCADA Test Bed Program, a partnership with Idaho National Laboratory,

---

[46] According to NCCIC officials, NCCIC is in the process of an organizational realignment. When completed, the United States Cyber Emergency Team and the Industrial Control Systems Cyber Emergency Team will be consolidated into a single entity within NCCIC.

[47] National Security Presidential Directive 54 (Homeland Security Presidential Directive/HSPD-23), issued on January 8, 2008, established the Comprehensive National Cybersecurity Initiative, which is aimed at safeguarding federal civilian executive branch government information systems. Pursuant to the directive, DHS established the NCCIC in October 2009.

[48] The Homeland Security Act of 2002, enacted in November 2002, established DHS, transferred TSA from DOT to DHS, and assigned DHS responsibility for protecting the nation from terrorism, which includes securing the nation's transportations systems. See Pub. L. No. 107-296, 116 Stat. 2135 (2002). Primary responsibility for regulating the safety of hazardous materials transportation via pipeline and the safety of pipeline systems remained with DOT. See e.g., 49 C.F.R. pts. 190-199.

[49] See Pub. L. No. 114-94, § 61003(c)(2), 129 Stat. 1312, 1779 (2015).

[50] DOE's Office of Cybersecurity, Energy Security and Emergency Response cybersecurity program for energy delivery systems is structured around three areas: (1) cybersecurity preparedness; (2) cyber incident response and recovery; and (3) research, development, and demonstration.

Sandia National Laboratories, and other national laboratories which addresses control system security challenges in the energy sector. Among its key functions, the program performs control systems testing, research, and development; control systems requirements development; and industry outreach.

Federal Energy Regulatory Commission (FERC)

FERC regulates the U.S. bulk electric power system, which is increasingly powered by natural gas pipeline systems.[51] FERC has regulatory authority over interstate natural gas pipelines under the Natural Gas Act.[52] However, its role is limited to natural gas pipeline siting and rate regulation. The North American Electric Reliability Corporation is the federally designated U.S. Electric Reliability Organization, and is overseen by FERC. The North American Electric Reliability Corporation, with approval from FERC, has developed mandatory critical infrastructure protection standards for protecting electric utility–critical and cyber-critical assets.

Private Sector

Although TSA has primary federal responsibility for overseeing interstate pipeline security, private sector pipeline operators are responsible for implementing asset-specific protective security measures. As we previously reported, operators have increased their attention on security by incorporating security practices and programs into their overall business operations.[53] Pipeline operators' interests and concerns are primarily represented by five major trade associations with ties to the pipeline industry—the Interstate Natural Gas Association of America (INGAA), American Gas Association (AGA), American Public Gas Association, American Petroleum Institute (API), and Association of Oil Pipe Lines. According to TSA officials, pipeline operators, and association representatives, these associations have worked closely with the federal government on a variety of pipeline security-related issues, including collaborating on TSA's voluntary standards and information sharing.

Federal and Nonfederal Pipeline Stakeholders Exchange Risk-Related Security Information

All of the pipeline operators and pipeline association representatives we interviewed reported receiving security information from federal and nonfederal entities. Pipeline operators also reported providing security-related information to federal agencies, including TSA, as incidents occur. Multiple federal entities exchange alerts of physical and cybersecurity incidents and other risk-related information with critical infrastructure partners, including pipeline operators. For example, DHS components including TSA's Intelligence and Analysis and NCCIC share security-related information on physical and cyber threats and

[51] FERC approved mandatory and enforceable cybersecurity standards in 2008 and physical security standards in 2014 for U.S. bulk electric operators. See 73 Fed. Reg. 7,368 (Feb. 7, 2008) (Order No. 706), 79 Fed. Reg. 70,069 (Nov. 25, 2014) (Order No. 802); see also 18 C.F.R. pt. 40.

[52] See 42 U.S.C. § 7172.

[53] GAO-10-867.

incidents with sector stakeholders. Specifically, Intelligence and Analysis provides quarterly intelligence briefings to pipeline operators. NCCIC also issues indicator bulletins, which can contain information related to cyber threat indicators, defensive measures, and cybersecurity risks and incidents.

Table 1. Federal Information Sharing Entities and Programs that Provide Information to Pipeline Stakeholders

Entity/Program	Product/service description
Department of Homeland Security (DHS)	
National Cybersecurity and Communications Integration Center (NCCIC)	NCCIC receives, triages, tracks, coordinates, and manages high volumes of threat, vulnerability, and incident information on a 24/7 basis. The watch floor disseminates this information to NCCIC analysts for resolution and shares alerts, reports, and other information products with the pipeline community. NCCIC also facilitates weekly teleconferences with private and public entities to discuss situational awareness and provide ongoing informational analysis related to current events. In addition, its Cyber Information Sharing and Collaboration Program bulletins provide incident analysis information derived from new cyber incidents or malicious code, threats, and vulnerabilities to, among others, pipeline operators.[a]
Transportation Security Administration (TSA) Transportation Security Operations Center (TSOC) TSA Intelligence and Analysis	The TSOC is the conduit with which TSA coordinates with DHS, the Federal Aviation Administration, the Federal Bureau of Investigation, and other law enforcement and security agencies to analyze and monitor security-related operations, incidents and crises in all transportation modes. In addition, pipeline operators are asked to voluntarily report security incidents to TSA via the TSOC. Intelligence and Analysis is to provide pipeline industry security professionals with timely and actionable information on terrorist threats to hazardous liquid and natural gas pipelines. For example, Intelligence and Analysis is to prepare quarterly and annual pipeline cyber and physical modal threat assessments and unclassified quarterly threat briefings based on analysis of primary threat actors, credible terrorist plots, and successful attacks, as well as tactics, techniques, procedures, and targets that could be employed in future attacks.
National Terrorism Advisory System (NTAS)	NTAS Bulletins—NTAS, DHS's system for communicating terrorist threats to the American public, issues bulletins that communicate terrorism information alerting sector stakeholders, including pipeline owners/operators, of any elevated (i.e., general information about timing and target) or imminent (i.e., credible, specific, and impending) threats.
Homeland Security Information Network (HSIN)	HSIN is the trusted network for homeland security mission operations to share sensitive but unclassified information. Federal, state, local, territorial, tribal, international, and private sector homeland security partners are to use HSIN to manage operations, analyze data, and send alerts and notices of cyber and physical security threats.
Protective Security Advisor (PSA) Program	PSAs are security subject matter experts who engage with state, local, tribal, and territorial government mission partners and members of the private sector stakeholder community to protect the nation's critical infrastructure. PSAs are to conduct voluntary, nonregulatory security surveys and assessments on critical infrastructure assets and facilities within their respective regions. PSAs also may conduct outreach activities with critical infrastructure owners and operators in support of DHS's infrastructure protection priorities.
Department of Transportation (DOT)	
Pipeline and Hazardous Materials Safety Administration (PHMSA)	PHMSA issues advisory bulletins to communicate safety-related conditions to pipeline operators and can issue advisory bulletins in coordination with TSA to notify pipeline operators of a security incident including identifying the affected operators, describing the threat, and providing information on federal resources for assistance. For example, in response to physical intrusions of pipelines and a coordinated campaign by domestic saboteurs, PHMSA issued an advisory bulletin, in coordination with TSA, to remind pipeline operators of the importance of safeguarding and securing their pipelines from physical and cyber intrusion or attack.

Entity/Program	Product/service description
Department of Energy (DOE)	
Cybersecurity Risk Information Sharing Program (CRISP)	CRISP is a public-private partnership to facilitate the timely sharing of cyber threat information and develop situational awareness tools to enhance the ability of the electricity sector, including electric companies or utilities that also own a natural gas pipeline(s), to identify, prioritize, and coordinate the protection of its critical infrastructure. DOE shares actionable cyber threat information with CRISP participants in near-real time via the Electricity ISAC.
Federal Energy Regulatory Commission (FERC)	
Office of Energy Infrastructure Security (OEIS)	OEIS conducts joint voluntary assessments of natural gas pipeline entities' information and operational technology systems and networks to assess their vulnerabilities to current threats and emerging exploits. According to FERC, under its Cybersecurity Architecture Assessment program, OEIS and TSA take a collaborative, nonregulatory approach to promote secure and resilient infrastructure through the sharing of information and best practices. The goal of the assessment program is to allow the assessed entity to gain a comprehensive understanding of its overall cybersecurity posture, identify potential areas of concern, articulate actionable recommendations and observations, and identify best practices that promote improvements to the security posture of the assessed entity.

Source: GAO analysis of agency documents | GAO-19-48.

[a]NCCIC sends Cyber Information Sharing and Collaboration Program bulletins generally to local and state government, critical infrastructure, private industry, or another country's computer emergency response team.

In addition, TSA and other federal entities have coordinated to address specific pipeline-related security incidents. For example, TSA officials coordinated with DOT, DOE, the Department of Justice, and FERC through the Oil and Natural Gas subsector SCC to address ongoing incidents of vandalism and sabotage of critical pipeline assets by environmental activists in 2016. In July 2017, according to DOT officials, PHMSA and TSA collaborated on a web-based portal to facilitate sharing sensitive but unclassified incident information among federal agencies with pipeline-related responsibilities. See Table 1 for the key federal information sharing entities and programs that exchange security-related or incident information with critical infrastructure stakeholders, including the pipeline sector.

Pipeline operators also share security-related information with TSA and the NCCIC. In its *Pipeline Security Guidelines*, TSA requests that pipeline operators report by telephone or email to its Transportation Security Operations Center (TSOC) any physical security incidents that are indicative of a deliberate attempt to disrupt pipeline operations or activities that could be considered precursors to such an attempt.[54] TSA's *Pipeline Security Guidelines* also request that operators report any actual or suspected cyber attacks that could impact pipeline industrial control systems or other information technology-based systems to the NCCIC. According to the TSOC's operating procedures, if a reported incident meets certain criteria, such as the incident was intended to or resulted in damage or requires a general evacuation of a facility, the TSOC watch officer is then to contact Office of Security and Industry Engagement officials. According to TSA officials, the TSOC does not conduct investigations of the specific security incidents that pipeline operators report. However, TSOC staff do analyze the incident information they receive for national trends and common threats. TSA officials stated that they share their observations with pipeline operators and other critical infrastructure asset owners during monthly and quarterly conference calls that TSA holds with pipeline operators.

[54] According to TSA officials, freight and passenger rail are the only two surface transportation modes whose operators are required to report incidents, potential threats, or significant security concerns. See 49 C.F.R. §§ 1580.105, 1580.203.

All the pipeline operators and association representatives we interviewed identified other nonfederal information sharing entities, including ISACs, fusion centers, industry associations, and SCCs, which provide forums for exchanging information about physical and cyber incidents throughout the pipeline sector. See Table 2 for nonfederal information sharing entities identified as available to pipeline operators.

Table 2. Nonfederal Information Sharing Entities

Entity	Product/service description
Downstream Natural Gas Information Sharing and Analysis Center (ISAC)	The Downstream Natural Gas ISAC serves natural gas utility (distribution) and pipeline (transmission) companies by facilitating communications between participants, the federal government, and other critical infrastructure. This ISAC is to disseminate threat information and indicators from government and other sources and provide analysis, coordination, and summarization of related industry-affecting information.
Oil and Natural Gas ISAC	The Oil and Natural Gas ISAC provides cyber threat information for the oil and natural gas industry. Its main goal is to assist in increasing the security posture of the industry's exploration and production, transportation, refining, and delivery systems from cyber-attacks through the analysis and sharing of cyber intelligence. As an industry owned and operated organization, it provides a mechanism for members to share information anonymously across its membership.
Fusion centers	Fusion centers are a collaborative effort of two or more federal, state, local, or tribal government agencies that combine resources, expertise, or information with the goal of maximizing the ability of such agencies to detect, prevent, investigate, apprehend, and respond to criminal or terrorist activity. For example, according to TSA officials, the New York State Intelligence Center shares threat data with pipeline operators.
Industry associations	Industry associations, such as the American Gas Association, the American Petroleum Institute, and the Interstate Natural Gas Association of America, representing companies delivering natural gas, exchange security-related information. Examples of such activities can include disseminating alerts from the National Cybersecurity and Communications Integration Center to their membership, hosting events to promote security awareness, and sharing security-related resources and guidance.
InfraGard	InfraGard, a partnership between the Federal Bureau of Investigation and the private sector, is to provide a vehicle for the timely exchange of information and promotes learning opportunities relevant to the protection of the nation's critical infrastructure.
Oil and Natural Gas Subsector Coordinating Council (SCC)	The Oil and Natural Gas SCC is to provide a private forum for coordination of oil and natural gas security strategies and activities, policy, and communication across the sector to support the nation's homeland security mission. This SCC provides a venue for industry owners and operators to mutually plan, implement, and execute sufficient and appropriate sector-wide security programs, procedures and processes, exchange information, and assess accomplishments and progress toward continuous improvement in the protection of the sector's critical infrastructure.

Source: GAO analysis of agency documents | GAO-19-48.

Operators and TSA officials reported that the current backlog in granting security clearances for some key pipeline operator employees was a significant factor affecting information sharing between TSA and pipeline operators. TSA officials acknowledged that some pipeline operators have had difficulty obtaining security clearances for key employees due to ongoing backlogs in processing requests by the Office of Personnel Management National Background Investigation Bureau, and that TSA's ability to share timely information with operators whose staff do not have a clearance may be hindered. Three of the 10 pipeline operators we interviewed identified receiving timely classified security information as a specific challenge due, in part, to difficulties staff have had obtaining security clearances. Further, 7 of the 10 pipeline operators that we interviewed reported experiencing delays in obtaining a security clearance or were aware of others who had experienced this issue. However, according to three operators we interviewed, TSA was helpful in facilitating approval of security clearances for the operators' personnel to access classified information when necessary.

This security clearance challenge is not faced by pipeline operators alone. In January 2018, we designated the backlog of investigations for the clearance process and the government-wide personnel security clearance process as a high-risk area. We will continue to monitor agencies' progress in reducing the backlog and improving the security clearance process.[55]

Pipeline Operators Use a Range of Guidelines and Standards to Address Risks, but TSA's Guidelines Lack Clear Definitions and a Process for Updating Them

Pipeline operators that we interviewed reported using a range of guidelines and standards to address their physical and cybersecurity risks, and all of them reported implementing TSA's voluntary *Pipeline Security Guidelines* that were applicable to their operations. TSA revised and issued its *Pipeline Security Guidelines* in March 2018, but the revised guidelines lack a defined process to consider updates to supporting guidance such as to the NIST *Framework for Improving Critical Infrastructure Cybersecurity* (Cybersecurity Framework). Furthermore, TSA has not clearly defined the terms within the criteria that pipeline operators are to use to determine the criticality of their facilities.

Pipeline Operators Use a Range of Guidelines and Standards to Address Security

Pipeline operators that we interviewed reported using a range of guidelines and standards to address their physical and cybersecurity risks. For example, all 10 of the pipeline operators we interviewed stated they had implemented the voluntary 2011 TSA Pipeline Security Guidelines the operators determined to be applicable to their operations.[56] The guidelines provide TSA's recommendations for pipeline industry security practices such as establishing a corporate security program and identifying critical facilities among others (see sidebar).[57] Five of the 10 pipeline operators we interviewed characterized the guidelines as generally or somewhat effective in helping to secure their operations, 1 was neutral on their effectiveness, and 4 did not provide an assessment of the guidelines' effectiveness. However, one operator pointed out that they had not adopted the guidelines' recommended interval of 36 months or

[55] See GAO press release "GAO Adds Government-wide Personnel Security Clearance Process to 'High Risk List'" (Washington, D.C., Jan. 25, 2018).

[56] Transportation Security Administration, *Pipeline Security Guidelines* (April 2011). TSA did not issue the revised guidelines until March 2018.

[57] According to industry association officials, AGA and INGAA members have made voluntary commitments to implement TSA's *Pipeline Security Guidelines*.

less for conducting security vulnerability assessments due to staffing limitations.[58] Also, another pipeline operator noted that they were working to implement the guidelines in the operations of a newly acquired asset that they determined was not using the guidelines in the same manner as their company.

Transportation Security Administration's *Pipeline Security Guidelines*

The Guidelines address the following areas:
1. Corporate Security Program
2. Corporate Security Plan
   a. Security Plan Elements
3. Risk Analysis
   a. Criticality Assessment
   b. Security Vulnerability Assessment
4. Criticality
a. Facility Criticality
5. Facility Security Measures
   a. Baseline and Enhanced Security Measures
   b. Site-Specific Security Measures
6. Pipeline Cyber Asset Security Measures
   a. Pipeline Cyber Assets Identification
   b. Security Measures for Pipeline Cyber Assets
   c. Cyber Security Planning and Implementation Guidance
7. Protective Measures for National Terrorism Advisory System Alerts

Source: Transportation Security Administration's *Pipeline Security Guidelines*, 2018. | GAO-19-48.

All of the pipeline operators we interviewed reported using other guidelines or standards to address pipeline systems' security risks. For example, pipeline operators reported using and industry association representatives reported that their members use INGAA's *Control Systems Cyber Security Guidelines for the Natural Gas Pipeline Industry*,[59] API's Pipeline SCADA Security standard,[60] and the NIST Cybersecurity Framework as sources of cybersecurity standards, guidelines, and practices that may be scaled and applied to address a pipeline operator's cybersecurity risks.[61]

Further, pipeline operators are required to adhere to regulations related to pipeline safety and, depending upon their assets, operations, and location, may be required to adhere to regulations for electrical utilities, chemical storage facilities, and locations near waterways. For example, all pipeline operators must adhere to DOT's PHMSA safety regulations.[62] In

[58] TSA's *Pipeline Security Guidelines* call for pipeline operators of critical facilities to conduct a security vulnerability assessment or the equivalent on a periodic basis, not to exceed 36 months, and within 12 months after completion of a significant enhancement or modification to the facility.

[59] Interstate Natural Gas Association of America, *Control Systems Cyber Security Guidelines for the Natural Gas Pipeline Industry Version 1.3* (Washington, D.C.: September 17, 2015).

[60] American Petroleum Institute, *Pipeline SCADA Security*, API Standard 1164 (June 2009).

[61] NIST, *Framework for Improving Critical Infrastructure Cybersecurity, Version 1.0* (Feb. 12, 2014). In response to Executive Order 13636, NIST issued the *Framework for Critical Infrastructure Cybersecurity*, which is intended to help organizations apply the principles and best practices of risk management to improving the security and resilience of critical infrastructure. The framework consists of five concurrent and continuous functions— identify, protect, detect, respond, and recover. When considered together, these functions provide a high-level, strategic view of the life-cycle of an organization's management of cybersecurity risk.

[62] See 49 C.F.R. pts. 190-199.

addition, pipeline operators whose systems include chemical facilities may be required to comply with DHS's Chemical Facility Anti-Terrorism Standards (CFATS).[63] Pipeline operators whose systems include a terminal located on a U.S. port may be required to comply with Maritime Transportation Security Act regulations.[64] For a listing of federal and industry guidelines identified as applicable to security by the pipeline operators, see appendix I.

TSA Does Not Have a Documented Process for Updating Its *Pipeline Security Guidelines* to Reflect Revisions to Supporting Standards

TSA's Pipeline Security Branch issued its revised *Pipeline Security Guidelines* in March 2018, but TSA has not established a documented process to ensure that revisions occur and fully capture updates to supporting standards and guidance. The guidelines were revised to, among other things, reflect the dynamic threat environment and to incorporate cybersecurity principles and practices from the NIST Cybersecurity Framework, which were initially issued in February 2014. To revise the guidelines and incorporate feedback, according to Pipeline Security Branch officials, they incorporated outcomes from pipeline modal threat assessments and best practices from security reviews, and collaborated with pipeline sector stakeholders—including industry associations and other federal agencies with a role in pipeline security. Officials from the industry associations we interviewed confirmed that they provided input to the revised pipeline guidelines, including meeting with and consolidating comments from member pipeline operators. See Figure 6 for a timeline of events pertinent to federal pipeline security guidelines.

TSA's *Pipeline Security Smart Practice Observations* for pipeline operators states that security plans should have a documented process to include security plan reviews and updates on a periodic and an as-needed basis.[65] *Standards for Internal Control in the Federal Government* states that periodic review of policies, procedures, and related control activities should occur to determine their continued relevance and effectiveness in achieving identified objectives or addressing related risks.[66] The NIPP and NIST also emphasize the need to provide updates on incident response guidance and security procedures, respectively. Moreover, other pipeline industry guidance cited by TSA's guidelines also has a prescribed interval for review and revision. For example, API reviews its standards at least every 5 years.

However, TSA has not instituted a documented process to consider the need to update the *Pipeline Security Guidelines* on a regular basis. Pipeline Security Branch officials acknowledged the value of having a defined process for reviewing and, if necessary, revising TSA's *Pipeline Security Guidelines* at regular defined intervals to ensure it includes, among other things, newly identified best practices and updated industry guidance that are relevant to pipeline operators, such as the elements of the latest version of NIST's Cybersecurity

---

[63] See 6 C.F.R. pt. 27. In 2007, DHS established the CFATS program to assess the risk posed by chemical facilities, place High Risk facilities in one of four risk-based tiers, require High Risk facilities to develop security plans, review these plans, and inspect the facilities to ensure compliance with regulatory requirements.

[64] Maritime Transportation Security Act of 2002, enacted to protect the nation's ports and waterways from a terrorist attack, regulates operators, including pipeline operators, with off shore or port facilities and requires certain protective measures such as vulnerability assessments and security plans. See generally Pub. L. No. 107-295, 116 Stat. 2064.

[65] Transportation Security Administration, *Pipeline Security Smart Practice Observations* (September 19, 2011).

[66] GAO-14-704G.

Framework. For example, TSA's revisions to its guidelines incorporated some, but not all of the elements of the NIST Cybersecurity Framework version 1. Specifically, to improve incident response, the NIST framework recommends implementing an incident response analysis and feedback function to a security program. However, TSA's *Pipeline Security Guidelines* do not include similar steps for pipelines operators to include in their pipeline security programs. Further, because NIST released version 1.1 of the Cybersecurity Framework in April 2018, the guidelines that TSA released in March 2018 do not incorporate cybersecurity elements that NIST added to the latest Cybersecurity Framework such as the Supply Chain Risk Management category.[67]

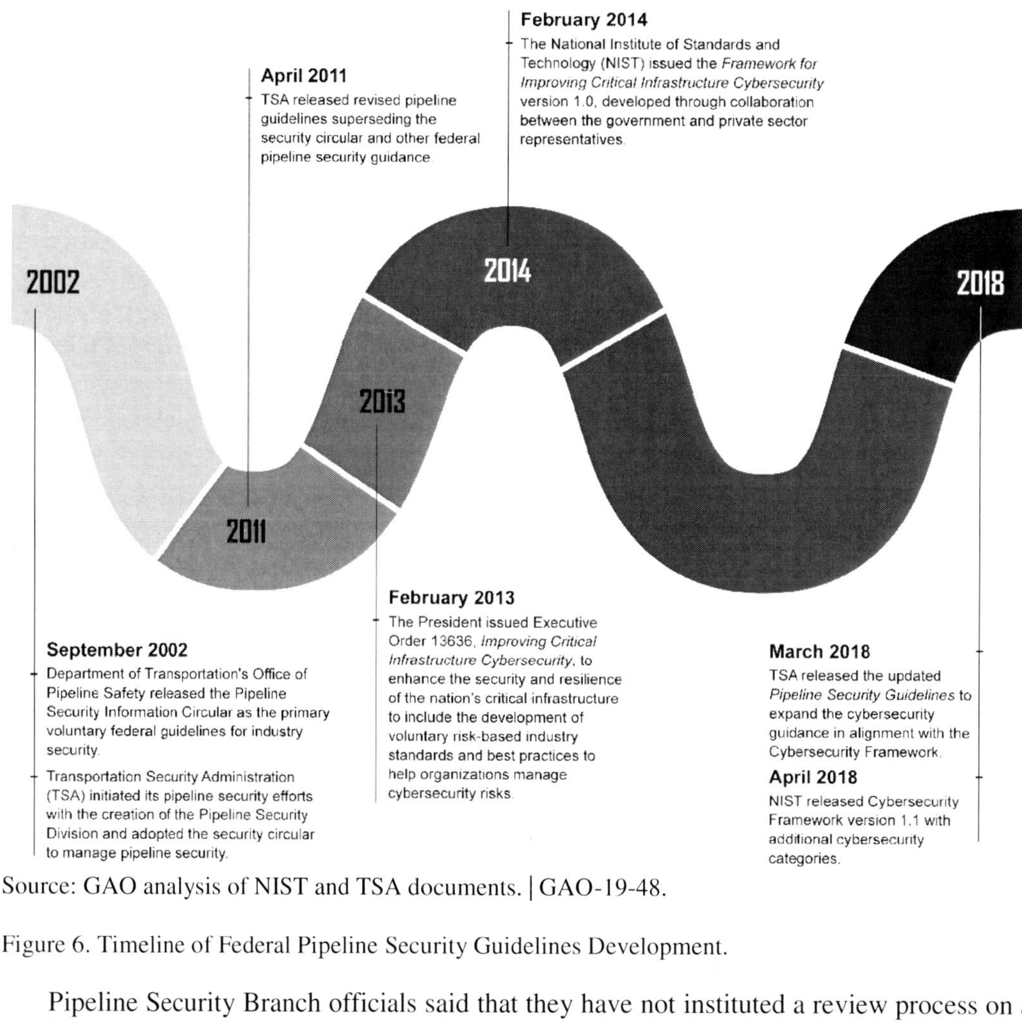

Source: GAO analysis of NIST and TSA documents. | GAO-19-48.

Figure 6. Timeline of Federal Pipeline Security Guidelines Development.

Pipeline Security Branch officials said that they have not instituted a review process on a regular basis because they intended to review and revise TSA's guidelines on an as-needed basis in response to updated supporting guidance, but could provide no timeline for doing so.

[67] NIST Special Publication 800-161, *Supply Chain Risk Management Practices for Federal Information Systems and Organizations* (April 2015). Supply chains begin with the sourcing of products and services and extend from the design, development, manufacturing, processing, handling, and delivery of products and services to the end user. Cyber supply chain risk management entails identifying, assessing, and mitigating "products and services that may contain potentially malicious functionality, are counterfeit, or are vulnerable due to poor manufacturing and development practices within the cyber supply chain."

Without a documented process defining how frequently Pipeline Security Branch staff are to review and revise its guidelines, TSA cannot ensure that its guidelines reflect the latest known standards and best practices for physical and cybersecurity, or address the persistent and dynamic security threat environment currently facing the nation's pipeline system.

Pipeline Security Guidelines Lack Clear Definitions to Ensure Pipeline Operators Consistently Apply TSA's Criteria for Identifying Critical Facilities

Under TSA's *Pipeline Security Guidelines*, pipeline operators are to self-identify the critical facilities within their system and report their critical facilities to TSA. TSA's Pipeline Security Branch conducts CFSRs at the critical facilities that pipeline operators have identified.

However, our analysis of TSA's data found that at least 34 of the top 100 critical pipeline systems deemed highest risk indicated that they had no critical facilities.[68] Accordingly, TSA would not conduct a CFSR at any of these systems' facilities because their operators identified none of them as critical.

Transportation Security Administration's Criteria for Determining Pipeline Facility Criticality

A facility or combination of facilities that, if damaged or destroyed, would have the potential to:

- Disrupt or significantly reduce required service or deliverability to installations identified as critical to national defense;
- Disrupt or significantly reduce required service or deliverability to key infrastructure (such as power plants or major airports) resulting in major economic disruption;
- Cause mass casualties or significant health effects;
- Disrupt or significantly reduce required service or deliverability resulting in a state or local government's inability to provide essential public services and emergency response for an extended period of time;
- Significantly damage or destroy national landmarks or monuments;
- Disrupt or significantly reduce the intended use of major rivers, lakes, or waterways (e.g., public drinking water for large populations or disruption of major commerce or public transportation routes);
- Disrupt or significantly reduce required service or deliverability to a significant number of customers or individuals for an extended period of time;
- Significantly disrupt pipeline system operations for an extended period of time (i.e., business critical facilities).

Source: Transportation Security Administration's *Pipeline Security Guidelines*, 2018. | GAO-19-48.

The fact that pipeline operators of about one third of the highest risk systems identified no critical facilities may be due, in part, to the Pipeline Security Branch not clearly defining the criteria outlined in the *Pipeline Security Guidelines* that pipeline operators are to use to determine the criticality of their facilities. Three of the 10 operators we interviewed stated

[68] Data on critical facility count for 10 of the 100 most critical pipeline systems were not present in the ranking.

that some companies reported to TSA that they had no critical facilities, and may possibly be taking advantage of the guidelines' lack of clarity. Accordingly, operators that report no critical facilities would avoid TSA's reviews of their facilities.

Our review of the eight criteria included in TSA's *Pipeline Security Guidelines* (see sidebar) found that no additional examples or clarification are provided to help operators determine criticality. Although we previously noted that 5 of the 10 operators we interviewed generally found TSA's *Guidelines* as a whole helpful in addressing pipeline security, more than half of the operators we interviewed identified TSA's criticality criteria as a specific area for improvement. Specifically, 3 of the 10 pipeline operators that we interviewed stated that TSA had not clearly defined certain terms within the criteria, and 3 additional operators of the 10 reported that additional consultation with TSA was necessary to appropriately apply the criteria and determine their facilities' criticality. For example, 2 operators told us that individual operators may interpret TSA's criterion, "cause mass casualties or significant health effect," differently. One of these operators that we interviewed stated that this criterion could be interpreted either as a specific number of people affected or a sufficient volume to overwhelm a local health department, which could vary depending on the locality. Another operator reported that because TSA's criteria were not clear, they created their own criteria which helped the operator identify two additional critical facilities.

Pipeline Security Branch officials acknowledged there are companies that report having no critical facilities in their pipeline systems. According to Pipeline Security Branch officials, pipeline operators are in the best position to determine which of their facilities are critical, and the companies that have determined that their pipeline systems have no critical facilities also have reported sufficient redundancies to make none of their facilities critical to the continuity of their operations. According to these officials, they have had extensive discussions with pipeline company officials to assess the validity of their criticality determinations, and have closely questioned companies to ensure they have properly applied TSA's criteria.

However, according to TSA's *Pipeline Security Guidelines*, operators should use a consistent set of criteria for determining the criticality of their facilities. In addition, *Standards for Internal Control in the Federal Government* states that management should define objectives clearly to enable the identification of risks.[69] To achieve this, management generally defines objectives in specific and measurable terms and ensures the terms are fully and clearly set forth so they can be easily understood.

Pipeline Security Branch officials acknowledged that the criticality definitions in the *Pipeline Security Guidelines* could be clarified to be more specific. Additionally, an industry association representative reported that the association, in consultation with TSA, has been developing supplementary guidance for its members to clarify certain terms in TSA's critical facility criteria. As of October 2018 this guidance is still under review at the association and has not been made available to the association's members. Pipeline Security Branch officials confirmed they worked with the industry association on its supplementary guidance, but also acknowledged that the supplementary guidance may only be distributed to the association's membership.

---

[69] GAO, *Standards for Internal Control in the Federal Government,* GAO-14-704G (Washington, D.C.: Sept. 10, 2014).

Without clearly defined criteria for determining pipeline facilities' criticality, TSA cannot ensure that pipeline operators are applying its guidance uniformly. Further, because TSA selects the pipeline facilities on which to conduct CFSRs based on operators' determinations, TSA cannot fully ensure that all of the critical facilities across the pipeline sector have been identified using the same criteria, or that their vulnerabilities have been identified and addressed.

TSA Assesses Pipeline Risk and Conducts Security Reviews, but Limited Workforce Planning and Shortfalls in Assessing Risk Present Challenges

TSA's Intelligence and Analysis identifies security risks to pipeline systems through various assessments. Additionally, TSA's Pipeline Security Branch conducts security reviews to assess pipeline operators' implementation of TSA's *Pipeline Security Guidelines*, but gaps in staffing and lack of a workforce plan may affect its ability to carry out effective reviews. The Pipeline Security Branch also developed a pipeline risk assessment to rank relative risk of the top 100 critical pipeline systems and to prioritize its security reviews of pipeline companies, but shortfalls in its calculations of threat, vulnerability, and consequence may limit its ability to accurately identify pipeline systems with the highest risk. Finally, the pipeline risk assessment has not been peer reviewed to validate the assessment's data and methodology, which we previously reported as a best practice in risk management.

TSA Conducts Assessments of Pipeline Security Risks

TSA's Intelligence and Analysis produces assessments related to pipeline security risks, including Pipeline Modal and Cyber Modal Threat Assessments and the Transportation Sector Security Risk Assessment. The Pipeline and Cyber Modal Threat Assessments are issued on a semiannual basis; TSA Intelligence and Analysis may also issue additional situation-based products on emerging threats. The Pipeline Modal and Cyber Modal Threat Assessments evaluate, respectively, physical and cyber threats to pipelines. The pipeline modal threat assessment evaluates terrorist threats to hazardous liquid and natural gas pipelines, and the cyber modal threat assessment evaluates cyber threats to transportation, including pipelines. Both assessments specifically analyze the primary threat actors, their capabilities, and activities—including attacks occurring internationally—as well as other characteristics of threat.

The Transportation Sector Security Risk Assessment assesses threat, vulnerability, and consequence for various attack scenarios across the five transportation modes for which TSA is responsible.[70] The scenarios define a type of threat actor—including homegrown violent

---

[70] According to TSA, the Transportation Sector Security Risk Assessment was developed both in response to requirements in statute to conduct risk assessments for the Transportation Systems sector and to fulfill TSA's operational and strategic need for a comprehensive risk assessment to aid in planning, risk-based decision making, and resource allocation. See, e.g., Pub. L. No. 110-53, § 1511, 121 Stat. 426-29 (2007); 6 U.S.C. § 1161 (requiring the submission of a nationwide risk assessment of a terrorist attack on railroad carriers). The

extremists and transnational extremists, such as al Qaeda and its affiliates—a target, and an attack mode. For example, a scenario might assess the risk of attacks using varying sizes of improvised explosive devices on pipeline system assets. As part of the assessment process, TSA engages with subject matter experts from TSA and industry stakeholder representatives to compile vulnerabilities for each mode, and TSA analyzes both direct and indirect consequences of the various attack scenarios. According to Pipeline Security Branch officials, the assessments produced by TSA's Intelligence and Analysis provide key information to inform the pipeline security program's efforts.

TSA Conducts Pipeline Security Reviews to Assess Implementation of Pipeline Guidelines, but Does Not Have a Strategic Workforce Plan to Address Staffing Challenges

According to TSA officials, TSA conducts pipeline security reviews— Corporate Security Reviews (CSRs) and Critical Facility Security Reviews (CFSRs)—to assess pipeline vulnerabilities and industry implementation of TSA's *Pipeline Security Guidelines*. However, as shown by Figure 7 below, the number of CSRs and CFSRs completed by TSA has varied during the last five fiscal years, ranging from zero CSRs conducted in fiscal year 2014 to 23 CSRs conducted in fiscal year 2018, as of July 31, 2018.[71]

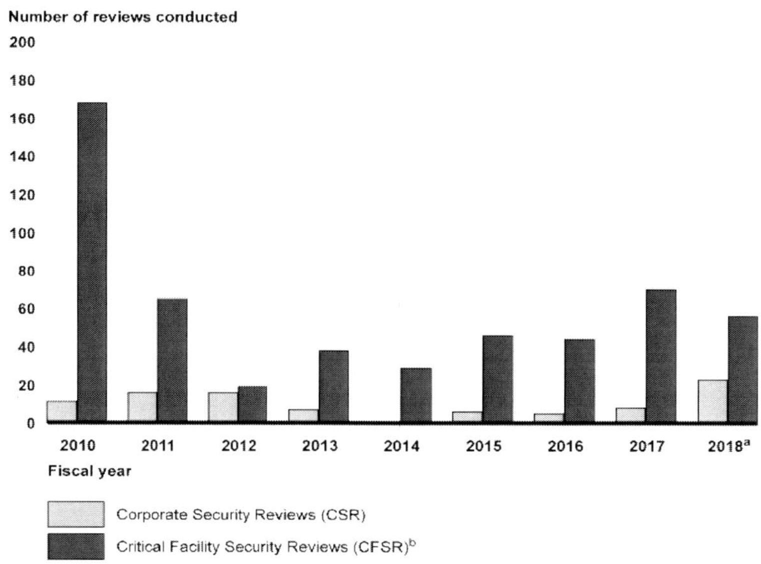

Source: GAO analysis of Transportation Security Administration-reported figures. | GAO-19-48.
[a]Fiscal year (FY) 2018 data are through July 31, 2018.
[b]Fiscal years 2010 and 2011 represent Critical Facility Inspections, which were the predecessor to CFSRs.

Figure 7. Pipeline Security Reviews Conducted, Fiscal Year 2010 through July 2018.

five transportation modes for which TSA is responsible are: Aviation; Freight Rail; Highway; Pipeline; and Mass Transit.

[71] According to TSA officials, the decline in CSRs from 2013 to 2015 was caused by travel restrictions during sequestration, as well a reorganization which moved the assessment function.

TSA officials reported that staffing limitations have prevented TSA from conducting more reviews. As shown in Table 3, TSA Pipeline Security Branch staffing levels (excluding contractor support) have varied significantly over the past 9 years ranging from 14 full-time equivalents (FTEs) in fiscal years 2012 and 2013 to one FTE in fiscal year 2014. They stated that, while contractor support has assisted with conducting CFSRs, there were no contractor personnel providing CSR support from fiscal years 2010 through 2017, but that has now increased to two personnel in fiscal year 2018.[72]

Table 3. TSA Pipeline Security Branch Staffing Levels, Fiscal Years 2010 through 2018

Fiscal Year	TSA Pipeline Security Branch Staffing[a]
2010	13
2011	13
2012	14
2013	14
2014	1
2015	6
2016	6
2017	6
2018	6

Source: Transportation Security Administration (TSA) documents. | GAO-19-48.
[a]TSA pipeline staffing numbers are in full-time equivalents.

TSA prioritizes reviewing and collecting information on the nation's top 100 critical pipeline systems. According to TSA officials, they would need to conduct 46 CSRs in order to review the top 100 critical pipeline systems. In July 2018, TSA officials stated that TSA's current target was to assess each pipeline company every 2 to 3 years; this would equate to about 15 to 23 CSRs per year.[73] TSA officials stated that they expect to complete 20 CSRs and 60 CFSRs per fiscal year with Pipeline Security Branch employees and contract support, and have completed 23 CSRs through July 2018 for fiscal year 2018.

Given the ever-increasing cybersecurity risks to pipeline systems, ensuring that the Pipeline Security Branch has the required cybersecurity skills to effectively evaluate pipeline systems' cybersecurity is essential. Pipeline operators we interviewed emphasized the importance of cybersecurity skills among TSA staff. Specifically, 6 of the 10 pipeline operators and 3 of the 5 industry representatives we interviewed reported that the level of cybersecurity expertise among TSA staff and contractors may challenge the Pipeline Security Branch's ability to fully assess the cybersecurity portions of its security reviews. TSA officials stated that Security Policy and Industry Engagement staff are working with DHS's National Protection and Programs Directorate to help address cyber-related needs, including identifying specific cybersecurity skills and competencies required for the pipeline security program. The officials were uncertain, however, whether TSA would use contractor support

[72] In addition to TSA pipeline personnel, pipeline security reviews received support from contractors and other personnel within TSA's Surface Division. TSA awards for contract support amounted to $2,443,634 on Critical Facility Inspections from fiscal years 2008 to 2011, $3,978,151 on CFSRs from fiscal years 2012 to 2016, $2,233,928 on CFSRs from fiscal years 2017 to 2021, and $2,366,481 on CSRs from fiscal years 2017 to 2021.

[73] To calculate the number of annual CSRs it would take to meet TSA's current target, we divided 46 CSRs by the number of years stated. For example, 46 CSRs divided by 2 years equals 23 CSRs per year; 46 CSRs divided by 3 years equals approximately 15 CSRs per year. This assumes that TSA does not review a pipeline company more than once in that time frame.

or support from the National Protection and Programs Directorate to provide identified skills and competencies. TSA officials also stated that Security Policy and Industry Engagement staff work with TSA's human resource professionals to identify critical skills and competencies needed for Pipeline Security Branch personnel, and helps its workforce maintain professional expertise by providing training and education for any identified skill or competency gaps.

Our previous work has identified principles that a strategic workforce planning process should follow including developing strategies tailored to address gaps in number, deployment, and alignment of human capital approaches for enabling and sustaining the contributions of all critical skills and competencies.[74] Workforce planning efforts, linked to an agency's strategic goals and objectives, can enable it to remain aware of and be prepared for its needs, including the size of its workforce, its deployment across the organization, and the knowledge, skills, and abilities needed for it to pursue its mission. Agencies should consider how hiring, training, staff development, performance management, and other human capital strategies can be aligned to eliminate gaps and improve the long-term contribution of skills and competencies identified as important for mission success.[75]

TSA has not established a workforce plan for its Security Policy and Industry Engagement or its Pipeline Security Branch that identifies staffing needs and skill sets such as the required level of cybersecurity expertise among TSA staff and contractors. When asked for TSA strategic workforce planning documents used to inform staffing allocations related to the pipeline security program, TSA officials acknowledged they do not have a strategic workforce plan. Rather, according to these officials, TSA determines agency-level staffing allocations through the Planning, Programming, Budgeting and Execution process, which is used to decide policy, strategy, and the development of personnel and capabilities to accomplish anticipated missions. According to TSA officials, when they use this process they look at existing resources and then set priorities based on the TSA Administrator's needs. However, a strategic workforce plan allows an agency to identify and prepare for its needs, such as the size of its workforce, its deployment across the organization, and the knowledge, skills, and abilities needed to pursue its mission. TSA officials stated that the agency has a detailed allocation plan for strategically aligning resources to screen passengers at TSA-regulated airports, but not for the entire agency.[76]

By establishing a strategic workforce plan, TSA can help ensure it has identified the knowledge, skills, and abilities that the future workforce of TSA's Pipeline Security Branch may need in order to meet its mission of reducing pipeline systems' vulnerabilities to physical and cybersecurity risks, especially in a dynamic and evolving threat environment. Further, as greater emphasis is placed on cybersecurity, determining the long-term staffing needs of the Pipeline Security Branch will be essential. Furthermore, a workforce plan could enable TSA to determine the number of personnel it needs to meet its stated goals for conducting CSRs and CFSRs.

---

[74] GAO, *Human Capital: Key Principles for Effective Strategic Workforce Planning,* GAO-04-39 (Washington, D.C.: Dec. 11, 2003).

[75] GAO, *Human Capital: A Guide for Assessing Strategic Development Efforts in the Federal Government*, GAO-04-546G (Washington, D.C.: Mar. 1, 2004).

[76] In 2018, we reported on TSA's airport staffing model and its use in assigning screening personnel to airports. See GAO, *Aviation Security: TSA Uses Current Assumptions and Airport-Specific Data for Its Staffing Process and Monitors Passenger Wait Times Using Daily Operations Data,* GAO-18-236 (Washington, D.C.: Feb. 1, 2018).

TSA Calculates Relative Risk of Pipeline Systems, but Its Ranking Tool Does Not Include Current Data or Align with DHS Priorities to Help Prioritize Security Reviews

After TSA identifies the top 100 critical pipeline systems based on throughput, the Pipeline Security Branch uses the Pipeline Relative Risk Ranking Tool (risk assessment), which it developed in 2007, to assess various security risks of those systems.[77] We previously reported, in 2010, that the Pipeline Security Branch was the first of TSA's surface transportation modes to develop a risk assessment model that combined all three components of risk—threat, vulnerability, and consequence—to generate a risk score.[78] The risk assessment generates a risk score for each of the 100 most critical pipeline systems and ranks them according to risk. The risk assessment calculates threat, vulnerability, and consequence for each pipeline system on variables such as the amount of throughput in the pipeline system and the number critical facilities. The risk assessment combines data collected from pipeline operators, as well as other federal agencies, such as the Departments of Transportation and Defense, to generate the risk score.

However, the last time the Pipeline Security Branch calculated relative risk among the top 100 critical pipeline systems using the risk assessment was in 2014. Pipeline Security Branch officials told us that they use the pipeline risk assessment to rank relative risk of the top 100 critical pipeline systems, and the standard operating procedures for conducting CSRs state the results of the risk ranking are the primary factor considered when prioritizing corporate security reviews of pipeline companies.[79] According to Pipeline Security Branch officials, the risk assessment has not changed since 2014 because the Pipeline Security Branch is still conducting CSRs based on the 2014 ranking of pipeline systems.

As outlined in Table 4 below, we identified several factors that likely limit the usefulness of the current risk assessment in calculating threat, vulnerability, and consequence to allow the Pipeline Security Branch to effectively prioritize reviews of pipeline systems. For example, because the risk assessment has not changed since 2014, information on threat may be outdated. Additionally, sources of data and underlying assumption and judgments regarding certain threat and vulnerability inputs to the assessment are not fully documented. For example, threats to cybersecurity are not specifically accounted for in the description of the risk assessment methodology, making it unclear if cybersecurity is part of the assessment's threat factor. Further, the risk assessment does not include information that is consistent with the NIPP and other DHS priorities for critical infrastructure risk mitigation, such as information on natural hazards and the ability to measure risk reduction (feedback data).

---

[77] According to DHS, a risk assessment is a product or process which collects information and assigns values to risks for the purpose of informing priorities, developing or comparing courses of action, and informing decision-making. A risk assessment is also considered the appraisal of the risks facing an entity, asset, system, network, geographic area or other grouping. See DHS Risk Lexicon, 2010.

[78] See GAO-10-867.

[79] In August 2010, we recommended, among other things, that the Pipeline Security Branch document a methodology for scheduling CSRs that considers a pipeline system's risk ranking as the primary scheduling criteria and to balance that with other practical considerations. As a result, the Pipeline Security Branch revised its CSR Standard Operating Procedures, as documented in a copy dated May 20, 2011, to state that the primary criteria for scheduling CSR visits is the pipeline system's relative risk (i.e., risk ranking), although other factors and considerations, such as operator availability and geographic location, will also play a role. Version 4.4, dated April 24, 2012, includes the same language. See GAO-10-867.

Table 4. Shortfalls in the Pipeline Security Branch's Risk Ranking Assessment

Identified Shortfalls in the Risk Assessment	Shortfall Description and Corresponding Risk Element Affected: Threat (T), Vulnerability (V), Consequence (C)		Why It Matters
Information may be outdated	• The Pipeline Security Branch has not updated the risk assessment since June 2014, because of competing priorities. Therefore, information used to determine calculations, such as threat information, may be outdated and not reflect threats to the industry that have emerged in recent years. • When the risk assessment was last updated in 2014, it used pipeline systems' throughput data from 2010 to assess relative risk and throughput may have changed since 2010.	T C	• Standards for Internal Control in the Federal Government calls for management to use quality information to achieve the entity's objectives, including using relevant data from reliable sources obtained in a timely manner. • Keeping the risk assessment updated with current information could help the Pipeline Security Branch ensure it is using its limited resources to review the pipeline systems with greater risk.
Data sources, underlying assumptions and judgments, and sources of uncertainty not always documented	• The Pipeline Security Branch ranked threat equally across pipeline systems because officials say they do not have enough threat information to distinguish threat by pipeline. However, this judgment is not documented in the risk assessment's methodology. • Threats to cybersecurity are not specifically accounted for in the description of the risk assessment methodology. • The number of critical facilities is part of a pipeline system's vulnerability score, but pipeline operators do not identify critical facilities consistently, leading to uncertainty in this input.	T T V	• According to the National Infrastructure Protection Plan (NIPP), a risk assessment's methodology must clearly document what information is used and how it is synthesized to generate a risk estimate, including any assumptions, judgments, sources of uncertainty, and any implications for interpreting the results from the assessment. • Documenting sources of data and agency assumptions, judgments, or decisions to exclude information could provide increased transparency to those expected to interpret or use the results.
Does not include risk information consistent with the NIPP or other Department of Homeland Security (DHS) priorities for critical infrastructure risk mitigation, such as: data on prior attacks	• The pipeline risk assessment includes a field that accounts for whether a pipeline experienced a previous security threat (including failed attacks). However, that field is not used in the risk assessment's calculation. Pipeline Security Branch officials acknowledged that prior attacks should be part of the threat calculation, but could not account for why they were not calculated for the systems in the risk assessment.	T	• Information provided by the Pipeline Security Branch suggests some pipeline systems have experienced such threats. According to the NIPP, judgments, such as deciding not to include information, should be articulated in the methodology. • Including past attacks on pipeline systems could help the Pipeline Security Branch better differentiate threat among pipeline systems.
Natural hazards	• The pipeline risk assessment does not account for natural hazards in its threat calculation. According to Pipeline Security Branch officials, there is not sufficient historical data available that would indicate a significant impact from natural disasters on pipeline infrastructure.	T	• According to the NIPP, threat includes natural hazards with the potential to harm life, information, operations, the environment, and/or property. As such, natural disasters are a key element of the DHS's critical infrastructure security and resilience mission.

Identified Shortfalls in the Risk Assessment	Shortfall Description and Corresponding Risk Element Affected: Threat (T), Vulnerability (V), Consequence (C)		Why It Matters
	• However, we identified possible sources of data for the Pipeline Security Branch to consider, including information from the Federal Emergency Management Agency.		• While there may not be historical data of natural hazard impact for every pipeline system, consulting other sources or experts could provide data or analysis for a more comprehensive threat picture.
Feedback data on pipeline system performance, including cybersecurity	• The risk assessment is unable to measure the progress a pipeline system made in addressing vulnerability gaps between reviews, because Pipeline Security Branch officials said their current measure—a vulnerability score—is unreliable for comparative and analytic purposes. However, they agree on the importance of a feedback mechanism tying results of reviews to a revised vulnerability metric. • The risk assessment does not include a measure of cybersecurity vulnerabilities. According to Pipeline Security Branch officials, absent data specific to pipelines on their cyber vulnerabilities, they are unable to include a pipeline's vulnerability to cyber attack in the risk assessment.	V V	• The NIPP and DHS's Risk Management fundamentals emphasize the important role that a feedback mechanism plays in risk management. • As pipeline operators implement increasing levels of network technologies to control their systems, the Pipeline Security Branch may not be fully accounting for pipeline systems' cybersecurity activities by not including the cybersecurity-related vulnerabilities in its risk assessment inputs. Developing a feedback mechanism based on implementation of TSA's Pipeline Security Guidelines-including those on cybersecurity-could be an important input to the risk assessment's vulnerability calculation. This information would also inform the amount of risk pipeline companies are reducing by implementing the guidelines and could be used to inform overall risk reduction.
Physical pipeline condition	• Pipeline physical condition is not accounted for in the current risk assessment. However, pipeline condition or location (such as above or below ground) could touch upon pipeline security as it relates to system vulnerability. According to the Transportation Systems Sector-Specific Plan, vulnerabilities to damage in aging transportation infrastructure—of which pipelines are a part—are projected to increase with continued climate change.	V	• DHS has listed the potential for catastrophic losses to dramatically increase the overall risk associated with failing infrastructure and highlighted risks due to climate change and natural hazards to pipelines. The NIPP defines vulnerability as a physical feature or operational attribute that renders an entity open to exploitation or susceptible to a given threat or hazard. • By considering additional information from DOT on the physical condition of a pipeline system, the Pipeline Security Branch could better inform its vulnerability calculations. Additionally, TSA could use the information to help pipeline operators identify security measures to help reduce vulnerability of an aging system because well-maintained, safe pipelines are more likely to tolerate a physical attack.

Table 4. (Continued)

Identified Shortfalls in the Risk Assessment	Shortfall Description and Corresponding Risk Element Affected: Threat (T), Vulnerability (V), Consequence (C)		Why It Matters
Cross-sector interdependencies	• The Pipeline Security Branch's pipeline risk assessment currently considers the effects of a pipeline system's ability to service assets such as major airports, the electric grid, and military bases. However, consequence is calculated on the loss or disruption of the pipeline system to these other assets and does not capture the dependency of the pipeline system on other energy sources, such as electricity. Pipeline Security Branch officials are considering cross-sector interdependencies and discuss these factors with operators as they relate to system resiliency, but did not see a direct link to pipeline security.	V	• According to the NIPP, understanding and addressing risks from cross-sector dependencies and interdependencies is essential to enhancing critical infrastructure security and resilience. • Considering interdependencies of sectors in both directions could improve the calculations in the pipeline risk assessment.

Source: GAO Analysis of Transportation Security Administration Pipeline Relative Risk Ranking Tool data | GAO-19-48.

According to Pipeline Security Branch officials, the risk ranking assessment is not intended to be a fully developed risk model detailing all pipeline factors influencing risk. Rather, officials said they are primarily interested in assessing risk data that impacts security. However, because TSA's Pipeline Security Program is designed to enhance the security preparedness of the pipeline systems, incorporating additional factors that enhance security into their risk calculation would better align their efforts with PPD-21. For example, PPD-21 calls for agencies to integrate and analyze information to prioritize assets and manage risks to critical infrastructure, as well as anticipate interdependencies and cascading impacts. For a more detailed discussion of the shortfalls we identified, refer to appendix II.

TSA's Pipeline Risk Assessment Has Not Been Peer Reviewed to Help Validate the Data and Methodology

In addition to the shortfalls identified above, the risk assessment has not been peer reviewed since its conception in 2007. In our past work, we reported that independent, external peer reviews are a best practice in risk management and that independent expert review panels can provide objective reviews of complex issues.[80] According to the National Research Council of the National Academies, external peer reviews should, among other

[80] See GAO, *Coast Guard: Security Risk Model Meets DHS Criteria, but More Training Could Enhance Its Use for Managing Programs and Operations*, GAO-12-14 (Washington, D.C.: Nov. 17, 2011); and *Aviation Security: Efforts to Validate TSA's Passenger Screening Behavior Detection Program Underway, but Opportunities Exist to Strengthen Validation and Address Operational Challenges*, GAO-10-763 (Washington, D.C.: May 20, 2011).

things, address the structure of the assessment, the types and certainty of the data, and how the assessment is intended to be used. The National Research Council has also recommended that DHS improve its risk analyses for infrastructure protection by validating the assessments and submitting them to independent, external peer review.[81]

Other DHS components have implemented our prior recommendations to conduct peer reviews of their risk assessments.[82] For example, in April 2013, we reported on DHS's management of its Chemical Facility Anti-Terrorism Standards (CFATS) program and found that the approach used to assess risk did not consider all of the elements of consequence, threat, and vulnerability associated with a terrorist attack involving certain chemicals.[83] The Infrastructure Security Compliance Division, which manages the CFATS program conducted a multiyear effort to improve their risk assessment methodology and included commissioning a peer review by the Homeland Security Studies and Analysis Institute, which resulted in multiple recommendations. As part of the implementation of some of the peer review's recommendations, DHS conducted peer reviews and technical reviews with government organizations and facility owners and operators, and worked with Sandia National Laboratories to verify and validate the CFATS program's revised risk assessment methodology, which was completed in January 2017.

According to Pipeline Security Branch officials, they are considering updates to the risk assessment methodology including changes to the vulnerability and consequence factors. These officials said the risk assessment was previously reviewed within the past 18 months by industry experts and they consider input from several federal partners including DHS, DOT, and the Department of Defense. Officials also said they will consider input from industry experts and federal partners while working on updating the risk assessment. However, most of the proposed changes to the risk assessment methodology officials described are ones that have been deliberated since our last review in 2010.[84] Therefore, an independent, external peer review would provide the opportunity for integration and analysis of additional outside expertise across the critical infrastructure community.

While independent, external peer reviews cannot ensure the success of a risk assessment approach, they can increase the probability of success by improving the technical quality of projects and the credibility of the decision-making process. According to the National Research Council of the National Academies, independent, external peer reviews should

---

[81] National Research Council of the National Academies, Review of the Department of Homeland Security's Approach to Risk Analysis (Washington, D.C., 2010).

[82] See GAO, *Critical Infrastructure Protection: DHS Efforts to Assess Chemical Security Risk and Gather Feedback on Facility Outreach Can Be Strengthened*, GAO-13-353 (Washington, D.C.: Apr. 5, 2013). See also GAO, *Critical Infrastructure Protection: DHS List of Priority Assets Needs to Be Validated and Reported to Congress*, GAO-13-296 (Washington, D.C.: Mar 25, 2013). In this March 2013 report, we found that changes to DHS's criteria for including assets on the National Critical Infrastructure Prioritization Program (NCIPP) list of the nation's highest-priority critical infrastructure could hinder DHS's ability to compare infrastructure across sectors and that a peer review would better position DHS to reasonably assure that the NCIPP list identifies the nation's highest priority critical infrastructure. DHS concurred with our recommendation, and in November 2013, DHS commissioned a seven-member panel to review the NCIPP process, which resulted in multiple observations, some of which DHS has taken steps to address. DHS's commissioning of a review panel satisfied the intent of our recommendation.

[83] See GAO-13-353.

[84] During our current review, Pipeline Security Branch officials reported that they are considering updates to the risk assessment methodology, including changes to vulnerability and consequence factors. However, the updates officials reported they were considering in 2018 are nearly identical to those that Pipeline Security Branch officials reported they were considering making in 2011 in response to our prior recommendation. These proposed changes were also present in the 2014 version of the risk assessment.

include validation and verification to ensure that the structure of the risk assessment is both accurate and reliable. Thus, an independent, external peer review would provide better assurance that the Pipeline Security Branch can rank relative risk among pipeline systems using the most comprehensive and accurate threat, vulnerability, and consequence information.

TSA HAS ESTABLISHED PERFORMANCE MEASURES, BUT LIMITATIONS HINDER TSA'S ABILITY TO DETERMINE PIPELINE SECURITY PROGRAM EFFECTIVENESS

TSA has established performance measures, as well as databases to monitor pipeline security reviews and analyze their results. However, weaknesses in its performance measures and its efforts to record pipeline security review recommendations limit its ability to determine the extent that its pipeline security program has reduced pipeline sector risks. Furthermore, we identified data reliability issues in the information that TSA collects to track the status of pipeline security review recommendations, such as missing data, inconsistent data entry formats, and data entry errors.

TSA Has Established Performance Measures but Faces Challenges in Assessing the Effectiveness of Its Efforts to Reduce Pipeline Security Risks

TSA has three sets of performance measures for its pipeline efforts: the Pipeline Security Plan in the 2018 Biennial National Strategy for Transportation Security (NSTS), a management measure in the DHS fiscal year 2019 congressional budget justification, and summary figures in their CSR and CFSR databases. As a result of our 2010 work, TSA established performance measures and linked them to Pipeline Security Plan goals within the Surface Security Plan of the 2018 NSTS.[85] See Table 5 below for the 2018 NSTS Pipeline Security Plan performance measures.

As shown in Table 6 below, DHS also included a management measure in its fiscal year 2019 congressional budget justification to track the annual number of completed pipeline security reviews.

Finally, TSA Pipeline Security Branch officials said they use summary figures in the CFSR status database and the CSR goals and priorities database as performance measures.[86]

---

[85] The NSTS provides biennial risk-based plans for transportation assets in the U.S. and identifies objectives which enhance the security of transportation infrastructure. The strategy includes a base plan, modal security plans, and an intermodal security plan. The Surface Security Plan includes four modal security plans: Mass Transit and Passenger Rail, Freight Rail, Highway and Motor Carrier, and Pipeline.

[86] TSA provided us with four databases containing CSR and CFSR information: Master CSR Recommendations Listing and Status (2010-2013), U-SSI CSR Data FY16-17 (10- 10-2017), U-SSI - CFSR Recommendations (10-10-2017) Data (2010-2017), and U-SSI- CFSR Recommendations Analysis. The first contained information on CSR recommendations and their most recent status. The second contained information on CSRs conducted on pipeline operators and their compliance with the guidelines arranged by strategic goals and priorities. The third contained information on CFSR recommendations made by TSA. Finally, the fourth contained information on the most recent status of those CFSR recommendations. In order to better

For example, these include the percentage of CFSR recommendations implemented and the average percentage compliance with the guidelines by fiscal year.

Table 5. 2018 NSTS Pipeline Security Plan Performance Measures, Goals 1 and 2

Goal	Objective	Outcome	Performance Measurement
NSTS Goal 1: Manage Risks to Transportation Systems from Terrorist Attack and Enhance System Resilience	Reduce the risks from a terrorist attack on pipeline systems through security plans addressing critical infrastructure protection, operational practices (to detect and deter), and cybersecurity.	Improvement of industry security plans and security planning through incorporation of TSA Pipeline Security Guidelines into existing security plans.	Percentage of critical pipeline systems implementing TSA Pipeline Security Guidelines as assessed through corporate and facility security reviews.
NSTS Goal 1: Manage Risks to Transportation Systems from Terrorist Attack and Enhance System Resilience	Conduct training of employees to identify, prevent, absorb, respond to, and recover from a terrorist attack.	Improved capability of the industry employees to identify, prevent, absorb, respond to, and recover from a physical and/or cyber terrorist attack.	Percentage of critical pipeline systems implementing TSA Pipeline Security Guidelines as assessed through corporate and facility security reviews.
NSTS Goal 1: Manage Risks to Transportation Systems from Terrorist Attack and Enhance System Resilience	Conduct exercises employing threat scenarios to evaluate and identify opportunities to improve security preparedness and resiliency.	Pipeline systems and public safety agencies are better prepared to respond and recover effectively in the event of security incidents.	Percentage of critical pipeline systems implementing TSA Pipeline Security Guidelines as assessed through corporate and facility security reviews.
NSTS Goal 2; Enhance Effective Domain Awareness of Transportation Systems and Threats	Maintain and enhance mechanisms for information and intelligence sharing between the pipeline industry and government.	Improved domain awareness through timely delivery of relevant intelligence and information products for pipeline industry to implement mitigation strategies to reduce risk.	Increased timely distribution of time sensitive intelligence products.
NSTS Goal 2; Enhance Effective Domain Awareness of Transportation Systems and Threats	Encourage industry engagement with first responders and the public to enhance understanding of community risks associated with pipeline systems.	Pipeline industry, first responders, and neighboring communities working collectively to plan and prepare for incidents that could disrupt pipeline operations and endanger the community.	Percentage of critical pipeline systems implementing TSA Pipeline Security Guidelines as assessed through corporate and facility security reviews.

Source: 2018 Biennial National Strategy for Transportation Security (NSTS) | GAO-19-48.

Table 6. Management Measure in DHS FY 2019 Congressional Budget Justification

Measure	Description
Number of High-Risk Pipeline Systems on Which Security Reviews Were Conducted.	Pipeline Security Reviews assess and elevate the security posture of the pipeline energy transportation mode. Information and recommendations from pipeline corporate headquarters and field site reviews inform critical energy facility operators of issues to enhance security from terrorism and criminal activity. The onsite security reviews develop firsthand knowledge of security planning and execution of the critical pipeline systems, establish communication with key pipeline security personnel, and identify and share smart practices. As industry wide security gaps are identified through the process, the TSA Surface Division develops programs to address gaps throughout the pipeline industry. Each pipeline corporation is assessed every 4 to 5 years.

Source: Department of Homeland Security (DHS) Transportation Security Administration (TSA) Fiscal Year (FY) 2019 Congressional Budget Justification | GAO-19-48.

---

distinguish their contents, from here on we refer to them as the CSR recommendations database, the CSR goals and priorities database, the CFSR recommendations database, and the CFSR status database.

We previously found that results-oriented organizations set performance goals to clearly define desired program outcomes and develop performance measures that are clearly linked to the performance goals.[87] Performance measures should focus on whether a program has achieved measurable standards toward achieving program goals, and allow agencies to monitor and report program accomplishments on an ongoing basis. Our previous work on performance metrics identified 10 attributes of effective performance.[88] Table 7 identifies each key attribute of effective performance measures along with its definition.

Table 7. Key Attributes of Effective Performance Measures

Attribute	Definition
Balance	A suite of measures ensures that an organization's various priorities are covered.
Clarity	Measure is clearly stated, and the name and definition are consistent with the methodology used to calculate it.
Core program activities	Measures cover the activities that an entity is expected to perform to support the intent of the program.
Government-wide priorities	Each measure covers a priority such as quality, timeliness, and cost of service.
Limited overlap	Measures provide new information beyond that provided by other measures.
Linkage	Measure is aligned with division-and agency-wide goals and mission and is clearly communicated throughout the organization.
Measurable target	Measure has a numerical goal.
Objectivity	Measure is reasonably free from significant bias or manipulation.
Reliability	Measure produces the same result under similar conditions.
Baseline and trend data	Measure has a baseline and trend data associated with it to identify, monitor, and report changes in performance and to help ensure that performance is viewed in context.

Source: GAO-17-542 | GAO-19-48.

We evaluated the current performance measures included in the 2018 NSTS, the DHS fiscal year 2019 congressional budget justification, the CSR goals and priorities database, and the CFSR status database related to TSA's Pipeline Security Branch.

We primarily focused on key attributes which could be applied to individual measures. These include clarity, linkage, measurable targets, objectivity, reliability, and baseline and trend data. Our prior work on performance measurement found that all performance measure attributes are not equal and failure to have a particular attribute does not necessarily indicate that there is a weakness in that area or that the measure is not useful; rather, it may indicate an opportunity for further refinement.[89]

Based on our evaluation, the TSA-identified measures do not possess attributes that we have identified as being key to successful performance measures. As a result, TSA cannot fully determine the extent to which the Pipeline Security Branch has achieved desired outcomes, including the effectiveness of its efforts to reduce risks to pipelines. Specifically, many of TSA's measures cover agency goals and mission, but they generally lack clarity and

---

[87] GAO, *Executive Guide: Effectively Implementing the Government Performance and Results Act*, GAO/GGD-96-118 (Washington, D.C.: June 1996); *Managing for Results: Enhancing Agency Use of Performance Information for Management Decision Making*, GAO-05-927 (Washington, D.C.: Sept. 9, 2005); and *Veterans Justice Outreach Program: VA Could Improve Management by Establishing Performance Measures and Fully Assessing Risks*, GAO-16-393 (Washington, D.C.: Apr. 28, 2016).

[88] GAO, *Military Personnel: DOD Needs to Establish Performance Measures for the Armed Forces Sports Program,* GAO-17-542 (Washington, D.C.: June 8, 2017).

[89] GAO, *Tax Administration: IRS Needs to Further Refine Its Tax Filing Season Performance Measures*, GAO-03-143 (Washington, D.C.: Nov. 22, 2002).

measurable targets, provide significantly overlapping information, and do not include baseline and trend data.

- Clarity. The pipeline-related measures in the 2018 NSTS are not clear because they do not describe the methodology used to calculate them, and the names and definitions are not clearly described. For example, NSTS goal 1 includes an objective to conduct training of employees responding to terrorist attacks. The desired outcome is to improve the capability of industry employees to respond and recover from terrorist attacks. However, the performance measure is the percentage of critical pipeline systems implementing the TSA *Pipeline Security Guidelines*. It is not clear if this measure is specific to the sections of the guidelines related to employee training or overall implementation of the guidelines. The CFSR status database measures include the percentage of recommendations implemented by topic, such as "Site Specific Security Measures," "Signage," or "Miscellaneous." However, the database does not specifically define these topics or explain the methodology for calculating the measures.[90] Unclear measures could be confusing and misleading to users.
- Core program activities. The pipeline-related measures in the 2018 NSTS cover some of the agency's core program activities, such as conducting security exercises with the pipeline industry and providing intelligence and information products to the industry. However, the NSTS Pipeline Security Plan measures do not specifically include some core program activities,[91] such as updating the TSA *Pipeline Security Guidelines* or the results of conducting CSRs and CFSRs in order to collect the information necessary for the existing performance measures. The CSR goals and priorities database and the CFSR status database include measures intended to track some of the results of pipeline security reviews, such as the average percentage compliance with the guidelines by fiscal year and the percentage of CFSR recommendations implemented. If core program activities are not covered, there may not be enough information available in those areas to managers and stakeholders.
- Limited overlap. The pipeline-related measures in the 2018 NSTS do not have limited overlap. As discussed previously, four of the five NSTS measures are based on the percentage of critical pipeline systems implementing TSA's *Pipeline Security Guidelines*. The management measure is based on the number of complete pipeline security reviews. The CFSR status database measures are based on the percentage of recommendations implemented overall and by groups. Finally, the CSR goals and priorities database measures are based on the average compliance percentage of companies that had CSRs conducted in fiscal years 2016 and 2017. This is similar to four of the five NSTS measures. Significantly overlapping measures may lead to redundant, costly information that does not add value for TSA management.

---

[90] Formula calculations provide some explanation of how the measures are calculated, although this may not be readily understood by users who are unfamiliar with spreadsheet formulas.

[91] For the purposes of this report, the core program activities were those described in the *Pipeline Security Guidelines* and the 2018 NSTS Pipeline Security Plan. These include developing and updating the guidelines; conducting CSRs and CFSRs; conducting exercises to evaluate preparedness for, response to, and recovery from physical and cyber security incidents; providing timely and relevant intelligence and information to industry; and promoting pipeline security awareness in communities surrounding critical pipeline assets and systems.

- Linkage. The pipeline-related measures in the 2018 NSTS generally exhibited this key attribute. For example, all of the NSTS measures were arranged by agency strategic goals and risk-based priorities. However, the management measure in DHS's fiscal year 2019 congressional budget justification and the CFSR status database measures did not specify the TSA goals and priorities to which they were aligned. If measures are not aligned with division and agency-wide goals and mission, the behaviors and incentives created by these measures do not support achieving those goals or mission.
- Measurable target. TSA's measures generally did not include measurable targets in the form of a numerical goal and none of the NSTS measures had measurable targets. For example, the NSTS measure under the Security Planning priority, which tracks the percentage of critical pipeline systems implementing TSA's *Pipeline Security Guidelines,* does not state what specific percentages would be considered an improvement in industry security plans. However, the management measure did include target numbers of pipeline security reviews by fiscal year. Both the CFSR status database measures and CSR goals and priorities database measures did not include measurable targets. Without measurable targets, TSA cannot tell if performance is meeting expectations.
- Objectivity. Because the pipeline-related measures in the 2018 NSTS, the CFSR status database, and the CSR goals and priorities database generally lack clarity and measurable targets, TSA cannot ensure its measures are free from bias or manipulation, and therefore, are not objective. If measures are not objective, the results of performance assessments may be systematically overstated or understated.
- Reliability. Because the pipeline-related measures in the 2018 NSTS, the CFSR status database, and the CSR goals and priorities database generally lack clarity, measurable targets, and baseline and trend data, it is not clear if TSA's measures produce the same result under similar conditions; therefore, the pipeline-related measures are unreliable. If measures are not reliable, reported performance data may be inconsistent and add uncertainty.
- Baseline and trend data. TSA's measures generally did not include baseline and trend data. For example, none of the NSTS measures included past results and compared them to measurable targets. TSA officials were unable to identify measures or goals to assess the extent to which pipeline operators have fully implemented the guidelines or increased pipeline security, but did say developing a feedback mechanism to measure progress in closing vulnerability gaps was important. However, the management measure did include the number of completed pipeline security reviews for each fiscal year from 2014 through 2017, as well as numerical goals. The CFSR status database includes information on CFSRs conducted from May 22, 2012, through June 29, 2017, but the measures are calculated for the entire time period rather than year-by-year. The CSR goals and priorities database measures include percentage compliance with the guidelines for CSRs conducted in fiscal years 2016 and 2017, as well as a combined measure. However, baseline and trend data are not tracked or reported in either database. Collecting, tracking, developing, and reporting baseline and trend data allows agencies to better evaluate progress being made and whether or not goals are being achieved.

Pipeline Security Branch officials explained that in addition to the measures reported in the 2018 NSTS Pipeline Security Plan, they primarily rely on measures assessing CSR and CFSR implementation for assessing the value of its pipeline security program. TSA officials reported that they collect and analyze data and information collected from CSRs and CFSRs to, among other things, determine strengths and weaknesses at critical pipeline facilities, areas to target for risk reduction strategies, and pipeline industry implementation of the voluntary *Pipeline Security Guidelines*. For example, TSA officials reported that they analyzed information from approximately 734 CFSR recommendations that were made during fiscal years 2012 through 2016. They found that pipeline operators had made the strongest improvements in security training, public awareness outreach and law enforcement coordination, and site specific security measures. The most common areas in need of improvement were 24x7 monitoring, frequency of security vulnerability assessments, and proper signage.

However, as described above, we found those measures also did not comport with key attributes for successful measures and we report below on reliability concerns for underlying data supporting those measures. In addition, while the Pipeline Security Branch may not rely on the measures included in the 2018 NSTS Pipeline Security Plan and the fiscal year 2019 congressional budget justification, they are important for reporting the status of pipeline security efforts to TSA as a whole and to external stakeholders such as Congress.

Taking steps to ensure that the pipeline security program performance measures exhibit key attributes of successful performance measures could allow TSA to better assess the program's effectiveness at reducing pipeline physical and cybersecurity risks. This could include steps such as modifying its suite of measures so they are clear, have measurable targets, and add baseline and trend data. Further examples include the following:

- Adding measurable targets consisting of numerical goals could allow TSA to better determine if the pipeline security program is meeting expectations. For example, measurable targets could be added to TSA's existing measures by developing annual goals for the percentage of recommendations implemented to the CFSR status database and then reporting annual results.
- To make measures clearer, TSA could verify that each measure has a clearly stated name, definition, and methodology for how the measure is calculated. For example, the NSTS objective for security training mentioned above could have more specific language explaining how the measure is calculated and whether it applies to pipeline operators' implementation of the training-related portions of the TSA *Pipeline Security Guidelines* or overall implementation.
- Finally, adding baseline and trend data could allow TSA to identify, monitor, and report changes in performance and help ensure that performance is viewed in context. For example, the NSTS measures, CFSR status database measures, and CSR goals and priorities database measures could have annual results from prior years. This could help TSA and external stakeholders evaluate the effectiveness of the pipeline security program and whether it is making progress toward its goals.

TSA Does Not Track the Implementation Status of Past CSR Recommendations, and Supporting Data Are Not Sufficiently Reliable

According to TSA officials, the primary means for assessing the effectiveness of the agency's efforts to reduce pipeline security risks is through conducting pipeline security reviews— Corporate Security Reviews (CSRs) and Critical Facility Security Reviews (CFSRs). However, TSA has not tracked the status of CSR recommendations for over 5 years and related security review data are not sufficiently reliable.

When conducting CSRs and CFSRs, TSA staff makes recommendations to operators, if appropriate. For example, a CSR recommendation might include a suggestion to conduct annual security-related drills and exercises, and a CFSR recommendation might include a suggestion to install barbed wire on the main gate of a pipeline facility. In response to recommendations that we made in our 2010 report, TSA developed three databases to track CSR and CFSR recommendations and their implementation status by pipeline facility, system, operator, and product type.[92] In addition, the agency recently developed a fourth database to collect and analyze information gathered from pipeline operators' responses to CSR questions. TSA officials reported that they use this database to assess the extent that TSA's pipeline security program has met NSTS goals and Pipeline Security Branch priorities. TSA officials stated that they use the CSR goals and priorities database for follow-up on recommendations, indications of improvement in pipeline security, and as an input into TSA performance goals and measures, including the performance measures for the 2018 NSTS Pipeline Security Plan.

We found several problems with the databases that indicate that the pipeline security program data are not sufficiently reliable and do not provide quality information that is current, complete, and accurate. First, the CSR recommendations database only included information for reviews conducted from November 2010 through February 2013. TSA officials stated that the agency stopped capturing CSR recommendations and status information in 2014. A TSA official stated that one factor was that the pipeline staffing level was one FTE in fiscal year 2014. However, the Pipeline Security Branch did not resume entering CSR recommendation-related information when staffing levels rose to 6 FTEs in the following year and beyond. As a result, TSA is missing over 5 years of data for the recommendations it made to pipeline operators when conducting CSRs.

The agency collected some information from CSRs conducted in fiscal years 2016 and 2017 in the separate CSR goals and priorities database. However, this database does not include all of the information that TSA collects when conducting CSRs. Specifically, the CSR goals and priorities database does not state which companies were reviewed, what specific recommendations were made, or the current status of those recommendations, and only records operators' responses to 79 of the 222 CSR questions.

Second, our review identified instances of missing data, inconsistent data entry formats, and data entry errors in the four databases. For example:

[92] GAO, *Pipeline Security: TSA Has Taken Actions to Help Strengthen Security, but Could Improve Priority-Setting and Assessment Processes,* GAO-10-867 (Washington, D.C.: Aug. 4, 2010).

- The CSR recommendations database had missing data in all 13 of the included fields and a data entry error shifted 50 observations into the wrong fields, impacting both the Status Date and Completion Code fields.[93]
- The CSR goals and priorities database had seven entries with inconsistent data formatting and five of those entries were not taken into account when calculating summary figures.[94]
- The CFSR recommendations database had missing data in 3 of 9 fields.[95] There was also inconsistent data entry formats in 3 fields.[96]
- The CFSR status database had missing data in 7 of 29 fields[97] and inconsistent data entry formats in 4 fields.[98]

Finally, TSA has not documented its data entry and verification procedures, such as in a data dictionary or user manual, and does not have electronic safeguards for out-of-range or inconsistent entries for any of the databases it uses to track the status of CSR or CFSR recommendations and analyze operator responses to the CSR. TSA Pipeline Security Branch officials told us that they had not documented data entry and verification procedures and did not have electronic safeguards. This was for two reasons. First, the officials stated that the databases are small and maintained in a commercial spreadsheet program that does not allow for electronic safeguards. However, based on our review of the databases, the spreadsheet program does allow for a variety of electronic safeguards. For example, entries can be restricted to only allow selections from a drop-down list or only allow dates to be entered. Second, only a small number of TSA employees enter information into these databases. TSA officials explained that typically one TSA employee is responsible for entering information from pipeline security reviews, and another individual, usually whoever conducted the review, is tasked to verify the accuracy of the data entered. As a result, according to the officials, any errors would be self-evident and caught during these TSA employees' reviews.

Our work has emphasized the importance of quality information for management to make informed decisions and evaluate agencies' performance in achieving key objectives and addressing risks. The *Standards for Internal Control in the Federal Government* states that management should use quality information to achieve agency objectives, where "quality" means, among other characteristics, current, complete, and accurate.[99] In addition, DHS's Information Quality Guidelines state that all DHS component agencies should treat information quality as integral to every step of the development of information, including

---

[93] For example, 3 fields had 1 percent or less missing data, 7 fields had approximately 2 percent, 2 fields had 17 percent, and 1 field had 18 percent. Further, we found that 6 out of 13 fields had inconsistent data entry formats or allowed unrestricted text entries. For example, the Status field describes the current status of TSA's recommendations and includes entries such as "1," "(1) Completed," and "Completed using alternative strategy."

[94] For example, in fiscal year 2017 under a CSR question related to elements addressed in the corporate security plan, Company 7 had a "1" entered for "Yes" under "Other." The entry does not include an explanation, and it is not included in the summary calculation for the company.

[95] For example, the City, Recommendation, and Group fields had approximately 1 percent missing data.

[96] For example, based on a legend included in the database, the Group field assigns values of 1 through 13 which represent different areas of physical security. However, there are three out-of-range entries of "0."

[97] For example, 1 field had 1 percent missing data, 3 fields had 5 percent, 2 fields had 32 percent, and 1 field had 46 percent.

[98] For example, the Status Date field included entries such as "4/11/2014," "Estimated Completion 12/31/2017," and "Evergreen/Annually."

[99] GAO-14-704G.

creation, collection, maintenance, and dissemination. The guidelines also state that agencies should substantiate the quality of the information disseminated through documentation or other appropriate means.[100]

Without current, complete, and accurate information, it is difficult for TSA to evaluate the performance of the pipeline security program. Until TSA monitors and records the status of these reviews' recommendations, it will be hindered in its efforts to determine whether its recommendations are leading to significant reduction in risk. By entering information on CSR recommendations and monitoring and recording their status, developing written documentation of its data entry and verification procedures and electronic safeguards, and improving the quality of its pipeline security program data, TSA could better ensure it has the information necessary to effectively monitor pipeline operators' progress in improving their security posture, and evaluate its pipeline security program's effectiveness in reducing security risks to pipelines.

CONCLUSION

A successful pipeline attack could have dire consequences on public health and safety, as well as the U.S. economy. Recent coordinated campaigns by environmental activists to disrupt pipeline operations, and the successful attempts by nation-state actors to infiltrate and obtain sensitive information from pipeline operators' business and operating systems, demonstrate the dynamic and continuous threat to the security of our nation's pipeline network.

To help ensure the safety of our pipelines throughout the nation, it is important for TSA to address weaknesses in the management of its pipeline security program. TSA's Pipeline Security Branch revised its security guidelines in March 2018 to, among other things, reflect the dynamic threat environment and incorporate NIST's Cybersecurity Framework cybersecurity principles and practices.[101] However, without a documented process defining how frequently TSA is to review and, if deemed necessary, revise its guidelines, TSA cannot ensure that its guidelines reflect the latest known standards and best practices for physical and cybersecurity, or address the persistent and dynamic security threat environment currently facing the nation's pipeline system. Further, without clearly defined criteria for determining pipeline facilities' criticality, TSA cannot ensure that pipeline operators are applying guidance uniformly and that all of the critical facilities across the pipeline sector have been identified; or that their vulnerabilities have been identified and addressed.

TSA could improve its ability to conduct pipeline security reviews and the means that it uses to prioritize which pipeline systems to review based on their relative risk ranking. Establishing a strategic workforce plan could help TSA ensure that it has identified the necessary skills, competencies, and staffing allocations that the Pipeline Security Branch needs to carry out its responsibilities, including conducting security reviews of critical pipeline companies and facilities, as well as their cybersecurity posture. Better considering threat, vulnerability, and consequence elements in its risk assessment and incorporating an

[100] Department of Homeland Security, *Information Quality Guidelines*, (Washington, D.C.: Mar. 2011).

[101] Five of the 10 pipeline operators we interviewed characterized the guidelines as effective in helping to secure their operations, one operator was neutral, and the remaining four did not comment on the guidelines' effectiveness.

independent, external peer review in its process would provide more assurance that the Pipeline Security Branch ranks relative risk among pipeline systems using comprehensive and accurate data and methods.

TSA could also improve its ability to assess the extent to which the Pipeline Security Branch has met its goals. Taking steps to ensure that the pipeline security program performance measures exhibit key attributes of successful performance measures could allow TSA to better assess the program's effectiveness at reducing pipeline physical and cybersecurity risks. Without current, complete, and accurate information, it is difficult for TSA to evaluate the performance of the pipeline security program. By monitoring and recording the status of CSR recommendations, developing written documentation of its data entry and verification procedures and electronic safeguards, and improving the quality of its pipeline security program data, TSA could better ensure it has the information necessary to effectively monitor pipeline operators' progress in improving their security posture, and evaluate its pipeline security program's effectiveness in reducing security risks to pipelines. Until TSA monitors and records the status of these reviews' recommendations, it will be hindered in its efforts to determine whether its recommendations are leading to significant reduction in risk.

RECOMMENDATIONS FOR EXECUTIVE ACTION

We are making 10 recommendations to TSA:

- The TSA Administrator should direct the Security Policy and Industry Engagement's Surface Division to implement a documented process for reviewing, and if deemed necessary, for revising TSA's *Pipeline Security Guidelines* at regular defined intervals. (Recommendation 1)
- The TSA Administrator should direct the Security Policy and Industry Engagement's Surface Division to clarify TSA's *Pipeline Security Guidelines* by defining key terms within its criteria for determining critical facilities. (Recommendation 2)
- The TSA Administrator should develop a strategic workforce plan for its Security Policy and Industry Engagement's Surface Division, which could include determining the number of personnel necessary to meet the goals set for its Pipeline Security Branch, as well as the knowledge, skills, and abilities, including cybersecurity, that are needed to effectively conduct CSRs and CFSRs. (Recommendation 3)
- The TSA Administrator should direct the Security Policy and Industry Engagement's Surface Division to update the Pipeline Relative Risk Ranking Tool to include up-to-date data to ensure it reflects industry conditions, including throughput and threat data. (Recommendation 4)
- The TSA Administrator should direct the Security Policy and Industry Engagement's Surface Division to fully document the data sources, underlying assumptions and judgments that form the basis of the Pipeline Relative Risk Ranking Tool, including sources of uncertainty and any implications for interpreting the results from the assessment. (Recommendation 5)

- The TSA Administrator should direct the Security Policy and Industry Engagement's Surface Division to identify or develop other data sources relevant to threat, vulnerability, and consequence consistent with the NIPP and DHS critical infrastructure risk mitigation priorities and incorporate that data into the Pipeline Relative Risk Ranking Tool to assess relative risk of critical pipeline systems, which could include data on prior attacks, natural hazards, feedback data on pipeline system performance, physical pipeline condition, and cross-sector interdependencies. (Recommendation 6)
- The TSA Administrator should direct the Security Policy and Industry Engagement's Surface Division to take steps to coordinate an independent, external peer review of its Pipeline Relative Risk Ranking Tool, after the Pipeline Security Branch completes enhancements to its risk assessment approach. (Recommendation 7)
- The TSA Administrator should direct the Security Policy and Industry Engagement's Surface Division to ensure that it has a suite of performance measures which exhibit key attributes of successful performance measures, including measurable targets, clarity, and baseline and trend data. (Recommendation 8)
- The TSA Administrator should direct the Security Policy and Industry Engagement's Surface Division to take steps to enter information on CSR recommendations and monitor and record their status. (Recommendation 9)
- The TSA Administrator should direct the Security Policy and Industry Engagement's Surface Division to improve the quality of its pipeline security program data by developing written documentation of its data entry and verification procedures, implementing standardized data entry formats, and correcting existing data entry errors. (Recommendation 10)

Agency Comments and Our Evaluation

We provided a draft of this chapter to DHS, DOE, DOT, and FERC. DHS provided written comments which are reproduced in appendix III. In its comments, DHS concurred with our recommendations and described actions planned to address them. DHS, DOE, DOT, FERC, also provided technical comments, which we incorporated as appropriate. We also provided draft excerpts of this product to the American Petroleum Institute (API), the Association of Oil Pipe Lines, the American Gas Association (AGA), the Interstate Natural Gas Association of America (INGAA), the American Public Gas Association, and the selected pipeline operators that we interviewed. For those who provided technical comments, we incorporated them as appropriate.

With regard to our first recommendation, that TSA implement a documented process for reviewing, and if deemed necessary, for revising its *Pipeline Security Guidelines* at regular defined intervals, DHS stated that TSA will implement a documented process for reviewing and revising its Pipeline Security Guidelines at regular defined intervals, as appropriate. DHS estimated that this effort would be completed by March 31, 2019. This action, if fully implemented, should address the intent of the recommendation.

With regard to our second recommendation, that TSA clarify its *Pipeline Security Guidelines* by defining key terms within its criteria for determining critical facilities, DHS stated that TSA will clarify its Pipeline Security Guidelines by defining key terms within its criteria for determining critical facilities. DHS estimated that this effort would be completed by May 31, 2019. This action, if fully implemented, should address the intent of the recommendation.

With regard to our third recommendation, that TSA develop a strategic workforce plan for its Security Policy and Industry Engagement's Surface Division, DHS stated that TSA will develop a strategic workforce plan for the division, which includes determining the number of personnel necessary to meet the goals set for the Pipeline Security Branch, as well as the knowledge, skills, and abilities, including cybersecurity, that are needed to effectively conduct CSRs and CFSRs. DHS estimated that this effort would be completed by June 30, 2019. This action, if fully implemented, should address the intent of the recommendation.

With regard to our fourth recommendation, that TSA update the Pipeline Relative Risk Ranking Tool to include up-to-date data in order to ensure it reflects industry conditions, including throughput and threat data, DHS stated that TSA will update the Pipeline Relative Risk Ranking Tool to include up-to-date data in order to ensure it reflects industry conditions, including throughput and threat data. DHS estimated that this effort would be completed by February 28, 2019. This action, if fully implemented, should address the intent of the recommendation.

With regard to our fifth recommendation, that TSA fully document the data sources, underlying assumptions, and judgements that form the basis of the Pipeline Relative Risk Ranking Tool, including sources of uncertainty and any implications for interpreting the results from the assessment, DHS stated that TSA will fully document the data sources, underlying assumptions, and judgements that form the basis of the Pipeline Relative Risk Ranking Tool. According to DHS, this will include sources of uncertainty and any implications for interpreting the results from the assessment. DHS estimated that this effort would be completed by February 28, 2019. This action, if fully implemented, should address the intent of the recommendation.

With regard to our sixth recommendation, that TSA identify or develop other data sources relevant to threat, vulnerability, and consequence consistent with the NIPP and DHS critical infrastructure risk mitigation priorities and incorporate that data into the Pipeline Relative Risk Ranking Tool to assess relative risk of critical pipeline systems, DHS stated that TSA will identify and/or develop other sources relevant to threat, vulnerability, and consequence consistent with the NIPP and DHS critical infrastructure risk mitigation priorities. DHS also stated that TSA will incorporate that data into the Pipeline Risk Ranking Tool to assess relative risk of critical pipeline systems, which could include data on prior attacks, natural hazards, feedback data on pipeline system performance, physical pipeline condition, and cross-sector interdependencies. DHS estimated that this effort would be completed by June 30, 2019. This action, if fully implemented, should address the intent of the recommendation.

With regard to our seventh recommendation, that TSA take steps to coordinate an independent, external peer review of its Pipeline Relative Risk Ranking Tool, after the Pipeline Security Branch completes enhancements to its risk assessment approach, DHS stated that, after completing enhancements to its risk assessment approach, TSA will take steps to coordinate an independent, external peer review of its Pipeline Relative Risk Ranking Tool. DHS estimated that this effort would be completed by November 30, 2019. This action, if fully implemented, should address the intent of the recommendation.

With regard to our eighth recommendation, that TSA ensure that the Security Policy and Industry Engagement's Surface Division has a suite of performance measures which exhibit key attributes of successful performance measures, including measurable targets, clarity, baseline, and trend data, DHS stated that TSA's Surface Division's Pipeline Section will develop both physical and cyber security performance measures, in consultation with pipeline stakeholders, to ensure that it has a suite of performance measures which exhibit key attributes of successful performance measures, including measurable targets, clarity, baseline, and trend data. DHS estimated that this effort would be completed by November 30, 2019. This action, if fully implemented, should address the intent of the recommendation.

With regard to our ninth recommendation, that TSA take steps to enter information on CSR recommendations and monitor and record their status, DHS stated that TSA will enter information on CSR recommendations and monitor and record their status. DHS estimated that this effort would be completed by October 31, 2019. This action, if fully implemented, should address the intent of the recommendation.

With regard to our tenth recommendation, that TSA take steps to improve the quality of its pipeline security program data by developing written documentation of its data entry and verification procedures, implementing standardized data entry formats, and correcting existing data entry errors, DHS stated that TSA will develop written documentation of its data entry and verification procedures, implementing standardized data entry formats, and correcting existing data entry errors. DHS estimated that this effort would be completed by July 31, 2019. This action, if fully implemented, should address the intent of the recommendation.

As agreed with your offices, unless you publicly announce the contents of this chapter earlier, we plan no further distribution until one day from the report date. At that time, we will send copies to the appropriate congressional committees; the Secretaries of Energy, Homeland Security, and Transportation; the Executive Director of the Federal Energy Regulatory Committee; and other interested parties.

Chris P. Currie
Director
Homeland Security and Justice Issues

Nick Marinos
Director
Cybersecurity and Data Protection Issues

List of Requesters

The Honorable Ron Johnson
Chairman

The Honorable Claire McCaskill
Ranking Member
Committee on Homeland Security and Governmental Affairs
Unites States Senate

The Honorable Maria Cantwell
Ranking Member
Committee on Energy and Natural Resources
United States Senate

The Honorable Michael McCaul
Chairman
Committee on Homeland Security
House of Representatives

The Honorable John Katko
Chairman
Subcommittee on Transportation and Protective Security
Committee on Homeland Security
House of Representatives

The Honorable Peter DeFazio
Ranking Member
Committee on Transportation and Infrastructure
House of Representatives

The Honorable Frank Pallone
Ranking Member
Committee on Energy and Commerce
House of Representatives

The Honorable Daniel Lipinski
Member of Congress
House of Representatives

APPENDIX I: FEDERAL AND INDUSTRY SECURITY GUIDELINES AND STANDARDS FOR THE PIPELINE SECTOR

This appendix lists security guidance and guidance-related tools that the pipeline operators and industry association officials we interviewed identified as adopted or available in order to secure their physical and cyber operations. This list should not be considered to include all physical and cybersecurity guidance that may be available or used by all pipeline operators nor do all operators use all guidance listed.

Table 8. Federal and Industry Guidelines and Regulations Identified as Applicable to Security by Selected Pipeline Operators

Document Title
American Gas Association (AGA), AGA and Interstate Natural Gas Association of America (INGAA), Security Practices Guidelines Natural Gas Industry Transmission and Distribution, May 2008
American National Standards Institute (ANSI)/International Society of Automation (ISA)-95.00.01-CDV3, Enterprise-Control System Integration Part 1: Models and Terminology (2008)
American Petroleum Institute (API), Security Guidelines for the Petroleum Industry, Third Edition, April 2005
API, Pipeline SCADA Security, API Standard 1164, Second Edition, October 2016
Canadian Standards Association (CSA) Z246.1-17: Security Management for Petroleum and Natural Gas Industry Systems, March 1,2017
CARVER (criticality, accessibility, recuperability, vulnerability, effect, and recognizability) + Shock Vulnerability Assessment Tool
Center for Internet Security Critical Security Controls
Department of Energy (DOE) ONG Cybersecurity Capability Maturity Model (ONG C2M2) program
Department of Homeland Security (DHS), Cyber Security Evaluation Tool (CSET)
DHS Chemical Facility Antiterrorism Standards (CFATS)
Department of Transportation, Federal Pipeline Safety Regulations
DHS Infrastructure Survey Tool
INGAA, Control System Cyber Security Guidelines for the Natural Gas Pipeline Industry, January 31, 2011
International Organization for Standardization (ISO) and International Electrochemical Commission (IEC), 17799/27001/27002, Information technology - Security techniques - Code of Practice for Information Security Management
ISO/ IEC 27001:2005: Information technology—Security Techniques—Information Security Management Systems—Requirements
ISO 31000—Risk Management
International Electrotechnical Commission 62443—Security for Industrial Automation and Control Systems
Maritime Transportation Security Act of 2002 (Public Law 107-295)
National Energy Board (NEB) Onshore Pipeline Regulations (OPR) SOR/99-294, June 19, 2016
National Institute of Standards and Technology (NIST), Special Publication (SP) 800-53: Security and Privacy Controls for Federal Information Systems and Organizations, April 2013
NIST, Framework for Improving Critical Infrastructure Cybersecurity Version 1.1, April 16, 2018
NIST, SP 800-82: Guide to Industrial Control Systems (ICS) Security Revision 2, May 2015
North American Electric Reliability Corporation, Critical Infrastructure Protection(CIP) standards

Source: GAO analysis of pipeline operator information. | GAO-19-48.

APPENDIX II: DESCRIPTION OF AREAS FOR IMPROVEMENT IN THE PIPELINE SECURITY BRANCH'S PIPELINE RELATIVE RISK RANKING TOOL

The Transportation Security Administration's (TSA) Pipeline Security Branch developed the Pipeline Relative Risk Ranking Tool (risk assessment) in 2007.[102] The risk assessment

[102] According to DHS, a risk assessment is a product or process which collects information and assigns values to risks for the purpose of informing priorities, developing or comparing courses of action, and informing

calculates threat, vulnerability, and consequence on variables such as the amount of throughput in the pipeline system (consequence input). Pipeline Security Branch officials told us that they use the pipeline risk assessment to rank relative risk of the top 100 critical pipeline systems, and the standard operating procedures for conducting Corporate Security Reviews (CSR) state the results of the risk ranking are the primary factor considered when prioritizing CSRs of pipeline companies.[103]

However, we identified several factors that likely limit the usefulness of the current assessment in calculating threat, vulnerability, and consequence to allow the Pipeline Security Branch to effectively prioritize reviews of pipeline systems. For example, because the risk assessment has not changed since 2014, information on threat may be outdated. Additionally, sources of data and underlying assumption and judgments regarding certain threat and vulnerability inputs to the assessment are not fully documented. For example, threats to cybersecurity are not specifically accounted for in the description of the risk assessment methodology, making it unclear if cybersecurity is part of the assessment's threat factor. Further, the risk assessment does not include information that is consistent with the National Infrastructure Protection Plan (NIPP) and other Department of Homeland Security (DHS) priorities for critical infrastructure risk mitigation, such as information on natural hazards and the ability to measure risk reduction (feedback data).

According to Pipeline Security Branch officials, the risk ranking assessment is not intended to be a fully developed risk model detailing all pipeline factors influencing risk. Rather, officials said they are primarily interested in assessing risk data that impacts security. However, because TSA's Pipeline Security Program is designed to enhance the security preparedness of the pipeline systems, incorporating additional factors that enhance security into their risk calculation of the most critical pipeline systems would better align their efforts with Presidential Policy Directive 21 (PPD-21). For example, PPD-21 calls for agencies to integrate and analyze information to prioritize assets and manage risks to critical infrastructure, as well as anticipate interdependencies and cascading impacts.

Below we present the various shortfalls in the risk assessment—outdated data, limited description of sources and methodology, and opportunities to better align with the NIPP and other DHS priorities for critical infrastructure risk mitigation—in the context of the components that comprise a risk assessment: threat, vulnerability, and consequence. Whereas in 2010 we made recommendations to improve the consequence component in the pipeline relative risk ranking tool, we have currently identified shortfalls that cut across all risk components: threat, vulnerability, and consequence.

---

decision making. A risk assessment is also considered the appraisal of the risks facing an entity, asset, system, network, geographic area or other grouping. See DHS Risk Lexicon, 2010.

[103] In August 2010, we recommended, among other things, that the Pipeline Security Branch document a methodology for scheduling CSRs that considers a pipeline system's risk ranking as the primary scheduling criteria and to balance that with other practical considerations. As a result, the Pipeline Security Branch revised its CSR Standard Operating Procedures, as documented in a copy dated May 20, 2011, to state that the primary criteria for scheduling CSR visits is the pipeline system's relative risk (i.e., risk ranking), although other factors and considerations, such as operator availability and geographic location, will also play a role. Version 4.4, dated April 24, 2012, includes the same language. See GAO-10-867.

Threat

We identified several shortfalls in the pipeline risk assessment's calculation of threat. First, while the risk assessment assesses consequence and vulnerability by pipeline system through use of multiple variables, it currently ranks threat for pipeline systems equally. Second, the evolving nature of threats to pipelines may not be reflected, since the risk assessment was last updated in 2014. Third, the threat calculation does not take into account natural hazards.

Pipeline Security Branch officials said they currently rank threat equally across pipeline systems because they do not have granular enough threat information to distinguish threat by pipeline. However, ranking threat equally effectively has no effect on the risk calculation for pipeline systems. Further, this judgment is not documented in the risk assessment's methodology. According to the NIPP, a risk assessment's methodology must clearly document what information is used and how it is synthesized to generate a risk estimate, including any assumptions and judgments. Additionally, our analysis of the pipeline risk assessment found that it includes at least one field that TSA could use to differentiate threat by pipeline. Specifically, the risk assessment includes a field that accounts for whether a pipeline experienced a previous security threat (including failed attacks), and information provided by Pipeline Security Branch suggests some pipeline systems have experienced such threats.

However, the Pipeline Security Branch did not capture these events in the risk assessment's calculation, which Pipeline Security Branch officials said should be part of the threat calculation, but could not account for why they were not calculated for the systems in the risk assessment. These officials also clarified that incidents such as suspicious photography or vandalism do not constitute an attack to be accounted for in the threat calculation. Documenting such assumptions, judgments, or decisions to exclude information could provide increased transparency to those expected to interpret or use the results.

Pipeline Security Branch officials also said that they ranked threat equally because TSA Intelligence and Analysis data show that threats to the oil and natural gas sector have been historically low, and Intelligence and Analysis does not conduct specific threat analysis against individual pipeline systems. However, the Pipeline Security Branch has not updated the risk assessment since June 2014; therefore, the threat information it used to determine threat calculations—and decide to rank threat equally—may be outdated and not reflect the threats to the industry that have emerged in recent years. In fact, pipeline operators we interviewed indicated that the types of threats that concern pipeline operators have evolved. For example, 5 of the 10 operators we interviewed indicated that environmental activists were an increased threat to the pipeline industry because they use sabotage techniques, such as valve turning and cutting in service pipelines with blow torches, against pipelines. Additionally, 6 of 10 pipeline operators we interviewed said cyber attacks from nation-state actors were a primary threat to their industry. Further, when TSA issued its revised *Pipeline Security Guidelines* in March 2018, it stated that its revisions to the guidelines were made to reflect the ever-changing threat environment in both the physical and cybersecurity realms. However, threats to cybersecurity are not specifically accounted for in the description of the risk assessment methodology. Recent Pipeline Modal and Cyber Modal Threat Assessments include cyber threats to the pipeline industry, but the description of the pipeline risk assessment's methodology does not specify what types of threat assessments (sources) are used to calculate its threat score. To better align with the guidance in the NIPP for documenting sources of information when conducting risk assessments, the Pipeline Security Branch should document the information used. Keeping the risk assessment updated with current information, as well as documenting those data sources, could help the Pipeline Security Branch ensure it is using its limited resources to review the pipeline systems with greater risk.

Natural Hazard Threats to Pipelines

The Transportation Systems Sector, of which pipelines are a part, is critical to the Pacific Northwest, but also at risk from natural hazards, like earthquakes. For example, according to the Department of Homeland Security, an earthquake in the Puget Sound region—which relies on the transportation of crude oil from Alaska—could cripple the ports of Seattle and Tacoma, as well as the Olympic and Williams Pipelines greatly impacting the Pacific Northwest Economic Region.

Hurricanes are the most frequent disruptive natural hazard for the oil and natural gas subsector and can cause the shutdown of facilities in an area, even when the facilities themselves are not directly affected by the storms. For example, according to the U.S. Energy Information Administration, the flow of petroleum into the New York area via pipeline from the Gulf Coast relies on the ability to move it through major terminals. In August 2017, Hurricane Harvey caused major disruptions to crude oil and petroleum product supply chains, including those to New York Harbor from Houston, Texas via the Colonial Pipeline. Due to the hurricane, decreased supplies of petroleum products available for the pipeline in Houston forced Colonial Pipeline to limit operations temporarily.

Source: GAO analysis of agency information. | GAO-19-48.

Finally, another shortfall in the current pipeline risk assessment methodology is that it does not account for natural hazards in its threat calculation, even though DHS's definition of threat includes natural hazards, and security and resilience of critical infrastructure are often presented in the context of natural hazards.[104] According to the NIPP, threat is a natural or manmade occurrence, individual, entity, or action that has or indicates the potential to harm life, information, operations, the environment, and/or property. As such, along with terrorism, criminal activity and cybersecurity, natural disasters are a key element of DHS's critical infrastructure security and resilience mission.

According to Pipeline Security Branch officials, there is not sufficient historical data available that would indicate a significant impact from natural disasters on specific pipeline systems. However, we identified possible sources of data for the Pipeline Security Branch to consider. For example, a 2016 RAND Corporation study examined national infrastructure systems' exposure to natural hazards, including pipelines.[105] Additionally, the Federal Emergency Management Agency (FEMA) has collaborated with stakeholders to develop the National Risk Index to, among other things, establish a baseline of natural hazards risk for the United States While there may not be historical data of natural hazard impact for every pipeline system, consulting other sources or experts could provide regional data or analysis to

[104] From the DHS Risk Lexicon, 2010 Edition, threat is a natural or man-made occurrence, individual, entity, or action that has or indicates the potential to harm life, information, operations, the environment, and/or property. Presidential Policy Directive/PPD-21, *Critical Infrastructure Security and Resilience* (Washington, D.C.: Feb. 12, 2013) also presents the security and resilience of critical infrastructure in the context of natural hazards.

[105] Henry H. Willis et al. *Current and Future Exposure of Infrastructure in the United States to Natural Hazards.* (Santa Monica, Calif.: RAND Corporation, 2016), https://www.rand.org/pubs/research_reports/RR1453.html.

build a more comprehensive threat picture to help distinguish threats by pipeline system. According to the NIPP, hazard assessments should rely not only on historical information, but also future predictions about natural hazards to assess the likelihood or frequency of various hazards.

Vulnerability

We also identified multiple shortfalls in the vulnerability factors used in the risk assessment methodology, such as the potential uncertainty of the number of critical facilities and incorporating a feedback mechanism to calculate overall risk reduction. Other considerations for vulnerability calculations include physical condition of the pipeline system, cybersecurity activities, and interdependencies among sectors.

The number of critical facilities a pipeline system has identified is used as an input for its vulnerability calculation in the Pipeline Security Branch's risk assessment methodology. As discussed earlier, we identified deficiencies in TSA's criteria for identifying critical facilities, and found that well-defined criteria and consistent application of the criteria for identifying critical facilities could improve the results of the Pipeline Security Branch's risk assessment. Nevertheless, communicating in the risk assessment the uncertainty that may be inherent in this self-reported information would better align the risk assessment with the NIPP.

Measuring Effectiveness in a Voluntary Environment

According to the National Infrastructure Protection Plan, the use of performance metrics is an important step in the critical infrastructure risk management process to enable assessment of improvements in critical infrastructure security and resilience. The metrics provide a basis for the critical infrastructure community to establish accountability, document actual performance, promote effective management, and provide a feedback mechanism to inform decision making.

By using metrics to evaluate the effectiveness of voluntary partnership efforts to achieve national and sector priorities, critical infrastructure partners can adjust and adapt their security and resilience approaches to account for progress achieved, as well as changes in the threat and other relevant environments. Metrics are used to focus attention on areas of security and resilience that warrant additional resources or other changes through an analysis of challenges and priorities at the national, sector, and owner/operator levels.

Metrics also serve as a feedback mechanism for other aspects of the critical infrastructure risk management approach.

Source: Department of Homeland Security. | GAO-19-48.

Another shortfall in the risk assessment is its inability to reliably measure the progress a pipeline system made in addressing vulnerability gaps between security reviews. The current risk assessment includes a CSR score as part of its vulnerability calculation, which was developed in part in response to our 2010 recommendation to use more reliable data to measure a pipeline system's vulnerability gap. However, during our review, Pipeline Security Branch officials said they plan to remove pipeline companies' CSR scores from the risk assessment calculations, because they and industry partners do not have confidence that the score appropriately measures a pipeline system's vulnerability. For example, Pipeline Security Branch officials explained that pipeline companies consider security factors differently, which can lead to variation in implementing risk reduction activities and by extension lead to different CSR scores. However, removing the CSR score eliminates the only feedback mechanism in the risk assessment from a pipeline company's actual security review conducted by the Pipeline Security Branch. The NIPP and DHS's Risk Management fundamentals emphasize the important role that such feedback mechanisms play in risk management. Officials from the Pipeline Security Branch agree on the importance of a feedback mechanism tying results of reviews to a revised vulnerability metric, but said they need a better measure than the current CSR score which is unreliable for comparative and analytic purposes. Developing a feedback mechanism based on implementation of TSA's *Pipeline Security Guidelines* could be an important input to the risk assessment's vulnerability calculation. This information would also inform the amount of risk pipeline companies are reducing by implementing the guidelines and could be used to inform overall risk reduction.

The physical and cyber environments in which the pipeline sector operates also present vulnerabilities not accounted for in the pipeline risk assessment. In recent years, DHS has listed the potential for catastrophic losses to dramatically increase the overall risk associated with failing infrastructure and highlighted risks due to climate change and natural hazards to pipelines.[106] For example, DHS reported extreme temperatures—such as higher and lower temperatures over prolonged periods of time—increase vulnerability to the critical infrastructure by causing elements to break and cease to function. Pipelines that freeze and then rupture can affect the energy and transportation systems sectors. As noted above, according to the NIPP, a natural or man-made occurrence or action with the potential to harm life is considered a threat, whereas vulnerability is defined as a physical feature or operational attribute that renders an entity open to exploitation or susceptible to a given threat or hazard. While pipeline physical condition is typically thought of in context of safety, pipeline condition or location (such as above or below ground) could touch upon pipeline security as it relates to system vulnerability. For example, a pipeline system or segment of a system with a compromised physical condition due to corrosion or age could affect the system's vulnerability to threats and affect its ability to recover from such threats by potentially increasing the time a system is offline.

According to the Transportation Systems Sector-Specific Plan, vulnerabilities to damage in aging transportation infrastructure—of which pipelines are a part—are projected to increase with the continued effects of climate change. Further, according to TSA's *Pipeline Security and Incident Recovery Protocol Plan*, pipeline integrity efforts—including the design, construction, operation, and maintenance of pipelines—are important to pipeline security because well-maintained, safe pipelines are more likely to tolerate a physical attack.[107] The Pipeline Security Branch already collects information from the Pipeline and Hazardous Materials Safety Administration (PHMSA) for its risk assessment, specifically information on High Consequence Area and High Threat Urban Area mileage.[108] By

---

[106] The Department of Homeland Security, *National Critical Infrastructure Protection and Resilience Annual Report 2011-2012,* Washington, D.C., Aug. 2013.

[107] Transportation Security Administration, *Pipeline Security and Incident Recovery Protocol Plan*, March 2010.

[108] PHMSA defines "high consequence areas" differently for gas and hazardous liquid. For gas, high consequence areas typically include highly populated or frequented areas, such as parks. See 49 C.F.R. § 192.903. For hazardous liquid, high consequence areas include highly populated areas, other populated areas, navigable waterways, and areas unusually sensitive to environmental damage. See 49 CFR § 195.450. TSA regulations

considering additional information PHMSA collects on pipeline integrity, the Pipeline Security Branch could also use the information to help pipeline operators identify security measures to help reduce the consequences related to the comparatively higher vulnerability of an aging or compromised system. This would align with the Pipeline Security Branch's efforts to improve security preparedness of pipeline systems and could better inform its vulnerability calculations for relative risk ranking of pipeline systems.

Capturing cybersecurity in the risk assessment is also an area for improvement. Pipeline Security Branch officials told us they consulted with the National Cybersecurity and Communications Integration Center to revise TSA's *Pipeline Security Guidelines* to align with the National Institute of Standards and Technology (NIST) Cybersecurity Framework and that absent data specific to pipelines on their cybersecurity vulnerabilities, they are unable to include a pipelines' vulnerability to cyber attack in the risk assessment. However, the Pipeline Security Branch recently updated the security review questions asked of pipeline operators during corporate and critical facility reviews based on the recently updated *Pipeline Security Guidelines*. Using these updated questions related to companies' cybersecurity posture, the Pipeline Security Branch could collect additional information on cybersecurity vulnerabilities which could inform the risk assessment. This could be an element of the feedback mechanism described above and emphasized in the NIPP. Additionally, NIST identified several supply chain vulnerabilities associated with cybersecurity, which are not currently accounted for in TSA's *Pipeline Security Guidelines*.[109] As pipeline operators implement increasing levels of network technologies to control their systems, the Pipeline Security Branch may not be fully accounting for pipeline systems' cybersecurity posture by not including the cybersecurity-related vulnerabilities in its risk assessment inputs.

Finally, we identified shortfalls in cross-sector interdependencies, which could affect vulnerability calculations. According to the NIPP, understanding and addressing risks from cross-sector dependencies and interdependencies is essential to enhancing critical infrastructure security and resilience. The Pipeline Security Branch's pipeline risk assessment currently considers the effects of a pipeline system's ability to service assets such as major airports, the electric grid, and military bases. However, consequence is calculated on the loss or disruption of the pipeline system to these other assets and does not capture the dependency of the pipeline system on other energy sources, such as electricity. Weather events such as Gulf of Mexico hurricanes and Superstorm Sandy highlighted the interdependencies between the pipeline and electrical sectors. Specifically, according to a 2015 DHS annual report on critical infrastructure, power failures during Superstorm Sandy in 2012 closed major pipelines for 4 days, reducing regional oil supplies by 35 to 40 percent. The report goes on to say that the interconnected nature of infrastructure systems can lead to cascading impacts and are

---

pertaining to rail transportation security define High Threat Urban Area as "an area comprising one or more cities and surrounding areas including a 10-mile buffer zone." See 49 C.F.R. § 1580.3.

[109] According to NIST's *Supply Chain Risk Management Practices for Federal Information Systems and Organizations*, NIST Special Publication 800-161 (April 2015), there are three principal vulnerabilities to identify: (1) Access paths within the supply chain that would allow malicious actors to gain information about the system and ultimately introduce components that could cause the system to fail at some later time; (2) Access paths that would allow malicious actors to trigger a component malfunction or failure during system operations; and (3) Dependencies on supporting or associated components that might be more accessible or easier for malicious actors to subvert than components that directly perform critical functions.

increasing in frequency.[110] Pipeline Security Branch officials are considering cross-sector interdependencies and said they discuss these factors with operators as they relate to system resiliency. Considering interdependencies of sectors in both directions—such as calculating the likelihood that an input like electricity could fail and cause disruptions to critical pipelines—could improve the calculations in the pipeline risk assessment.

Consequence

As previously discussed, the Pipeline Security Branch last calculated relative risk among the top 100 pipeline systems in 2014. When doing so, it used pipeline systems' throughput data from 2010 to assess relative risk. According to Pipeline Security Branch officials, the amount of throughput in pipeline systems does not change substantially year to year. However, Standards for Internal Control in the Federal Government calls for management to use quality information to achieve the entity's objectives, including using relevant data from reliable sources obtained in a timely manner. The Pipeline Security Branch uses throughput data as a consequence factor in the risk assessment to determine a pipeline system's relative risk score.[111] Throughput changes could affect relative risk ranking and the Pipeline Security Branch's ability to accurately prioritize reviews based on relative risk.

APPENDIX III: COMMENTS FROM THE DEPARTMENT OF HOMELAND SECURITY

U.S. Department of Homeland Security
Washington, DC 20528

Homeland
Security

November 29, 2018

Chris P. Currie
Director, Homeland Security and Justice
U.S. Government Accountability Office
441 G Street, NW
Washington, DC 20548

Nick Marinos
Director, Cybersecurity & Data Protection Issues
U.S. Government Accountability Office
441 G Street, NW
Washington, DC 20548

---

[110] The DHS report highlighted this element of risk management stating while sectors understand the direct impacts (i.e., loss of life and economic consequences) from damaged or failing infrastructure, the dependencies and interdependencies associated with related service disruptions are not as well known.

[111] A pipeline system with higher throughput would be considered to have a higher consequence score.

Re: Management Response to Draft Report GAO-19-48, "CRITICAL INFRASTRUCTURE PROTECTION: Actions Needed to Address Significant Weaknesses in TSA's Pipeline Security Program Management"

Dear Messrs. Currie and Marinos:

Thank you for the opportunity to review and comment on the draft report. The U.S. Department of Homeland Security (DHS) appreciates the U.S. Government Accountability Office's (GAO) work in planning and conducting its review and issuing this report.

The Department remains committed to working with our Federal and private sector partners in the security and resilience of our Nation's critical pipeline infrastructure. As noted in the National Infrastructure Protection Plan (NIPP 2013), "[v]oluntary collaboration between private sector owners and operators (including their partner associations, vendors, and others) and their government counterparts has been and will remain the primary mechanism for advancing collective action toward national critical infrastructure security and resilience."

DHS is extremely proud of the work the Transportation Security Administration (TSA) has done to foster collaboration with the pipeline industry and significantly improve physical security and cybersecurity. This has included the publication of security guidelines, extensive information sharing, and the conduct and analysis of individual security reviews. For example, TSA conducted 62 Critical Facility Security Reviews (CFSRs) and 23 Corporate Security Reviews (CSRs) during fiscal year (FY) 2018.

In March 2018, TSA published an update to the TSA "Pipeline Security Guidelines," which included considerable input and collaboration with Federal and industry partners, and a complete update to the recommended cybersecurity measures. GAO's draft report notes, "[a]ll operators that GAO interviewed stated that they had implemented TSA's Pipeline Security Guidelines," and many indicated "the Guidelines were effective in helping to secure their operations." This is consistent with TSA's observations and data collected during CSRs and CFSRs.

Additionally, we were pleased to note that GAO's report recognized pipeline operators are receiving security information from a variety of sources including TSA, the National Cyber Security and Communications Integration Center, Information Sharing and Analysis Centers, fusion centers, industry associations, and the pipeline Sector Coordinating Council.

DHS and TSA recognize the challenging and evolving nature of the threat, particularly with regard to cybersecurity. DHS recently inaugurated the National Risk Management Center and one of its first projects is to partner with TSA to conduct 10 in-depth cybersecurity reviews with pipeline companies during FY 2019. Ongoing CSRs and these assessments will provide valuable insights on the status of cybersecurity measures in the industry.

GAO's report also determined the pipeline sector to be "resilient and versatile," and that pipeline operators have been able to rapidly respond to the adverse consequences of an incident and quickly restore pipeline service. Likewise, the report noted pipeline infrastructure includes redundancies that make the national system resilient.

All Federal programs, regardless of size, have room for improvement, and we appreciate GAO's efforts to identify areas for improvement in the TSA Pipeline Security program. However, the use of "significant weaknesses" in the report title is an unfortunate mischaracterization that does not accurately convey the overall program effectiveness or account for the substantial work TSA has accomplished.

The draft report contained 10 recommendations, with which the Department concurs. Attached find our detailed response to each recommendation. Technical comments were previously provided under separate cover.

Again, thank you for the opportunity to review and comment on this draft report. Please feel free to contact me if you have any questions. We look forward to working with you again in the future.

Sincerely,

JIM H. CRUMPACKER, CIA, CFE
Director
Departmental GAO-OIG Liaison Office

Attachment: Management Response to Recommendations Contained in GAO-19-48

GAO recommended that the Administrator of the Transportation Security Administration:

Recommendation 1: Direct the Security Policy and Industry Engagement's Surface Division to implement a documented process for reviewing, and if deemed necessary, for revising TSA's "Pipeline Security Guidelines" at regular defined intervals.

Response: Concur. TSA Surface Division, Pipeline Section personnel will implement a documented process for reviewing and personnel revising TSA's "Pipeline Security Guidelines" at regular defined intervals, as appropriate. Estimated Completion Date (ECD): March 31, 2019.

Recommendation 2: Direct the Security Policy and Industry Engagement's Surface Division to clarify its TSA's "Pipeline Security Guidelines" by defining key terms within its criteria for determining critical facilities.

Response: Concur. TSA Surface Division, Pipeline Section personnel will clarify TSA's "Pipeline Security Guidelines" by defining key terms within TSA criteria for determining critical facilities. ECD: May 31, 2019.

Recommendation 3: Develop a strategic workforce plan for its Security Policy and Industry Engagement's Surface Division, which could include determining the number of personnel necessary to meet the goals set for its Pipeline Security Branch, as well as the knowledge, skills, and abilities, including cybersecurity, that are needed to effectively conduct CSRs and CFSRs.

Response: Concur. TSA Surface Division personnel will develop a Strategic Workforce Plan for the Division, which includes determining the number of personnel necessary to meet the goals set for our Pipeline Security Branch, as well as the knowledge, skills, and abilities, including cybersecurity, that are needed to effectively conduct CSRs and CFSRs. ECD: June 30, 2019.

Recommendation 4: Direct the Security Policy and Industry Engagement's Surface Division to update the Pipeline Relative Risk Ranking Tool to include up-to-date data in order to ensure it reflects industry conditions, including throughput and threat data.

Response: Concur. TSA Surface Division, Pipeline Section personnel will update the Pipeline Relative Risk Ranking Tool to include up-to-date data in order to ensure it reflects industry conditions, including throughput and threat data. ECD: February 28, 2019.

Recommendation 5: Direct the Security Policy and Industry Engagement's Surface Division to fully document the data sources, underlying assumptions and judgements that form the basis of the Pipeline Relative Risk Ranking Tool, including sources of uncertainty and any implications for interpreting the results from the assessment.

Response: Concur. TSA Surface Division, Pipeline Section personnel will fully document the data sources, underlying assumptions, and judgements that form the basis of the Pipeline Relative Risk Ranking Tool, including sources of uncertainty and any implications for interpreting the results from the assessment. ECD: February 28, 2019.

Recommendation 6: Direct the Security Policy and Industry Engagement's Surface Division to identify or develop other data sources relevant to threat, vulnerability, and consequence consistent with the NIPP and DHS critical infrastructure risk mitigation priorities and incorporate that data into the Pipeline Relative Risk Ranking Tool to assess relative risk of critical pipeline systems, which could include data on prior attacks natural hazards, feedback data on pipeline system performance, physical pipeline condition, and cross-sector interdependencies.

Response: Concur. TSA Surface Division, Pipeline Section personnel will identify and/or develop other sources relevant to threat, vulnerability, and consequence consistent with the NIPP and DHS critical infrastructure risk mitigation priorities. and incorporate that data into the Pipeline Risk Ranking Tool to assess relative risk of critical pipeline systems, which could include data on prior attacks, natural hazards, feedback data on pipeline system performance, physical pipeline condition, and cross-sector interdependencies. ECD: June 30, 2019.

Recommendation 7: Direct the Security Policy and Industry Engagement's Surface Division to take steps to coordinate an independent, external peer review of its Pipeline Relative Risk Ranking Tool, after the Pipeline Security Branch completes enhancements to its risk assessment approach.

Response: Concur. TSA Surface Division personnel will take steps to coordinate an independent, external peer review of its Pipeline Relative Risk Ranking Tool, after the Pipeline Security Branch completes enhancements to its risk assessment approach. Given this is an unfunded requirement, the necessary work on the other recommendations made in the report, the identification of an independent, external peer organization, and the potential need to develop a services contract for this review, completion of this recommendation may require up to a year. ECD: November 30, 2019.

Recommendation 8: Direct the Security Policy and Industry Engagement's Surface Division to ensure that it has a suite of performance measures which exhibit key attributes of successful performance measures, including measurable targets, clarity, baseline, and trend data.

Response: Concur. TSA Surface Division, Pipeline Section personnel will ensure there is a suite of performance measures which exhibit key attributes of successful performance measures, including measurable targets, clarity, baseline, and trend data. Given the challenge in developing both physical and cyber security performance measures in consultation with pipeline stakeholders, the development of these performance measures will take one year. ECD: November 30, 2019.

Recommendation 9: Direct the Security Policy and Industry Engagement's Surface Division to take steps to enter information on CSR recommendations and monitor and record their status.

Response: Concur. TSA Surface Division, Pipeline Section personnel will enter information on CSR recommendation and monitor and record TSA status. Since this is an unfunded requirement, the resourcing for this recommendation requires the completion and execution of the strategic workforce plan (Recommendation 3), which will not be completed until June 30, 2019. ECD: October 31, 2019.

Recommendation 10: Direct the Security Policy and Industry Engagement's Surface Division to take steps to improve the quality of its pipeline security program data by developing written documentation of its data entry and verification procedures, implementing standardized data entry formats, and correcting existing data entry errors.

Response: Concur. TSA Surface Division, Pipeline Section personnel will improve the quality of its pipeline security program data by developing written documentation of its data entry and verification procedures, implementing standardized data entry formats, and correcting existing data entry errors.
ECD: July 31, 2019.

In: Top 10 Reports and Testimonies in December 2018
Editor: Sarah J. Nygaard
ISBN: 978-1-53615-507-5

Chapter 4

IMPROPER PAYMENTS: ADDITIONAL GUIDANCE NEEDED TO IMPROVE OVERSIGHT OF AGENCIES WITH NONCOMPLIANT PROGRAMS*

United States Government Accountability Office

ABBREVIATIONS

AFR	Agency Financial Report
CFO	Chief Financial Officer
CFO Act	Chief Financial Officers Act of 1990
DHS	Department of Homeland Security
DOD	Department of Defense
DOL	Department of Labor
Education	Department of Education
EITC	Earned Income Tax Credit
FNS	Food and Nutrition Service
Ginnie Mae	Government National Mortgage Association
HHS	Department of Health and Human Services
IG	Inspector General
IPERA	Improper Payments Elimination and Recovery Act of 2010
IPERIA	Improper Payments Elimination and Recovery Improvement Act of 2012
IPIA	Improper Payments Information Act of 2002
IRS	Internal Revenue Service
OIG	Office of Inspector General
OMB	Office of Management and Budget
PAR	Performance and Accountability Report
SSA	Social Security Administration

* This is an edited, reformatted and augmented version of the United States Government Accountability Office Report to Congressional Committees, Publication No. GAO-19-14, dated December 2018.

Treasury	Department of the Treasury
USDA	U.S. Department of Agriculture

WHY GAO DID THIS STUDY

Government-wide estimated improper payments totaled almost $1.4 trillion from fiscal year 2003 through fiscal year 2017. IPERA requires IGs to annually assess and report on whether executive branch agencies complied with the six criteria to (1) publish an agency financial report or performance accountability report, (2) conduct program-specific improper payment risk assessments, (3) publish improper payment estimates, (4) publish corrective action plans, (5) publish and meet annual improper payment reduction targets, and (6) report a gross improper payment rate of less than 10 percent.

This chapter examines the extent to which

1. CFO Act agencies complied with IPERA criteria for fiscal years 2016 and 2017, and the trends evident since 2011, as reported by their IGs;
2. CFO Act agencies addressed requirements for programs reported as noncompliant with IPERA criteria for 3 or more consecutive years, as of fiscal year 2016, and communicated their strategies to Congress for reducing improper payments and achieving compliance; and
3. OMB made determinations regarding whether additional funding would help CFO Act agency programs reported as noncompliant with IPERA criteria for 2 consecutive years, as of fiscal years 2016 and 2017, come into compliance.

GAO analyzed the IGs' fiscal years 2016 and 2017 IPERA compliance reports; reviewed prior GAO reports on agencies' IPERA compliance; reviewed agency information submitted to Congress; and made inquiries to OMB, applicable agencies, and IGs; and assessed such information based on relevant IPERA provisions and OMB and other guidance.

WHAT GAO RECOMMENDS

GAO recommends that OMB update its guidance to specify other types of quality information that agencies with programs noncompliant for 3 or more consecutive years should include in their notifications to Congress, such as significant matters related to risks, issues, root causes, measurable milestones, designated senior officials, accountability mechanisms, and corrective actions or strategies planned or taken by agencies to achieve compliance.

GAO provided a draft of this chapter to OMB and requested comments, and OMB said that it had no comments. GAO also provided a draft of this chapter to the 24 CFO Act agencies and their IGs and requested comments. In its written comments, the Social Security Administration (SSA) stated that it provided information on measurable milestones, designated senior officials, and accountability mechanisms in its agency financial report. However, SSA did not provide this information in its notifications to Congress for programs reported as noncompliant under IPERA as of fiscal year 2016. GAO believes that OMB should take steps to update OMB's guidance to help ensure that agencies report such significant information and include it in their notifications to Congress. In addition, several agencies and IGs provided technical comments, which were incorporated in the report as appropriate.

WHAT GAO FOUND

Over half of the 24 Chief Financial Officers Act of 1990 (CFO Act) agencies were reported by their inspectors general (IG) as noncompliant with one or more criteria under the Improper Payments Elimination and Recovery Act of 2010 (IPERA) for fiscal years 2016 and 2017. Nine CFO Act agencies have been reported as noncompliant in one or more programs every year since the implementation of IPERA in fiscal year 2011, totaling 7 consecutive years of noncompliance.

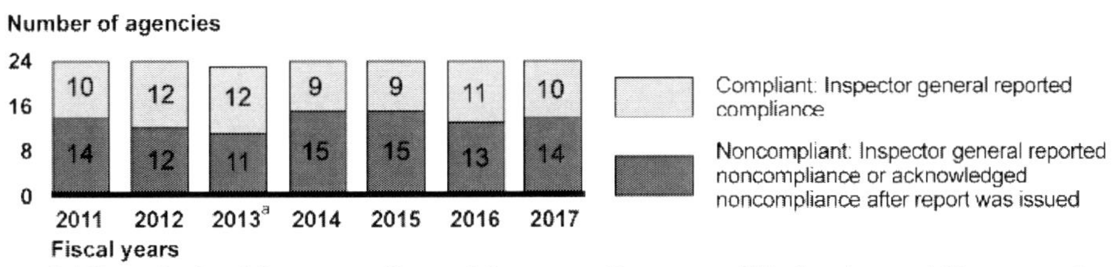

Source: GAO analysis of Inspector General Improper Payments Elimination and Recovery Act of 2010 (PERA) copliance reports from fiscal years 2011 through 2017. | GAO-19-14.

Number of Chief Financial Officers Act Agencies Compliant under IPERA, as Reported or Acknowledged by Their Inspectors General

The IGs of the 14 noncompliant agencies reported that a total of 58 programs were responsible for the identified instances of noncompliance in fiscal year 2017. Further, 18 of the 58 programs at 9 agencies were reported as noncompliant for 3 or more consecutive years. Fourteen of these 18 programs accounted for an estimated $74.4 billion of the $141 billion total estimated improper payments for fiscal year 2017; the other 4 programs did not report improper payment estimates. This sum may include estimates that are of unknown reliability. The $74.4 billion is primarily composed of estimates reported for two noncompliant programs, the Department of Health and Human Services' Medicaid program and the Department of the Treasury's (Treasury) Earned Income Tax Credit program; estimated improper payments for these two programs are also a central part of certain high-risk areas in GAO's 2017 High-Risk List.

Agencies with any program reported as noncompliant for 3 or more consecutive years are required to notify Congress of their program's consecutive noncompliance and submit a proposal for reauthorization or statutory change to bring that program into compliance. GAO found that three agencies with one or more programs reported as noncompliant for 3 or more consecutive years, as of fiscal year 2016, did not notify Congress or submit the required proposals. The Departments of Labor and the Treasury submitted proposed legislative changes in response to their programs being previously reported as noncompliant, but did not notify Congress of the programs' continued noncompliance as of fiscal year 2016. The U.S. Department of Agriculture (USDA) has not notified Congress despite prior GAO and USDA

IG recommendations to do so. To address these issues, in June 2018 the Office of Management and Budget (OMB) updated its guidance to clarify the notification requirements for each consecutive year a program is reported as noncompliant.

GAO found that five agencies did notify Congress as required, and included additional quality information that is not specifically required, but could be useful in updating Congress on their compliance efforts. For example, all five agencies provided information on the root causes, risks, changes, or issues affecting their efforts and corrective actions or strategies to address them; three agencies provided other quality information on accountability mechanisms, designated senior officials, and measurable milestones.

Additional Information Included in Notifications to Congress by Five Agencies with Programs Reported by Their Inspectors General as Noncompliant under the Improper Payments Elimination and Recovery Act of 2010 for 3 or More Consecutive Years, as of Fiscal Year 2016

Agency	Additional information included					
	Root causes	Risks/ issues/ changes	Corrective actions/ strategies	Measurable milestones	Designated senior officials	Accountability mechanisms
Dept. of Defense	Yes	Yes	Yes	Yes	Yes	Yes
Dept. of Education	Yes	Yes	Yes	Yes	Yes	Yes
Dept. of Health Human Services	Yes	Yes	Yes	No	No	No
Dept. of Homeland Security	Yes	Yes	Yes	Yes	Yes	Yes
Social Security Administration	Yes	Yes	Yes	No	No	No
Total	5	5	5	3	3	3

Source: GAO analysis of Chief Financial Officers Act of 1990 agencies' notifications to Congress for programs with 3 or more consecutive years of noncompliance with the Improper Payments Elimination and Recovery Act of 2010 as of fiscal year 2016. | GAO-19-14.

In June 2018, OMB updated its guidance to clarify agency reporting requirements for programs reported as noncompliant for 3 or more consecutive years. However, the updated guidance does not direct agencies to include the types of quality information included in these five agencies' notifications for fiscal year 2016. GAO's *Standards for Internal Control in the Federal Government* emphasizes the importance of communicating quality information, such as significant matters affecting agencies' efforts to achieve compliance objectives. Such information could be useful in understanding the current challenges of these programs and is essential for assessing agency efforts to address high-risk and other issues. As a result, Congress could have more complete information to effectively oversee agency efforts to address program noncompliance for 3 or more consecutive years.

When programs are reported as noncompliant for 2 consecutive years, IPERA gives OMB authority to determine whether additional funding is needed to help resolve the noncompliance. In April 2018, OMB staff stated that they determined that no additional funding was needed for the 15 programs that were reported as noncompliant for 2 consecutive years, as of fiscal year 2016, and that they primarily rely on the IGs' recommendations in their annual IPERA compliance reports when making funding determinations. OMB staff subsequently stated that they no longer need to conduct a detailed review of the IGs' IPERA compliance reports to identify recommendations related to additional funding needs. Instead, OMB updated its guidance in June 2018 to direct agencies to submit proposals to OMB regarding additional funding needs to help address IPERA noncompliance and clarified that the funding determination process will unfold as part of the annual development of the President's Budget. As of September 2018, OMB was in the process of making funding determinations for 12 programs that were reported as noncompliant as of fiscal year 2017 and stated that any determinations made would be developed in the President's Budget for fiscal year 2020.

December 7, 2018

The Honorable Ron Johnson
Chairman

The Honorable Claire McCaskill
Ranking Member
Committee on Homeland Security and Governmental Affairs
United States Senate

The Honorable Trey Gowdy
Chairman

The Honorable Elijah Cummings
Ranking Member
Committee on Oversight and Government Reform
House of Representatives

Improper payments—payments that should not have been made or were made in incorrect amounts—have been estimated to total almost $1.4 trillion government-wide from fiscal years 2003 through 2017.[1] Estimates of total improper payments have increased over the years— from $35 billion for 27 programs in fiscal year 2003 to approximately $141 billion for 90 programs in fiscal year 2017. It is important to note that these estimates themselves may not be accurate, reliable, or complete, because, as we have reported, the federal government is unable to determine the full extent to which improper payments occur and reasonably assure that appropriate actions are taken to reduce them.[2] In addition, certain

[1] As required by the Improper Payments Information Act of 2002, Pub. L. No. 107-300, 116 Stat. 2350 (Nov. 26, 2002), *codified as amended at* 31 U.S.C. § 3321 note, certain agencies were required to start reporting improper payment estimates beginning for fiscal year 2003. An improper payment is defined as any payment that should not have been made or that was made in an incorrect amount (including overpayments and underpayments) under statutory, contractual, administrative, or other legally applicable requirements. It includes any payment to an ineligible recipient, any payment for an ineligible good or service, any duplicate payment, any payment for a good or service not received (except for such payments where authorized by law), and any payment that does not account for credit for applicable discounts. Office of Management and Budget guidance also instructs agencies to report as improper payments any payments for which insufficient or no documentation was found. It is important to note that improper payment totals are estimated and may or may not represent a loss to the government.

[2] GAO, Financial Audit: Fiscal Years 2017 and 2016 Consolidated Financial Statements of the U.S. Government, GAO-18-316R (Washington, D.C.: Feb. 15, 2018).

inspectors general (IG) have reported issues with their agencies' reported improper payment estimates that were caused by insufficient sampling methods and flawed estimation methodologies for calculating and reporting improper payment estimates.

Fiscal year 2017 marked the seventh year of the implementation of the Improper Payments Elimination and Recovery Act of 2010 (IPERA), which, among other things, requires federal agencies' IGs to annually assess and report on whether the agencies under their jurisdiction have complied with six IPERA criteria.[3] The IGs' annual IPERA compliance reports serve a key function to reasonably assure that improper payment estimates are accurate, reliable, and complete and that Congress has information on agencies' efforts to address improper payments. We previously reported on agencies' IPERA compliance for fiscal years 2011 through 2015, as reported by the IGs.[4]

We performed our work under the authority of the Comptroller General to conduct evaluations on his own initiative and to assist Congress with its oversight responsibilities.[5] We conducted this audit to summarize and evaluate agency compliance under IPERA for fiscal years 2016 and 2017, as reported by their IGs.[6] Specifically, this chapter discusses the extent to which (1) agencies listed in the Chief Financial Officers Act of 1990, as amended,[7] (CFO Act) complied with the six criteria listed in IPERA for fiscal years 2016 and 2017, and the trends evident since fiscal year 2011, as reported by their IGs; (2) CFO Act agencies addressed the requirements for programs and activities reported as noncompliant with IPERA criteria for 3 or more consecutive years, as of fiscal year 2016, and communicated their strategies to Congress for reducing improper payments and achieving compliance; and (3) the Office of Management and Budget (OMB) made determinations regarding whether additional funding would help CFO Act agency programs and activities reported as noncompliant with IPERA criteria for 2 consecutive years to come into compliance, as of fiscal years 2016 and 2017. We focused on the 24 agencies listed in the CFO Act because estimates of their improper payments represent over 99 percent of the total reported estimated improper payments for fiscal years 2016 and 2017.

To determine the extent to which CFO Act agencies were reported as compliant with the six criteria listed in IPERA for fiscal years 2016 and 2017, and trends evident since fiscal year 2011, we reviewed the IGs' IPERA compliance reports issued for fiscal years 2016 and 2017 and identified trends in agencies' compliance, and their respective programs' and activities' compliance, since fiscal year 2011 based on results summarized in our prior reports.[8]

To determine the extent to which CFO Act agencies addressed the requirements for programs and activities reported as noncompliant for 3 or more consecutive years as of fiscal

---

[3] IGs are required to issue compliance reports as indicated in IPERA, Pub. L. No. 111-204, § 3, 124 Stat. 2224, 2232 (July 22, 2010), *codified at* 31 U.S.C. § 3321 note.

[4] GAO, Improper Payments: CFO Act Agencies Need to Improve Efforts to Address Compliance Issues, GAO-16-554 (Washington, D.C.: June 30, 2016), and Improper Payments: Additional Guidance Could Provide More Consistent Compliance Determinations and Reporting by Inspectors General, GAO-17-484 (Washington, D.C.: May 31, 2017).

[5] 31 U.S.C. § 717(b).

[6] The IGs' IPERA compliance reports for fiscal years 2016 and 2017 were due in May 2017 and 2018, respectively.

[7] The CFO Act, Pub. L. No. 101-576, 104 Stat. 2838 (Nov. 15, 1990), among other things, established chief financial officers to oversee financial management activities at 23 major executive departments and agencies. The list now includes 24 entities, which are often referred to collectively as CFO Act agencies, and is codified, as amended, in section 901 of Title 31, United States Code.

[8] GAO-16-554 and GAO-17-484.

year 2016, we requested and reviewed the applicable agencies' notifications to Congress provided by the respective agencies.[9] In addition, we reviewed the content of agencies' notifications to evaluate their efforts to communicate quality information to Congress, consistent with Principle 15 of *Standards for Internal Control in the Federal Government*, which emphasizes the need for an entity's management to externally communicate the necessary, quality information—such as significant matters related to risks, changes, or issues concerning their strategies for achieving compliance.[10] We did not evaluate the sufficiency and completeness of the agency-provided information.

To determine the extent to which OMB made determinations regarding whether additional funding would help CFO Act agency programs and activities reported as noncompliant for 2 consecutive years come into compliance, as of fiscal years 2016 and 2017, we interviewed key OMB staff on their process for determining additional funding needs for noncompliant programs and activities and reviewed the applicable agencies' IG compliance reports that OMB staff stated they relied on when making such determinations. Lastly, we corroborated our findings with OMB, the 24 CFO Act agencies, and their IGs. Appendix I provides additional information on our scope and methodology.

We conducted this performance audit from November 2017 to December 2018 in accordance with generally accepted government auditing standards. Those standards require that we plan and perform the audit to obtain sufficient, appropriate evidence to provide a reasonable basis for our findings and conclusions based on our audit objectives. We believe that the evidence obtained provides a reasonable basis for our findings and conclusions based on our audit objectives.

BACKGROUND

In November 2002, Congress passed and the President signed the Improper Payments Information Act of 2002 (IPIA), which was later amended by IPERA and the Improper Payments Elimination and Recovery Improvement Act of 2012 (IPERIA).11 The amended legislation requires executive branch agencies to (1) review all programs and activities and identify those that may be susceptible to significant improper payments (commonly referred to as a risk assessment), (2) publish improper payment estimates for those programs and activities that the agency identified as being susceptible to significant improper payments, (3) implement corrective actions to reduce improper payments and set reduction targets, and (4) report on the results of addressing the foregoing requirements.[12]

[9] Under IPERA, when programs are reported as noncompliant for 3 or more consecutive years, the respective agencies are required to submit to Congress within 30 days of the IG's report either (1) a reauthorization proposal for the program or (2) the proposed statutory changes necessary to bring the program or activity into compliance. GAO has previously recommended that agencies also notify Congress if they determine that such proposals are not necessary. We reviewed agency notifications submitted to Congress after the IGs' fiscal year 2016 IPERA compliance results in May 2017 because the IGs' reporting triggers the agency reporting requirements.

[10] GAO, Standards for Internal Control in the Federal Government, GAO-14-704G (Washington, D.C.: September 2014).

[11] Pub. L. No. 112-248, 126 Stat. 2390 (Jan. 10, 2013).

[12] For fiscal year 2014 and beyond, "significant improper payments" are defined as gross annual improper payments in a program that may have exceeded either (1) 1.5 percent of program outlays and $10 million or (2) $100 million (regardless of the improper payment rate). Additionally, the Disaster Relief Appropriations Act, 2013,

In addition to the agencies' identifying programs and activities that are susceptible to significant improper payments, OMB designates as high priority the programs with the most egregious cases of improper payments. Specifically, under a provision added to IPIA by IPERIA, OMB is required to annually identify a list of high-priority federal programs in need of greater oversight and review. In general, for fiscal years 2014 through 2017, OMB implemented this requirement by designating high-priority programs based on a threshold of $750 million in estimated improper payments for a given fiscal year.[13] OMB also plays a key role in implementing laws related to improper payment reporting. Specifically, OMB is directed by statute to provide guidance to federal agencies on estimating, reporting, reducing, and recovering improper payments.

IPERA also requires executive agencies' IGs to annually determine and report on whether their respective agencies complied with certain IPERArelated criteria. If an agency does not meet one or more of the six IPERA criteria for any of its programs or activities, the agency is considered noncompliant overall. The six criteria are as follows:

1. *publish a report* in the form and content required by OMB—typically an agency financial report (AFR) or a performance and accountability report (PAR)—for the most recent fiscal year, and post that report on the agency website;
2. *conduct a program-specific risk assessment,* if required, for each program or activity that conforms with IPIA as amended;[14]
3. *publish improper payment estimates* for all programs and activities deemed susceptible to significant improper payments under the agency's risk assessments;
4. *publish corrective action plans* for those programs and activities assessed to be at risk for significant improper payments;
5. *publish and meet annual reduction targets* for all programs and activities assessed to be at risk for significant improper payments; and
6. *report a gross improper payment rate of less than 10 percent* for each program and activity for which an improper payment estimate was published.

Under IPERA, agencies reported by their IG as not in compliance with any of these criteria in a fiscal year are required to submit a plan to Congress describing the actions they will take to come into compliance, and such plans shall include measureable milestones, the designation of senior accountable officials, and the establishment of accountability

---

Pub. L. No. 113-2, div. A, § 904(b), 127 Stat. 4, 17 (Jan. 29, 2013), required that all programs receiving funds appropriated by that act be deemed susceptible to significant improper payments, which consequently requires the agencies responsible for these programs to estimate improper payments, implement corrective actions, and report on their results for these programs.

[13] Office of Management and Budget, *Appendix C to Circular No. A-123, Requirements for Effective Estimation and Remediation of Improper Payments*, OMB Memorandum M-15- 02 (Washington, D.C.: October 2014). OMB updated its guidance in June 2018, and effective for fiscal year 2018 reporting, the threshold for high-priority program determinations is increased to $2 billion in estimated improper payments. Office of Management and Budget, *Appendix C to Circular No. A-123, Requirements for Payment Integrity Improvement*, OMB Memorandum M-18-20 (Washington, D.C.: June 2018).

[14] IPIA requires that program and activity risk assessments be conducted at least once every 3 fiscal years.

mechanisms to achieve compliance. OMB guidance states that agencies are required to submit these plans to Congress and OMB in the first year of reported noncompliance.[15]

When agency programs are reported as noncompliant for consecutive years, IPERA and OMB guidance requires agencies and OMB to take additional actions.[16] Specifically, an agency with a program reported as noncompliant for 3 or more consecutive years is required to submit to Congress within 30 days of the IG's report either (1) a reauthorization proposal for the program or (2) the proposed statutory changes necessary to bring the program or activity into compliance.[17] We previously recommended that when agencies determine that reauthorization or statutory changes are not necessary to bring the programs into compliance, the agencies should state so in their notifications to Congress. Effective starting with fiscal year 2018 reporting, OMB updated its guidance to instruct agencies with programs reported as noncompliant for 3 consecutive years to explain what the agency is doing to achieve compliance if a reauthorization proposal or proposed statutory change will not bring a program into compliance with IPERA. The updated guidance also instructs agencies with programs reported as noncompliant for 4 or more consecutive years to submit a report to Congress and OMB (within 30 days of the IG's determination of noncompliance) detailing the activities taken and still being pursued to prevent and reduce improper payments.[18]

If agency programs are reported as noncompliant under IPERA for 2 consecutive years, and the Director of OMB determines that additional funding would help the agency come into compliance, the head of the agency must obligate additional funding in the amount determined by the Director to intensify compliance efforts.[19]

IPERA directs the agency to exercise any reprogramming or transfer authority that the agency may have to provide additional funding to meet the level determined by OMB and, if necessary, submit a request to Congress for additional reprogramming or transfer authority to meet the full level of funding determined by OMB. Table 1 summarizes agency and OMB requirements related to agency programs that are noncompliant under IPERA, as reported by their IGs.

---

[15] Office of Management and Budget, Appendix C to Circular No. A-123, Requirements for Effective Estimation and Remediation of Improper Payments, OMB Memorandum M-15- 02, and Office of Management and Budget, Appendix C to Circular No. A-123, Requirements for Payment Integrity Improvement, OMB Memorandum M-18-20. OMB M15-02 was effective for fiscal years 2016 and 2017 reporting, the years included in our audit. OMB M-15-02 was superseded by OMB M-18-20, which was issued June 26, 2018, and will be effective beginning with fiscal year 2018 reporting. Unless noted otherwise, the requirements in OMB M-15-02 and OMB M-18-20 referenced in this report are the same.

[16] Hereafter in this report, programs represents both programs and activities, as applicable.

[17] While IPERA states that these procedures are required of agencies with programs reported as noncompliant more than 3 consecutive years, OMB M-15-02 adds to this by instructing agencies with exactly 3 consecutive years of reported noncompliance to also take these steps.

[18] Office of Management and Budget, Appendix C to Circular No. A-123, Requirements for Payment Integrity Improvement, OMB Memorandum M-18-20.

[19] OMB interprets this requirement as applying only to agencies and programs with exactly 2 consecutive years of noncompliance findings. According to OMB staff, the annual budget process allows agencies to continue submitting budget requests that support achieving IPERA compliance in subsequent years.

Table 1. Overview of OMB and Agency Requirements for Agency Programs Not in Compliance under IPERA as Reported by Their Igs

Years program reported as noncompliant	Requirements for applicable agencies and OMB	Fiscal years effective[a]	
		2016 and 2017	2018
One year[b]	Agency: Within 90 days of the IG's determination of noncompliance, the agency should submit a plan to Congress and OMB describing the actions that the agency will take to come into compliance that includes measurable milestones, senior agency officials, and accountability mechanisms.	X	X
Two consecutive years[c]	OMB: The Director of OMB has authority to determine if additional funding for intensified compliance efforts would help the agency program(s) come into compliance.	X	X
Two consecutive years[c]	Agency: If OMB determines that additional funding for intensified compliance efforts is warranted, the agency shall (1) exercise reprogramming or transfer authority to provide additional funding to meet the level determined by OMB; and (2) submit a request to Congress for additional re-programming or transfer authority if additional funding is needed to meet the full level of funding determined by OMB.	X	X
	Agency: The agency should create a proposal and submit it to OMB during its next budget submission that will bring the agency into compliance.	—	X
Three or more consecutive years[d]	Agency: Within 30 days of the IG's determination of noncompliance, the agency is required to submit to Congress either (1) a reauthorization proposal or (2) proposed statutory changes necessary to bring the program or activity into compliance.	X	X
	Agency: If the proposals are not deemed necessary, then the agency must state so and explain what the agency is doing to achieve compliance.	—	X
Four or more consecutive years	Agency: Within 30 days of the IG's determination of noncompliance, agencies are required to submit a report to Congress and OMB detailing the activities taken to complete the requirements for 1 year, 2 years, 3 years, 4 years, and so forth of noncompliance and include a description of any of the requirements that were fulfilled in years one, two, or three that are still relevant and being pursued as a means to prevent and reduce improper payments.	—	X

Sources: IPERA and OMB memorandums. | GAO-19-14.

Legend: X = requirement was applicable to agencies or OMB in the fiscal year(s) indicated. — = requirement was not applicable to agencies or OMB in the fiscal year(s) indicated. IG = inspector general. IPERA = Improper Payments Elimination and Recovery Act of 2010. OMB = Office of Management and Budget.

[a] OMB Circular No. A-123, Appendix C (M-15-02) was issued in October 2014 and was effective for agencies reporting for fiscal years 2016 and 2017, the years included in our audit. In June 2018, OMB issued revised guidance (OMB Circular No. A-123, Appendix C (M-18-20)), which included additional agency reporting requirements that are effective for fiscal year 2018.

[b] OMB guidance states that agencies are required to submit these plans to Congress and OMB in the first year of reported noncompliance.

[c] OMB interprets this requirement as applying only to agencies and programs with exactly 2 consecutive years of noncompliance findings. According to OMB staff, the annual budget process allows agencies to continue submitting budget requests that support achieving IPERA compliance in subsequent years.

[d] While IPERA states that these procedures are required of agencies with more than 3 consecutive years of noncompliance findings by their IGs, OMB Circular No. A-123, Appendix C (M-15-02), adds to this by instructing agencies with exactly 3 consecutive years of reported noncompliance to also take these steps.

Over Half of the CFO Act Agencies Were Reported as Noncompliant under IPERA for Fiscal Years 2016 and 2017, and Consecutive Years of Noncompliance Continue for Certain Programs

Over Half of the Agencies Were Reported as Noncompliant for Fiscal Years 2016 and 2017

Seven years after the initial implementation of IPERA, over half of the 24 CFO Act agencies were reported as noncompliant by their IGs for fiscal years 2016 and 2017. Specifically, 13 agencies were reported as noncompliant with one or more IPERA criteria for fiscal year 2016, and 14 agencies were reported as noncompliant for fiscal year 2017 (see fig. 1). Nine of these agencies have been reported as noncompliant in one or more programs every year since IPERA was implemented in 2011 (see app. II for additional details on CFO Act agencies' compliance under IPERA for fiscal years 2011 through 2017, as reported by their IGs).

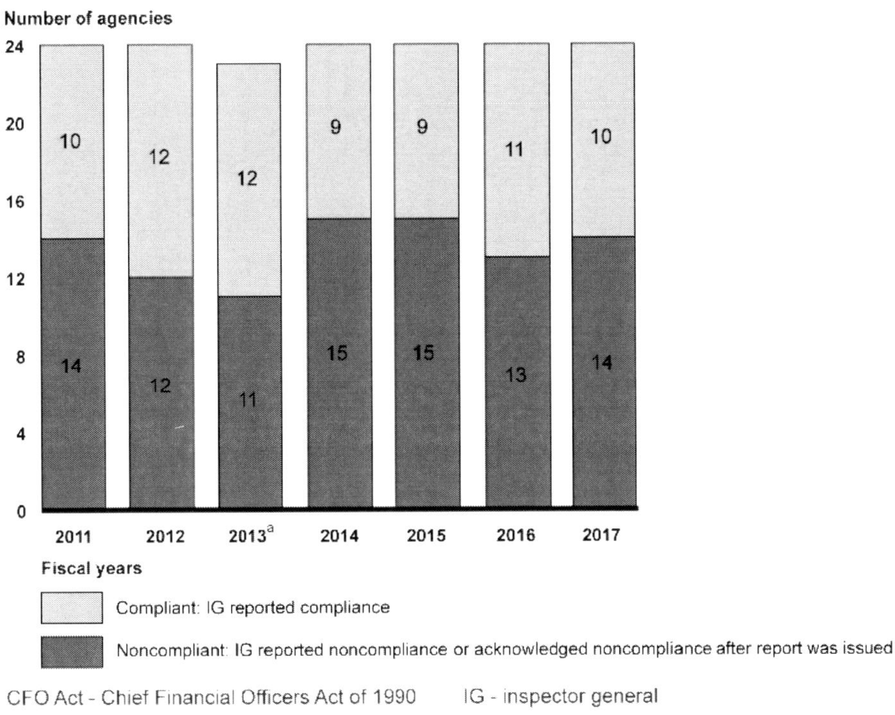

Source: GAO analysis of CFO Act agencies' IG IPERA reports for fiscal years 2011 through 2017. | GAO-19-14.

[a] For fiscal year 2013, one inspector general did not issue a compliance report because the agency did not publish improper payment information.

Figure 1. Number of CFO Act Agencies Compliant under IPERA for Fiscal Years 2011 through 2017, as Reported or Acknowledged by Their Inspectors General.

Although the number of agencies reported as noncompliant under IPERA has varied slightly since fiscal year 2011, the total instances of noncompliance for all six criteria substantially improved after fiscal year 2011, when IPERA was first implemented. As shown in figure 2, the total instances decreased from 38 instances (for 14 noncompliant agencies) for fiscal year 2011 to 26 instances (for 14 noncompliant agencies) for fiscal year 2017.[20]

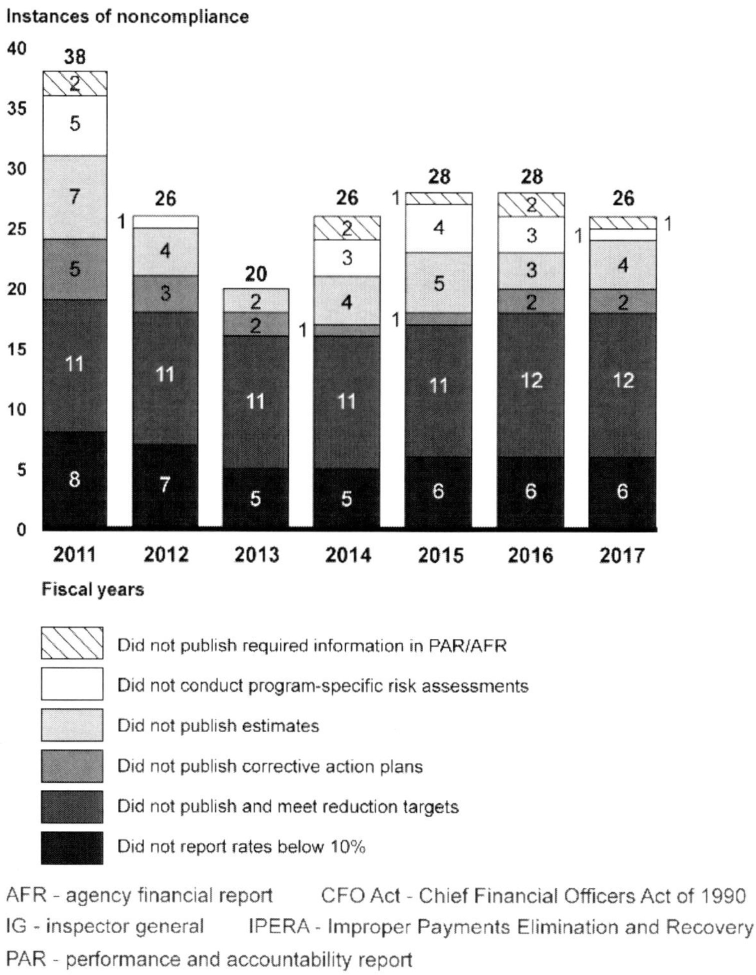

Source: GAO analysis of CFO Act agencies' IG IPERA reports for fiscal years 2011 through 2017. | GAO-19-14.

Figure 2. Total Instances of CFO Act Agencies' Noncompliance with IPERA Criteria, for Fiscal Years 2011 through 2017, as Reported or Acknowledged by Their Inspectors General.

Also, for fiscal year 2017, 7 of 14 agencies were reported as noncompliant for only one criterion per noncompliant program. Of these, 6 agencies—the Departments of Homeland Security (DHS), Education (Education), Commerce, and Transportation; the General Services

[20] See app. III for additional details on agencies' and programs' compliance for each criterion, as reported by their IGs, for fiscal years 2016 and 2017. Total reported instances of noncompliance exceed the number of noncompliant agencies because certain agencies were reported as noncompliant with more than one IPERA criterion.

Administration; and the Social Security Administration (SSA)—were only reported as noncompliant with the IPERA criterion that requires agencies to publish and meet reduction targets. In addition, the Department of the Treasury (Treasury) was only reported as noncompliant with the IPERA criterion that requires agencies to report improper payment rates below 10 percent.

Furthermore, the programs reported as noncompliant for fiscal year 2017 accounted for a significantly smaller portion of the total reported estimated improper payments as compared to the noncompliant programs for fiscal year 2015. Specifically, we previously reported that 52 noncompliant programs accounted for $132 billion (or about 96 percent) of the $137 billion total reported estimated improper payments for fiscal year 2015, whereas 58 noncompliant programs accounted for $80 billion (or about 57 percent) of the $141 billion total reported estimated improper payments for fiscal year 2017.[21] Although improper payment estimates associated with noncompliant programs vary from year to year, this decrease (approximately $52 billion) was primarily due to two programs. Specifically, the Department of Health and Human Services' (HHS) Medicare Fee-for-Service (Parts A and B) and Medicare Part C programs were reported as noncompliant and accounted for approximately $43 billion and $14 billion, respectively, of estimated improper payments for fiscal year 2015. These programs were reported as compliant for fiscal year 2017 and accounted for approximately $36 billion and $14 billion, respectively, or about 36 percent of the $141 billion total reported improper payments for fiscal year 2017.

Certain Programs Continue to Be Reported as Noncompliant for Consecutive Years

Almost a third (18 programs) of the 58 programs that contributed to 14 CFO Act agencies' noncompliance under IPERA, as of fiscal year 2017, were reported as noncompliant for 3 or more consecutive years. The number of programs noncompliant for 3 or more consecutive years has continually increased since fiscal year 2015, as shown in figure 3. Specifically, 12 programs (associated with 7 agencies) were reported as noncompliant for 3 or more consecutive years, as of fiscal year 2015, and the number increased to 14 programs (associated with 8 agencies) and 18 programs (associated with 9 agencies), as of fiscal years 2016 and 2017, respectively.

These programs accounted for a substantial portion of the $141 billion total estimated improper payments for fiscal year 2017. As shown in table 2, 14 of the 18 programs that were reported as noncompliant for 3 or more consecutive years reported improper payment estimates that accounted for an estimated $74.4 billion (about 53 percent) of the $141 billion, while the other 4 programs did not report improper payment estimates for fiscal year 2017 and were reported by their respective IGs as noncompliant with the IPERA criterion to publish improper payment estimates.

[21] GAO-17-484.

Table 2. Fiscal Year 2017 Reported Improper Payment Estimates for 18 Programs Reported as Noncompliant under IPERA for 3 or More Consecutive Years

Agency	Program	Estimate[a] (dollars in millions)
U.S. Department of Agriculture	1.Food and Nutrition Service (FNS) Child and Adult Care Food Program[b]	Not reported
	2. FNS National School Lunch Program[b]	1,875
	3. FNS School Breakfast Program[b]	958
	4.FNS Special Supplemental Nutrition Program for Women, Infants, and Children[b]	197
	5. FNS Supplemental Nutrition Assistance Program	Not reported
Department of Defense	6. Travel Pay	263
Department of Health and Human Services	7. Temporary Assistance for Needy Families[b]	Not reported
	8. Children's Health Insurance Program	1,236
	9. Medicaid	36,731
Department of Housing and Urban Development	10. Rental Housing Assistance Programs[c]	Not reported
Department of Labor	11. Unemployment Insurance Benefit[b]	4,066
Department of the Treasury	12. Earned Income Tax Credit[b]	16,232
Department of Veterans Affairs	13.CommunityCare	5,258
	14. Purchased Long Term Service and Support	1,890
	15. Beneficiary Travel	224
	16. Supplies and Materials	480
Social Security Administration	17. Supplemental Security Income[b]	5,020
Department of Homeland Security	18.U.S. Customs and Border Protection –Refund & Drawback	15
Total for 18 programs reported as noncompliant for 3 or more consecutive years, as of fiscal year 2017		74,445

Source: GAO analysis of Office of Management and Budget data and Chief Financial Officers Act of 1990 agencies' inspector general Improper Payments Elimination and Recovery Act of 2010 (IPERA) reports for fiscal year 2017. | GAO-19-14.

[a] Reported estimates of improper payments totaled approximately $141 billion for fiscal year 2017, attributable to 90 programs across 21 agencies. It is important to note that these estimates themselves may not be accurate, reliable, or complete, because, as we have reported, the federal government is unable to determine the full extent to which improper payments occur and reasonably assure that appropriate actions are taken to reduce them. See GAO, Financial Audit: Fiscal Years 2017 and 2016 Consolidated Financial Statements of the U.S. Government, GAO-18-316R (Washington, D.C.: Feb. 15, 2018). In addition, certain inspectors general have reported issues with their agencies' reported improper payment estimates that were caused by insufficient sampling methods and flawed estimation methodologies for calculating and reporting improper payment estimates.

[b] These programs have been reported as noncompliant since the implementation of the Improper Payments Elimination and Recovery Act of 2010 in fiscal year 2011.

[c] The Department of Housing and Urban Development ceased reporting an estimate of improper payments for certain of its Rental Housing Assistance Programs in fiscal year 2017.

The $74.4 billion is primarily composed of estimates reported for 2 noncompliant programs—HHS's Medicaid program ($36.7 billion) and Treasury's Earned Income Tax Credit program ($16.2 billion)— totaling $52.9 billion (or approximately 71 percent of the $74.4 billion). Improper payments associated with these two noncompliant programs are also a central part of two areas included in our 2017 High-Risk List, which includes federal programs and operations that are especially vulnerable to waste, fraud, abuse, and mismanagement, or that need transformative change.[22]

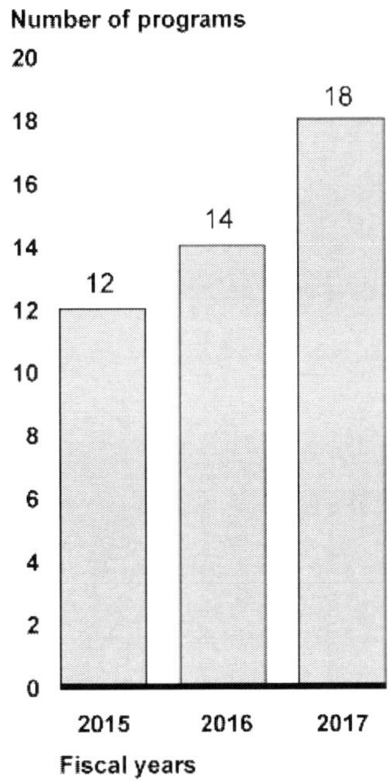

Source: GAO analysis of Chief Financial Act of 190 (CFO Act) agencies' inspector general (IG) Improper Payments elimination and Recovery At of 2010 (IPERA) report for fiscal years 2015 through 2017. | GAO-19-14.

Figure 3. Number of CFO Act Agency Programs Noncompliant under IPERA for 3 or More Consecutive Years, for Fiscal Years 2015 through 2017, as Reported or Acknowledged by Their IGs.

Eight of the 18 noncompliant programs have been reported as noncompliant since the implementation of IPERA in fiscal year 2011, for a total of 7 consecutive years, as shown in table 2. Reported compliance for Treasury's Earned Income Tax Credit improved from being reported as noncompliant with multiple IPERA criteria in fiscal year 2013 to noncompliance with only one criterion for the last 4 years (fiscal years 2014 through 2017).

CFO Act Agencies Did Not Always Notify Congress, and They Provided Varying Information on Programs Reported as Noncompliant for 3 or More Consecutive Years

Eight CFO Act agencies' programs were reported as noncompliant under IPERA for 3 or more consecutive years, as of fiscal year 2016.[23] Three of these agencies did not notify

[22] GAO, *High-Risk Series: Progress on Many High-Risk Areas, While Substantial Efforts Needed on Others*, GAO-17-317 (Washington, D.C.: Feb. 15, 2017). Improper payments associated with these two programs are a central part of the Medicaid Program and Enforcement of Tax Laws high-risk areas.

Congress of their program's continued noncompliance as required.[24] In addition to submitting the required notifications for their noncompliant programs, the other five agencies also included additional information in their notifications—such as measurable milestones, designation of senior officials, and accountability mechanisms—useful for assessing their efforts to achieve compliance. In June 2018, OMB updated its guidance to clarify agency reporting requirements for each consecutive year a program is reported as noncompliant. However, OMB's updated guidance did not direct agencies to include other types of quality information in their notifications for programs reported as noncompliant for 3 or more consecutive years that could help Congress to more effectively assess their efforts to address long-standing challenges and other issues affecting these programs and to achieve compliance.

CFO Act Agencies with Programs Reported as Noncompliant for 3 or More Consecutive Years Did Not Always Notify Congress

Of the eight agencies with programs reported as noncompliant under IPERA for 3 or more consecutive years as of fiscal year 2016, we found that five agencies notified Congress of their noncompliance as required. Specifically, the Department of Defense (DOD), Education, HHS, DHS, and SSA notified Congress of their programs' reported noncompliance for 3 or more consecutive years as of fiscal year 2016 as required by IPERA and OMB guidance. The remaining three agencies—the U.S. Department of Agriculture (USDA), the Department of Labor (DOL), and Treasury— did not notify Congress as required.

Additional information regarding the three agencies that did not submit their required notifications to Congress is summarized below:

- *USDA:* In May 2017, the USDA IG reported that four USDA Food and Nutrition Service programs—Child and Adult Care Food Program; National School Lunch Program; School Breakfast Program; and Special Supplemental Nutrition Program for Women, Infants, and Children—had been noncompliant for 6 consecutive years, as of fiscal year 2016. However, USDA has not notified Congress of these programs' continued noncompliance with IPERA as of fiscal year 2016, despite prior

---

[23] See app. IV for a list of CFO Act agencies and programs reported as noncompliant for 3 or more consecutive years, as of fiscal year 2016. We limited our review to agency notifications submitted to Congress after the IGs reported the fiscal year 2016 IPERA compliance results in May 2017 because the IGs' reporting triggers the agency reporting requirements. In addition, we did not review the notifications for programs reported as noncompliant as of fiscal year 2017 (with IPERA compliance results reported in May 2018), because of timing limitations.

[24] IPERA and OMB require agencies to submit a request for program reauthorization or a proposal for statutory changes necessary to bring programs into compliance with IPERA. While IPERA states that this requirement is for agencies with more than 3 consecutive years of noncompliance findings by their IGs, OMB M-15-02 adds to this by instructing agencies with exactly 3 consecutive years of reported noncompliance to also take these steps. We previously reported that when an agency determines that a reauthorization or statutory change proposal is not needed to bring a program into compliance, the agency should indicate such in its notifications to Congress.

recommendations that we, and the USDA IG, made to USDA to do so.[25] USDA staff stated in May 2018 that USDA drafted, but had not submitted, a letter to Congress regarding these programs' noncompliance.

- *DOL:* In June 2017, the DOL IG reported that the Unemployment Insurance Benefit program had been noncompliant for 6 consecutive years, as of fiscal year 2016. In October 2016, DOL included proposed legislation in its last notification to Congress regarding this program, approximately 8 months prior to the DOL IG's IPERA compliance report. However, because the requirement for agencies to notify Congress is triggered by IG reporting of programs that are noncompliant for 3 or more consecutive years, DOL should have also notified Congress regarding the program's continued noncompliance in fiscal year 2016 after the IG's report was issued in June 2017. DOL staff stated in August 2018 that the proposed legislation included in its October 2016 notification had not been enacted and that DOL is currently working to develop a new report to Congress and OMB detailing corrective actions taken to bring the program into compliance.
- *Treasury:* In May 2017, the Treasury IG reported that the Earned Income Tax Credit (EITC) program had been noncompliant for 6 consecutive years, as of fiscal year 2016. We previously reported that Treasury submitted proposed statutory changes to Congress for this program in August 2014 and in June 2015.[26] As stated in the Treasury IG's fiscal year 2016 IPERA compliance report, the proposed statutory changes would help prevent the improper issuance of billions of dollars in refunds as it would provide the Internal Revenue Service (IRS) with expanded authority to systematically correct erroneous claims that are identified when tax returns are processed and allow IRS to deny erroneous EITC refund claims before they are paid. Further, Treasury stated that IRS has repeatedly requested authority to correct such errors in subsequent fiscal year budgets, including its fiscal year 2019 budget submission. In June 2018, Treasury staff stated that the Consolidated Appropriations Act, 2016 provided IRS with additional tools for reducing EITC improper payments; however, the act did not expand IRS's authority to systematically correct the erroneous claims that are identified when tax returns are processed.[27]

  Treasury staff also stated that the department has continued to coordinate with OMB on required reporting for the EITC program because of the program's complexity, and that OMB has not requested additional actions or documentation regarding the program's noncompliance. Although continued coordination with OMB is important, Treasury did not notify Congress regarding the EITC program's continued noncompliance as required.

In summary, despite reporting requirements in IPERA and OMB guidance, one agency (USDA) has not notified Congress about four programs being reported as noncompliant for 6

---

[25] See GAO recommendations in GAO-16-554 and GAO-17-484. See the USDA IG recommendation in, U.S. Department of Agriculture, Office of Inspector General, *USDA'S Fiscal Year 2016 Compliance with Improper Payment Requirements,* Audit Number 50024-0011-11 (Washington, D.C.: May 2017).

[26] GAO-16-554 and GAO-17-484.

[27] The Protecting Americans from Tax Hikes Act of 2015, which was enacted as part of the Consolidated Appropriations Act, 2016, included reforms, that among other things, allow IRS earlier access to Form W-2s, which enables IRS to systemically verify more wage data and return information. Pub. L. No. 114-113, div. Q, § 201, 129 Stat. 2242, 3076 (Dec. 18, 2015).

consecutive years, as of fiscal year 2016. The remaining two agencies (DOL and Treasury) that did not notify Congress of their programs' consecutive noncompliance, as of fiscal year 2016, submitted notifications to Congress prior to their respective IGs' fiscal year 2016 compliance results. However, IPERA requires agencies to notify Congress when programs are reported as noncompliant for more than 3 consecutive years and thus DOL and Treasury should have also notified Congress about their programs' being reported as noncompliant for 6 consecutive years, as of fiscal year 2016.

It is important that agencies continue to notify Congress of their programs' consecutive noncompliance each year after the third consecutive year as the information related to their proposals or regarding their IPERA compliance efforts included in prior years' notifications to Congress may significantly change over time. Unless agencies continue to notify Congress in subsequent years, Congress may lack the current and relevant information needed to effectively assess agencies' proposals or monitor their efforts to address problematic programs in a timely manner. OMB updated its guidance in June 2018 to provide more clarity regarding the notification requirements for each consecutive year a program is reported as noncompliant. Effective implementation of this guidance may help ensure that agencies consistently provide required information to Congress on these programs in future years.

Certain Agencies Provided Additional Quality Information on IPERA Compliance Efforts in Their Notifications to Congress

We found that the five agencies—DOD, DHS, Education, HHS, and SSA—that notified Congress regarding their programs' reported noncompliance for 3 or more consecutive years, as of fiscal year 2016, also included additional information about their efforts to achieve IPERA compliance. Although IPERA does not specifically require that agency proposals for reauthorization or other statutory change provide such information, including it could help Congress to better assess the agencies' proposals included in these notifications and to oversee agency efforts to address long-standing challenges and compliance issues associated with these programs.

In many instances, the types of additional information provided by these agencies are similar to information that agencies are required to provide to Congress or OMB in other required notifications or other reports, such as annual AFRs or PARs. For example, all improper payment estimates reported under IPIA, as amended, must be accompanied by information on what the agency is doing to reduce improper payments, including a description of root causes and the steps the agency has taken to ensure accountability. Further, IPERA and OMB guidance require agencies to provide corrective action plans to Congress for programs reported as noncompliant for 1 year. Such plans should include actions planned or taken to address the program's noncompliance, measurable milestones, a senior official designated to oversee progress, and the accountability mechanisms in place to hold the senior official accountable.[28]

[28] IPERA requires agencies to submit corrective action plans to Congress when programs are reported as noncompliant for a fiscal year. As noted above, OMB guidance interprets this requirement as applying only to agencies with exactly 1 year of reported noncompliance.

In addition, GAO's *Standards for Internal Control in the Federal Government* emphasizes the importance of communicating quality information, such as significant matters related to risks, changes, or issues affecting agencies' efforts to achieve compliance objectives, to external parties—such as legislators, oversight bodies, and the general public.[29] Furthermore, in our fiscal year 2017 High-Risk Update, we also highlight the importance of these types of information when assessing agency efforts to address issues associated with programs included on our High-Risk List.[30] Examples of such information include (1) action plans that are accessible and transparent with clear milestones and metrics, including established goals and performance measures to address identified root causes; (2) leadership commitment of top (or senior) officials to establish long-term priorities and goals and continued oversight and accountability; (3) monitoring progress against goals, assessing program performance, or reporting potential risks; and (4) demonstrated progress, through recommendations implemented, actions taken for improvement, and effectively addressing identified root causes and managing high-risk issues.

Table 3. Additional Information Included in Notifications to Congress by Five Agencies with Programs Reported as Noncompliant under the Improper Payments Elimination and Recovery Act of 2010 for 3 or More Consecutive Years, as of Fiscal Year 2016

Agency	Additional information included[a]					
	Root causes	Risks, issues, or changes	Corrective actions or strategies	Measurable milestones	Designated senior officials	Accountability mechanisms
Department of Defense	Yes	Yes	Yes	Yes	Yes	Yes
Department of Education	Yes	Yes	Yes	Yes	Yes	Yes
Department of Health and Human Services	Yes	Yes	Yes	No	No	No
Department of Homeland Security	Yes	Yes	Yes	Yes	Yes	Yes
Social Security Administration	Yes	Yes	Yes	No	No	No
Total	5	5	5	3	3	3

Source: GAO analysis of Chief Financial Officers Act of 1990 agencies' notifications to Congress for programs with 3 or more consecutive years of noncompliance as of fiscal year 2016. | GAO-19-14

[a] Descriptions of the additional types of information shown above are as follows:

Root causes: Underlying issues or causes that directly lead to an improper payment or hinder the program's ability to achieve compliance and, if corrected, would prevent the improper payments. Risks, issues, or changes: Internal or external risk factors in an agency's environment, significant changes that have (or may) occur, and internal control issues in their systems or processes that may adversely affect their ability to achieve compliance. Corrective actions or strategies: Specific action items or strategies planned, developed, implemented, or taken to address a program's noncompliance. Measurable milestones: Key action items in the agency's efforts to achieve compliance that are measurable and include specific target dates. Designated senior officials: Senior agency official designated to oversee and be held accountable for the agency's efforts and related progress for each of its programs or activities to achieve compliance. Accountability mechanisms: Appropriate incentives and consequences for the senior official designated to oversee the agency's efforts to achieve compliance.

---

[29] GAO-14-704G. Such significant matters could include internal or external risk factors in an agency's environment—including significant related changes that have (or may) occur, such as complex organizational or program structures, new or existing legal requirements, or natural disasters, and internal control issues in the design, implementation, or operating effectiveness of a system or related processes, which may adversely affect the entity's ability to achieve compliance and its reporting objectives.

[30] GAO-17-317. Every 2 years at the start of a new Congress, GAO calls attention to agencies and program areas that are at high risk because of their vulnerabilities to fraud, waste, abuse, and mismanagement or that are most in need of transformation. Two programs, HHS's Medicaid and Treasury's EITC, were reported as noncompliant under IPERA for 3 or more consecutive years, as of fiscal years 2016 and 2017. As noted in table 2, these two programs accounted for approximately $52.9 billion (or 37.5 percent) of the $141 billion of the total reported improper payments estimates for fiscal year 2017. Improper payments associated with these two noncompliant programs are also a central part of two areas included in our 2017 High-Risk List.

Table 3 summarizes the types of additional information described above that the five agencies provided in their fiscal year 2016 notifications to Congress to address programs with 3 or more consecutive years of noncompliance. All five agencies informed Congress of (1) root causes that directly lead to improper payments or hindered the program's ability to achieve compliance; (2) certain risks, significant changes, or issues affecting their efforts; and (3) their corrective actions or strategies to achieve compliance. Three of the five agencies—DOD, Education, and DHS—also included the other types of additional information described above in their notifications, including measurable milestones, designated senior officials to oversee progress, and accountability mechanisms established to help achieve compliance. For example, all three agencies designated their chief financial officers (CFO) to oversee progress toward achieving measurable milestones and expanded their official roles and responsibilities to hold them accountable. Education and DHS stated that these responsibilities were added to their respective CFOs' individual performance plans. Although OMB updated its guidance in June 2018 to clarify agency reporting requirements related to programs reported as noncompliant for 3 or more consecutive years, the updated guidance did not direct agencies to include other types of quality information in their notifications, such as those described above. In addition, information related to measurable milestones, corrective actions, risks, issues, or other items affecting agencies' efforts may change significantly over time. With this additional information, Congress could have more complete information to effectively oversee agency efforts to address long-standing challenges and other issues that have contributed to programs being reported as noncompliant for 3 or more consecutive years.

OMB Updated Guidance for Determining Additional Funding Needs for Programs Reported as Noncompliant for 2 Consecutive Years

Fifteen programs in seven agencies and 12 programs in six agencies were reported as noncompliant for 2 consecutive years as of fiscal years 2016 and 2017, respectively.[31] For agencies reported as noncompliant under IPERA for 2 consecutive years for the same program, IPERA gives the Director of OMB the authority to determine whether additional funding would help the agencies come into compliance.[32] If the OMB Director determines that such funding would help, the agency is required to use any available reprogramming or transfer authority to meet the funding level that the OMB Director specified and, if such authorities are not sufficient, submit a request to Congress for additional reprogramming or transfer authority. According to OMB staff, OMB determined that no additional funding was needed for programs reported as noncompliant for 2 consecutive years as of fiscal year 2016. As of September 2018, OMB was in the process of making funding determinations for 12

[31] See app. IV for all agencies and programs with 2 consecutive years of noncompliance as reported by their IGs, as of fiscal years 2016 and 2017.

[32] As noted above, OMB interprets this requirement as applying only to agencies and programs with exactly 2 consecutive years of noncompliance findings. According to OMB staff, the annual budget process allows agencies to continue submitting budget requests that support achieving IPERA compliance in subsequent years.

programs that were reported as noncompliant as of fiscal year 2017 and stated that any determinations made would be developed in the President's Budget for fiscal year 2020.

Table 4. CFO Act Agency Programs Reported as Noncompliant for 2 Consecutive Years by Their IGs and Noncompliance Determinations for Each IPERA Criterion, as of Fiscal Year 2017

Agencies and programs	Published information in PAR/AFR	Conducted program-specific risk assessment(s)	Published estimate(s)	Published corrective action plan(s)	Published and met reduction target(s)	Reported rate(s) below 10 percent
Department of Defense						
1. Navy Commercial Bill Pay Office -Naples	X	*	*	*	*	*
2. Defense Finance and Accounting Services - Commercial Pay	X	*	X	*	*	*
3. U.S. Army Corps of Engineers -Travel Pay	X	*	*	*	X	*
4. Military Health Benefits	X	*	X	X	*	*
5. Military Pay	X	*	*	X	*	*
6. Civilian Pay	X	*	*	*	*	*
7. Military Retiree and Annuitant Benefit Payments	X	*	*	X	X	*
Department of Education						
8. Pell Grant	*	*	*	*	X	*
Department of Health and Human Services						
9. Foster Care	*	*	*	*	X	*
Department of Veterans Affairs						
10. Civilian Health and Medical Program of the Department of Veterans Affairs	*	*	*	*	X	*
General Services Administration						
11. Rental of Space Program	*	*	*	*	X	*
12. Section 7(a) Loan Guaranty Purchases	*	*	*	*	X	*

Source: GAO analysis of CFO Act agencies' IG IPERA compliance reports for fiscal years 2017. | GAO-19-14.

Note: These12 programs were determined to be noncompliant with IPERA for 2 consecutive years as of fiscal year 2017. The specific IPERA criterion (or criteria) with which each program was noncompliant in fiscal year 2017, as shown in this table, may differ from the criterion the program was noncompliant with in a prior year. For agencies reported as noncompliant under IPERA for 2 consecutive years for the same program, IPERA gives the Director of OMB the authority to determine whether additional funding would help the agency come into compliance. OMB interprets this requirement as applying only to agencies and programs with exactly 2 consecutive years of noncompliance findings. According to OMB staff, the annual budget process allows agencies to continue submitting budget requests that support achieving IPERA compliance in subsequent years.

Legend: X = Program was noncompliant with IPERA criterion, as reported by the agencies' IG. * = Program was not reported by the IG as noncompliant with IPERA criterion. AFR = agency financial report. CFO Act = Chief Financial Officers Act of 1990 IG = inspector general. IPERA = Improper Payments Elimination and Recovery Act of 2010. OMB = Office of Management and Budget. PAR = performance and accountability report

The 12 programs reported as noncompliant for 2 consecutive years, as of fiscal year 2017, accounted for approximately $3 billion (2 percent) of the $141 billion total improper payment estimate for that year. Of these 12 programs, more than half (or 7 of the 12) were attributable to DOD; however, Education's Pell Grant program accounted for $2.2 billion (or 74 percent) of the $3 billion in improper payment estimates for programs reported as noncompliant programs for 2 consecutive years, for fiscal year 2017. In addition, as shown in table 4, the 12 programs reported as noncompliant for 2 consecutive years, as of fiscal year 2017, were primarily noncompliant with the IPERA criteria that required agencies to publish information in their PAR or AFR or publish and meet reduction targets.

As noted previously, IPERA gives OMB authority to determine whether additional funding for intensified compliance efforts would help the agency come into compliance under IPERA. Therefore, an established process for making timely, well-informed funding determinations is an essential part of ensuring that agencies have sufficient resources and take steps to intensify their compliance efforts in a timely manner. In April 2018, OMB staff stated that when making funding determinations, they primarily rely on the IGs' recommendations in their annual IPERA compliance reports. OMB staff also stated that for its fiscal year 2016 determinations, OMB determined that additional funding was not needed because the IGs' recommendations did not specify that additional funding was needed to help resolve the programs' noncompliance.

The IGs' annual reports provide information on agencies' IPERA compliance and may be useful to OMB as a tool to help them make determinations for additional funding. However, IPERA does not require IGs to address funding levels in their annual compliance reports, and OMB's guidance does not inform the IGs that their work might be relied upon in this manner. We reviewed the IGs' fiscal years 2016 and 2017 IPERA compliance reports for the agencies with programs reported as noncompliant for 2 consecutive years and found that the IGs did not make any recommendations regarding additional funding needed to bring these programs into compliance. In addition, as specifically stated by the IGs for Education and USDA in their IPERA reports, OMB has the statutory responsibility to make these funding determinations. Education IG's fiscal year 2017 IPERA compliance report stated that "If OMB recommends that the Department needs additional funding or should take any other actions to become compliant with IPERA, we recommend that the Department implement OMB's recommendations." Also, the USDA IG's fiscal year 2016 IPERA compliance report stated, "For agencies that are not compliant for 2 consecutive years for the same program, the Director of OMB will determine if additional funding would help these programs come into compliance." As a result, OMB's reliance on IG recommendations as the source of information to support additional funding determinations may not provide sufficient information to effectively assess agencies' funding needs to address noncompliance.

OMB staff subsequently stated that they no longer need to conduct a detailed review of the IGs' IPERA compliance reports to identify recommendations related to additional funding needs. Instead, OMB Memorandum M-18-20, issued in June 2018, updated OMB Circular No. A-123, Appendix C, and clarified that the funding determination process will unfold as part of the annual development of the President's Budget, as described in OMB Circular No.

A-11.[33] This updated guidance also directs agencies to submit proposals to OMB regarding additional funding needs that may help them address IPERA noncompliance.

To illustrate, under this new guidance, the IGs' fiscal year 2018 IPERA compliance reports will be due in May 2019, and any funding needs to address noncompliance would be incorporated in the next annual budget preparation process, the results of which are due to be submitted to Congress in February 2020 for the President's Budget for fiscal year 2021. Once OMB's determinations have been made and communicated to agencies, agencies would respond by performing the required reprogramming and making transfers under existing authority, where available. Any requests for additional transfer authority may be incorporated into subsequent appropriations legislation.[34]

Conclusion

Estimated improper payments reported government-wide total almost $1.4 trillion from fiscal year 2003 through fiscal year 2017. The number of programs reported as noncompliant under IPERA for 3 or more consecutive years has continued to increase, from 12 programs (associated with 7 agencies) to 18 programs (associated with 9 agencies) as of fiscal years 2015 and 2017, respectively. Including additional useful, up-to-date information—such as measurable milestones, risks, or other issues affecting agency efforts to achieve compliance—in notifications to Congress, which are required when programs are reported as noncompliant for 3 or more consecutive years, could help Congress better assess agency efforts to address long-standing challenges and other issues associated with them. Although certain agencies included certain types of additional information in their notifications as of fiscal year 2016, OMB guidance does not require agencies to include such information in their notifications. As a result, Congress may lack sufficient information to effectively oversee agency efforts and take prompt action to help address long-standing challenges or other issues associated with these programs.

Recommendation for Executive Action

The Director of OMB should take steps to update OMB guidance to specify other types of quality information that agencies with programs noncompliant for 3 or more consecutive years should include in their notifications to Congress, such as significant matters related to risks, issues, root causes, measurable milestones, designated senior officials, accountability mechanisms, and corrective actions or strategies planned or taken by agencies to achieve compliance. (Recommendation 1)

---

[33] Office of Management and Budget, Appendix C to Circular No. A-123, Requirements for Payment Integrity Improvement, OMB Memorandum M-18-20, and Preparation, Submission, and Execution of the Budget, OMB Circular No. A-11 (Washington, D.C.: June 2018).

[34] A full timeline for preparation of the annual President's Budget can be found in OMB Circular No. A-11 § 10.5.

AGENCY COMMENTS AND OUR EVALUATION

We provided a draft of this chapter to OMB and requested comments, and OMB said that it had no comments. We also provided a draft of this chapter to the 24 CFO Act agencies and their IGs and requested comments. We received letters from the DHS Office of Inspector General (OIG), SSA, and the United States Agency for International Development. These letters are reproduced in appendixes V through VII. We also received technical comments from DOL, the Department of Veterans Affairs, the General Services Administration, HHS, the Department of Housing and Urban Development, and the Treasury OIG, which we incorporated in the report as appropriate. The remaining agencies and OIGs either did not provide comments or notified us via email that they had no comments.

In its comments, SSA stated that it provided information to Congress on measurable milestones, designated senior officials, and accountability mechanisms in its AFR. In the report, we acknowledge that these types of additional information are similar to information that agencies are required to provide to Congress or OMB in other reports, such as annual AFRs. However, our analysis was based on SSA's fiscal year 2016 notifications to Congress for programs reported as noncompliant under IPERA, in which this specific information was not reported. As such, we continue to believe that OMB should take steps to update OMB guidance to help ensure that agencies report such significant information and include it in their notifications to Congress.

We are sending copies of this chapter to the appropriate congressional committees, the Director of the Office of Management and Budget, and other interested parties.

Beryl H. Davis
Director
Financial Management and Assurance

APPENDIX I: OBJECTIVES, SCOPE, AND METHODOLOGY

Our objectives were to determine the following:

1. The extent to which the 24 agencies listed in the Chief Financial Officers Act of 1990, as amended (CFO Act),[35] complied with the six criteria listed in the Improper Payments Elimination and Recovery Act of 2010 (IPERA),[36] for fiscal years 2016 and 2017, and the trends evident since 2011, as reported by their inspectors general (IG).
2. The extent to which CFO Act agencies addressed requirements for programs and activities reported as noncompliant with IPERA criteria for 3 or more consecutive

[35] The CFO Act, Pub. L. No. 101-576 104 Stat. 2838 (Nov. 15, 1990), established, among other things, chief financial officers to oversee financial management activities at 23 major executive departments and agencies. The list now includes 24 entities, which are often referred to collectively as CFO Act agencies, and is codified, as amended, in section 901 of Title 31, United States Code.

[36] Pub. L. No. 111-204, 124 Stat. 2224 (July 22, 2010), *codified as amended at* 31 U.S.C. § 3321 note.

years, as of fiscal year 2016, and communicated their strategies to Congress for reducing improper payments and achieving compliance.

3. The extent to which the Office of Management and Budget (OMB) made determinations regarding whether additional funding would help CFO Act programs and activities reported as noncompliant with IPERA criteria for 2 consecutive years, as of fiscal years 2016 and 2017, come into compliance.

Although the responsibility for complying with provisions of improper payment-related statutes rests with the head of each executive agency, we focused on the 24 agencies listed in the CFO Act because estimates of their improper payments represent over 99 percent of the total reported estimated improper payments for fiscal years 2016 and 2017. Our work did not include validating or retesting the data or methodologies that the IGs used to determine and report compliance. We corroborated all of our findings with OMB and all 24 CFO Act agencies and IGs.

To address our first objective, we identified the requirements that agencies must meet by reviewing the Improper Payments Information Act of 2002 (IPIA),[37] IPERA, and OMB guidance. We reviewed the CFO Act agency IGs' IPERA compliance reports for fiscal years 2016 and 2017, which were the most current reports available at the time of our review.

We summarized the overall agency and program-specific compliance determinations with the six IPERA criteria, as reported by the IGs. For fiscal years 2011 through 2015, we relied on and reviewed prior year supporting documentation and analyses of CFO Act agencies' IPERA compliance, as reported in our prior reports, in order to identify compliance trends since 2011, as reported by the IGs.[38] Based on these reports, we summarized the programs and the number of consecutive years that they were reported as noncompliant. For each IG report that did not specifically state that the agency had programs noncompliant for consecutive years, we compared the list of programs reported as noncompliant for fiscal years 2016 and 2017 to the list of programs reported as noncompliant for fiscal years 2014 and 2015 in our prior reports. Lastly, we corroborated our findings with OMB and all 24 CFO Act agencies and IGs.

To address our second objective, we determined if the agencies responsible for programs and activities reported as noncompliant for 3 or more consecutive years as of fiscal year 2016 had submitted the required proposals (reauthorizations or statutory changes) to Congress by requesting and reviewing documentation of the required submissions and relevant notifications to Congress obtained from each applicable agency. Further, we reviewed the content of each agency notification to evaluate agencies' efforts to communicate quality information to Congress concerning their strategies for achieving compliance consistent with *Standards for Internal Control in the Federal Government*.[39] Principle 15 of these standards emphasizes the need for an entity's management to communicate necessary quality information,

[37] Pub. L. No. 107-300, 116 Stat. 2350 (Nov. 26, 2002), *codified as amended at* 31 U.S.C. § 3321 note.

[38] GAO, *Improper Payments: CFO Act Agencies Need to Improve Efforts to Address Compliance Issues*, GAO-16-554 (Washington, D.C.: June 30, 2016), and *Improper Payments: Additional Guidance Could Provide More Consistent Compliance Determinations and Reporting by Inspectors General*, GAO-17-484 (Washington, D.C.: May 31, 2017).

[39] GAO, *Standards for Internal Control in the Federal Government*, GAO-14-704G (Washington, D.C.: September 2014).

such as significant matters related to risks, changes, or issues affecting agencies' efforts, to achieve compliance objectives, to external parties—such as legislators, oversight bodies, and the general public. To identify other types of information useful for this purpose, we reviewed IPIA, as amended; IPERA; and OMB guidance for information agencies are required to provide to Congress or OMB in other notifications and reports, such as their corrective action plans or strategies, measurable milestones, designated senior officials, and accountability mechanisms for achieving compliance. We also reviewed information used to assess agency efforts to address issues associated with programs on our High-Risk List.[40]

To determine the extent to which agencies' notifications to Congress included these additional types of useful information for their applicable program(s), we used a data collection instrument to document our determinations regarding the additional types of quality information included in each notification. In addition, two GAO analysts independently reviewed each agency's notification and documented their determinations regarding the types of information included in the notifications. Differences between the analysts' determinations were identified and resolved to ensure that the types of additional information were consistently identified and categorized. We did not evaluate the sufficiency and completeness of the agency-provided information. Lastly, we corroborated our findings with the respective agencies and IGs.

To address our third objective, we identified provisions in IPIA, IPERA, and OMB guidance that are applicable to OMB for programs reported as noncompliant for 2 consecutive years.[41] To determine if OMB made additional funding determinations for agency programs and activities reported as noncompliant for 2 consecutive years as of fiscal years 2016 and 2017, we requested relevant information and communications from OMB and the applicable agencies and IGs. We also interviewed key OMB staff on their process for determining additional funding needs for noncompliant programs and activities as of fiscal years 2016 and 2017 and related results. In addition, we reviewed the applicable fiscal years 2016 and 2017 CFO Act agency IG IPERA compliance reports, which OMB staff stated they relied on for determining whether noncompliant programs and activities required additional funding. We also asked the agencies whether they coordinated with OMB regarding their need for additional funding for programs and activities reported as noncompliant for 2 consecutive years as of fiscal years 2016 and 2017. Lastly, we corroborated our findings with OMB and the respective agencies and IGs.

We conducted this performance audit from November 2017 to December 2018 in accordance with generally accepted government auditing standards. Those standards require that we plan and perform the audit to obtain sufficient, appropriate evidence to provide a reasonable basis for our findings and conclusions based on our audit objectives. We believe that the evidence obtained provides a reasonable basis for our findings and conclusions based on our audit objectives.

---

[40] [6]GAO, *High-Risk Series: Progress on Many High-Risk Areas, While Substantial Efforts Needed on Others*, GAO-17-317 (Washington, D.C.: February 2017).

[41] Office of Management and Budget, Appendix C to Circular No. A-123, Requirements for Effective Estimation and Remediation of Improper Payments, OMB Memorandum M-15- 02, and Appendix C to Circular No. A-123, Requirements for Payment Integrity Improvement, OMB Memorandum M-18-20.

APPENDIX II: CFO ACT AGENCIES' OVERALL IPERA COMPLIANCE FOR FISCAL YEARS 2011 THROUGH 2017, AS REPORTED OR ACKNOWLEDGED BY THEIR IGS

Figure 4 details the 24 Chief Financial Officers Act of 1990 (CFO Act) agencies' overall compliance under the Improper Payments Elimination and Recovery Act of 2010 (IPERA), as reported by their inspectors general, for fiscal years 2011 through 2017. We previously reported on CFO Act agencies' overall reported compliance for fiscal years 2011 through 2015.[42]

	Fiscal year							
Agency	2011	2012	2013	2014	2015	2016	2017	Number of years reported as noncompliant
Department of Agriculture	X	X	X	X	X	X	X	7
Department of Commerce	✓	✓	✓	✓	✓	✓	X	1
Department of Defense	✓	X	X	X	X	X	X	6
Department of Education	✓	✓	✓	X	X	X	X	4
Department of Energy	X	✓	✓	✓	✓	✓	✓	1
Department of Health and Human Services	X	X	X	X	X	X	X	7
Department of Homeland Security	X	X	X	X	X	X	X	7
Department of Housing and Urban Development	✓	✓	X	X	X	X	X	5
Department of the Interior	X	✓	✓	X	X	✓	✓	3
Department of Justice	✓	✓	✓	✓	✓	✓	✓	0
Department of Labor	X	X	X	X	X	X	X	7
Department of State	X	✓	✓	✓	✓	✓	✓	1
Department of Transportation	X	X	X	X	X	X	X	7
Department of the Treasury	X	X	X	X	X	X	X	7
Department of Veterans Affairs	X	X	X	X	X	X	X	7
Environmental Protection Agency	✓	X	✓	✓	✓	✓	✓	1
General Services Administration	✓	✓	✓	X	X	X	X	4
National Aeronautics and Space Administration	X	✓	✓	✓	✓	✓	✓	1
National Science Foundation	✓	X	NR	X	✓	✓	✓	2
Nuclear Regulatory Commission	✓	✓	✓	✓	✓	✓	✓	0
Office of Personnel Management	X	✓	✓	✓	X	✓	✓	2
Small Business Administration	X	X	X	X	X	X	X	7
Social Security Administration	X	X	X	X	X	X	X	7
U.S. Agency for International Development	✓	✓	✓	✓	✓	✓	✓	0
Total not reported	0	0	1	0	0	0	0	
Total compliant agencies	10	12	12	9	9	11	10	
Total noncompliant agencies	14	12	11	15	15	13	14	

✓ Compliant: IG reported compliance

X Noncompliant: IG reported noncompliance or acknowledged noncompliance after report was issued

NR Not reported: IG did not issue compliance report because agency did not publish improper payment information

CFO Act - Chief Financial Officers Act of 1990

IG - inspector general

IPERA - Improper Payments Elimination and Recovery Act of 2010

Source: GAO analysis of CFO agencies' IG PERA reports for fiscal years 2011 through 2017. | GAO-19-14.

Figure 4. CFO Act Agencies' Overall IPERA Compliance for Fiscal Years 2011 through 2017, as Reported or Acknowledged by Their Igs.

[42] GAO, Improper Payments: Additional Guidance Could Provide More Consistent Compliance Determinations and Reporting by Inspectors General, GAO-17-484 (Washington, D.C.: May 31, 2017).

Appendix III: CFO Act Agencies and Programs Reported as Noncompliant with IPERA for Fiscal Years 2016 and 2017

Tables 5 and 6 detail the Chief Financial Officers Act of 1990 (CFO Act) agencies and programs reported by their inspectors general as noncompliant with the six criteria specified by the Improper Payments Elimination and Recovery Act of 2010 (IPERA), for fiscal years 2016 and 2017. We previously reported on CFO Act agencies' reported compliance with the six IPERA criteria for fiscal year 2015.[43]

Table 5. CFO Act Agency Programs That IGs Reported as Noncompliant with IPERA Criteria for Fiscal Year 2016

Agencies and programs	Published information in PAR/AFR	Conducted program-specific risk assessment(s)	Published estimate(s)	Published corrective action plan(s)	Published and met reduction target(s)	Reported rate(s) below 10 percent
U.S. Department of Agriculture						
1. Food and Nutrition Service (FNS) Supplemental Nutrition Assistance Program	*	*	X	*	*	*
2. FNS Child and Adult Care Food Program	*	*	X	*	*	*
3. FNS National School Lunch Program	*	*	*	*	X	X
4. FNS School Breakfast Program	*	*	*	*	X	X
5. FNS Special Supplemental Nutrition Program for Women, Infants, and Children	*	*	*	*	X	*
6. Farm Service Agency (FSA) Loan Deficiency Payment	*	*	*	*	X	*
7. FSA Livestock Forage Disaster Program	*	*	*	*	X	*
8. FSA Livestock Indemnity Program	*	*	*	*	X	X

[43] GAO, Improper Payments: Additional Guidance Could Provide More Consistent Compliance Determinations and Reporting by Inspectors General, GAO-17-484 (Washington, D.C.: May 31, 2017).

Agencies and programs	Published information in PAR/AFR	Conducted program-specific risk assessment(s)	Published estimate(s)	Published corrective action plan(s)	Published and met reduction target(s)	Reported rate(s) below 10 percent
9. FSA Supplemental Revenue Assistance Payments	*	*	*	*	X	X
Department of Defense[a]						
10. Navy Commercial Bill Pay Office - Naples	X	*	*	X	*	*
11. Defense Finance and Accounting Service Commercial Pay	X	*	*	X	*	*
12. U.S. Army Corps of Engineers Travel Pay	X	*	X	X	X	*
13. Military Health Benefits	X	*	*	X	*	*
14. Military Pay	X	*	*	X	*	*
15. Civilian Pay	X	*	*	X	*	*
16. Military Retiree and Annuitant Benefit Payments	X	*	*	X	*	*
17. Travel Pay	X	*	X	X	X	*
18. Navy Enterprise Resource Planning Commercial Pay	X	*	*	X	*	*
19. Navy Commercial Bill Pay Office - Singapore	X	X	*	*	*	*
Department of Education						
20. Pell Grant	*	*	*	*	X	*
21. Department-managed grant programs	*	X	*	*	*	*
22. Federal Student Aid - managed contracting activities	*	X	*	*	*	*
23. Direct Loan	*	*	*	*	X	*
Department of Health and Human Services						
24. Temporary Assistance for Needy Families (TANF)[b]	*	*	X	X	X	X
25. Medicaid	*	*	*	*	*	X

Table 5. (Continued)

Agencies and programs	Published information in PAR/AFR	Conducted program-specific risk assessment(s)	Published estimate(s)	Published corrective action plan(s)	Published and met reduction target(s)	Reported rate(s) below 10 percent
26. Children's Health Insurance Program	*	*	*	*	X	*
27. Foster Care	*	*	*	*	X	*
28. Medicare Advantage (Part C)	*	*	*	*	X	*
29. Medicare Fee-for-Service (Parts A and B)	*	*	*	*	*	X
Department of Homeland Security						
30. U.S. Customs and Border Protection -Refund & Drawback	*	*	*	*	X	*
31. Federal Emergency Management Agency (FEMA) - Assistance to Firefighters Grant	*	*	*	*	X	*
32. FEMA -Flood Risk Map-Flood Hazard Mapping & Risk Analysis	*	*	*	*	X	*
33. FEMA -Public Assistance	*	*	*	*	X	*
34. FEMA -Port Security Grant Program	*	*	*	*	X	*
35. FEMA -Vendor Pay	*	*	*	*	X	*
36. Office of Inspector General - Hurricane Sandy Payroll & Travel	*	*	*	*	X	*
37. FEMA -Federal Insurance and Mitigation Administration - Non Claims Loss Payments	X	*	*	*	*	*
38. FEMA -Flood Risk Map Program – Grants	X	*	*	*	*	*
39. Non Disaster Relief Fund Travel	X	*	*	*	*	*

Agencies and programs	Published information in PAR/AFR	Conducted program-specific risk assessment(s)	Published estimate(s)	Published corrective action plan(s)	Published and met reduction target(s)	Reported rate(s) below 10 percent
Department of Housing and Urban Development						
40. Rental Housing Assistance Programs	*	*	*	*	X	*
41. Government National Mortgage Association programsc	*	X	*	*	*	*
42. Payments to Federal employees for all program offices	*	X	*	*	*	*
43. Federal Housing Administration (FHA) Single Family Notes	*	X	*	*	*	*
44. FHA -Other Disbursements	*	X	*	*	*	*
Department of Labor						
45. Unemployment Insurance Benefit	*	*	*	*	X	X
46. Federal Employees' Compensation Act	*	*	*	*	X	*
Department of Transportation						
47. Federal Aviation Administration Facilities and Equipment - Disaster Relief Appropriations Act	*	*	*	*	X	*
48. Federal Railroad Administration's High-Speed Intercity Passenger Rail	*	*	*	*	X	*
49. Federal Transit Administration's Formula Grants and Passenger Rail Investment and Improvement Act	*	*	*	*	X	*
Department of the Treasury						
50. Earned Income Tax Credit	*	*	*	*	*	X
Department of Veterans Affairs						
51. Civilian Health and Medical Program of the Department of Veterans Affairs	*	*	*	*	X	*

Table 5. (Continued)

Agencies and programs	Published information in PAR/AFR	Conducted program-specific risk assessment(s)	Published estimate(s)	Published corrective action plan(s)	Published and met reduction target(s)	Reported rate(s) below 10 percent
52. Community Care	*	*	*	*	X	X
53.Purchased Long Term Service and Support	*	*	*	*	X	X
54. Beneficiary Travel	*	*	*	*	X	*
55.Supplies and Materials	*	*	*	*	X	*
56. State Home Per Diem Grants	*	*	*	*	X	*
General Services Administration						
57. Rental of Space Program	*	*	*	*	X	*
Small Business Administration						
58. Section 7(a) Loan Guaranty Purchases	*	*	*	*	X	*
59.Disbursements for Goods and Services	*	*	*	*	*	X
Social Security Administration						
60. Supplemental Security Income	*	*	*	*	X	*
61.Old-Age, Survivors, and Disability Insurance	*	*	*	*	X	*
Total agencies noncompliant with criterion (marked X)	2	3	3	2	12	6
Total noncompliant programs as of fiscal year 2016	13	7	5	10	38	12

Source: GAO analysis of CFO Act agencies' IG IPERA compliance reports for fiscal year 2016. | GAO-19-14.

[a] The Department of Defense (DOD) published the Improper Payment and Payment Recapture Programs section of its fiscal year 2016 AFR on November 15, 2016. However, it did not publish the AFR by March 1, 2017; therefore, the DOD IG determined the agency to be noncompliant with this IPERA criterion, as reported in the fiscal year 2016 IPERA compliance report.

[b] The Department of Health and Human Services (HHS) does not agree with its IG's assessment of 2 criteria for the TANF program—published and met reduction target(s) and reported rate(s) below 10 percent—which were reported by HHS IG as noncompliant for fiscal year 2016.

[c] The Department of Housing and Urban Development does not agree with its IG's assessment of the criterion to conduct program-specific risk assessments for the Government National Mortgage Association (Ginnie Mae) programs. The agency stated that although some of Ginnie Mae's programs were noncompliant with this criterion in fiscal year 2016, not all of its programs were noncompliant.

Legend: X = Program was noncompliant with IPERA criterion, as reported by the agency's IG. * = IG did not report the program as noncompliant with IPERA criterion. AFR = agency financial report. CFO Act = Chief Financial Officers Act of 1990. IG = inspector general. IPERA = Improper Payments Elimination and Recovery Act of 2010. PAR = performance and accountability report

Table 6. CFO Act Agency Programs That IGs Reported as Noncompliant with IPERA Criteria for Fiscal Year 2017

Agencies and programs	Published information in PAR/AFR	Conducted program-specific risk assessment(s)	Published estimate(s)	Published corrective action plan(s)	Published and met reduction target(s)	Reported rate(s) below 10 percent
U.S. Department of Agriculture						
1. Farm Service Agency Noninsured Crop Disaster Assistance Program	*	*	*	*	X	*
2. Food and Nutrition Service (FNS) Supplemental Nutrition Assistance Program	*	*	X	*	*	*
3. FNS Child and Adult Care Food Program	*	*	X	*	*	*
U.S. Department of Agriculture						
4. FNS National School Lunch Program	*	*	*	*	X	X
5. FNS School Breakfast Program	*	*	*	*	X	X
6. FNS Special Supplemental Nutrition Program for Women, Infants, and Children	*	*	*	*	X	*
Department of Commerce						
7. Disaster Relief Appropriations Act	*	*	*	*	X	*
Department of Defense[a]						
8. U.S. Army Corps of Engineers (USACE) Commercial Pay	X	*	X	X	X	*
9. Navy Commercial Bill Pay Office - Naples	X	*	*	*	*	*
10. Defense Finance and Accounting Service Commercial Pay	X	*	X	*	*	*
11. USACE Travel Pay	X	*	*	*	X	*
12. Military Health Benefits	X	*	X	X	*	*
13. Military Pay	X	*	*	X	*	*
14. Civilian Pay	X	*	*	*	*	*
15. Military Retiree and Annuitant Benefit Payments	X	*	*	X	X	*
16. Travel Pay	X	*	X	X	X	*
Department of Education						
17. Pell Grant	*	*	*	*	X	*
Department of Health and Human Services						
18. Temporary Assistance for Needy Families	*	*	X	X	*	*
19. Medicaid	*	*	*	*	X	X
20. Children's Health Insurance Program	*	*	*	*	X	*
21. Foster Care	*	*	*	*	X	*
Department of Homeland Security						
22. U.S. Customs and Border Protection Refund & Drawback	*	*	*	*	X	*
23. U.S. Coast Guard Acquisition, Construction, and Improvement and Operating Expense: Hurricane Sandy Disbursements	*	*	*	*	X	*
Department of Housing and Urban Development						
24. Rental Housing Assistance Programs	*	*	X	*	*	*

Table 6. (Continued)

Agencies and programs	Published information in PAR/AFR	Conducted program-specific risk assessment(s)	Published estimate(s)	Published corrective action plan(s)	Published and met reduction target(s)	Reported rate(s) below 10 percent
25. Community Development Block Grant entitlement grant	*	*	X	*	*	*
26. Federal Housing Administration Single Family Insurance Claims Program	*	*	X	*	*	*
27. Disaster -Federal Emergency Management Agency, Disaster Housing Assistance Program	*	X	*	*	*	*
28. U.S. Department of Transportation Surface Transportation Project	*	X	*	*	*	*
29. HOME Investment Partnerships Program (HOME)	*	X	X	*	*	*
30. Housing Trust Fund	*	X	*	*	*	*
31. Hurricane Ike, Other Disasters	*	X	*	*	*	*
32. Self-Help and Assistance Homeownership	*	X	*	*	*	*
33. Master Subservicer Default Activity	*	X	*	*	*	*
34. American Recovery and Reinvestment Act - Energy and Green Retrofit Loan Financing	*	X	*	*	*	*
35. Emergency Home Loan Program (EHLP)	*	X	*	*	*	*
36. EHLP -Direct Loan Financing Account	*	X	*	*	*	*
37. Homeownership and Rental Housing Solutions Grant Assistance, Section 236	*	X	*	*	*	*
38. Housing Counseling	*	X	*	*	*	*
39. Housing for Special Populations - Capital Advance Portion of Expenditures, Section 202	*	X	*	*	*	*
40. Housing for the Elderly and Handicapped	*	X	*	*	*	*
Department of Labor						
41. Unemployment Insurance Benefit	*	*	*	*	X	X
Department of Transportation						
42. Federal Transit Administration Emergency Relief Program - Disaster Relief Appropriations Act, 2013 (DRAA) Program	*	*	*	*	X	*
43. Office of Inspector General DRAA Activity	*	*	*	*	X	*
Department of the Treasury						
44. Earned Income Tax Credit	*	*	*	*	*	X
Department of Veterans Affairs						
45. Civilian Health and Medical Program of the Department of Veterans Affairs	*	*	*	*	X	*
46. Community Care	*	*	*	*	X	X
47. Purchased Long Term Service and Support	*	*	*	*	X	X
48. Beneficiary Travel	*	*	*	*	X	X
49. Supplies and Materials	*	*	*	*	X	X
50. Communications, Utilities, and Other Rents	*	*	*	*	*	X

Agencies and programs	Published information in PAR/AFR	Conducted program-specific risk assessment(s)	Published estimate(s)	Published corrective action plan(s)	Published and met reduction target(s)	Reported rate(s) below 10 percent
51. Prosthetics	*	*	*	*	*	X
52. Post-9/11 GI Bill	*	*	*	*	X	*
53. Pension	*	*	*	*	X	*
54. Medical Care Contracts and Agreements	*	*	*	*	*	X
General Services Administration						
55. Rental of Space Program	*	*	*	*	X	*
Small Business Administration						
56. Section 7(a) Loan Guaranty Purchases	*	*	*	*	X	*
57. Disaster Direct Loan Program	*	*	*	*	X	X
Social Security Administration						
58. Supplemental Security Income	*	*	*	*	X	*
Total agencies noncompliant with criterion (marked X)	1	1	4	2	12	6
Total noncompliant programs as of fiscal year 2017	9	14	11	6	29	13

Source: GAO analysis of CFO Act agencies' IG IPERA compliance reports for fiscal year 2017. | GAO-19-14.

[a] The Department of Defense (DOD) published a Payment Integrity section in its fiscal year 2017 AFR. However, it did not publish all required information; therefore, the DOD IG determined the agency to be noncompliant with this IPERA criterion, as reported in the fiscal year 2017 IPERA compliance report. Legend: X = Program was noncompliant with IPERA criterion, as reported by the agency's IG. * = IG did not report the program as noncompliant with IPERA criterion. AFR = agency financial report. CFO Act = Chief Financial Officers Act of 1990. IG = inspector general. IPERA = Improper Payments Elimination and Recovery Act of 2010. PAR = performance and accountability report

Appendix IV: CFO Act Agencies with Programs Reported by Their IGs as Noncompliant for 2 or More Consecutive Years, as of Fiscal Years 2016 and 2017

Table 7 details the Chief Financial Officers Act of 1990 (CFO Act) agencies and programs reported by their inspectors general as noncompliant under the Improper Payments Elimination and Recovery Act of 2010 (IPERA) for 2 or more consecutive years, as of fiscal years 2016 and 2017. We previously reported on CFO Act agencies' reported compliance for fiscal year 2015.[44]

Table 7. CFO Act Agencies and Programs Reported or Acknowledged by Their IGs as Noncompliant for 2 or More Consecutive Years, as of Fiscal Years 2016 and 2017

		Consecutive years of reported noncompliance as of fiscal year	
Agencies	**Noncompliant programs**	**2016**	**2017**
U.S. Department of Agriculture	Food and Nutrition Service (FNS) Supplemental Nutrition Assistance Program	2	3
	Farm Service Agency (FSA) Livestock Forage Disaster Program	2	NA
	FSA Supplemental Revenue Assistance Payments	2	NA
U.S. Department of Agriculture	FNS Child and Adult Care Food Program	6	7

[44] GAO, Improper Payments: Additional Guidance Could Provide More Consistent Compliance Determinations and Reporting by Inspectors General, GAO-17-484 (Washington, D.C.: May 31, 2017).

Table 7. (Continued)

		Consecutive years of reported noncompliance as of fiscal year	
Agencies	**Noncompliant programs**	**2016**	**2017**
U.S. Department of Agriculture	FNS National School Lunch Program	6	7
	FNS School Breakfast Program	6	7
	FNS Special Supplemental Nutrition Program for Women, Infants, and Children	6	7
Department of Defense	Defense Finance and Accounting Service Commercial Pay	1	2
	Civilian Pay	1	2
	Military Health Benefits	1	2
	Military Pay	1	2
	Military Retiree and Annuitant Benefit Payments	1	2
	U.S. Army Corps of Engineers Travel Pay	1	2
	Navy Commercial Bill Pay Office - Naples	1	2
	Travel Pay	5	6
Department of Education	Pell Grant	1	2
	Direct Loan	3	NA
Department of Health and Human Services	Foster Care	1	2
	Medicare Advantage (Part C)	2	NA
	Children's Health Insurance Program	2	3
	Medicaid	3	4
	Medicare Fee-for-Service (Parts A and B)	5	NA
	Temporary Assistance for Needy Families	6	7
Department of Homeland Security	U.S. Customs and Border Protection Refund & Drawback	2	3
	Federal Emergency Management Agency (FEMA) - Assistance to Firefighters Grant	2	NA
	FEMA - Public Assistance	3	NA
	FEMA - Vendor Pay	3	NA
Department of Housing and Urban Development	Government National Mortgage Association programs[a]	2	NA
	Rental Housing Assistance Programs	2	3
Department of Labor	Unemployment Insurance Benefit	6	7
Department of the Treasury	Earned Income Tax Credit	6	7
Department of Veterans Affairs	Civilian Health and Medical Program of the Department of Veterans Affairs	1	2
	Community Care	2	3
	Purchased Long Term Service and Support	2	3
	Beneficiary Travel	2	3
	Supplies and Materials	2	3
Small Business Administration	Section 7(a) Loan Guaranty Purchases	1	2
	Disbursements for Goods and Services	2	NA
General Services Administration	Rental of Space Program	1	2
Social Security Administration	Old-Age, Survivors, and Disability Insurance	2	NA
	Supplemental Security Income	6	7
Total programs reported noncompliant for 2 consecutive years, as of fiscal years 2016 and 2017		15	12
Total programs reported noncompliant for 3 or more consecutive years, as of fiscal years 2016 and 2017		14	18

Source: GAO analysis of CFO Act agencies' IG IPERA compliance reports for fiscal years 2016 and 2017. | GAO-19-14.

[a] The Department of Housing and Urban Development does not agree with its IG's reporting of the Government National Mortgage Association programs as noncompliant for 2 consecutive years, as of fiscal year 2016. Legend: CFO Act = Chief Financial Officers Act of 1990. IG = inspector general. IPERA = Improper Payments Elimination and Recovery Act of 2010. NA = Not applicable because IGs did not report program as noncompliant as of fiscal year 2016 or noncompliant as of fiscal year 2017.

Appendix V: Comments from the Department of Homeland Security Office of Inspector General

OFFICE OF INSPECTOR GENERAL
Department of Homeland Security

Washington, DC 20528 / www.oig.dhs.gov

October 25, 2018

Beryl Davis
Director, Financial Management and Assurance
U.S. Government Accountability Office
441 G Street, NW,
Washington, DC 20226

Dear Ms. Davis:

Thank you for the opportunity to review and comment on the draft report, "Improper Payments – *Additional Guidance Needed to Improve Oversight of Agencies with Noncompliant Programs.*" The Department of Homeland Security (DHS) Office of Inspector General appreciates the Government Accountability Office's work to review agencies' compliance under the *Improper Payments Elimination and Recovery Act of 2010* (IPERA).

Through our audits and recommendations, the Department has improved its processes and procedures and implemented more effective internal controls to reduce improper payments. As your office reported, DHS properly notified Congress of its programs' noncompliance for 3 or more consecutive years as of FY 2016 as required by IPERA and Office of Management and Budget guidance. Through DHS' continued hard work, all of these programs met their reduction targets in FY 2017 and are now compliant. As of FY 2017, U.S. Customs and Border Protection - Refund and Drawback is the only DHS program non-compliant for 3 consecutive years.

Sincerely,

Sondra F. McCauley
Assistant Inspector General for Audits

Appendix VI: Comments from the Social Security Administration

SOCIAL SECURITY
Office of the Commissioner

October 31, 2018

Ms. Beryl Davis
Director, Financial Management and Assurance
United States Government Accountability Office
441 G Street, NW
Washington, DC 20548

Dear Ms. Davis:

Thank you for the opportunity to review the draft report, "IMPROPER PAYMENTS: Additional Guidance Needed to Improve Oversight of Agencies with Noncompliant Programs" (GAO-19-14). We support the finding that we notified Congress of three or more consecutive years of noncompliance under the Improper Payments Elimination and Recovery Act (IPERA) of 2010 for fiscal years (FY) 2016 and 2017 because we did not meet our reduction targets for the Supplemental Security Income (SSI) program.

In your report, you indicated that we provided some additional information to Congress, along with four other agencies, but did not include measurable milestones, designated senior officials, or accountability mechanisms. We did in fact provide this information and addressed each in our Agency Financial Report as follows.

- Measurable Milestones – We conduct Continuing Disability Reviews and SSI redeterminations and identified these workloads as measurable milestones to address improper payments. Our annual budget determines these workload volumes.
- Designated Senior Officials – We designated the Chair of our Improper Payments Oversight Board as our Senior Official.
- Accountability Mechanisms – Effective in FY 2012, as required by IPERA, we hold managers, program officials, and senior executives accountable for reducing improper payments. For these employees, their annual performance plans reflect their responsibility to support efforts to maintain sufficient internal controls to prevent, detect, and recover improper payments and meet targets to reduce improper payments. Rating officials hold these employees accountable for the content of their performance plans.

Sincerely,

Stephanie Hall

Stephanie Hall
Acting Deputy Chief of Staff

SOCIAL SECURITY ADMINISTRATION BALTIMORE, MD 21235-0001

APPENDIX VII: COMMENTS FROM THE UNITED STATES AGENCY FOR INTERNATIONAL DEVELOPMENT

USAID
FROM THE AMERICAN PEOPLE

Beryl Davis
Director, Financial Management and Assurance
U.S. Government Accountability Office
441 G Street, NW
Washington, DC 20226

Re: Draft Report "GAO-19-14 (Code 102476) Improper Payments, Additional Guidance Needed to Improve Oversight of Agencies with Noncompliant Programs"

Dear Ms. Davis:

I am pleased to provide the United States Agency for International Development's (USAID) formal response to the draft report of the U. S. Government Accountability Office (GAO) entitled, *"Improper Payments, Additional Guidance Needed to Improve Oversight of Agencies with Noncompliant Programs"*.

USAID is proud to be one of only three Federal Departments and Agencies identified in the report as having complied with all reporting requirements that concern improper payments from Fiscal Year (FY) 2011 through FY 2017. This record of compliance has significant, since the Office of the Inspector General audits and verifies it annually.

USAID has a rigorous payment process supported by extensive core financial-system and procedural controls which has led to a consistently low rate of erroneous payments. As a result, the Office of Management and Budget granted USAID relief from related reporting requirements for three years, starting with the FY 2015 Agency Financial Report. Even with this relief, USAID has maintained our readiness and expertise in finding and reporting on improper payments by continuing to perform risk assessments annually to identify programs that could be susceptible to significant improper payments. In the FY 2018 Agency Financial Report, USAID will again publish our improper payments rate, which will demonstrate our continued prudent and diligent stewardship of taxpayer dollars.

Thank you for the opportunity to respond to your draft report, and for the courtesies extended by your staff while conducting this engagement. We appreciate the opportunity to participate in the evaluation of our compliance with IPERA.

Sincerely,

Angelique M. Crumbly
Acting Assistant Administrator
Bureau for Management

In: Top 10 Reports and Testimonies in December 2018
Editor: Sarah J. Nygaard
ISBN: 978-1-53615-507-5

Chapter 5

INFORMATION SECURITY: AGENCIES NEED TO IMPROVE IMPLEMENTATION OF FEDERAL APPROACH TO SECURING SYSTEMS AND PROTECTING AGAINST INTRUSIONS*

United States Government Accountability Office

ABBREVIATIONS

BOD	Binding Operational Directive
CAP	Cross-Agency Priority
CDM	Continuous Diagnostics and Mitigation
CFO	Chief Financial Officer
CIO	Chief Information Officer
CSIP	*Cybersecurity Strategy and Implementation Plan*
DEFEND	Dynamic and Evolving Federal Enterprise Network Defense
DHS	Department of Homeland Security
DNS	Domain Name System
FISMA	*Federal Information Security Modernization Act*
IG	Inspectors General
IPv6	Internet Protocol Version 6
NCPS	National Cybersecurity Protection System
NSD	Network Security Deployment
NIST	National Institute of Standards and Technology
OMB	Office of Management and Budget
SCADA	Supervisory Control and Data Acquisition
SIEM	Security Information and Event Management
SP	Special Publication

* This is an edited, reformatted and augmented version of United States Government Accountability Office; Report to Congressional Committees, Publication No. GAO-19-105, dated December 2018.

TIC	Trusted Internet Connection
US-CERT	United States Computer Emergency Readiness Team

Why GAO Did This Study

Federal agencies are dependent on information systems to carry out operations. The risks to these systems are increasing as security threats evolve and become more sophisticated. To reduce the risk of a successful cyberattack, agencies can deploy intrusion detection and prevention capabilities on their networks and systems.

GAO first designated federal information security as a government-wide high-risk area in 1997. In 2015, GAO expanded this area to include protecting the privacy of personally identifiable information. Most recently, in September 2018, GAO updated the area to identify 10 critical actions that the federal government and other entities need to take to address major cybersecurity challenges.

The federal approach and strategy for securing information systems is grounded in the provisions of the *Federal Information Security Modernization Act of 2014* and Executive Order 13800. The act requires agencies to develop, document, and implement an agency-wide program to secure their information systems. The Executive Order, issued in May 2017, directs agencies to use the National Institute of Standards and Technology's cybersecurity framework to manage cybersecurity risks.

The *Federal Cybersecurity Enhancement Act of 2015* contained a provision for GAO to report on the effectiveness of the government's approach and strategy for securing its systems. GAO determined (1) the reported effectiveness of agencies' implementation of the government's approach and strategy; (2) the extent to which DHS and OMB have taken steps to facilitate the use of intrusion detection and prevention capabilities to secure federal systems; and (3) the extent to which agencies reported implementing capabilities to detect and prevent intrusions.

To address these objectives, GAO analyzed OMB reports related to agencies' information security practices including OMB's annual report to Congress for fiscal year 2017. GAO also analyzed and summarized agency-reported security performance metrics and IG-reported information for the 23 civilian CFO Act agencies. In addition, GAO evaluated plans, reports, and other documents related to DHS intrusion detection and prevention programs, and interviewed OMB, DHS, and agency officials.

What GAO Recommends

GAO is making two recommendations to DHS, to among other things, coordinate with agencies to identify additional needs for training and guidance. GAO is also making seven recommendations to OMB to, among other things, direct the Federal CIO to update the mandated report with required information, such as detecting advanced persistent threats. DHS concurred with GAO's recommendations. OMB did not indicate whether it concurred with the recommendations or not.

What GAO Found

The 23 civilian agencies covered by the *Chief Financial Officers Act of 1990* (CFO Act) have often not effectively implemented the federal government's approach and strategy for securing information systems (see figure below). Until agencies more effectively implement the government's approach and strategy, federal systems will remain at risk. To illustrate:

- As required by Office of Management and Budget (OMB), inspectors general (IGs) evaluated the maturity of their agencies' information security programs using performance measures associated with the five core security functions—identify, protect, detect, respond, and recover. The IGs at 17 of the 23 agencies reported that their agencies' programs were not effectively implemented.
- IGs also evaluated information security controls as part of the annual audit of their agencies' financial statements, identifying material weaknesses or significant deficiencies in internal controls for financial reporting at 17 of the 23 civilian CFO Act agencies.
- Chief information officers (CIOs) for 17 of the 23 agencies reported not meeting all elements of the government's cybersecurity cross-agency priority goal. The goal was intended to improve cybersecurity performance through, among other things, maintaining ongoing awareness of information security, vulnerabilities, and threats; and implementing technologies and processes that reduce malware risk.
- Executive Order 13800 directed OMB, in coordination with the Department of Homeland Security (DHS), to assess and report on the sufficiency and appropriateness of federal agencies' processes for managing cybersecurity risks. Using performance measures for each of the five core security functions, OMB determined that 13 of the 23 agencies were managing overall enterprise risks, while the other 10 agencies were at risk. In assessing agency risk by core security function, OMB identified a few agencies to be at high risk (see figure at the top of next page).

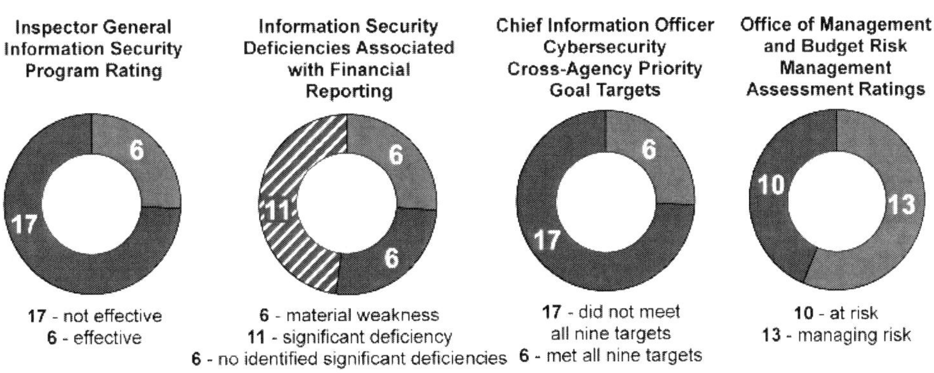

Source: GAO analysis of agency fiscal year 2017 Federal Information Security Modernization Act of 2014 and agency financial reports for fiscal year 2017. | GAO-19-105.

Fiscal Year 2017 Indicators of the 23 Selected Civilian Agencies' Effectiveness in Implementing the Federal Approach and Strategy for Securing Information Systems.

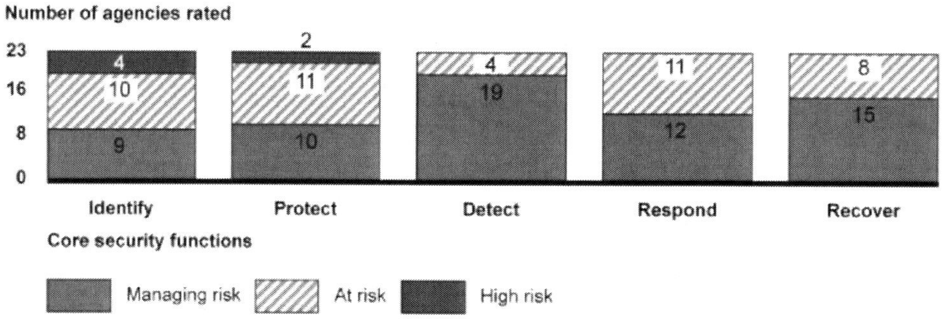

Source: GAO analysis of Office of Management and Budget Fiscal Year 2017 Federal Information Security Modernization Act of 2014 Annual Report to Congress. | GAO-19-105.

Risk Management Assessment Ratings by Core Security Function for the 23 Civilian *Chief Financial Officers Act of 1990* Agencies, Fiscal Year 2017.

DHS and OMB facilitated the use of intrusion detection and prevention capabilities to secure federal agency systems, but further efforts remain. For example, in response to prior GAO recommendations, DHS had improved the capabilities of the National Cybersecurity Protection System (NCPS), which is intended to detect and prevent malicious traffic from entering agencies' computer networks. However, the system still had limitations, such as not having the capability to scan encrypted traffic. The department was also in the process of enhancing the capabilities of federal agencies to automate network monitoring for malicious activity through its Continuous Diagnostics and Mitigation (CDM) program. However, the program was running behind schedule and officials at most agencies indicated the need for additional training and guidance. Further, the Federal CIO issued a mandated report assessing agencies' intrusion detection and prevention capabilities, but the report did not address required information, such as the capability of NCPS to detect advanced persistent threats, and a cost/benefit comparison of capabilities to commercial technologies and tools.

Selected agencies had not consistently implemented capabilities to detect and prevent intrusions into their computer networks. Specifically, the agencies told GAO that they had not fully implemented required actions for protecting email, cloud services, host-based systems, and network traffic from malicious activity. For example, 21 of 23 agencies had not, as of September 2018, sufficiently enhanced email protection through implementation of DHS' directive on enhanced email security. In addition, less than half of the agencies that use cloud services reported monitoring these services. Further, most of the selected 23 agencies had not fully implemented the tools and services available through the first two phases of DHS's CDM program. Until agencies more thoroughly implement capabilities to detect and prevent intrusions, federal systems and the information they process will be vulnerable to malicious threats.

December 18, 2018

The Honorable Ron Johnson
Chairman

The Honorable Claire McCaskill
Ranking Member
Committee on Homeland Security and Governmental Affairs
United States Senate

The Honorable Michael McCaul
Chairman

The Honorable Bennie G. Thompson Ranking Member
Committee on Homeland Security
House of Representatives

Federal agencies are dependent on computerized (cyber) information systems and electronic data to carry out operations and to process, maintain, and report essential information. Virtually all federal operations are supported by computer systems and electronic data, and agencies would find it difficult, if not impossible, to carry out their missions and account for their resources without these information assets. Hence, the security of these systems and data is vital to public confidence and the nation's safety, prosperity, and well-being. Further, many of these systems contain vast amounts of personally identifiable information,[1] thus, making it imperative to protect the confidentiality, integrity, and availability of this information and effectively respond to data breaches and security incidents when they occur.

The risks to information systems supporting the federal government are increasing as security threats continue to evolve and become more sophisticated. These risks include escalating and emerging threats from around the globe, steady advances in the sophistication of attack technology, and the emergence of new and more destructive attacks.

Compounding these risks, computer networks and systems used by federal agencies are often riddled with security vulnerabilities—both known and unknown. These systems are often interconnected with other internal and external systems and networks, including the Internet, thereby increasing the number of avenues of attack and expanding their attack surface.

Our previous reports, and those by federal inspectors general, describe persistent information security weaknesses that place federal agencies at risk of disruption or inappropriate disclosure of sensitive information. Accordingly, GAO made more than 3,000 recommendations to agencies since 2010 aimed at addressing cybersecurity shortcomings. Although many of these recommendations have been addressed, approximately 700 had not been implemented as of November 2018.

The federal approach and strategy for securing information systems is grounded in the provisions of the *Federal Information Security Modernization Act of 2014* (FISMA)[2] and

[1] Personally identifiable information is any information that can be used to distinguish or trace an individual's identity, such as name, date and place of birth, or Social Security number, and other types of personal information that can be linked to an individual, such as medical, educational, financial, and employment information.

[2] The *Federal Information Security Modernization Act of 2014* (FISMA 2014), enacted as Pub. L. No. 113-283, 128 Stat. 3073 (Dec. 18, 2014), largely superseded the *Federal Information Security Management Act of 2002* (FISMA 2002), enacted as *Title III, E-Government Act of 2002*, Pub. L. No. 107-347, 116 Stat. 2899, 2946

Executive Order 13800.[3] FISMA requires agencies to develop, document, and implement an agency-wide information security program to secure federal information systems, and assigns oversight responsibilities to the Department of Homeland Security (DHS) and the Office of Management and Budget (OMB). The executive order establishes a policy for managing cybersecurity risk and directs agencies to use the National Institute of Standards and Technology (NIST) cybersecurity framework[4] to manage these risks.

GAO first designated federal information security as a government-wide high-risk area almost 22 years ago in 1997.[5] In 2003,[6] we expanded this area to include computerized systems supporting the nation's critical infrastructure and, in 2015,[7] we further expanded this area to include protecting the privacy of personally identifiable information. We continued to identify federal information security as a government-wide high-risk area in our February 2017 high-risk update report.[8]

Most recently, in September 2018,[9] we provided an update to the information security high-risk area by identifying four major cybersecurity challenges facing the nation and 10 critical actions that the federal government and other entities needed to take to address them. These actions included developing and executing a more comprehensive federal strategy for national cybersecurity and global cyberspace. In this update, we noted that establishing a comprehensive cybersecurity strategy and performing effective oversight were a major challenge.

The *Federal Cybersecurity Enhancement Act of 2015*,[10] which was enacted December 18, 2015, included a provision for GAO to report on the effectiveness of the federal government's approach and strategy for securing agency information systems, including intrusion detection and prevention capabilities.[11] Our specific objectives were to assess: (1) the reported effectiveness of selected agencies' implementation of the federal government's approach and strategy to securing agency information systems; (2) the extent to which OMB and DHS have facilitated the use of intrusion detection and prevention capabilities to secure federal agency information systems; and (3) the extent to which selected agencies reported implementing capabilities to detect and prevent intrusions.

To address the first objective, we reviewed annual reports from OMB and the 23 civilian agencies covered by the *Chief Financial Officers Act of 1990* (CFO Act).[12] These reports

---

(Dec. 17, 2002). As used in this report, FISMA refers both to FISMA 2014 and to those provisions of FISMA 2002 that were either incorporated into FISMA 2014 or were unchanged and continue in full force and effect.

[3] The White House, *Strengthening the Cybersecurity of Federal Networks and Critical Infrastructure*, Executive Order 13800 (Washington, D.C.: May 11, 2017), 82 Fed. Reg. 22391 (May 16, 2017).

[4] National Institute of Standards and Technology, *Framework for Improving Critical Infrastructure Cybersecurity*, Version 1.1 (Gaithersburg, MD: Apr. 16, 2018).

[5] GAO, *High-Risk Series: An Overview*, GAO-HR-97-1 (Washington, D.C.: February 1997) and GAO, *High-Risk Series: Information Management and Technology*, GAO-HR-97-9 (Washington, D.C.: February 1997).

[6] GAO, *High Risk Series: An Update,* GAO-03-119 (Washington, D.C.: January 2003).

[7] GAO, *High-Risk Series: An Update,* GAO-15-290 (Washington, D.C.: Feb. 11, 2015).

[8] GAO, *High-Risk Series: Progress on Many High-Risk Areas, While Substantial Efforts Needed on Others,* GAO-17-317 (Washington, D.C.: Feb. 15, 2017).

[9] GAO, *High-Risk Series: Urgent Actions Are Needed to Address Cybersecurity Challenges Facing the Nation,* GAO-18-622, (Washington, D.C.: Sep. 6, 2018).

[10] The act is a part of the *Consolidated Appropriations Act, 2016*, Pub. L. No. 114-113, div. N, title II, subtitle B, 129 Stat. 2242, 2963-2975 (Dec. 18, 2015).

[11] According to NIST, intrusions are defined as attempts to bypass the security mechanisms of a computer or network or to compromise the confidentiality, integrity and availability of the information they contain.

[12] The 23 civilian *Chief Financial Officers Act of 1990* agencies are the Departments of Agriculture, Commerce, Education, Energy, Health and Human Services, Homeland Security, Housing and Urban Development, the

were related to the implementation of FISMA for fiscal year 2017, which was the most recent fiscal year for which the reports were available. In addition, we examined performance metrics related to the cybersecurity cross-agency priority (CAP) goal[13] for fiscal years 2016 and 2017 for the 23 agencies. We also reviewed the financial statement audit reports for the 23 civilian agencies for fiscal years 2016 and 2017. Because we focused our work on the 23 civilian agencies, results from these reviews are not generalizable to the entire federal government.

For the second objective, we collected and reviewed information security-related documents from OMB and DHS and compared them to requirements of the *Federal Cybersecurity Enhancement Act of 2015*. We also interviewed knowledgeable officials from OMB and DHS regarding their agencies' efforts to fulfill requirements of the act.

In addition, we assessed the extent to which DHS had improved the capabilities of the National Cybersecurity Protection System (NCPS).[14] To do this, we assessed the department's actions to implement nine recommendations GAO previously made to, among other things, enhance the system and better define requirements for future capabilities.[15] We also reviewed documents and interviewed DHS officials to determine other actions, beyond those related to our recommendations, that the department had taken to improve the system. Further, we held semi-structured interviews[16] with knowledgeable officials from the 23 civilian CFO Act agencies to obtain their views on the intrusion detection and prevention capabilities made available by DHS. The results of these interviews are not generalizable to all federal agencies.

To address the third objective, we summarized information from our semi-structured interviews about reported capabilities implemented at the 23 civilian CFO Act agencies to detect and prevent intrusions. We also analyzed security status reports from DHS. See appendix I for additional details on our objectives, scope, and methodology.

We conducted this performance audit from December 2017 to December 2018 in accordance with generally accepted government auditing standards. Those standards require that we plan and perform the audit to obtain sufficient, appropriate evidence to provide a reasonable basis for our findings and conclusions based on our audit objectives. We believe that the evidence obtained provides a reasonable basis for our findings and conclusions based on our audit objectives.

Interior, Justice, Labor, State, Transportation, the Treasury, and Veterans Affairs; the Environmental Protection Agency; General Services Administration; National Aeronautics and Space Administration; National Science Foundation; Nuclear Regulatory Commission; Office of Personnel Management; Small Business Administration; Social Security Administration; and the U.S. Agency for International Development. We did not include the Department of Defense in the scope of our audit because the *Federal Cybersecurity Enhancement Act of 2015* only applies to civilian agencies.

[13] The cybersecurity CAP goal was established by the prior administration as part of implementing the requirement in the *GPRA Modernization Act of 2010*, Pub. L. No. 111- 352, § 5, 124 Stat. 3866, 3873 (Jan. 4, 2011) codified at 31 U.S.C. § 1120(a)(1)(B).

[14] NCPS, designed and operated by DHS, was developed to be one of the tools to aid federal agencies in mitigating information security threats. The system is to provide DHS with the capability to provide four cyber-related services to federal agencies: intrusion detection, intrusion prevention, analytics, and information sharing.

[15] GAO, *Information Security: DHS Needs to Enhance Capabilities, Improve Planning, and Support Greater Adoption of Its National Cybersecurity Protection System*, GAO-16-294 (Washington, D.C.: Jan. 28, 2016).

[16] A semi-structured interview methodology generally involves asking a similar subset of questions of multiple interviewees. We used a semi-structured interview format with both closed- and open-ended questions. The intent of our open-ended questions was to engage the agency officials in a conversation about the topics being discussed.

BACKGROUND

Cybersecurity incidents continue to impact federal entities and the information they maintain. According to OMB's 2018 annual FISMA report to Congress, agencies reported 35,277 information security incidents to DHS's U.S. Computer Emergency Readiness Team (US-CERT)[17] in fiscal year 2017. As shown in Figure 1, these incidents involved threat vectors, such as web-based attacks, phishing attacks,[18] and the loss or theft of computer equipment, among others.[19]

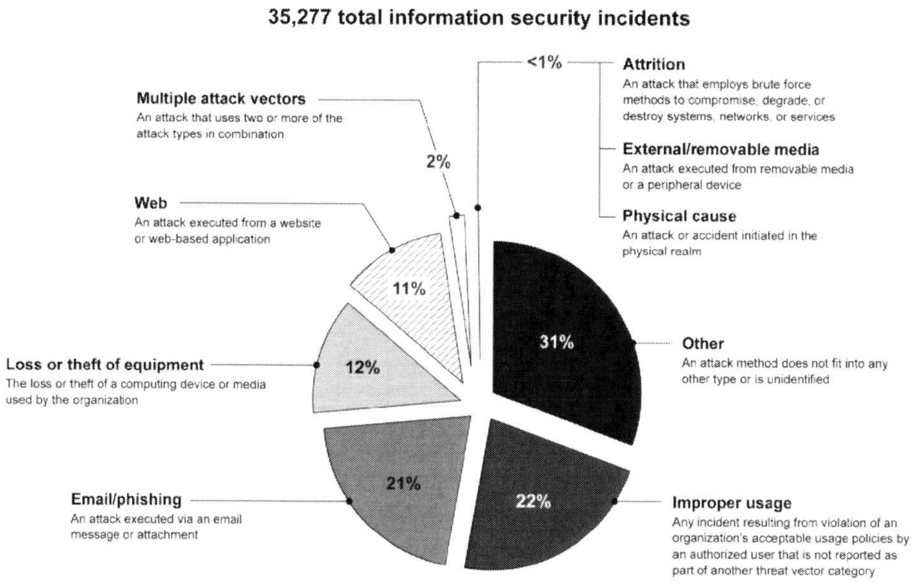

Source: GAO analysis of United States Computer Emergency Readiness Team and Office of Management and Budget data for fiscal year 2017. | GAO-19-105.

Figure 1. Federal Information Security Incidents by Threat Vector Category, Fiscal Year 2017.

These incidents and others like them can pose a serious challenge to economic, national, and personal privacy and security. The following examples highlight the impact of such incidents:

- In March 2018, the Department of Justice reported that it had indicted nine Iranians for conducting a massive cybersecurity theft campaign on behalf of the Islamic Revolutionary Guard Corps. According to the department, the Iranians allegedly stole more than 31 terabytes of documents and data from more than 140 American universities, 30 U.S. companies, and 5 federal government agencies, among other entities.

[17] Within DHS, US-CERT is a component of the National Cybersecurity and Communications Integration Center. It serves as the central federal information security incident center specified by FISMA.

[18] Phishing is a digital form of social engineering that uses authentic-looking, but fake, emails to request information from users or direct them to a fake website that requests information.

[19] A threat vector (or avenue of attack) specifies the conduit or means used by the source or attacker to initiate a cyberattack.

- In March 2018, a joint alert from DHS and the Federal Bureau of Investigation stated that, since at least March 2016, Russian government actors had targeted U.S. government entities and critical infrastructure sectors, including the energy, nuclear, water, aviation, and critical manufacturing sectors.
- In June 2015, the Office of Personnel Management reported that an intrusion into its systems had affected the personnel records of about 4.2 million current and former federal employees. Then, in July 2015, the agency reported that a separate but related incident had compromised its systems and the files related to background investigations for at least 21.5 million individuals.

Federal Law and Policy Prescribe the Federal Approach and Strategy for Securing Information Systems

The federal approach and strategy for securing information systems is prescribed by federal law and policy. FISMA sets requirements for effectively securing federal systems and information. In addition, the *Federal Cybersecurity Enhancement Act of 2015* requires protecting federal networks through the use of federal intrusion prevention and detection capabilities. Further, Executive Order 13800, *Strengthening the Cybersecurity of Federal Networks and Critical Infrastructure*,[20] directs agencies to manage cybersecurity risks to the federal enterprise by, among other things, using the NIST *Framework for Improving Critical Infrastructure Cybersecurity*[21] (cybersecurity framework).

The Federal Information Security Modernization Act of 2014 Sets Requirements for Securing Federal Systems and Information

FISMA was enacted to improve federal cybersecurity and clarify government-wide responsibilities. The law is intended to provide for improved oversight of federal agencies' information security programs. Specifically, the law provides a comprehensive framework for ensuring the effectiveness of information security controls over information resources that support federal operations and assets. The law is also intended to ensure the effective oversight of information security risks, including those throughout civilian, national security, and law enforcement agencies.

FISMA assigns OMB and DHS oversight roles in ensuring federal agencies' compliance with the law. Among other things, FISMA requires OMB to develop and oversee the implementation of policies, principles, standards, and guidelines on information security in federal agencies, except with regard to national security systems. The law also assigns OMB the responsibility of requiring agencies to identify and provide information security protections commensurate with assessments of risk to their information and information systems. The law further requires DHS to administer the implementation of agency information security policies and practices for non-national security information systems, in consultation with OMB, by developing, issuing, and overseeing implementation of binding

---

[20] The White House, *Strengthening the Cybersecurity of Federal Networks and Critical Infrastructure*, Executive Order 13800 (Washington, D.C.: May 11, 2017), 82 Fed. Reg. 22391 (May 16, 2017).

[21] National Institute of Standards and Technology, *Framework for Improving Critical Infrastructure Cybersecurity*, Version 1.1 (Gaithersburg, MD: Apr. 16, 2018).

operational directives;[22] monitoring agency implementation of information security policies and practices; and convening meetings with senior agency officials to help ensure their effective implementation of information security policies and practices, among other things.

FISMA assigned to NIST the responsibility for developing standards and guidelines that include minimum information security requirements. To this end, NIST has issued several publications to provide guidance for agencies in implementing an information security program. For example, NIST Special Publication (SP) 800-53[23] provides guidance to agencies on the selection and implementation of information security and privacy controls for systems.

FISMA also assigns to the head of each executive branch agency, responsibility for providing information security protections commensurate with the risk and magnitude of harm resulting from unauthorized access, use, disclosure, disruption, modification, or destruction of information systems used or operated by an agency or by a contractor of an agency or other organization on behalf of an agency. The law also delegates to the agency chief information officer (CIO), or comparable official, the authority to ensure compliance with FISMA requirements. The CIO is responsible for designating a senior agency information security officer whose primary duty is information security.

In addition, the law requires agencies to develop, document, and implement an agency-wide information security program to secure federal information systems. Specifically, these information security programs are to provide risk-based protections for the information and information systems that support the operations and assets of the agency. Further, FISMA requires agencies to comply with DHS binding operational directives, OMB policies and procedures, and NIST federal information processing standards.

FISMA also has reporting requirements for OMB and federal agencies. Specifically, OMB is to report annually, in consultation with DHS, on the effectiveness of agency information security policies and practices, including a summary of major agency information security incidents and an assessment of agency compliance with NIST standards. Further, the law requires agencies to report annually to OMB, DHS, certain congressional committees, and the Comptroller General of the United States on the adequacy and effectiveness of their information security policies, procedures, and practices, as well as their compliance with FISMA.

The Federal Cybersecurity Enhancement Act of 2015 Articulates Requirements for Protecting Federal Networks through the Use of Federal Intrusion Prevention and Detection Capabilities

The *Federal Cybersecurity Enhancement Act of 2015*, among other things, sets forth authority for enhancing federal intrusion prevention and detection capabilities among federal entities. The act contains several provisions for DHS and OMB. Specifically, the act requires that DHS deploy, operate, and maintain capabilities to prevent and detect cybersecurity risks

---

[22] Binding operational directives are compulsory directions to agencies in order to safeguard federal information and information systems, are in accordance with OMB guidelines, and may be revised or repealed by the OMB Director. FISMA authorizes DHS to develop and issue binding operational directives to federal agencies and oversee their implementation by agencies. DHS has developed and issued seven binding operational directives, instructing agencies to, among other things, enhance e-mail security by removing certain insecure protocols.

[23] National Institute of Standards and Technology, *Security and Privacy Controls for Federal Information Systems and Organizations*, Special Publication 800-53, Revision 4 (Gaithersburg, MD: April 2013).

in network traffic traveling to or from an agency's information system. DHS is to make these capabilities available for use by any agency.

In addition, the act requires DHS to improve intrusion detection and prevention capabilities, as appropriate, by regularly deploying new technologies and modifying existing technologies. The act also requires OMB and DHS, in consultation with appropriate agencies, to review and update government-wide policies and programs to ensure appropriate prioritization and use of network security monitoring tools within agency networks, and to brief appropriate congressional committees.

The Executive Order on Strengthening the Cybersecurity of Federal Networks and Critical Infrastructure Directs Agencies to Use the Cybersecurity Framework for Managing Risks

In May 2017, the President signed Executive Order 13800, which sets policy for managing cybersecurity risk as an executive branch enterprise. Specifically, it outlines actions to enhance cybersecurity across federal agencies and critical infrastructure to improve the nation's cyber posture and capabilities against cybersecurity threats. To this end, the order states that the President will hold executive agency heads accountable for managing agency-wide cybersecurity risk and directs each executive agency to use the NIST cybersecurity framework to manage those risks.

The cybersecurity framework, which provides guidance for cybersecurity activities, is based on five core security functions:

- Identify: Develop an organizational understanding to manage cybersecurity risk to systems, people, assets, data, and capabilities.
- Protect: Develop and implement appropriate safeguards to ensure delivery of critical services.
- Detect: Develop and implement appropriate activities to identify the occurrence of a cybersecurity event.[24]
- Respond: Develop and implement appropriate activities to take action regarding a detected cybersecurity incident.
- Recover: Develop and implement appropriate activities to maintain plans for resilience and to restore capabilities or services that were impaired due to a cybersecurity incident.

According to NIST, these five functions should be performed concurrently and continuously to address cybersecurity risk. In addition, when considered together, they provide a high-level, strategic view of the life cycle of an organization's management of cybersecurity risk. Within the five functions are 23 categories and 108 subcategories that include controls for achieving the intent of each function.[25] Appendix II provides a description of the cybersecurity framework categories and subcategories of controls.

---

[24] Cybersecurity events are cybersecurity changes that may have an impact on the organizational operations (including mission, capabilities, or reputation).

[25] For example, "risk assessment" is one of five categories that comprise the "identify" function. The risk assessment category is divided into six subcategories that involve activities such as identifying and documenting internal and external threats; identifying potential business impacts and likelihoods; and determining risk based on threats, vulnerabilities, likelihoods, and impacts. Each subcategory activity cross-

GAO Has Reported on Challenges Related to Establishing a Comprehensive Cybersecurity Strategy

In February 2013, we reported that the government had issued a variety of strategy-related documents that addressed priorities for enhancing cybersecurity within the federal government, as well as for encouraging improvements in the cybersecurity of critical infrastructure within the private sector. However, we noted that no overarching cybersecurity strategy had been developed that articulated priority actions, assigned responsibilities for performing them, and set time frames for their completion.[26] Accordingly, we recommended that the White House Cybersecurity Coordinator[27] in the Executive Office of the President develop an overarching federal cybersecurity strategy that included all key elements of the desirable characteristics of a national strategy.[28] These characteristics would include, among other things, milestones and performance measures for major activities to address stated priorities; cost and resources needed to accomplish stated priorities; and specific roles and responsibilities of federal organizations related to the strategy's stated priorities.

Since that time, the executive branch has made progress toward outlining a federal strategy for confronting cyber threats. For example, in September 2018,[29] we reported that recent executive branch initiatives that identify cybersecurity priorities for the federal government provide a good foundation toward establishing a more comprehensive strategy. Nevertheless, we pointed out that additional efforts were needed to address all of the desirable characteristics of a national strategy that we recommended.

Specifically, recently issued executive branch strategy documents[30] did not include key elements of desirable characteristics that can enhance the usefulness of a national strategy as guidance for decision makers in allocating resources, defining policies, and helping to ensure accountability. For example, these strategy documents did not generally include:

- milestones and performance measures to gauge results;
- resources needed to carry out the goals and objectives; and
- clearly defined roles and responsibilities for key agencies, such as DHS, the Department of Defense, and OMB.

---

references information system controls from various information security publications, including NIST Special Publication 800-53.

[26] GAO, *Cybersecurity: National Strategy, Roles, and Responsibilities Need to Be Better Defined and More Effectively Implemented,* GAO-13-187 (Washington, D.C.: Feb. 14, 2013).

[27] In December 2009, a Special Assistant to the President was appointed as Cybersecurity Coordinator to address the recommendations made in the Cyberspace Policy Review, including coordinating interagency cybersecurity policies and strategies and developing a comprehensive national strategy to secure the nation's digital infrastructure.

[28] In 2004, we developed a set of desirable characteristics that can enhance the usefulness of national strategies in allocating resources, defining policies, and helping to ensure accountability. See GAO, *Combating Terrorism: Evaluation of Selected Characteristics in National Strategies Related to Terrorism*, GAO-04-408T (Washington, D.C.: Feb. 3, 2004).

[29] GAO-18-622.

[30] These initiatives include Executive Order 13800, the National Security Strategy, and DHS Cybersecurity Strategy.

Ultimately, we determined that a more clearly defined, coordinated, and comprehensive approach to planning and executing an overall strategy would likely lead to significant progress in furthering strategic goals and lessening persistent weaknesses.

Subsequent to our September 2018 report, the President issued the *National Cyber Strategy* on September 20, 2018.[31] The strategy builds upon Executive Order 13800 and describes actions that federal agencies and the administration are to take to, among other things, secure federal information systems. For example, the strategy states that the administration is expected to further enable DHS to secure federal department and agency networks, to include ensuring that DHS has appropriate access to agency information systems for cybersecurity purposes and can take and direct action to safeguard systems. In addition, the strategy states that the administration plans to continue with its existing efforts underway to transition agencies to shared services and infrastructure and that DHS is to have appropriate visibility into those services and infrastructure to improve cybersecurity posture.[32]

DHS Offers Federal Agencies Capabilities Intended to Detect and Prevent Intrusions to Federal Information Systems

DHS's Network Security Deployment (NSD) division manages cybersecurity programs that are intended to improve the cybersecurity posture of the federal government. Among these programs, NCPS provides a capability to detect and prevent potentially malicious network traffic from entering agencies' networks. In addition, the Continuous Diagnostics and Mitigation (CDM) program provides tools to agencies intended to identify and resolve cyber vulnerabilities on an ongoing basis.

DHS's National Cybersecurity Protection System Is Intended to Detect and Prevent Cyber Intrusions

Operated by DHS's US-CERT, NCPS is intended to detect and prevent cyber intrusions into agency networks, analyze network data for trends and anomalous data, and share information with agencies on cyber threats and incidents. Deployed in stages, this system, operationally known as EINSTEIN, has provided increasing capabilities to detect and prevent potential cyberattacks involving the network traffic entering or exiting the networks of participating federal agencies. Table 1 provides an overview of the EINSTEIN deployment stages to date.

In January 2016, we reported the projected total life-cycle cost of the program was approximately $5.7 billion through fiscal year 2018.[33] In addition, according to the Federal CIO, Congress appropriated $468 million in fiscal year 2017 and $402 million in fiscal year 2018 for NCPS.

---

[31] The White House, *National Cyber Strategy* (Washington, D.C.: Sept. 20, 2018).

[32] Evaluating the *National Cyber Strategy* to determine if it included the key elements of desirable characteristics discussed in GAO-18-622 was not within the scope of this review.

[33] GAO-16-294.

Table 1. Overview of the National Cybersecurity Protection System (NCPS) Deployment, 2003-2013

Operational name	Deployment year	NCPS objective	Description
EINSTEIN 1	2003	Intrusion detection	Provides an automated process for collecting, correlating, and analyzing agencies' computer network traffic information from sensors installed at their Internet connections.[a]
EINSTEIN 2	2009	Intrusion detection	Monitors federal agency Internet connections for specific predefined signatures of known malicious activity and alerts DHS's U.S. Computer Emergency Readiness Team (US-CERT) when specific network activity matching the predetermined signatures is detected.[b]
EINSTEIN 3 Accelerated	2013	Intrusion detection Intrusion prevention	Automatically blocks malicious traffic from entering or leaving federal civilian agency networks. This capability is managed by Internet service providers, who administer intrusion prevention and threat-based decision making using DHS-developed indicators of malicious cyber activity to develop signatures.[c]

Source: GAO analysis of Department of Homeland Security (DHS) data. | GAO-19-105.

[a]The network traffic information includes source and destination Internet Protocol addresses used in the communication, source and destination ports, the time the communication occurred, and the protocol used to communicate.

[b]Signatures are recognizable, distinguishing patterns associated with cyberattacks, such as a binary string associated with a computer virus or a particular set of keystrokes used to gain unauthorized access to a system.

[c]An indicator is defined by DHS as human-readable cyber data used to identify some form of malicious cyber activity. These data may be related to Internet Protocol addresses, domains, e-mail headers, files, and character strings. Indicators can be either classified or unclassified.

In that report, we also noted that NCPS was partially, but not fully, meeting most of its stated system objectives.[34] Although the system's intrusion detection capabilities provided the ability to detect known patterns of malicious activity on agency networks, it was limited in its capabilities to identify potential threats using anomaly-based detection. We also reported that although DHS had developed metrics for measuring the performance of NCPS, the metrics did not gauge the quality, accuracy, or effectiveness of the system's intrusion detection and prevention capabilities.

The department had also identified needs for future capabilities, but had not defined requirements for the capability to detect threats entering and exiting cloud service providers. Further, DHS had not considered specific vulnerability information for agency information systems in making risk-based decisions about future intrusion prevention capabilities.

Accordingly, we made nine recommendations to DHS to, among other things, enhance the NCPS capabilities for meeting its objectives and better define requirements for future capabilities. DHS agreed with each of our nine recommendations and indicated that it would take steps to address them.

DHS's Continuous Diagnostics and Mitigation Program Provides Agencies with Tools and Services Intended to Secure Agency Systems

DHS's CDM program provides federal agencies with tools and services that have the intended capability to automate network monitoring, correlate and analyze security-related information, and enhance risk-based decision making at agency and government-wide levels. These tools include sensors that perform automated scans or searches for known cyber

[34] GAO-16-294.

vulnerabilities, the results of which can feed into a dashboard that, at an agency level, is intended to alert network managers and enable the agency to allocate resources based on the risk. Summary data from each participating agency's dashboard is expected to be transmitted to the Federal Dashboard where the data can be used to inform decisions about cybersecurity risks across the federal government. There are four phases of CDM implementation:

- Phase 1—involves deploying products to automate hardware and software asset management, configuration settings, and common vulnerability management capabilities. According to the *Cybersecurity Strategy and Implementation Plan*,[35] DHS purchased phase 1 tools and integration services for all participating agencies in fiscal year 2015. DHS plans to have all phase 1 tools deployed at participating agencies by the end of the second quarter of fiscal year 2019.
- Phase 2—intends to address privilege management and infrastructure integrity by allowing agencies to monitor users on their networks and to detect whether users are engaging in unauthorized activity. According to the *Cybersecurity Strategy and Implementation Plan*, DHS was to provide agencies with additional phase 2 capabilities throughout fiscal year 2016, with the full suite of CDM phase 2 capabilities delivered by the end of that fiscal year. However, according to the OMB FISMA *Annual Report to Congress for Fiscal Year 2017*, the CDM program began deploying Phase 2 tools and sensors during fiscal year 2017.[36] DHS plans to have all phase 2 tools deployed at participating agencies by the end of fiscal year 2019.
- Phase 3—includes detection capabilities that are intended to assess agency network activity and identify any anomalies that may indicate a cybersecurity compromise.[37] Full operating capability[38] for phases 1, 2, and 3 is planned to be achieved by the end of fiscal year 2022.[39]
- Phase 4—intends to provide tools to (1) protect data at rest, in transit, and in use; (2) prevent loss of data; and (3) manage and mitigate data breaches. According to CDM program officials, phase 4 has not been approved and no tools have been selected.

---

[35] Office of Management and Budget, *Cybersecurity Strategy and Implementation Plan (CSIP) for the Federal Civilian Government*, Memorandum M-16-04 (Washington, D.C.: Oct. 30, 2015). CSIP identified objectives, key actions, responsibilities, and timeframes for completing actions that were intended to strengthen cybersecurity at federal civilian agencies.

[36] Office of Management and Budget, *Federal Information Security Modernization Act of 2014, Annual Report to Congress Fiscal Year 2017* (Washington, D.C.: Mar. 2018).

[37] CDM phase 3 also includes, among other things, completing remaining required phase 1 activities and integrating all deployed phase 2 tools into agency and federal dashboards.

[38] DHS's NSD division considers an agency to have reached full operating capability for a given CDM phase when the full set of capabilities for the phase has been fully deployed across the agency (i.e., the capabilities have been installed, configured, integrated, and data is feeding into the agency's dashboard).

[39] According to CDM program officials, initial operational capability—a project milestone attained when the capabilities for a phase have been fully deployed to at least five agencies—for phase 3 is planned by the end of fourth quarter fiscal year 2019.

NIST Recommends That Federal Agencies Deploy Intrusion Detection and Prevention Capabilities

An approach for protecting systems against cybersecurity compromise is for federal agencies to build successive layers of defense mechanisms at strategic points in their information technology infrastructures. This approach, commonly referred to as defense in depth, entails implementing a series of protective mechanisms so that if one mechanism fails to detect and prevent an attack, another will provide a backup defense. By utilizing defense in depth, federal agencies can reduce the risk of a successful cyberattack by implementing intrusion detection and prevention capabilities.

NIST has developed guidelines for protecting agency information systems using intrusion detection and prevention capabilities. For example, NIST SP 800-53 recommends that agencies strategically deploy capabilities and perform monitoring of their systems to include observation of events occurring on their network and at the external boundary of their network. In addition, NIST SP 800-94 provides agencies with guidance in designing, implementing, configuring, securing, monitoring, and maintaining such capabilities.[40]

As part of their defense-in-depth approach and, as recommended by the NIST guidelines, agencies can deploy the following list of capabilities, among others, on their networks to detect and prevent an attack:

- Protecting email from intrusions: According to OMB,[41] email, by way of phishing attacks, remains one of the most common threat vectors across the government. Methods for protecting email include encryption, false email alerts, and anti-spear-phishing training.[42]
- Monitoring cloud services: Cloud vendors provide services to agencies, including Software as a Service,[43] Platform as a Service,[44] and Infrastructure as a Service.[45] As agencies increasingly rely on cloud services, monitoring traffic to and from their cloud service providers helps to ensure that agencies detect malicious traffic.
- Using host-based intrusion prevention: Host-based intrusion prevention systems provide defense at an individual system or device level by protecting against

---

[40] National Institute of Standards and Technology, *Guide to Intrusion Detection and Prevention Systems*, Special Publication 800-94 (Gaithersburg, MD: February 2007).

[41] Office of Management and Budget, *Federal Cybersecurity Risk Determination Report and Action Plan* (Washington, D.C.: May 2018).

[42] Spear phishing represents a digital form of social engineering that uses authentic looking emails, websites, or instant messages that are closely tailored to their intended audience to get users to download malware, open malicious attachments, or open links that direct them to a website that requests information or executes malicious code.

[43] In Software as a Service, the agency uses the service provider's applications, which are accessible from various client devices through an interface such as a web browser (e.g., web-based e-mail system). The agency does not manage or control the underlying infrastructure or the individual application capabilities.

[44] In Platform as a Service, the agency deploys its own or acquired applications created using programming languages and tools supported by the provider. The agency does not manage or control the underlying infrastructure, but controls and configures the deployed applications.

[45] In Infrastructure as a Service, the agency has the capability to provision processing, storage, networks, and other fundamental computing resources and run its own software, including operating systems and applications. The agency does not manage or control the underlying infrastructure but controls and configures operating systems, storage, deployed applications, and possibly, selected networking components (e.g., host firewalls).

malicious activities. Host-based capabilities include memory-based protection[46] and application whitelisting.[47]

- Monitoring external and internal traffic: Agencies can monitor external and internal traffic, including: encrypted traffic, traffic between workstations and servers on the network, and direct connections to outside entities such as universities. Monitoring traffic helps to ensure that agencies detect malicious activity.
- Using security information and event management: A security information and event management capability produces real-time alerts and notifications of significant security events. Security alerts and notifications can provide the agency with better situational awareness regarding possible intrusion activity.

SELECTED AGENCIES WERE NOT EFFECTIVELY IMPLEMENTING THE FEDERAL GOVERNMENT'S APPROACH AND STRATEGY TO SECURING INFORMATION SYSTEMS

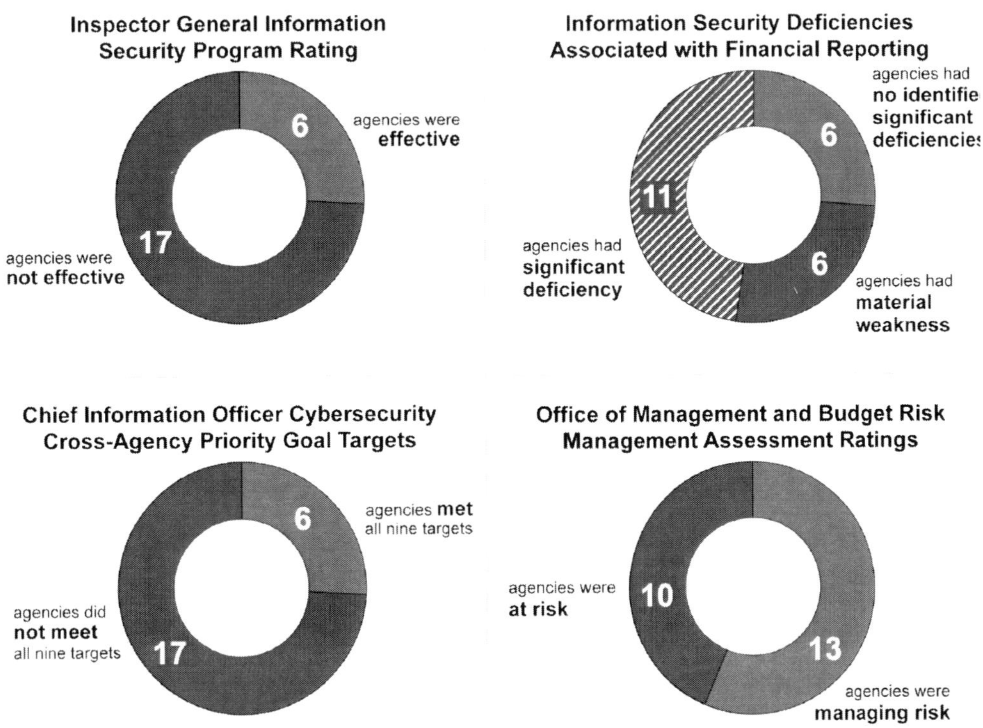

Source: GAO analysis of agency fiscal year 2017 Federal Information Security Modernization Act of 2014 and agency financial reports for fiscal year 2017. | GAO-19-105.

Figure 2. Fiscal Year 2017 Indicators of the 23 Civilian *Chief Financial Officers Act of 1990* Agencies' Effectiveness in Implementing the Federal Approach and Strategy for Securing Information Systems.

[46] Memory based protections are safeguards that protect memory from unauthorized code execution.

[47] An application whitelist is a list of applications and application components that an agency has authorized for use on its hosts.

According to inspectors general, agency CIOs, and OMB reports on federal information security practices, many agencies were not effectively implementing the federal government's approach and strategy to securing information systems as of fiscal year 2017. Agencies' inspectors general determined that most of the 23 civilian CFO Act agencies did not have effective agency-wide information security programs. They also reported that agencies did not have effective information security controls in place, leading to deficiencies in internal control over financial reporting. In addition, the CIOs demonstrated that, during fiscal years 2016 and 2017, most agencies had not met all targets for the cybersecurity CAP goal for improving cybersecurity performance. Further, based on FISMA metrics reported for fiscal year 2017, OMB determined that 13 of the 23 agencies were managing risks to their enterprise, while the other 10 agencies were at risk of ineffectively identifying, protecting, detecting, responding to, and if necessary, recovering from cyber intrusions. Figure 2 summarizes agencies' efforts to implement the government's approach and strategy for securing information systems as of fiscal year 2017.

Appendix III includes a table that provides an additional overview of the effectiveness of each agency's implementation of the government's approach and strategy to securing information systems.

Inspectors General Determined That Most Selected Agencies Did Not Have Effective Information Security Programs or Controls in Place as of Fiscal Year 2017

Inspectors general determined that more than half of the 23 civilian CFO Act agencies did not have effective agency-wide information security programs as of fiscal year 2017. Further, in agency financial statement audit reports for fiscal year 2017, inspectors general reported that, despite improvements being made in information security practices, most of the civilian CFO Act agencies continued to exhibit deficiencies in information security controls. As a result of these deficiencies, inspectors general reported material weaknesses or significant deficiencies in internal control over financial reporting.

Inspectors General Indicate That Few Agencies Had Effective Information Security Programs

FISMA requires inspectors general to determine the effectiveness of their respective agencies' information security programs. To do so, FISMA reporting instructions[48] direct inspectors general to provide a maturity rating for agency information security policies, procedures, and practices related to the five core security functions established in the NIST cybersecurity framework, as well as for the agency-wide information security program.

The ratings used to evaluate the effectiveness of agencies' information security programs are based on a five-level maturity model, as described in Table 2.

---

[48] Inspectors general FISMA metrics and reporting instructions were developed as a collaborative effort amongst OMB, DHS, and the Council of the Inspectors General on Integrity and Efficiency, in consultation with the Federal CIO Council. The FISMA metrics and reporting instructions provide reporting requirements across key areas to be addressed in the independent assessment of agencies information security programs. See *Fiscal Year 2017 Inspector General Federal Information Security Modernization Act of 2014 Reporting Metrics* (April 17, 2017).

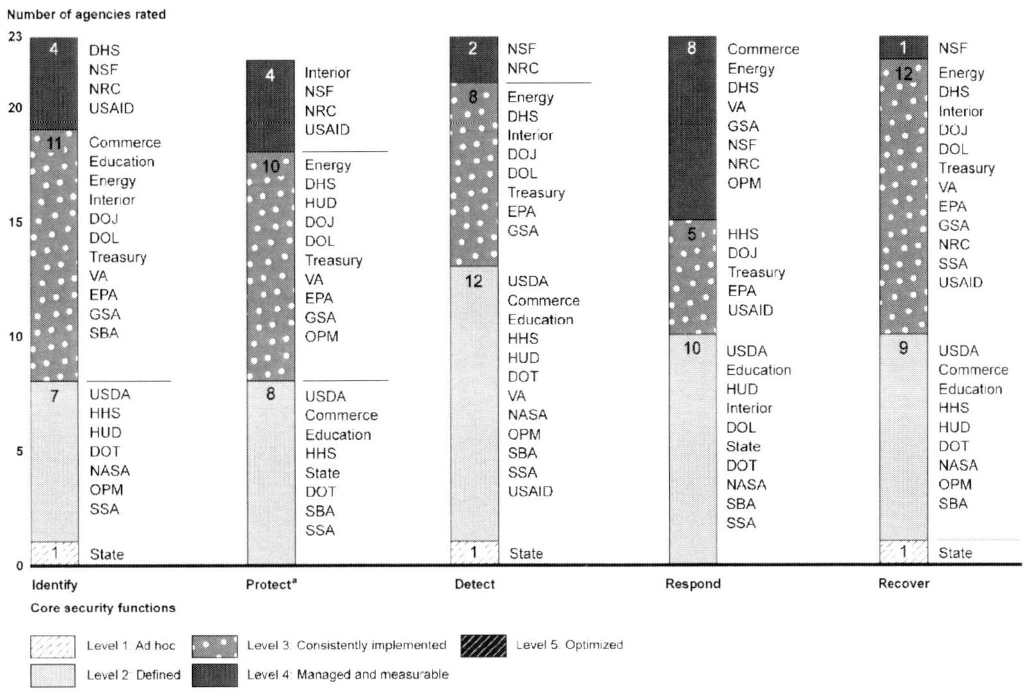

DHS (Department of Homeland Security), NSF (National Science Foundation), NRC (Nuclear Regulatory Commission), USAID (United States Agency for International Development), Commerce (Department of Commerce), Education (Department of Education), Energy (Department of Energy), Interior (Department of the Interior), DOJ (Department of Justice), DOL (Department of Labor), Treasury (Department of the Treasury), VA (Department of Veterans Affairs), EPA (Environmental Protection Agency), GSA (General Services Administration), SBA (Small Business Administration), USDA (United States Department of Agriculture), HHS (Department of Health & Human Services), HUD (Department of Housing and Urban Development), DOT (Department of Transportation), NASA (National Aeronautics and Space Administration), OPM (Office of Personnel Management), SSA (Social Security Administration), State (Department of State)

Source: GAO analysis of agency fiscal year 2017 Federal Information Security Modernization Act of 2014 reports. | GAO-19-105.

[a]Only 22 agencies are listed because the NASA inspector general did not provide a rating for the Protect function.

Figure 3. Inspector General Ratings of Agencies' Information Security Policies, Procedures, and Practices Related to the Five Core Security Functions, as of Fiscal Year 2017.

According to this maturity model, Level 4 (managed and measurable) represents an effective level of security.[49] Therefore, if an inspector general rates the agency's information security program at Level 4 or Level 5, then that agency is considered to have an effective information security program.[50]

For fiscal year 2017, the inspectors general for 6 of the 23 civilian CFO Act agencies reported that their agencies had an effective agency-wide information security program. More specifically, for the 5 core security functions, most inspectors general reported that their agency was at Level 3 (consistently implemented) for the *identify*, *protect*, and *recover* functions, and at Level 2 (defined) for the *detect* and *respond* functions, as shown in Figure 3.

---

[49] NIST defines security control effectiveness as the extent to which security controls are implemented correctly, operate as intended, and produce the desired outcome with respect to meeting the security requirements for the information system and are in compliance with established security policies.

[50] *Fiscal Year 2017 Inspector General Federal Information Security Modernization Act of 2014 Reporting Metrics* (April 17, 2017).

Table 2. Inspector General Reporting Metrics Maturity Model

Maturity level	Description
Level 1: Ad hoc	Policies, procedures, and strategy are not formalized; activities are performed in an ad hoc, reactive manner.
Level 2: Defined	Policies, procedures, and strategy are formalized and documented, but not consistently implemented.
Level 3: Consistently Implemented	Policies, procedures, and strategy are consistently implemented, but quantitative and qualitative effectiveness measures are lacking.
Level 4: Managed and Measurable	Quantitative and qualitative measures on the effectiveness of policies, procedures, and strategy are collected across the organization and used to assess those policies procedures, and strategy, and make necessary changes.
Level 5: Optimized	Policies, procedures, and strategy are fully institutionalized, repeatable, self-generating, consistently implemented, and regularly updated based on a changing threat and technology landscape and business/mission needs.

Source: GAO analysis of Fiscal Year 2017 Inspector General *Federal Information Security Modernization Act of 2014* Reporting Metrics, April 17, 2017. | GAO-19-105.

Inspectors General Continued to Identify Significant Security Control Deficiencies in Controls over Financial Reporting at Most Selected Agencies

Inspectors general report on the effectiveness of agencies' information security controls as part of the annual audits of the agencies' financial statements. The reports resulting from these audits include a description of information security control deficiencies related to the five major control categories defined by the *Federal Information System Controls Audit Manual* (FISCAM)—access controls, configuration management, segregation of duties, contingency planning, and security management.[51] The reports also identify the inspectors general's designation of information security as a significant deficiency[52] or material weakness in internal control over financial reporting systems.[53]

For fiscal year 2017, inspectors general continued to identify information security control deficiencies in each of the five major control categories across the 23 civilian CFO Act agencies. The number of agencies with deficiencies in the access control and contingency

[51] FISCAM is GAO's audit methodology for performing information system control audits in accordance with generally acceptable government auditing standards. The five control categories defined by this manual include: (1) access controls that limit or detect access to computer resources, thereby protecting them against unauthorized modification, loss, and disclosure; (2) configuration management controls that prevent unauthorized changes to information system resources and to assure that software is current and known vulnerabilities are patched; (3) segregation of duties controls that prevent an individual from controlling all critical stages of a process by splitting responsibilities between two or more organizational groups; (4) contingency planning controls that help avoid significant disruptions in computer-dependent operations; (5) and security management controls that provide a framework for ensuring that risks are understood and that effective controls are selected, implemented, and operating as intended. See GAO, *Federal Information System Controls Audit Manual* (FISCAM), GAO-09-232G (Washington, D.C.: February 2009).

[52] A significant deficiency is a deficiency, or a combination of deficiencies, in internal control over financial reporting that is less severe than a material weakness, yet important enough to merit attention by those charged with governance. A deficiency in internal control exists when the design or operation of a control does not allow management or employees, in the normal course of performing their assigned functions, to prevent, or detect and correct, misstatements on a timely basis.

[53] A material weakness is a deficiency, or combination of deficiencies, in internal control over financial reporting, such that there is a reasonable possibility that a material misstatement of the entity's financial statements will not be prevented, or detected and corrected, on a timely basis.

planning information security control categories decreased between fiscal years 2016 and 2017, according to the inspectors general.

Nevertheless, the inspectors general reported that agencies continued to exhibit deficiencies in these two control categories. In addition, the number of agencies with deficiencies in the security management and segregation of duties control categories increased from the prior year. The number of agencies reported as having deficiencies in the configuration management control category remained the same. Figure 4 shows the number of agencies that reported deficiencies in each of the information security control categories for fiscal years 2016 and 2017.

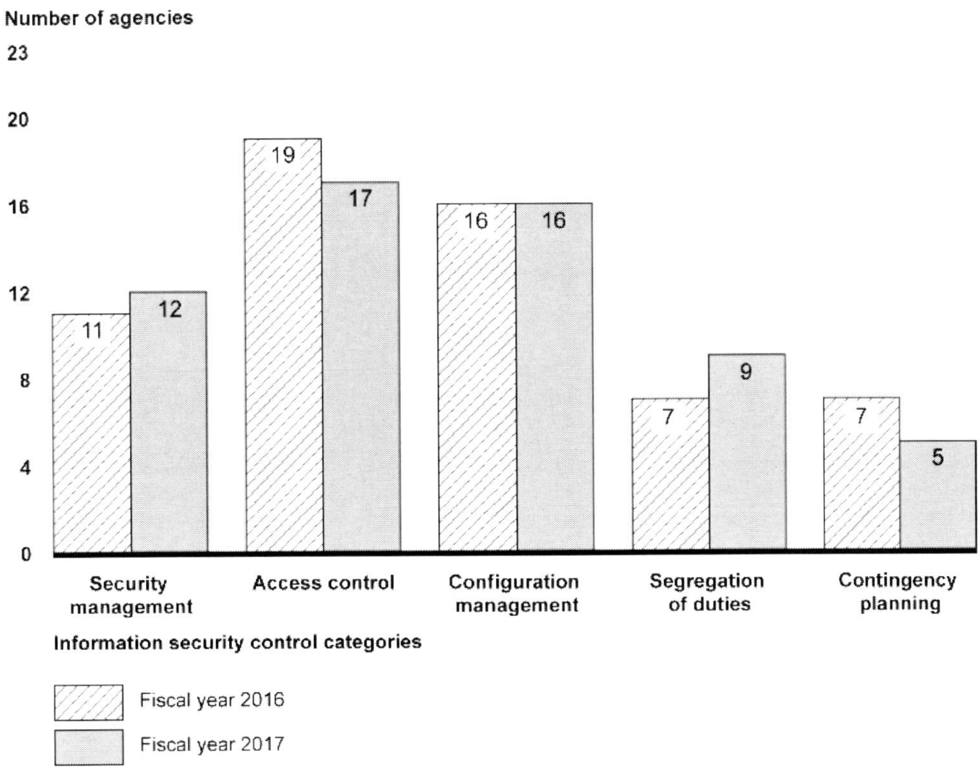

Source: GAO analysis of agency financial reports for fiscal years 2016 and 2017. | GAO-19-105.

Figure 4. Number of Civilian *Chief Financial Officers Act of 1990* Agencies Reporting Deficiencies in Information Security Control Categories for Fiscal Years 2016 and 2017.

Overall, inspectors general for the 23 civilian CFO Act agencies reported progress in agencies' information security practices for fiscal year 2017. Specifically, during that time, 17 inspectors general designated information security as either a significant deficiency (11) or material weakness (6) in internal control over financial reporting systems for their agencies. This is a decrease from the previous fiscal year when 19 inspectors general designated information security as a significant deficiency (12) or material weakness (7).

Most Agencies Reported Not Meeting All Targets for the Cybersecurity Cross-Agency Priority Goal in Fiscal Years 2016 and 2017

Reporting instructions contained in the fiscal year 2017 FISMA metrics[54] directed CIOs to assess their agencies' progress toward achieving outcomes that strengthen federal cybersecurity. To do this, CIOs evaluated their agencies' performance in reaching targets for specific FISMA reporting metrics. According to the reporting instructions, certain metrics were selected to represent the administration's cybersecurity CAP goal. These selected metrics allowed CIOs to evaluate their agencies progress in meeting targets for that goal.

Table 3. Priority Areas, Performance Indicators, and Targets for the Cybersecurity Cross-Agency Priority Goal, Fiscal Years 2015–2017

Priority area	Performance indicator	Target
Information security continuous monitoring is the provision that covers ongoing observation, assessment, analysis, and diagnosis of an organization's cybersecurity posture, hygiene, and operational readiness.	Hardware asset management	Implemented at 95 percent for the agency
	Software asset management	Implemented at 95 percent for the agency
	Vulnerability management	Implemented at 95 percent for the agency
	Secure configuration management	Implemented at 95 percent for the agency
Identity, credential, and access management is the implementation of a set of capabilities that are intended to ensure users must authenticate their identities in order to use information technology resources and have access to only those resources that are required for their job function.	Implementation of personal identity verification for unprivileged users	Implemented at 85 percent for unprivileged users
	Implementation of personal identity verification for privileged users	Implemented at 100 percent for privileged users
Anti-phishing and malware defense is the implementation of technologies, processes, and training that are intended to reduce the risk of malware introduced through email and malicious or compromised web sites.	Anti-phishing defense	Implemented at 90 percent for 5 of the top 7 anti-phishing defenses
	Malware defenses	Implemented at 90 percent for 3 of the top 5 malware defenses
	Other defenses	Implemented at 90 percent for 2 of the top 4 other defenses

Source: GAO analysis of Office of Management and Budget Fiscal Year 2017 Federal Information Security Modernization Act of 2014 Annual Report to Congress. | GAO-19-105.

The cybersecurity CAP goal for fiscal years 2015 through 2017[55] was to improve cybersecurity performance by having an ongoing awareness of information security, vulnerabilities, and threats impacting the operating information environment; ensuring that only authorized users have access to resources and information; and implementing technologies and processes that reduce the risk of malware. The cybersecurity CAP goal consisted of three priority areas with a total of nine performance indicators. Each of the nine performance indicators had an expected level of performance, or target, for implementation.

---

[54] Each year, OMB and DHS work with an interagency group to develop the CIO FISMA metrics. These metrics are organized around the five cybersecurity framework core security functions and track agencies' progress in implementing cybersecurity capabilities.

[55] Although the CAP goal was in place for fiscal years 2015 through 2017, the scope of our review was for fiscal years 2016 and 2017.

Table 3 shows the three priority areas and related performance indicators and targets of the cybersecurity CAP goal for fiscal years 2015 through 2017.

According to agency CIO assessments for fiscal year 2017, 6 of the 23 agencies met all 9 targets for the cybersecurity CAP goal. More specifically,

- 8 agencies met all four targets for the information security continuous monitoring priority area;
- 16 agencies met the two targets for the identity, credential, and access management priority area; and
- 17 agencies met all three targets for the anti-phishing and malware defense priority area.

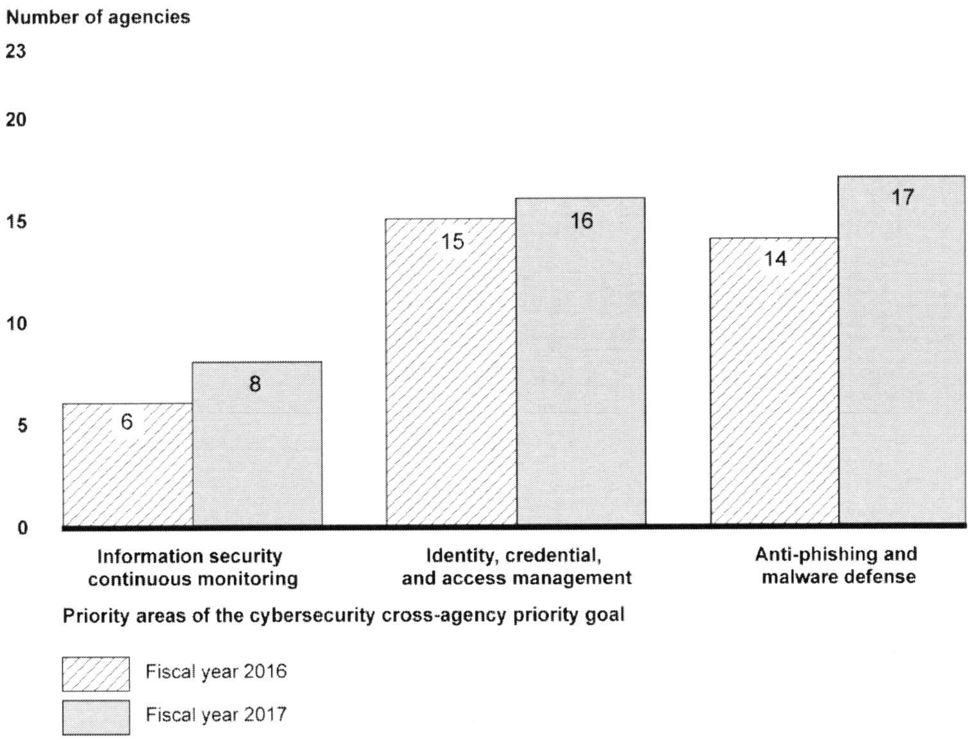

Source; GAO analysis of agency reported data. | GAO-19-105.

The 23 selected civilian agencies are the Departments of Agriculture, Commerce, Education, Energy, Health and Human Services, Homeland Security, Housing and Urban Development, the Interior, Justice, Labor, State, Transportation, the Treasury, and Veterans Affairs; the Environmental Protection Agency; General Services Administration; National Aeronautics and Space Administration; National Science Foundation; Nuclear Regulatory Commission; Office of Personnel Management; Small Business Administration; Social Security Administration; and the U.S. Agency for International Development.

Figure 5. Number of the 23 Selected Civilian Agencies That Reported Meeting Targets for the Cybersecurity Cross-Agency Priority Goal Priority Areas, Fiscal Years 2016 and 2017.

In addition, CIOs reported that agencies were making progress in meeting the targets for the nine performance indicators for fiscal years 2016 and 2017, with increases in the number of agencies meeting the targets within each of the three priority areas.

However, although the number of agencies that met the targets in individual priority areas showed a net increase, not all agencies maintained their status. For example, the CIO for one agency reported meeting all three targets for the anti-phishing and malware defense priority area in fiscal year 2016, but reported that the agency only met two of the three targets in fiscal year 2017. Figure 5 shows the number of agencies that reported meeting each of the targets within the individual cybersecurity CAP goal priority areas for fiscal years 2016 and 2017.

Although the CIOs for only six agencies reported meeting each of the targets associated with all nine performance indicators for the three cybersecurity CAP goal priority areas, the CIOs at an additional eight agencies reported meeting each target for two of the three priority areas. Specifically,

- one CIO reported that its agency met each of the targets for the (1) information security continuous monitoring and (2) identity, credential, and access management priority areas;
- another CIO reported that its agency met each of the targets for the (1) information security continuous monitoring and (2) anti-phishing and malware defense priority areas; and
- the CIOs at six other agencies met each of the targets for the (1) identity, credential, and access management and (2) anti-phishing and malware defense priority areas.

In fiscal year 2018, the President's Management Agenda[56] replaced the three cybersecurity-focused CAP goal priority areas with updated performance indicators, most of which are to be met by 2020:

1) the manage asset security priority area is similar to the information security continuous monitoring priority area from the previous CAP goal and has a focus on understanding the assets and users on agency networks. In addition to hardware asset and software asset management, this priority area includes performance indicators for authorization and mobile device management.
2) the limit personnel access priority area focuses on issues of access management. This area includes performance indicators for using automated access management and managing access for privileged network and high-impact system users. The privileged network access management performance indicator is a continuation of the identity, credential, and access management priority area of the previous cybersecurity CAP goal. Therefore, agencies are expected to complete this metric by the end of the fiscal year 2018 FISMA reporting year.
3) the protect networks and data priority area, which is similar to the anti-phishing and malware defense priority area from the previous cybersecurity CAP goal, has three

[56] The President's Management Agenda is intended to lay out a long-term vision for modernizing the federal government in key areas that will improve the ability of agencies to deliver mission outcomes, provide excellent service, and effectively steward taxpayer dollars on behalf of the American people.

new performance indicators: intrusion detection and prevention, exfiltration and enhanced defenses, and data protection.

Appendix IV describes the updated cybersecurity-focused CAP priority areas and performance indicators in more detail.

OMB Determined That 13 of the 23 Civilian CFO Act Agencies Were Managing Cybersecurity Risk

In Executive Order 13800, the President directed OMB, in coordination with DHS, to assess and report to the executive branch on the sufficiency and appropriateness of federal agencies' processes for managing cybersecurity risks. For these risk management assessments,[57] OMB leveraged the FISMA metrics reported by agency CIOs and inspectors general for fiscal year 2017. The metrics addressed domains that correspond with the five core security functions identified in the cybersecurity framework. Table 4 lists these domains and their relationship to the core functions.

Table 4. ***Federal Information Security Modernization Act*** **Reporting Metric Domains Leveraged by OMB to Assess Agency Risk Management Processes**

Core security functions	Domains
Identify	Asset management and authorization Comprehensive risk management
Protect	Remote access protection Credentialing and authorization Network protection
Detect	Anti-phishing capabilities Malware defense capabilities Exfiltration and other capabilities
Respond	Planning and processes Evaluation and Improvement
Recover	Planning and testing personal impact process Back-up capacity

Source: GAO analysis of Office of Management and Budget Fiscal Year 2017 Federal Information Security Modernization Act of 2014 Annual Report to Congress. | GAO-19-105.

Based on OMB's evaluation of these domains, agency risk management processes related to the five core security functions and overall agency enterprise fell into one of the following three rating categories:

- managing risk: required cybersecurity policies, procedures, and tools are in use and the agency actively manages cybersecurity risks;
- at risk: some essential policies, processes, and tools are in place to mitigate overall cybersecurity risk, but significant gaps remain; and
- high risk: key fundamental cybersecurity policies, processes, and tools are either not in place or not deployed sufficiently.

For fiscal year 2017, OMB reported that not all agencies were managing risk. When considering each of the five core security functions, OMB reported that most of the 23 agencies were at risk or at high risk with regard to the *identify* and *protect* core security

[57] Office of Management and Budget, *Federal Information Security Modernization Act of 2014, Annual Report to Congress Fiscal Year 2017* (Washington, D.C.: Mar. 2018).

functions. Less than half of the 23 agencies were at risk with regard to the *detect*, *respond*, and *recover* core security functions. Overall, OMB determined that 13 agencies were managing risk and that the remaining 10 agencies were at risk of not effectively identifying, protecting, detecting, responding to, and if necessary, recovering from cyber intrusions. Figure 6 shows OMB's risk management assessment ratings by core security function across the 23 agencies for fiscal year 2017.

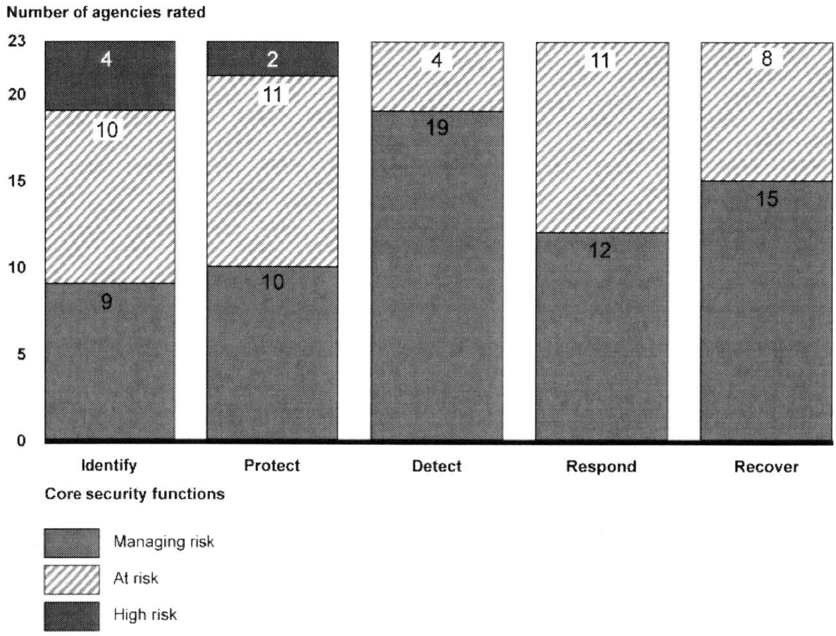

Source: GAO analysis of Office of Management and Budget Fiscal Year 2017 Federal Information Security Modernization Act of 2014 Annual Report to Congress. | GAO-19-105.

The 23 civilian agencies covered by the *Chief Financial Officers Act of 1990* are the Departments of Agriculture, Commerce, Education, Energy, Health and Human Services, Homeland Security, Housing and Urban Development, the Interior, Justice, Labor, State, Transportation, the Treasury, and Veterans Affairs; the Environmental Protection Agency; General Services Administration; National Aeronautics and Space Administration; National Science Foundation; Nuclear Regulatory Commission; Office of Personnel Management; Small Business Administration; Social Security Administration; and the U.S. Agency for International Development.

Figure 6. Risk Management Assessment Ratings by Core Security Function for the 23 Civilian *Chief Financial Officers Act of 1990* Agencies, Fiscal Year 2017.

DHS and OMB Facilitated the Use of Intrusion Detection and Prevention Capabilities to Secure Federal Agency Systems, but Further Efforts Remain

DHS and OMB, as required by law and policy, have taken various actions to facilitate the agencies' use of intrusion detection and prevention capabilities to secure federal systems. For example, DHS has developed an intrusion assessment plan, deployed NCPS to offer intrusion detection and prevention capabilities to agencies, and is providing tools and services to agencies to monitor their networks through its CDM program. However, NCPS still had limitations in detecting certain types of traffic and agencies were not sending all appropriate traffic through the system. Further, CDM was behind at meeting planned implementation dates, and agencies have requested additional training and guidance for these services. OMB has taken steps to improve upon agencies' capabilities, but has not completed a policy and strategy to do so, or fully reported on its assessment of agencies' capabilities.

DHS Has Taken Actions to Facilitate the Use of Intrusion Detection and Prevention Capabilities and to Make Improvements to Those Capabilities

The *Federal Cybersecurity Enhancement Act of 2015* requires DHS, in coordination with OMB, to develop and implement an intrusion assessment plan to proactively detect, identify, and remove intruders in agency information systems on a routine basis. The act also requires that the plan be updated, as necessary.

In December 2016, DHS documented its *Intrusion Assessment Plan*.[58] In the plan, DHS outlined tools, platforms, resources, and ongoing work that the department provides, and that are intended to help agencies detect, identify, and remove intruders on their networks and systems. The intrusion assessment plan also outlines a defense-in-depth strategy, which utilizes multiple layers of cybersecurity and deploys multiple capabilities in combination, to secure agencies' networks and information systems. For example, the plan calls for DHS to implement NCPS to provide a perimeter defense for the networks of federal civilian executive branch agencies, while the agencies are to deploy their own intrusion detection and prevention capabilities inside their networks. DHS submitted its intrusion assessment plan to OMB in January 2017.

DHS Has Worked to Improve NCPS, but Agencies Did Not Route All Traffic through Intrusion Detection and Prevention Capabilities Offered by this System

The *Federal Cybersecurity Enhancement Act of 2015* also requires DHS to deploy, operate, and maintain a capability to detect cybersecurity risks and prevent network traffic associated with such risks from transiting to or from an agency information system. In addition, the act requires that DHS make regular improvements to intrusion detection and prevention capabilities by deploying new technologies and modifying existing technologies. Further, the act requires agencies to use this capability on all information traveling between their information systems and any information system other than an agency information system.

DHS developed NCPS, operationally known as EINSTEIN, to provide the capabilities to detect and prevent potentially malicious network traffic from entering agency networks.

[58] Department of Homeland Security, *Intrusion Assessment Plan: Fiscal Year 2016 Report to Congress* (Washington, D.C.: Dec. 22, 2016).

Consistent with recommendations we made to DHS in January 2016, DHS has taken actions to improve these capabilities and has other actions underway.[59] For example, the department

- determined that enhancing NCPS's current intrusion detection approach to include functionality that would detect deviations from normal network behavior baselines would be feasible. In addition, according to DHS officials, the department was operationalizing functionality intended to identify malicious activity in network traffic otherwise missed by signature-based methods.
- determined that developing enhancements to current intrusion detection capabilities to facilitate the scanning of Internet Protocol Version 6 (IPv6)[60] traffic would be feasible. According to DHS officials, the department has developed plans to fully support IPv6 for several of its NCPS intrusion detection capabilities. Further, the department has developed implementation schedules and begun roll-out of the enhancements.
- updated the tool it uses to manage and deploy intrusion detection signatures to include a mechanism to clearly link signatures to publicly available, open-source information.
- developed clearly defined requirements for detecting threats on agency internal networks and at cloud service providers to help better ensure effective support of information security activities. According to DHS officials, the department was also continuing pilot activities with cloud service providers to enhance protections of agency assets.
- developed processes and procedures for using vulnerability information, such as data from the CDM program as it becomes available, to help ensure the department is using a risk-based approach for the selection/development of future NCPS intrusion prevention capabilities.

Nevertheless, NCPS continues to have known limitations in its ability to identify potential threats. For example:

- NCPS does not have the ability to effectively detect intrusions across multiple types of traffic. Specifically, DHS determined that developing enhancements to current intrusion detection capabilities to facilitate the scanning of traffic related to supervisory control and data acquisition (SCADA)[61] control systems would not be

---

[59] GAO-16-294.

[60] In September 2010, the federal chief information officer issued a memorandum for agency chief information officers stating that the federal government is committed to the operational deployment and use of IPv6, and in July 2012, the Federal Chief Information Officer Council Strategy and Planning Committee issued a roadmap toward IPv6 adoption within the government. The roadmap stated that though both IPv4 (the legacy version of IP) and IPv6 are being used on the Internet, IPv4 is, by far, still the dominate protocol because of its legacy deployment. However, IPv6 traffic growth is inevitable due to the current state of IPv4 address exhaustion, creating an extreme supply and demand curve required to support communications between the U.S. government and its citizens and business partners worldwide.

[61] SCADA is one type of control system, which is a computer-based system used within many infrastructures and industries to monitor and control sensitive processes and physical functions. Control systems perform functions that range from simple to complex. They can be used to simply monitor processes—for example, the environmental conditions in a small office building—or to manage the complex activities of a municipal water

feasible. However, according to DHS officials, the department is exploring capabilities that are intended to provide critical, cross-sector, real-time visibility into critical infrastructure companies that utilize SCADA systems. In addition, DHS determined that the scanning of encrypted traffic would not be feasible. Nevertheless, according to its officials, the department performed research on potential architectural, technical, and policy mitigation strategies that could provide both the protection and situational awareness for encrypted traffic. The department has actions under way to continue its research in this area.

- DHS does not always explicitly ask agencies for feedback or confirmation of receipt of NCPS-related notification. While the department had drafted a standard operating procedure related to its incident notification process, the policy did not instruct DHS analysts specifically to include a solicitation of feedback from agencies within the notification. Further, US-CERT could not provide any information regarding the timetable for when these procedures would take effect.
- Metrics for NCPS, as provided by DHS, do not provide information about how well the system is enhancing government information security or the quality, efficiency and accuracy of supporting actions. Without the deployment of comprehensive measures, DHS cannot appropriately articulate the value provided by NCPS. While the department had taken actions to develop new measures, these measures did not provide a qualitative or quantitative assessment of the system's ability to fulfill the system's objectives.
- NSD did not provide guidance to agencies on how to securely route their information to their Internet service providers. Without providing network routing guidance, NSD has no assurance that the traffic it sees constitutes all or only a subset of the traffic the customer agencies intend to send.

As shown in Table 5, as of October 2018, the department had implemented five of the nine recommendations and was in the process of implementing the remainder. However, until DHS completes implementation of the remaining recommendations, the effectiveness of NCPS's intrusion detection and prevention capabilities may be hindered.

In addition, the 23 civilian CFO Act agencies had implemented NCPS capabilities to varying degrees. In a March 2018 report, OMB reported that 21 (about 91 percent) of the 23 agencies had implemented the first two iterations of the NCPS capabilities.[62] In addition, 15 (about 65 percent) of the 23 agencies had implemented all three NCPS capabilities, as shown in Table 6 below.[63]

However, agencies did not route all network traffic for all information traveling between their information systems and any information system other than an agency information system through NCPS sensors.

---

system or a nuclear power plant. Control systems are vulnerable to cyberattack from inside and outside the control system network.

[62] Office of Management and Budget, *Federal Information Security Modernization Act of 2014, Annual Report to Congress Fiscal Year 2017* (Washington, D.C.: Mar. 2018).

[63] While the March 2018 report shows that DHS reported 17 of the 23 civilian CFO Act agencies implementing all three NCPS capabilities, two of the 17 agencies had not fully implemented the EINSTEIN 3 Accelerated Email Filtering capability. Accordingly, we have adjusted this number to reflect the number of agencies that have fully implemented all three capabilities.

Table 5. Status of GAO 2016 Recommendations to Improve the National Cybersecurity Protection System (NCPS) Capabilities as of October 2018[a]

Recommendation	Status	
	Implemented	In process
Determine the feasibility of enhancing NCPS's current intrusion detection approach to include functionality that would detect deviations from normal network behavior baselines.	✓	
Determine the feasibility of developing enhancements to current intrusion detection capabilities to facilitate the scanning of traffic not currently scanned by NCPS.	✓	
Update the tool the U.S. Computer Emergency Readiness Team uses to manage and deploy intrusion detection signatures to include the ability to more clearly link signatures to publicly available, open-source data repositories.	✓	
Consider the viability of using vulnerability information, such as data from the Continuous Diagnostics and Mitigation program as it becomes available, as an input into the development and management of intrusion detection signatures.		✓
Develop a timetable for finalizing the incident notification process, to ensure that customer agencies are being sent notifications of potential incidents, which clearly solicit feedback on the usefulness and timeliness of the notification.		✓
Develop metrics that clearly measure the effectiveness of NCPS's efforts, including the quality, efficiency, and accuracy of supporting actions related to detecting and preventing intrusions, providing analytic services, and sharing cyber-related information.		✓
Develop clearly defined requirements for detecting threats on agency internal networks and at cloud service providers to help better ensure effective support of information security activities.	✓	
Develop processes and procedures for using vulnerability information, such as data from the Continuous Diagnostics and Mitigation program as it becomes available, to help ensure DHS is using a risk-based approach for the selection/development of future NCPS intrusion prevention capabilities.	✓	
Work with customer agencies and the Internet service providers to document secure routing requirements in order to better ensure the complete, safe, and effective routing of information to NCPS sensors.		✓

Legend: ✓ A checkmark indicates that the recommendation was either implemented or in the process of being implemented, as designated by the column heading.

Source: GAO analysis of Department of Homeland Security data. | GAO-19-105.

[a]Recommendations are found in *Information Security: DHS Needs to Enhance Capabilities, Improve Planning, and Support Greater Adoption of its National Cybersecurity Protection System*. GAO-16-294 (Washington, D.C.: Jan. 28, 2016).

For example, officials at 13 of 23 agencies stated that not all of their agency external network traffic flowed through NCPS.[64] To illustrate, officials at one agency estimated that 20 percent of their external network traffic did not flow through the system. In addition, 4 of the agencies in our review previously cited several challenges in routing all of their traffic through NCPS intrusion detection sensors, including capacity limitations of the sensors, agreements with external business partners that use direct network connections, interagency network connections that do not route through Internet gateways, use of encrypted communications mechanisms, and backup network circuits that are not used regularly. NSD officials stated that agencies are responsible for routing their traffic to the intrusion detection sensors, and DHS does not have a role in that aspect of NCPS implementation. As a result,

[64] External network traffic (traffic that is routed through agency's external connections) must be routed through a Trusted Internet Connection. External connections include those connections between an agency's information system or network and the globally-addressable Internet or a remote information system or network and networks located on foreign territory.

potential cyberattacks may not be detected or prevented for a portion of the external traffic at federal agencies. As noted above, we previously recommended that DHS work with agencies to better ensure the complete routing of information to NCPS sensors.

Table 6. Number of Civilian *Chief Financial Officers Act of 1990* Agencies[a] that Had Implemented the National Cybersecurity Protection System Capabilities through EINSTEIN, by Implementation Status, as of September 2017

Capability	Implemented	In progress	Deferred[b]	Not implemented
EINSTEIN 1 / EINSTEIN 2	21	2	0	0
EINSTEIN 3 Accelerated (DNS Sinkholing)[c]	23	0	0	0
EINSTEIN 3 Accelerated (Email Filtering)[d]	15	6	2	0

Source: Office of Management and Budget Federal Information Security Modernization Act of 2014 Annual Report to Congress Fiscal Year 2017. | GAO-19-105.

[a]These summary implementation data aggregate the status for parent agencies based on the lowest implementation status of all of their components.

[b]An agency with a deferred status faced a technical challenge to implement email filtering for its third-party, cloud-based email service. DHS continues to work with the affected agencies and their EINSTEIN 3 Accelerated service provider to engineer solutions.

[c]The Domain Name System (DNS) Sinkholing capability, used to detect and prevent malicious traffic from federal civilian networks, redirects malicious traffic to "safe servers," also known as "sinkhole" servers."

[d]The email filtering capability, used to protect against the use of email to deliver malware or induce users to download malware to infect agency networks, scans email destined for federal civilian networks for malicious attachments and other potential cyber threats before being delivered to end-users. According to DHS officials, as of November 2018, the completed number greatly increased since the September 2017 report, with the CFO Act agencies being at 99 percent completed.

DHS Has Taken Steps to Provide Advanced Network Security Tools, but Has Not Met Planned Implementation Dates

The *Federal Cybersecurity Enhancement Act of 2015* requires DHS to include, in the efforts of the department to continuously diagnose and mitigate cybersecurity risks, advanced network security tools to improve the visibility of network activity and to detect and mitigate intrusions and anomalous activity.

According to DHS officials, the department is addressing the requirement to improve the visibility of network activity by including advanced network security tools as a part of CDM phase 3. In April 2018, we testified that DHS had previously planned to provide 97 percent of federal agencies with the services they needed for CDM phase 3 in fiscal year 2017.[65] In

[65] GAO, *Cybersecurity: DHS Needs to Enhance Efforts to Improve and Promote the Security of Federal and Private-Sector Networks*, GAO-18-520T (Washington, D.C.: Apr. 24, 2018).

addition, according to OMB's annual FISMA report for fiscal year 2017, the CDM program was to continue to incorporate additional capabilities, including phase 3, in fiscal year 2018.[66]

However, DHS now expects initial operational capabilities[67] to be in place for phase 3 in fiscal year 2019. The department has awarded contracts of approximately $3.26 billion to support its Dynamic and Evolving Federal Enterprise Network Defense (also known as DEFEND) aspect of the CDM program, which is to include phase 3. DEFEND also is to provide coverage for existing agency deployments. According to DHS documentation, the task orders associated with DEFEND are to be issued between the second quarter of fiscal year 2018 and the second quarter of fiscal year 2024.

Agencies Indicated the Need for Additional Training and Guidance Related to NCPS and CDM

FISMA requires that DHS provide operational and technical assistance to agencies in implementing policies, principles, standards, and guidelines on information security. Toward this end, DHS has available training and guidance related to the implementation of the capabilities of NCPS (i.e., EINSTEIN) and CDM. Specifically:

- According the DHS officials, the department offers training and guidance to agencies on EINSTEIN 1 implementation. For example, DHS established a program in which the Software Engineering Institute will provide training and mentoring to agencies looking to enhance their understanding of, and proficiency with, the EINSTEIN 1 capability (e.g., network traffic information).[68] NCPS program officials stated that agencies can use this service, which is available at no charge to them, on an unlimited basis as long as the requests relate to EINSTEIN 1. According to the officials, training and guidance related to EINSTEIN 2 and EINSTEIN 3 Accelerated is limited because DHS intentionally restricts the amount of data provided to agencies.
- According to DHS officials, the department also offers training and guidance to assist agencies with the implementation and use of resources associated with the CDM program, including webinars, guides, and computer-based training. The DEFEND contracts that the department awarded also include a mechanism for agencies to procure specialized tailored training, such as on the use of CDM tools. The department also offers customer advisory forums every other month that agencies are invited to attend. According to CDM program officials, the program's governance, among other topics, is commonly discussed during these forums. Further, the department provides agencies with guidance, such as various governance documents, best practices, and frequently asked questions, through a web portal that

---

[66] Office of Management and Budget, *Federal Information Security Modernization Act of 2014, Annual Report to Congress Fiscal Year 2017* (Washington, D.C.: Mar. 2018).

[67] Initial operational capability is a DHS-defined project milestone that is attained when the capabilities for a phase have been fully deployed to at least five agencies.

[68] The Software Engineering Institute is a federally funded research and development center at Carnegie Mellon University. The institute works with DHS to strengthen the nation's resistance to cyber threats and improve the practice of cybersecurity.

is made available by OMB. In addition, US-CERT offers the CDM training program, which is to provide CDM implementation resources.

Nevertheless, most agencies told us that they wanted DHS to provide more training and guidance as it relates to their implementation of the capabilities made available by NCPS and CDM. Specifically,

- Officials from 16 of 23 agencies reported that they wanted to receive additional training on NCPS capabilities. For example, officials at 5 agencies stated that they would like to receive training related to using network traffic information, understanding alerts, or implementing capabilities for cloud services. The officials also stated that they wanted training specific to agency security personnel.
- Officials from 19 of 23 agencies stated that they wanted to receive additional guidance related to NCPS's capabilities, but not all of the 19 provided specific details. For example, officials from at least 3 agencies stated that they wanted additional guidance such as, "how to" documents, descriptions of architecture details, or guidance documents that explain NCPS's capabilities so that agencies can gauge the gap between the security that the system provides and the security being provided by their own agency's capabilities.
- Officials from 21 of 23 agencies reported that they wanted to receive additional training on implementing CDM at their agencies. For example, officials from 7 agencies suggested that additional training on the use of the tools would be beneficial.
- Officials from 22 of 23 agencies stated that they wanted additional guidance as it relates to CDM implementation. For example, officials from one agency stated that they would like examples of best practices and successful deployments.

These requests for additional training and guidance demonstrate that agencies are either unaware of the available training and guidance, or that the training may not meet their needs. Until DHS coordinates with agencies to determine if additional training and guidance are needed, agencies may not be able to fully realize the benefits of the capabilities provided by the NCPS and CDM programs.

OMB Took Actions to Oversee Agency Implementation of Intrusion Detection and Prevention Capabilities and Report to Congress, but Did Not Fully Complete Required Actions

Although OMB took steps to report on agencies' implementation of intrusion detection and prevention capabilities, it did not report on all required actions. For example, the office did not submit DHS's intrusion plan to Congress as required by the *Federal Cybersecurity Enhancement Act of 2015*. In addition, OMB provided various reports to Congress that described agencies' intrusion detection and prevention capabilities, but the reports did not always include all information required by the act. Further, OMB developed a draft policy and strategy that were intended to improve agency capabilities, but it had not finalized these documents.

OMB Did Not Submit the Intrusion Assessment Plan to Congress or Fully Describe the Plan's Implementation in Other Reports

The *Federal Cybersecurity Enhancement Act of 2015* requires OMB to submit the intrusion assessment plan developed by DHS to the appropriate congressional committees no later than 6 months after the date of enactment of the act. The act also required OMB to submit to Congress a description of the implementation of the intrusion assessment plan and the findings of the intrusion assessments[69] conducted pursuant to the intrusion assessment plan no later than 1 year after the date of enactment of the act, and annually thereafter.

Although DHS developed and documented an intrusion assessment plan, which described a defense-in-depth approach to security, OMB did not submit the plan to Congress, as called for in the act. Even though DHS submitted the plan to OMB in January 2017, OMB had not submitted it to Congress as of October 2018 (21 months after DHS submitted the plan and 28 months past the due date).

On the other hand, OMB did submit its own reports to Congress which generally described elements of the implementation of DHS's intrusion assessment plan and intrusion assessment findings. In September 2017, OMB issued its analysis of agencies' implementation of intrusion detection and prevention capabilities, or more specifically, agencies' implementation of the various versions of NCPS.[70] In addition, the office's annual FISMA report, issued most recently in March 2018,[71] generally covered elements of the intrusion assessment plan. OMB personnel within the Office of the Federal CIO believed that these two reports, along with a process the office had initiated to validate incidents across the government, addressed the requirement for OMB to submit to Congress a description of the implementation of the intrusion assessment plan and the findings of the intrusion assessments conducted pursuant to the plan.

However, the September 2017 and March 2018 reports did not address other elements described in DHS's intrusion assessment plan. For example, OMB did not describe agency roles associated with segmenting their networks, identifying key servers based on threat and impact, ensuring all applications are appropriately tracked and configured, and categorizing and tagging data based on threat and impact. While OMB has provided important information to congressional stakeholders through its own reports, until it submits the plan and addresses all elements described in DHS's intrusion assessment plan, it will continue to be remiss in providing timely and sufficiently detailed information regarding the intrusion assessment plan to congressional stakeholders to support their oversight responsibilities.

---

[69] Intrusion assessments, as defined by the *Federal Cybersecurity Enhancement Act of 2015*, refer to actions taken under the intrusion assessment plan to identify and remove intruders in agency information systems.

[70] Office of Management and Budget, *Agency Application of the National Cybersecurity Protection System and Intrusion Detection and Prevention Capabilities* (Washington, D.C.: September 2017).

[71] Office of Management and Budget, *Federal Information Security Modernization Act of 2014, Annual Report to Congress Fiscal Year 2017* (Washington, D.C.: Mar. 2018).

OMB Submitted Its Analysis of Agencies' Application of Intrusion Detection and Prevention Capabilities, but Did Not Include the Degree to Which the Capabilities Had Been Applied

The *Federal Cybersecurity Enhancement Act of 2015* also required that OMB submit an analysis of agencies' application of the intrusion detection and prevention capabilities to Congress no later than 18 months after the date of enactment of the act, and annually thereafter. OMB was to include a list of federal agencies and the degree to which each agency had applied the intrusion detection and prevention capabilities in this analysis.

As discussed previously in this chapter, OMB issued its analysis of agencies' implementation of intrusion detection and prevention capabilities in September 2017. However, the analysis did not include the degree to which agencies had applied the intrusion detection and prevention capabilities. For example, the analysis did not reflect that not all agencies were using this capability on all information traveling between their systems and any system other than an agency system, as required by the act. Until OMB includes the degree to which agencies have applied intrusion detection and prevention capabilities in its analysis, it cannot provide congressional stakeholders with an accurate portrayal of the extent to which the capabilities are detecting and preventing potential intrusions.

The Federal Chief Information Officer Reported on Intrusion Detection and Prevention Capabilities, but Did Not Address All Elements Required by the Federal Cybersecurity Enhancement Act of 2015

The *Federal Cybersecurity Enhancement Act of 2015* further required that the Federal Chief Information Officer, within OMB, submit a report to Congress no earlier than 18 months after the date of enactment, but no later than 2 years after that date, assessing the intrusion detection and intrusion prevention capabilities that DHS made available to agencies. The act required that the report address (1) the effectiveness of DHS's system used for detecting, disrupting, and preventing cyber-threat actors, including advanced persistent threats, from accessing agency information and agency information systems; (2) whether the intrusion detection and prevention capabilities, continuous diagnostics and mitigation, and other systems deployed are effective in securing federal information systems; (3) the costs and benefits of the intrusion detection and prevention capabilities, including as compared to commercial technologies and tools, and including the value of classified cyber threat indicators; and (4) the capability of agencies to protect sensitive cyber threat indicators and defensive measures if they were shared through unclassified mechanisms for use in commercial technologies and tools.

In a report issued in September 2018 (about 8 months past the required due date), the Federal Chief Information Officer provided Congress an assessment of intrusion detection and intrusion prevention capabilities across the federal enterprise. The report pointed out, among other things, that agencies did not possess or properly deploy capabilities to detect or prevent intrusions or minimize the impact of intrusions when they occur. In addition, the report acknowledged the need to improve the effectiveness of intrusion detection and intrusion prevention capabilities and stated that OMB would track performance through the CAP goal and annual FISMA reports.

However, the report did not address all of the requirements specified in the act. For example, the report did not address whether DHS's system (i.e., NCPS) was effective in detecting advanced persistent threats. In addition, the report did not include a comparison of the costs and benefits of the intrusion detection and prevention capabilities versus commercial technologies and tools, or the value of classified cyber threat indicators. Further, the report did not address the capability of agencies to protect sensitive cyber threat indicators and defensive measures. Until OMB updates the Federal CIO report to address all of the requirements specified in the act, it will continue to be remiss in providing timely and sufficiently detailed information, such as that related to costs and benefits, among other elements in the act, to congressional stakeholders to support their oversight responsibilities.

OMB Initiated Plans for Improving Agencies' Implementation of Intrusion Detection and Prevention Capabilities, but Has Not Completed a Policy and Strategy

In addition to OMB's responsibilities in the *Federal Cybersecurity Enhancement Act of 2015*, OMB has initiated plans for further improving agencies' intrusion detection and prevention capabilities. In response to a tasking in Executive Order 13800, the Director of the American Technology Council coordinated the development of a report to the President from the Secretary of DHS, the Director of OMB, and the Administrator of the General Services Administration, regarding the modernization of federal information technology (IT).

The report, *Report to the President on Federal IT Modernization*, identified actions that OMB should take for (1) prioritizing the modernization of high-risk, high-value assets and (2) modernizing the Trusted Internet Connection (TIC) program[72] and NCPS to improve protections,[73] remove barriers, and enable commercial cloud migration. For example, OMB was to take the following actions subsequent to the December 13, 2017 report issuance date:

- Within 60 days: Update a TIC policy to address challenges with agencies' perimeter-based architectures, such as the modernization of NCPS. In addition, introduce a "90 day sprint" during which approved projects would pilot proposed changes in TIC requirements.
- Within 90 days: Update the annual FISMA and CAP goal metrics to focus on those critical capabilities that were most commonly lacking among agencies and focus oversight assessments on high-value assets.
- Within 120 days: In conjunction with DHS, develop a strategy for optimally realigning resources across agencies to reduce the risk to high-value assets and respond to cybersecurity incidents for those assets.

OMB has taken steps toward implementing several, but not all, of these actions. For example, it introduced a "90 day sprint" and, according to knowledgeable OMB staff, the outcomes of this action are directly informing changes in TIC requirements. In addition,

---

[72] In November 2007, OMB issued M-08-05 that announced the Trusted Internet Connections Initiative, which is intended to improve the federal government's security posture by reducing and consolidating external network connections, including Internet connections, currently in use by the government, and by centrally monitoring the traffic passing through these connections for potentially malicious activity. All federal agencies in the executive branch, except for the Department of Defense, are required to implement the initiative. Although the initiative is intended to secure connections to the Internet, other external connections to potentially unsecured systems must also be routed through an approved TIC access point, even if they do not pass through the Internet.

[73] The modernization report notes that TIC gateways apply common security protections for agencies, as well as common intrusion detection, information sharing, and prevention capabilities under DHS's NCPS.

OMB updated the annual FISMA and CAP goal metrics by including several metrics that focus on high-value assets. The updated FISMA and CAP goal metrics went into effect in April 2018.

However, while OMB had taken steps toward updating the TIC policy and developing a strategy for optimally realigning resources, the policy and strategy were in draft and had not yet been finalized as of October 2018. The agency did not specify a time frame for finalizing the policy and strategy. Until OMB finalizes the TIC policy and the strategy for optimally realigning resources, the enhancements offered through the policy and strategy are unlikely to be realized.

SELECTED AGENCIES HAD NOT CONSISTENTLY IMPLEMENTED CAPABILITIES TO DETECT AND PREVENT INTRUSIONS

FISMA requires agencies to provide information security protections to prevent unauthorized access to their systems and information. Officials from the 23 selected agencies reported to us that they generally took steps to meet this requirement by augmenting the tools and services provided by DHS with their own intrusion detection and prevention capabilities. However, agencies did not consistently implement five key capabilities specified by DHS and NIST guidance. In addition, most of the agencies did not fully implement any of the phases of DHS's CDM program that is intended to improve their capabilities to detect and prevent intrusions.

Few Agencies Had Fully Implemented Required Email Protections

Binding Operational Directive (BOD) 18-01 instructs agencies to enhance email security.[74] These enhancements include enabling encrypted email transmission, ensuring that receiving mail servers know what actions the agency would like taken when an email falsely claims to have originated from the agency, and removing certain insecure protocols, among others.[75] The final deadline for implementing all BOD 18-01 requirements was October 16, 2018. Additionally, NIST SP 800-53 Revision 4 recommends that security awareness training include training on how to recognize and prevent spear-phishing attempts.

As of September 2018, only 2 of the 23 agencies reported implementing all of the email requirements. For the remaining 21 agencies:

- 9 agencies stated that their agency had plans to implement all enhancements by the October 2018 deadline,

---

[74] According to OMB, email, by way of phishing attacks, remains one of the most common threat vectors (or avenues of attack) across the government. See *Federal Cybersecurity Risk Determination Report and Action Plan* (Washington, D.C.: May 2018).

[75] Department of Homeland Security, *Enhance Email and Web Security*, BOD 18-01 (Washington, D.C.: Oct. 16, 2017).

- 1 agency was uncertain whether it would meet the deadline, and
- 11 stated they would not be able to meet the deadline.[76]

By contrast, the majority of agencies (22 of 23) reported that they had trained staff on spear-phishing exercises, as recommended by NIST SP 800-53 Revision 4. Officials at the remaining agency told us that the agency planned to have spear-phishing exercises in fiscal year 2019. Such training should help ensure that phishing will be a less effective attack vector against the majority of agencies. While agencies benefit from secure protocols and spear-phishing training, implementing the remaining BOD 18-01 email requirements would provide additional protection to agency information systems.

Agencies Informed GAO That They Often Had Not Implemented Four Key Capabilities

NIST recommends that federal agencies deploy intrusion detection and prevention capabilities. These capabilities include monitoring cloud services, using host-based intrusion prevention systems, monitoring external and internal network traffic, and using a security information and event management (SIEM) system. However, in our semi-structured interviews of the 23 agencies, officials told us that they often had not implemented many of these capabilities. Such inconsistent implementation exposes federal systems and the information they contain to additional risk. As part of their continuing oversight efforts, OMB and DHS can use the information below to work with agencies to identify obstacles and impediments affecting the agencies' abilities to implement these capabilities.

Less Than Half of the Selected Agencies That Used Cloud Services Monitored Their Cloud-Related Traffic

NIST SP 800-53 Revision 4 states that agencies should monitor and control communications at the external boundary of the network. However, as of June 2018, fewer than half of the agencies that used cloud computing services were monitoring cloud traffic. Specifically:

- 10 of 22 agencies that used Infrastructure as a Service were monitoring inbound and outbound Infrastructure as a Service traffic,
- 7 of 21 agencies that used Platform as a Service were monitoring inbound and outbound Platform as a Service traffic, and
- 10 of 23 agencies that used Software as a Service were monitoring inbound and outbound Software as a Service traffic.

---

[76] In September 2018, DHS issued a temporary policy exception notice to federal agencies for BOD 18-01's weak email cipher requirement. The notice requested that agencies impacted by the notice submit to DHS preventive security measures and a mitigation strategy that would be in place until these matters would be resolved. Evaluating DHS's temporary policy exception notice and agency actions taken as a result of the notice was not within the scope of this review. Of the 11 agencies that said they would not meet the October 2018 deadline, 4 stated that they could not meet the weak email cipher requirement due to their reliance on external email vendors. Two of the 4 said they were unable to meet other requirements as well.

Without monitoring traffic to and from cloud service providers, agencies risk a greater chance of malicious cloud activity detrimentally affecting agency information security.

Several Selected Agencies Had Not Fully Deployed Host-Based Capabilities

NIST SP 800-53 Revision 4 states that agency internal monitoring may be achieved by utilizing intrusion prevention capabilities. These capabilities include using host-based intrusion prevention systems to provide defense at an individual system or device level by protecting against malicious activities. Host-based capabilities include memory-based protection[77] and application whitelisting.[78]

As of June 2018, officials at the 23 agencies reported the following to us:

- 16 agencies used host-based intrusion prevention capabilities,
- 15 agencies used memory-based protection, and
- 8 agencies used host-based application whitelisting.

Until host-based intrusion protections are fully deployed, agencies will be at greater risk of malicious activity adversely affecting agency operations.

Not All Selected Agencies Monitored External and Internal Traffic

NIST SP 800-53 Revision 4 also states that agencies should monitor and control communications at the external boundary of the network and at key internal boundaries (e.g., network traffic). NIST guidance also stated that an agency should deploy monitoring devices strategically within the network to detect essential information.

However, the agencies in our review did not always monitor external and internal traffic. For example, of the 23 agencies:

- 5 reported that they were not monitoring inbound or outbound direct connections to outside entities.
- 11 reported that they were not persistently monitoring inbound encrypted traffic.
- 8 reported that they were not persistently monitoring outbound encrypted traffic.

In addition, 13 agencies reported they were not using a network-based session capture solution.[79] Of the 10 agencies that reported using this solution, officials from 2 agencies stated that they were not capturing workstation-to-workstation connections. Without thorough monitoring of external and internal traffic, agencies will have less assurance that they are aware of compromised or potentially compromised traffic within their network.

Most Agencies Reported Using a Security Information and Event Management Capability, but Did Not Always Use this Capability to Analyze Potential Threats

NIST SP 800-53 Revision 4 states that agencies should establish enhanced monitoring capabilities. Such capabilities should include automated mechanisms that collect and analyze

---

[77] Memory-based protections are safeguards that protect memory from unauthorized code execution.

[78] An application whitelist is a list of applications and application components that an agency has authorized for use on its hosts.

[79] A network-based session capture solution records information exchanged across an agency's network.

incident data for increased threat and situational awareness. According to NIST, a security information and event management (SIEM) system analyzes data from different sources and identifies and prioritizes significant events. Sources of data used by SIEM systems include logs from database systems, network devices, security systems, web applications, and workstation operating systems.[80]

Of the 23 agencies that we reviewed, 21 reported using a SIEM capability. Over half of the agencies employing a SIEM used one or more of their logs to match against known vulnerabilities and advanced persistent threats, as well as to create real-time alerts. For example, of the 21 agencies:

- 14 agencies reported collecting database logs, but only 7 agencies reported using the logs to match against known vulnerabilities and persistent threats and to create real-time alerts;
- 20 agencies reported collecting network logs, but only 13 agencies reported using them to match against known vulnerabilities and persistent threats and to create real-time alerts;
- 21 agencies reported collecting security logs, but only 13 reported using them to match against known vulnerabilities and persistent threats and to create real-time alerts;
- 15 agencies reported collecting web application logs, but only 9 agencies reported using them to match against known vulnerabilities and persistent threats and to create real-time alerts; and
- 13 agencies reported collecting workstation logs, but only 8 agencies reported using them to match against known vulnerabilities and persistent threats and to create real-time alerts.
- Only 5 agencies collected all 5 types of logs and used them to match against known vulnerabilities and persistent threats and to create real-time alerts.

By not fully using SIEM capabilities, agencies will have less assurance that relevant personnel will be aware of possible weaknesses or intrusions.

Agencies Are in the Process of Implementing DHS' CDM Program, but Most Agencies Have Not Fully Implemented Any of the Program Phases

To further enhance their intrusion detection and prevention capabilities, the 23 civilian CFO Act agencies were in the process of implementing DHS's CDM program. As previously discussed, Phase 1 of the program involves deploying products to automate hardware and software asset management, configuration settings, and common vulnerability management capabilities. Phase 2 intends to address privilege management and infrastructure integrity by allowing agencies to monitor users on their networks and to detect whether users are engaging

[80] According to NIST, logs are records of the events occurring within an organization's systems and networks. Logs from security software, operating systems, and applications typically contain information that includes security-related data.

in unauthorized activity. Phase 3 is intended to assess agency network activity and identify any anomalies that may indicate a cybersecurity compromise.

As of June 2018, most agencies had not fully implemented any of the three phases. As shown in Figure 7, 15 agencies had partially implemented phase 1, 21 had partially or not yet begun to implement phase 2, and none of thc agencies had fully implemented phase 3.

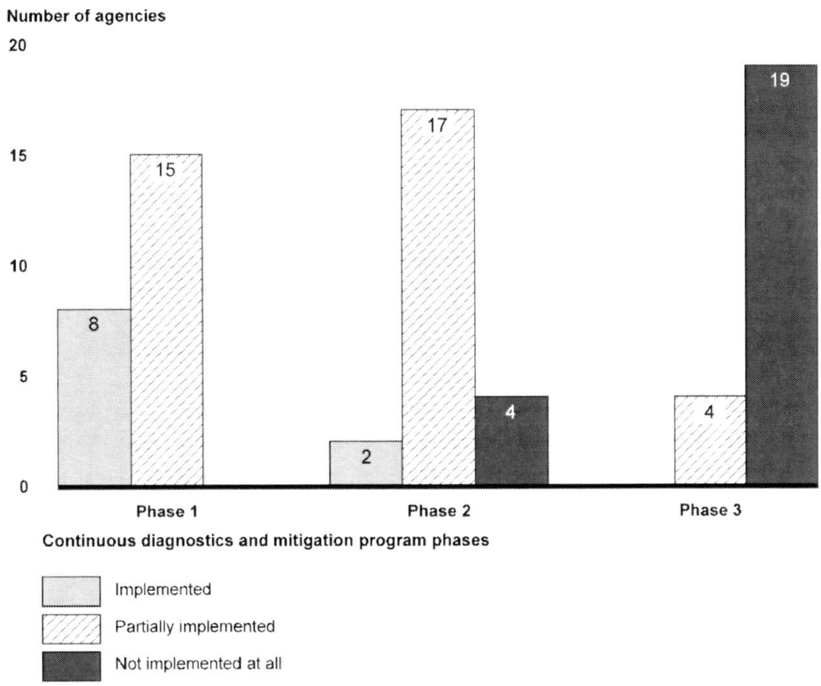

Source: GAO analysis based on agency provided data. | GAO-19-105.

Figure 7. Civilian *Chief Financial Officers Act of 1990* Agencies' Implementation of DHS's Continuous Diagnostics and Mitigation Program Phases, as of June 2018.

Agencies' implementation status has been affected, at least in part, due to delays in DHS's deployment of the program phases. As a result, federal systems will remain at risk until the program is fully deployed.

CONCLUSION

Many agencies have not effectively implemented the federal approach and strategy for securing information systems. For example, the inspectors general for 17 of the 23 selected agencies reported that their agencies had not effectively implemented their information security programs and had significant information security deficiencies associated with internal control over financial reporting. In addition, CIOs for 17 agencies reported not meeting all nine targets for the cybersecurity cross-agency priority goal. Further, OMB determined that that only 13 of the 23 agencies were managing risks to their overall enterprise, while the other 10 agencies were at risk. Until agencies more effectively implement the government's approach and strategy, federal systems will remain at risk.

DHS and OMB have initiatives underway that are intended to further improve agencies' security posture. However, although DHS had provided training and guidance for NCPS and CDM, agencies expressed the need for more. In addition, OMB had also not finalized its policy and strategy aimed at addressing challenges with perimeter security and protecting high value assets, respectively. OMB had also not provided useful information to Congress, such as a description of agencies' implementation of DHS's intrusion assessment plan, the degree to which agencies are using NCPS, a complete analysis of agencies' implementation of DHS's intrusion assessment plan, or the costs and benefits of using commercial tools.

Although agencies' officials reported various efforts underway to enhance their agency's intrusion detection and prevention capabilities, implementation efforts across the federal government were not consistent. OMB and DHS can use the information provided in this chapter to work with agencies to identify obstacles and impediments affecting the agencies' abilities to implement these capabilities.

Recommendations for Executive Action

We are making a total of nine recommendations, including two to DHS and seven to OMB. Specifically:

- The Secretary of DHS should direct the Network Security Deployment division to coordinate further with federal agencies to identify training and guidance needs for implementing NCPS and CDM. (Recommendation 1)
- The Secretary of DHS should direct the appropriate staff to work with OMB to follow up with agencies to identify obstacles and impediments affecting their abilities to implement intrusion detection and prevention capabilities. (Recommendation 2)
- The Director of OMB should submit the intrusion assessment plan to the appropriate congressional committees. (Recommendation 3)
- The Director of OMB should report on implementation of the defense-in-depth strategy described in the intrusion assessment plan, including all elements described in the plan. (Recommendation 4)
- The Director of OMB should update the analysis of agencies' intrusion detection and prevention capabilities to include the degree to which agencies are using NCPS. (Recommendation 5)
- The Director of OMB should direct the Federal CIO to update her report to Congress to include required information, such as detecting advanced persistent threats, a comparison of the costs and benefits of the capabilities versus commercial technologies and tools, and the capability of agencies to protect sensitive cyber threat indicators and defense measures. (Recommendation 6)
- The Director of OMB should establish a time frame for finalizing the Trusted Internet Connections policy intended to address challenges with agencies' perimeter-based architectures and issue it when finalized. (Recommendation 7)

- The Director of OMB should establish a time frame for finalizing the strategy for realigning resources across agencies to protect high-value assets and issue it when finalized. (Recommendation 8)
- The Director of OMB should direct the Federal CIO to work with DHS to follow-up with agencies to identify obstacles and impediments affecting their abilities to implement intrusion detection and prevention capabilities. (Recommendation 9)

AGENCY COMMENTS AND OUR EVALUATION

We provided a draft of this chapter to OMB and the 23 civilian CFO Act agencies, including DHS, covered by our review. In response, OMB provided comments via email, and DHS and three other agencies (the Department of Commerce, Social Security Administration, and U.S. Agency for International Development) provided written comments, which are reprinted in appendices V through VIII, respectively. The 19 remaining agencies (the Departments of Agriculture, Education, Energy, Health and Human Services, Housing and Urban Development, the Interior, Justice, Labor, State, Transportation, the Treasury, and Veterans Affairs; as well as the Environmental Protection Agency, General Services Administration, National Aeronautics and Space Administration, National Science Foundation, Nuclear Regulatory Commission, Office of Personnel Management, and Small Business Administration) stated via email that they had no comments.

In its comments, which the OMB liaison provided to GAO via email on December 7, 2018, OMB did not state whether it agreed or disagreed with the seven recommendations that we made to it. Rather, according to the liaison, OMB agreed with the facts in our draft report, but found that the report did not reflect the agency's rationale for not submitting the DHS intrusion assessment plan to Congress and a report on the implementation of the plan, as required by the *Federal Cybersecurity Enhancement Act of 2015*. The liaison stated that OMB is working closely with DHS to provide strategic direction in assessing gaps in, and modernizing, the manner in which intrusion detection and prevention capabilities are delivered to the federal government. Further, in a subsequent email on December 10, 2018, OMB said it believes the Federal CIO's September 2018 report to Congress, along with data provided in OMB's fiscal year 2017 FISMA report to Congress, achieves the outcomes sought by the *Federal Cybersecurity Enhancement Act of 2015* and demonstrates OMB's continuous engagement with DHS across the evolution of the intrusion detection and prevention program.

As stated in our report, we acknowledge that OMB has provided important information to congressional stakeholders through its reports. However, OMB's reports did not cover all outcomes described in the act. For example, as we pointed out, these reports did not fully address implementation of the defense-in-depth strategy described in DHS's intrusion assessment plan. In addition, although OMB reported on several elements required by the *Federal Cybersecurity Enhancement Act of 2015*, it did not report on all of the required elements. For example, the reports did not address whether DHS's NCPS was effective in detecting advanced persistent threats. The reports also did not include a comparison of the costs and benefits of the intrusion detection and prevention capabilities versus commercial technologies and tools, or the value of classified cyber threat indicators. Further, the reports did not address the capability of agencies to protect sensitive cyber threat indicators and defensive measures. Accordingly, we maintain that our recommendations for OMB to report on required elements in the *Federal Cybersecurity Enhancement Act of 2015* are warranted.

In addition, OMB suggested that we revise our recommendations to the agency to include a shared responsibility with DHS to help drive desired outcomes. However, six of the seven recommendations we are making to OMB are related to specific OMB responsibilities cited in either the *Federal Cybersecurity Enhancement Act of 2015* or the *Report to the President on Federal IT Modernization*. As such, we believe the recommendations are appropriately addressed to OMB. Furthermore, our recommendations do not prevent OMB from working with DHS to implement them. Our seventh recommendation to OMB—to work with DHS to follow up with agencies to identify obstacles and impediments affecting their abilities to implement intrusion detection and prevention capabilities—includes a shared responsibility with DHS. OMB also provided technical comments, which we incorporated into the report, as appropriate.

Subsequent to providing initial comments on our draft report, OMB issued a memorandum intended to provide a strategy for realigning resources across agencies to protect high-value assets.[81] This action addresses our recommendation 8, which called for the Director of OMB to establish a time frame for finalizing the strategy for realigning resources across agencies to protect high-value assets, and to issue the strategy when finalized.

In its comments, DHS stated that it concurred with the two recommendations we made to the department. DHS stated that it expects to implement the recommendations in 2019.

The Department of Commerce commented that the report was reasonable and that the department agreed with the findings and recommendations.

In its comments, the Social Security Administration stated that protecting its networks and information is a critical priority. According to the agency, it continued to make improvements in fiscal year 2018, such as improvements and progress in securing applications, leveraging the cloud, managing its assets and vulnerabilities, strengthening its network and incident response capabilities, improving its security training, and enhancing the overall effectiveness of its cybersecurity program.

Finally, the U.S. Agency for International Development commented that its inspector general had improved the agency's capability maturity ratings for core security functions in fiscal year 2018. The agency also pointed out that it was the only selected agency in which fiscal year 2017 indicators of effectiveness in implementing the federal approach and strategy for securing information systems were all positive (as noted in Appendix III).

We are sending copies of this chapter to appropriate congressional committees, the Director of OMB, the heads of the 23 civilian CFO Act agencies and their inspectors general, and other interested congressional parties.

Gregory C. Wilshusen
Director, Information Security Issues

---

[81] Office of Management and Budget, *Strengthening the Cybersecurity of Federal Agencies by Enhancing the High Value Asset Program*, M-19-03 (Washington, D.C.: Dec. 10, 2018).

Appendix I: Objectives, Scope, and Methodology

The *Federal Cybersecurity Enhancement Act of 2015*, which was enacted December 18, 2015, included a provision for GAO to report on the effectiveness of the federal government's approach and strategy for securing agency information systems, including intrusion detection and prevention capabilities.[82] The objectives of our review were to assess: (1) the reported effectiveness of selected agencies' implementation of the federal government's approach and strategy to securing agency information systems; (2) the extent to which the Office of Management and Budget (OMB) and the Department of Homeland Security (DHS) have facilitated the use of intrusion detection and prevention capabilities to secure federal agency information systems; and (3) the extent to which selected agencies reported implementing intrusion detection and prevention capabilities.

Selected agencies for our review were the 23 civilian agencies covered by the *Chief Financial Officers Act of 1990* (CFO Act).[83] We did not include the Department of Defense because the *Federal Cybersecurity Enhancement Act of 2015* only pertains to civilian agencies. Because we focused our work on the 23 civilian agencies, results from these reviews are not generalizable to the entire federal government.

To assess the reported effectiveness of agencies' implementation of the federal government's approach and strategy to securing agency information systems, we

- described the federal government's approach and strategy by summarizing the Federal Information Security Modernization Act of 2014 (FISMA),[84] Executive Order 13800, Strengthening the Cybersecurity of Federal Networks and Critical Infrastructure,[85] and the National Institute of Standards and Technology's (NIST) Framework for Improving Critical Infrastructure Cybersecurity[86] (cybersecurity framework).
- assessed the reported effectiveness of agencies' implementation of the approach and strategy by reviewing annual reports from OMB and the inspectors general (IG) of the 23 civilian CFO Act agencies regarding the reported implementation of FISMA for fiscal year 2017. We described the IG reported maturity levels, including the Office of Inspectors General FISMA Reporting Metrics definition of "effectiveness." These maturity levels are based on security domains aligned with the five core

[82] The act is a part of the *Consolidated Appropriations Act*, 2016, Pub. L. No. 114-113, div. N, title II, subtitle B, 129 Stat. 2242, 2963 -2975 (Dec. 18, 2015).

[83] The 23 civilian *Chief Financial Officers Act of 1990* agencies are the Departments of Agriculture, Commerce, Education, Energy, Health and Human Services, Homeland Security, Housing and Urban Development, the Interior, Justice, Labor, State, Transportation, the Treasury, and Veterans Affairs; the Environmental Protection Agency; General Services Administration; National Aeronautics and Space Administration; National Science Foundation; Nuclear Regulatory Commission; Office of Personnel Management; Small Business Administration; Social Security Administration; and the U.S. Agency for International Development.

[84] The *Federal Information Security Modernization Act of 2014* (FISMA 2014), enacted as Pub. L. No. 113-283, 128 Stat. 3073 (Dec. 18, 2014), largely superseded the *Federal Information Security Management Act of 2002* (FISMA 2002), enacted as *Title III, E-Government Act of 2002*, Pub. L. No. 107-347, 116 Stat. 2899, 2946 (Dec. 17, 2002). As used in this report, FISMA refers both to FISMA 2014 and to those provisions of FISMA 2002 that were either incorporated into FISMA 2014 or were unchanged and continue in full force and effect.

[85] The White House, *Strengthening the Cybersecurity of Federal Networks and Critical Infrastructure,* Executive Order 13800 (Washington, D.C.: May 11, 2017), 82 Fed. Reg. 22391 (May 16, 2017).

[86] National Institute of Standards and Technology, *Framework for Improving Critical Infrastructure Cybersecurity*, Version 1.1 (Gaithersburg, MD: Apr. 16, 2018).

functions in NIST's cybersecurity framework. We also summarized IG reported conclusions on the effectiveness of agencies' information security programs for fiscal year 2017.

- reviewed the fiscal year 2016 and 2017 financial statement audit reports for each of the 23 civilian CFO Act agencies to identify the extent to which any significant deficiencies or material weaknesses related to information security over financial systems had been reported and to identify information security control weaknesses reported by the IGs.
- identified whether agencies had met the targets for the cybersecurity focused cross-agency priority goal for fiscal years 2016 and 2017 by examining agency-reported performance metrics for fiscal years 2016 and 2017.
- evaluated OMB's agency risk management assessment ratings to make a determination on how agencies were managing risk to their enterprise. These conclusions were based on FISMA metrics, and are aligned with the five core security functions defined in the cybersecurity framework.
- interviewed knowledgeable OMB officials and staff to obtain their views on the reported effectiveness of the federal government's approach and strategy to securing agency information systems.

To assess the extent to which OMB and DHS have facilitated the use of intrusion detection and prevention capabilities to secure federal agency information systems, we

- determined the extent OMB and DHS fulfilled their requirements described in the *Federal Cybersecurity Enhancement Act of 2015* by collecting and reviewing artifacts from OMB and DHS and comparing them to the provisions outlined in the act. We also interviewed knowledgeable officials from OMB and DHS regarding their efforts to fulfill their requirements described in the act.
- determined the effectiveness of corrective actions taken by DHS to address nine previously reported recommendations we made in our report related to NCPS.[87] Specifically, we collected appropriate artifacts and assessed the artifacts against the criteria used in that report, and determined the extent to which the actions taken by DHS met the intent of the recommendations, and we met with DHS staff responsible for the remediation activities and obtained their views of the status of actions taken to address the recommendations.
- held semi-structured interviews[88] with knowledgeable officials from the 23 civilian CFO Act agencies. During these interviews, we obtained the agency's views on whether they need more training and guidance from DHS for NCPS and CDM. We also interviewed knowledgeable officials and staff at DHS to obtain their views on how DHS had improved the intrusion detection and prevention capabilities it

---

[87] GAO, *Information Security: DHS Needs to Enhance Capabilities, Improve Planning, and Support Greater Adoption of Its National Cybersecurity Protection System*, GAO-16-294 (Washington, D.C.: Jan. 28, 2016).

[88] A semi-structured interview methodology generally involves asking a similar subset of questions of multiple interviewees. We used a semi-structured interview format with both closed- and open-ended questions. The intent of our open-ended questions was to engage the agency officials in a conversation about the topics being discussed.

provides to federal agencies. We also interviewed DHS officials to obtain their views on the training and guidance that the department makes available to agencies.

To assess the extent to which selected agencies reported implementing intrusion detection and prevention capabilities, we described the reported intrusion detection and prevention capabilities implemented by the 23 civilian CFO Act civilian agencies by

- summarizing implemented intrusion detection and prevention capability information obtained from the semi-structured interviews at the 23 civilian CFO Act agencies described above;
- identifying the extent to which the 23 civilian CFO Act agencies were in compliance with DHS's binding operating directive (BOD) pertaining to enhanced email and web security (BOD 18-01) by collecting and summarizing *Cyber Hygiene Trustworthy Email* reports from the 23 agencies and determining the extent to which the agencies had taken required actions to implement the BOD.

During the semi-structured interviews, we also obtained the agency's views and experiences with other programs and services provided by DHS, including the extent to which agencies had implemented the tools offered by the department's Continuous Diagnostics and Mitigation (CDM) program.

To determine the reliability of submitted data and obtain clarification about agencies' processes to ensure the accuracy and completeness of data used in their respective FISMA reports, we analyzed documents and conducted interviews with officials from 6 of the 23 civilian CFO Act agencies. To select these six agencies, we sorted agency fiscal year 2017 information technology budget data from highest to lowest amount and then divided the data into three tiers: high spending, medium spending, and low spending. We then randomly selected two agencies from each of the three tiers. The selected agencies were the Departments of Agriculture, Commerce, Housing and Urban Development, Transportation, and Veterans Affairs, and the U.S. Agency for International Development. While not generalizable to all agencies, the information we collected and analyzed about the six selected agencies provided insights into various processes in place to produce FISMA reports. Based on this assessment, we determined that the data were sufficiently reliable for the purposes of our reporting objectives.

We conducted this performance audit from December 2017 to December 2018 in accordance with generally accepted government auditing standards. Those standards require that we plan and perform the audit to obtain sufficient, appropriate evidence to provide a reasonable basis for our findings and conclusions based on our audit objectives. We believe that the evidence obtained provides a reasonable basis for our findings and conclusions based on our audit objectives.

APPENDIX II: CYBERSECURITY FRAMEWORK

The National Institute of Standards and Technology established the cybersecurity framework to provide guidance for cybersecurity activities within the private sector and government agencies at all levels.[89] The cybersecurity framework consists of five core functions: identify, protect, detect, respond, and recover. Within the five functions are 23 categories and 108 subcategories that define discrete outcomes for each function, as described in Table 7.

Table 7. National Institute of Standards and Technology Framework for Improving Critical Infrastructure Cybersecurity

Category	Subcategory
Identify (ID) core function	
Asset Management (ID.AM): The data, personnel, devices, systems, and facilities that enable the organization to achieve business purposes are identified and managed consistent with their relative importance to organizational objectives and the organization's risk strategy.	ID.AM-1: Physical devices and systems within the organization are inventoried.
	ID.AM-2: Software platforms and applications within the organization are inventoried.
	ID.AM-3: Organizational communication and data flows are mapped.
	ID.AM-4: External information systems are catalogued.
	ID.AM-5: Resources (e.g., hardware, devices, data, time, personnel, and software) are prioritized based on their classification, criticality, and business value.
	ID.AM-6: Cybersecurity roles and responsibilities for the entire workforce and third-party stakeholders (e.g., suppliers, customers, partners) are established.
Business Environment (ID.BE): The organization's mission, objectives, stakeholders, and activities are understood and prioritized; this information is used to inform cybersecurity roles, responsibilities, and risk management decisions	ID.BE-1: The organization's role in the supply chain is identified and communicated.
	ID.BE-2: The organization's place in critical infrastructure and its industry sector is identified and communicated.
	ID.BE-3: Priorities for organizational mission, objectives, and activities are established and communicated.
	ID.BE-4: Dependencies and critical functions for delivery of critical services are established.
	ID.BE-5: Resilience requirements to support delivery of critical services are established for all operating states (e.g., under duress/attack, during recovery, normal operations).
Governance (ID.GV): The policies, procedures, and processes to manage and monitor the organization's regulatory, legal, risk, environmental, and operational requirements are understood and inform the management of cybersecurity risk.	ID.GV-1: Organizational cybersecurity policy is established and communicated.
	ID.GV-2: Cybersecurity roles and responsibilities are coordinated and aligned with internal roles and external partners.
	ID.GV-3: Legal and regulatory requirements regarding cybersecurity, including privacy and civil liberties obligations, are understood and managed.
	ID.GV-4: Governance and risk management processes address cybersecurity risks.
Risk Assessment (ID.RA): The organization understands the cybersecurity risk to organizational operations (including mission, functions, image, or reputation), organizational assets, and individuals.	ID.RA-1: Asset vulnerabilities are identified and documented.
	ID.RA-2: Cyber threat intelligence is received from information sharing forums and sources.
	ID.RA-3: Threats, both internal and external, are identified and documented.
	ID.RA-4: Potential business impacts and likelihoods are identified.
	ID.RA-5: Threats, vulnerabilities, likelihoods, and impacts are used to determine risk.

[89] National Institute of Standards and Technology, *Framework for Improving Critical Infrastructure Cybersecurity*, Version 1.1 (Gaithersburg, MD: Apr. 16, 2018).

Category	Subcategory
Identify (ID) core function	
	ID.RA-6: Risk responses are identified and prioritized.
Risk Management Strategy (ID.RM): The organization's priorities, constraints, risk tolerances, and assumptions are established and used to support operational risk decisions.	ID.RM-1: Risk management processes are established, managed, and agreed to by organizational stakeholders.
	ID.RM-2: Organizational risk tolerance is determined and clearly expressed.
	ID.RM-3: The organization's determination of risk tolerance is informed by its role in critical infrastructure and sector specific risk analysis.
Supply Chain Risk Management (ID.SC): The organization's priorities, constraints, risk tolerances, and assumptions are established and used to support risk decisions associated with managing supply chain risk. The organization has established and implemented the processes to identify, assess and manage supply chain risks.	ID.SC-1: Cyber supply chain risk management processes are identified, established, assessed, managed, and agreed to by organizational stakeholders.
	ID.SC-2: Suppliers and third party partners of information systems, components, and services are identified, prioritized, and assessed using a cyber supply chain risk assessment process.
	ID.SC-3: Contracts with suppliers and third-party partners are used to implement appropriate measures designed to meet the objectives of an organization's cybersecurity program and Cyber Supply Chain Risk Management Plan.
	ID.SC-4: Suppliers and third-party partners are routinely assessed using audits, test results, or other forms of evaluations to confirm they are meeting their contractual obligations.
	ID.SC-5: Response and recovery planning and testing are conducted with suppliers and third-party providers.
Protect (PR) core function	
Identity Management, Authentication and Access Control (PR.AC): Access to physical and logical assets and associated facilities is limited to authorized users, processes, and devices, and is managed consistent with the assessed risk of unauthorized access to authorized activities and transactions.	PR.AC-1: Identities and credentials are issued, managed, verified, revoked, and audited for authorized devices, users and processes.
	PR.AC-2: Physical access to assets is managed and protected.
	PR.AC-3: Remote access is managed.
	PR.AC-4: Access permissions and authorizations are managed, incorporating the principles of least privilege and separation of duties.
	PR.AC-5: Network integrity is protected (e.g., network segregation, network segmentation).
	PR.AC-6: Identities are proofed and bound to credentials and asserted in interactions.
	PR.AC-7: Users, devices, and other assets are authenticated (e.g., single-factor, multi-factor) commensurate with the risk of the transaction (e.g., individuals' security and privacy risks and other organizational risks)
Awareness and Training (PR.AT): The organization's personnel and partners are provided cybersecurity awareness education and are trained to perform their cybersecurity-related duties and responsibilities consistent with related policies, procedures, and agreements.	PR.AT-1: All users are informed and trained.
	PR.AT-2: Privileged users understand their roles and responsibilities.
	PR.AT-3: Third-party stakeholders (e.g., suppliers, customers, partners) understand their roles and responsibilities.
	PR.AT-4: Senior executives understand their roles and responsibilities.
	PR.AT-5: Physical and cybersecurity personnel understand their roles and responsibilities.
Data Security (PR.DS): Information and records (data) are managed consistent with the organization's risk strategy to protect the confidentiality, integrity, and availability of information.	PR.DS-1: Data-at-rest is protected.
	PR.DS-2: Data-in-transit is protected.
	PR.DS-3: Assets are formally managed throughout removal, transfers, and disposition.
	PR.DS-4: Adequate capacity to ensure availability is maintained.
	PR.DS-5: Protections against data leaks are implemented.
	PR.DS-6: Integrity checking mechanisms are used to verify software, firmware, and information integrity.
	PR.DS-7: The development and testing environment(s) are separate from the production environment.
	PR.DS-8: Integrity checking mechanisms are used to verify hardware integrity.

Table 7. (Continued)

Category	Subcategory
Protect (PR) core function	
Information Protection Processes and Procedures (PR.IP): Security policies (that address purpose, scope, roles, responsibilities, management commitment, and coordination among organizational entities), processes, and procedures are maintained and used to manage protection of information systems and assets.	PR.IP-1: A baseline configuration of information technology/industrial control systems is created and maintained incorporating security principles (e.g., concept of least functionality).
	PR.IP-2: A System Development Life Cycle to manage systems is implemented.
	PR.IP-3: Configuration change control processes are in place.
	PR.IP-4: Backups of information are conducted, maintained, and tested.
	PR.IP-5: Policy and regulations regarding the physical operating environment for organizational assets are met.
	PR.IP-6: Data is destroyed according to policy.
	PR.IP-7: Protection processes are improved.
	PR.IP-8: Effectiveness of protection technologies is shared.
	PR.IP-9: Response plans (Incident Response and Business Continuity) and recovery plans (Incident Recovery and Disaster Recovery) are in place and managed.
	PR.IP-10: Response and recovery plans are tested.
	PR.IP-11: Cybersecurity is included in human resources practices (e.g., deprovisioning, personnel screening).
	PR.IP-12: A vulnerability management plan is developed and implemented.
Maintenance (PR.MA): Maintenance and repairs of industrial control and information system components are performed consistent with policies and procedures.	PR.MA-1: Maintenance and repair of organizational assets are performed and logged, with approved and controlled tools.
	PR.MA-2: Remote maintenance of organizational assets is approved, logged, and performed in a manner that prevents unauthorized access.
Protective Technology (PR.PT): Technical security solutions are managed to ensure the security and resilience of systems and assets, consistent with related policies, procedures, and agreements.	PR.PT-1: Audit/log records are determined, documented, implemented, and reviewed in accordance with policy.
	PR.PT-2: Removable media is protected and its use restricted according to policy.
	PR.PT-3: The principle of least functionality is incorporated by configuring systems to provide only essential capabilities.
	PR.PT-4: Communications and control networks are protected.
	PR.PT-5: Mechanisms (e.g., failsafe, load balancing, hot swap) are implemented to achieve resilience requirements in normal and adverse situations.
Detect (DE) core function	
Anomalies and Events (DE.AE): Anomalous activity is detected and the potential impact of events is understood.	DE.AE-1: A baseline of network operations and expected data flows for users and systems is established and managed.
	DE.AE-2: Detected events are analyzed to understand attack targets and methods.
	DE.AE-3: Event data are collected and correlated from multiple sources and sensors.
	DE.AE-4: Impact of events is determined.
	DE.AE-5: Incident alert thresholds are established.
Security Continuous Monitoring (DE.CM): The information system and assets are monitored to identify cybersecurity events and verify the effectiveness of protective measures.	DE.CM-1: The network is monitored to detect potential cybersecurity events.
	DE.CM-2: The physical environment is monitored to detect potential cybersecurity events.
	DE.CM-3: Personnel activity is monitored to detect potential cybersecurity events.
	DE.CM-4: Malicious code is detected.
	DE.CM-5: Unauthorized mobile code is detected.
	DE.CM-6: External service provider activity is monitored to detect potential cybersecurity events.

Category	Subcategory
Detect (DE) core function	
	DE.CM-7: Monitoring for unauthorized personnel, connections, devices, and software is performed.
	DE.CM-8: Vulnerability scans are performed.
Detection Processes (DE.DP): Detection processes and procedures are maintained and tested to ensure awareness of anomalous events.	DE.DP-1: Roles and responsibilities for detection are well defined to ensure accountability.
	DE.DP-2: Detection activities comply with all applicable requirements.
	DE.DP-3: Detection processes are tested.
	DE.DP-4: Event detection information is communicated.
	DE.DP-5: Detection processes are continuously improved.
Respond (RS) core function	
Response Planning (RS.RP): Response processes and procedures are executed and maintained, to ensure response to detected cybersecurity incidents.	RS.RP-1: Response plan is executed during or after an incident.
Communications (RS.CO): Response activities are coordinated with internal and external stakeholders (e.g., external support from law enforcement agencies).	RS.CO-1: Personnel know their roles and order of operations when a response is needed.
	RS.CO-2: Incidents are reported consistent with established criteria.
	RS.CO-3: Information is shared consistent with response plans.
	RS.CO-4: Coordination with stakeholders occurs consistent with response plans.
	RS.CO-5: Voluntary information sharing occurs with external stakeholders to achieve broader cybersecurity situational awareness.
Analysis (RS.AN): Analysis is conducted to ensure effective response and support recovery activities.	RS.AN-1: Notifications from detection systems are investigated.
	RS.AN-2: The impact of the incident is understood.
	RS.AN-3: Forensics are performed.
	RS.AN-4: Incidents are categorized consistent with response plans.
	RS-AN-5: Processes are established to receive, analyze and respond to vulnerabilities disclosed to the organization from internal and external sources (e.g., internal testing, security bulletins, or security researchers).
Mitigation (RS.MI): Activities are performed to prevent expansion of an event, mitigate its effects, and resolve the incident.	RS.MI-1: Incidents are contained.
	RS.MI-2: Incidents are mitigated.
	RS.MI-3: Newly identified vulnerabilities are mitigated or documented as accepted risks.
Improvements (RS.IM): Organizational response activities are improved by incorporating lessons learned from current and previous detection/response activities.	RS.IM-1: Response plans incorporate lessons learned.
	RS.IM-2: Response strategies are updated
Recovery Planning (RC.RP): Recovery processes and procedures are executed and maintained to ensure restoration of systems or assets affected by cybersecurity incidents.	RC.RP-1: Recovery plan is executed during or after a cybersecurity incident.
Improvements (RC.IM): Recovery planning and processes are improved by incorporating lessons learned into future activities.	RC.IM-1: Recovery plans incorporate lessons learned.
	RC.IM-2: Recovery strategies are updated.
Communications (RC.CO): Restoration activities are coordinated with internal and external parties (e.g., coordinating centers, Internet Service Providers, owners of attacking systems, victims, other CSIRTs, and vendors).	RC.CO-1: Public relations are managed.
	RC.CO-2: Reputation is repaired after an incident.
	RC.CO-3: Recovery activities are communicated to internal and external stakeholders as well as executive and management teams.

Source: National Institute of Standards and Technology. | GAO-19-105.

Appendix III: Reported Effectiveness of Agencies' Implementation of the Federal Approach for Securing Information Systems

The federal approach and strategy for securing information systems is prescribed by federal law and policy, including the *Federal Information Security Modernization Act of 2014*[90] and the presidential executive order on *Strengthening the Cybersecurity of Federal Networks and Critical Infrastructure*.[91] Accordingly, federal reports describing agency implementation of this law and policy, and reports of related agency information security activities, indicated the effectiveness of agencies' efforts to implement the federal approach and strategy. Table 8 summarizes the reported effectiveness of the 23 civilian *Chief Financial Officers Act of 1990* agencies to implement the government's approach and strategy to securing information systems.

Table 8. Fiscal Year 2017 Indicators of the 23 Selected Civilian *Chief Financial Officers Act of 1990* Agencies' Effectiveness in Implementing the Federal Approach and Strategy for Securing Information Systems

Agency	Inspector General Information Security Program Ratings	Inspector General Internal Control Deficiencies over Financial Reporting	CIO Cybersecurity Cross-Agency Priority Goal Targets	OMB Risk Management Assessment Ratings
US Department of Agriculture	Not effective	Material weakness	Not met	At risk
Department of Commerce	Not effective	Significant deficiency	Not met	At risk
Department of Education	Not effective	Significant deficiency	Met	Managing risk
Department of Energy	Effective	—	Not met	At risk
Department of Health and Human Services	Not effective	Material weakness	Not met	At risk
Department of Homeland Security	Effective	Material weakness	Not met	Managing risk
Department of Housing and Urban Development	Not effective	Significant deficiency	Met	Managing risk
Department of the Interior	Not effective	Significant deficiency	Not met	Managing risk
Department of Justice	Not effective	—	Not met	Managing risk
Department of Labor	Not effective	Significant deficiency	Not met	Managing risk
Department of State	Not effective	Significant deficiency	Not met	At risk
Department of Transportation	Not effective	—	Not met	At risk
Department of the Treasury	Not effective	Material weakness	Not met	Managing risk
Department of Veterans Affairs	Not effective	Material weakness	Not met	At risk
Environmental Protection Agency	Effective	Significant deficiency	Not met	At risk

[90] The *Federal Information Security Modernization Act of 2014*, enacted as Pub. L. No. 113-283, 128 Stat. 3073 (Dec. 18, 2014), largely superseded the *Federal Information Security Management Act of 2002*, enacted as *Title III, E-Government Act of 2002*, Pub. L. No. 107-347, 116 Stat. 2899, 2946 (Dec. 17, 2002).

[91] The White House, *Strengthening the Cybersecurity of Federal Networks and Critical Infrastructure*, Executive Order 13800 (Washington, D.C.: May 11, 2017), 82 Fed. Reg. 22391 (May 16, 2017).

Agency	Inspector General Information Security Program Ratings	Inspector General Internal Control Deficiencies over Financial Reporting	CIO Cybersecurity Cross-Agency Priority Goal Targets	OMB Risk Management Assessment Ratings
General Services Administration	Not effective	Significant deficiency	Met	Managing risk
National Aeronautics and Space Administration	Not effective	Significant deficiency	Not met	At risk
National Science Foundation	Effective	—	Not met	Managing risk
Nuclear Regulatory Commission	Effective	—	Not met	Managing risk
Office of Personnel Management	Not effective	Material weakness	Met	Managing risk
Small Business Administration	Not effective	Significant deficiency	Not met	At risk
Social Security Administration	Not effective	Significant deficiency	Met	Managing risk
US Agency for International Development	Effective	—	Met	Managing risk
Totals[a]	17[b]	17c	17d	10e

Legend: "—" means that information security was not designated as a significant deficiency or material weakness for that agency.

Source: GAO analysis based on agency and Office of Management and Budget fiscal year 2017 *Federal Information Security Modernization Act* data and agency financial reports for fiscal year 2017. | GAO-19-105.

[a]Although the totals for some of the columns are the same, the agencies included in the totals are not.

[b]The inspector general for 17 agencies reported that their agency did not have an effective information security program.

[c]The inspector general for 17 agencies designated information security as a significant deficiency or material weakness.

[d]The chief information officers for 17 agencies reported that their agencies did not meet all nine targets for the cybersecurity cross-agency priority goal.

[e]OMB reported that 10 agencies had enterprises that were at risk.

Appendix IV: Updated Cybersecurity-Focused Cross-Agency Priority Goal

The President's Management Agenda identifies cross-agency priority (CAP) goals to target areas where multiple agencies must collaborate to effect change.[92] The agenda issued in fiscal year 2018 established an information technology modernization goal that includes a cybersecurity objective with specific priority areas and performance indicators. This cybersecurity-focused goal is intended to drive progress in the government's efforts to modernize information technology to increase productivity and security. Figure 8 describes the 3 updated cybersecurity-focused cross-agency priority areas and 10 performance indicators. Each federal agency is expected to meet one of the 10 new performance indicators by the end of fiscal year 2018 and the remainder by 2020.

[92] The President's Management Agenda is intended to lay out a long-term vision for modernizing the federal government in key areas that will improve the ability of agencies to deliver mission outcomes, provide excellent service, and effectively steward taxpayer dollars on behalf of the American people.

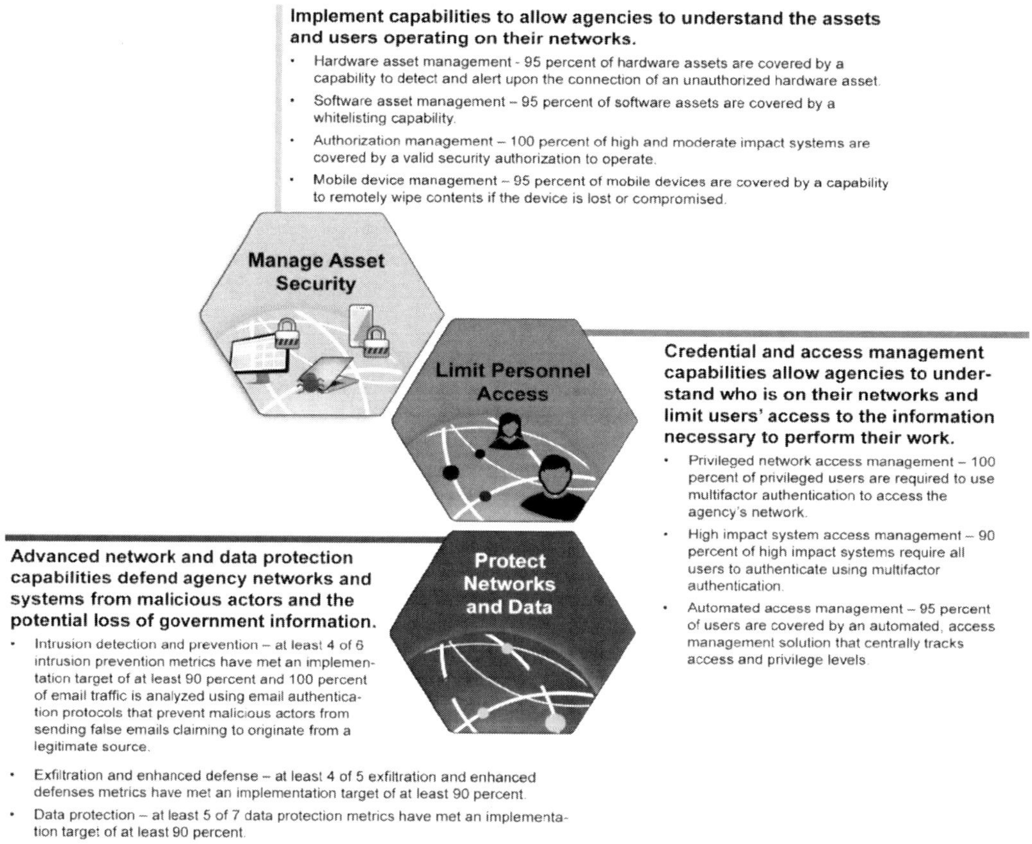

Source: Performance.gov. | GAO-19-105.

Figure 8. Cybersecurity-Focused Cross-Agency Priority Goal Priority Areas and Performance Indicators, Fiscal Years 2018– 2022.

APPENDIX V: COMMENTS FROM THE DEPARTMENT OF HOMELAND SECURITY

U.S. Department of Homeland Security
Washington, DC 20528

Homeland Security

December 11, 2018

Gregory C. Wilshusen
Director, Information Security Issues
U.S. Government Accountability Office
441 G Street, NW
Washington, DC 20548

Re: Management Response to Draft Report GAO-19-105, "INFORMATION SECURITY: Agencies Need to Improve Implementation of Federal Approach to Securing Systems and Protecting Against Intrusions" (Job Code 102490)

Dear Mr. Wilshusen,

Thank you for the opportunity to review and comment on this draft report. The U.S. Department of Homeland Security (DHS) appreciates the U.S. Government Accountability Office's (GAO) work in planning and conducting its review and issuing this report.

The Department is pleased to note GAO's positive recognition of DHS initiatives being taken to further secure agency information systems. These include the development of an in-depth "Intrusion Assessment Plan" that outlines tools, platforms, and resources; development of the National Cybersecurity Protection System (NCPS); and providing tools and services to agencies to monitor their networks through the Continuous Diagnostic and Mitigation (CDM) program. DHS is committed to helping agencies, which are responsible for their own cybersecurity, reduce the risk of successful cyber-attacks.

The draft report contained nine recommendations including two for DHS with which the Department concurs. Attached find our detailed response to each recommendation. Technical comments were previously provided under separate cover.

Again, thank you for the opportunity to review and comment on this draft report. Please feel free to contact me if you have any questions. We look forward to working with you again in the future.

Sincerely,

JIM H. CRUMPACKER, CIA, CFE
Director
Departmental GAO-OIG Liaison Office

Attachment: Management Response to the Recommendations Contained in GAO-19-105

GAO recommended that the Secretary of Homeland Security:

Recommendation 1: Direct the Network Security Deployment division to coordinate further with federal agencies to identify training and guidance needs for implementing NCPS and CDM.

Response: Concur. The Cybersecurity and Infrastructure Security Agency's (CISA) NCPS Program Office will work with the CISA's Federal Network Resilience (FNR) Division to ensure a broader dissemination of existing training materials and offerings to all federal agencies. In addition, the NCPS Program Office will explore options for improving the training offerings that are available. Estimated Completion Date (ECD): November 30, 2019.

Recommendation 2: Direct the appropriate staff to work with Office of Management and Budget (OMB) to follow-up with agencies to identify obstacles, and impediments affecting their abilities to implement intrusion detection and prevention capabilities.

Response: Concur. The CISA NCPS Program Office and FNR Division will continue to work with OMB and federal agencies to identify obstacles and impediments to effectively implementing NCPS capabilities. The NCPS Program Office meets with representatives from OMB on a bi-weekly basis to discuss the status of agency efforts. As part of these bi-weekly meetings, CISA staff will work with OMB to develop an approach to better engage on follow-up activities. ECD: September 30, 2019.

APPENDIX VI: COMMENTS FROM THE DEPARTMENT OF COMMERCE

UNITED STATES DEPARTMENT OF COMMERCE
Chief Information Officer
Washington, D.C. 20230

DEC 1 0 2018

Mr. Gregory C. Wilshusen
Director, Information Security Issues
Government Accountability Office
441 G Street NW
Washington, DC 20548

Dear Mr. Wilshusen:

Thank you for the opportunity to review and comment on the Government Accountability Office's (GAO) draft report entitled *Information Security: Agencies Need to Improve Implementation of Federal Approach to Securing Systems and Protecting Against Intrusions* (GAO-19-105).

On behalf of the Department of Commerce, I have enclosed our comments on the report. We concur and have no comments on the draft report.

Sincerely,

RODNEY TURK

Digitally signed by RODNEY TURK
Date: 2018.12.10 09:50:11 -05'00'

Rodney W. Turk
Acting Chief Information Officer

Department of Commerce
Office of the Chief Information Officer
Office of the Secretary

Technical and Editorial Comments on the GAO Report Entitled Information Security: Agencies Need to Improve Implementation of Federal Approach to Securing Systems and Protecting Against Intrusions (GAO-19-105).

The Office of the Chief Information Officer has reviewed the report and provides general comments are below. The OCIO has no technical and editorial comments, also reflected below. Page numbers refer to page numbers in the report unless otherwise stated.

General Comments
The report is reasonable, and we concur with its findings and recommendations.

Recommended Changes for Factual/Technical Information.

None

Editorial Comments

None

APPENDIX VII: COMMENTS FROM THE SOCIAL SECURITY ADMINISTRATION

SOCIAL SECURITY
Office of the Commissioner

December 10, 2018

Mr. Gregory C. Wilshusen
Director, Information Security Issues
United States Government Accountability Office
441 G Street, NW
Washington, DC 20548

Dear Mr. Wilshusen:

Thank you for the opportunity to review the draft report, "INFORMATION SECURITY: Agencies Need to Improve Implementation of Federal Approach to Securing Systems and Protecting Against Intrusions" (GAO-19-105). Please see our enclosed comments.

Sincerely,

Stephanie Hall
Acting Deputy Chief of Staff

SSA COMMENTS ON THE GOVERNMENT ACCOUNTABILITY OFFICE (GAO) DRAFT REPORT, "INFORMATION SECURITY: AGENCIES NEED TO IMPROVE IMPLEMENTATION OF FEDERAL APPROACH TO SECURING SYSTEMS AND PROTECTING AGAINST INTRUSIONS" (GAO-19-105)

Protecting our networks and the information we use to administer our programs is a critical priority. We can never rest in our efforts to keep the public's data secure. We address this challenge proactively with an integrated, multi-layered, risk-based program that continually adds new defenses. We work with the Department of Homeland Security and third-party assessors to test the effectiveness of our program and identify areas of improvement. We are making ongoing improvements to our information security protocols to keep pace with changes in the operating environment and to mitigate known risks.

We continually improve our processes and capabilities to address the ever-changing threat environment and escalating risks. In fiscal year 2018, we made improvements and progress in securing applications, leveraging the cloud, managing our assets and vulnerabilities, strengthening our network and incident response capabilities, improving our security training, and enhancing the overall effectiveness of our cybersecurity program. We are confident that our proactive planning, coupled with our responsiveness to external assessments and continuous improvement processes, should provide the foundation for achieving a higher Federal Information Security Management Act compliance maturity level.

Appendix VIII: Comments from the U.S. Agency for International Development

USAID
FROM THE AMERICAN PEOPLE

Gregory C. Wilshusen
Director, Information Security Issues
United States Government Accountability Office
441 G Street, N.W.
Washington, D.C. 20548

Re: INFORMATION SECURITY: Agencies Need to Improve Implementation of Federal Approach to Securing Systems and Protecting Against Intrusions (GAO-19-105)

Dear Mr. Wilshusen:

I am pleased to provide the formal response of the U. S. Agency for International Development (USAID) to the draft report produced by the U. S. Government Accountability Office (GAO) entitled, *"INFORMATION SECURITY: Agencies Need to Improve Implementation of Federal Approach to Securing Systems and Protecting Against Intrusions" (GAO-19-105).*

As the report indicates, USAID has a successful approach to securing our information-technology (IT) systems and protecting against intrusion. Table 8 in the report (pages 62-63) lists USAID as the only Department or Agency within the Federal Government rated as effectively meeting the Inspector General Information-Security Program Ratings, targets of the Chief Information Officer's Cybersecurity Cross-Agency Priority Goal, and the Office of Management and Budget's Risk-Management Assessment Ratings.

The Agency continues to mature its cybersecurity posture, as shown by the improvements seen in the USAID 2018 Office of Inspector General Annual Federal Information Security Management Act (FISMA) Metrics Report, based on 2018 data. Since then, USAID has improved in three Core Security Functions of the Inspector General Ratings of Agencies' Information-Security Policies, Procedures, and Practices (pg. 22):

- For Fiscal Year (FY) 2018, USAID was rated at a 5 for "Identify";
- For FY 2018, USAID was rated at a 4 for "Detect"; and
- For FY 2018, USAID was rated at a 4 for "Recover."

I am transmitting this letter for inclusion in the GAO's final report. Thank you for the opportunity to respond to the draft report, and for the courtesies extended by your staff while conducting this engagement.

Sincerely,

Angelique M. Crumbly
Acting Assistant Administrator
Bureau for Management

In: Top 10 Reports and Testimonies in December 2018
Editor: Sarah J. Nygaard
ISBN: 978-1-53615-507-5

Chapter 6

National Security: Long-Range Emerging Threats Facing the United States As Identified by Federal Agencies*

United States Government Accountability Office

Abbreviations

AI	Artificial Intelligence
DHS	Department of Homeland Security
DIA	Defense Intelligence Agency
DOD	Department of Defense
ICBM	Intercontinental ballistic missile
IoT	Internet of Things
ISR	Intelligence, surveillance, and reconnaissance
NATO	North Atlantic Treaty Organization
ODNI	Office of the Director of National Intelligence
State	Department of State

Why GAO Did This Study

The United States faces a complex array of threats to our national security, including our political, economic, military, and social systems. These threats will continue to evolve as new and resurgent adversaries develop politically and militarily, as weapons and technology advance, and as environmental and demographic changes occur. A House committee report accompanying a bill for the National Defense Authorization Act for Fiscal Year 2018 included a provision for GAO to identify emerging threats of high national security consequence. This chapter focuses on long-range emerging threats—those that may occur in

* This is an edited, reformatted and augmented version of the United States Government Accountability Office Report to congressional committees, Publication No. GAO-19-204SP, dated December 2018.

approximately 5 or more years, or those that may occur during an unknown timeframe—as identified by various respondents at the Department of Defense (DOD), Department of State (State), Department of Homeland Security (DHS), and the Office of the Director of National Intelligence (ODNI).

To identify long-range emerging threats, GAO administered a questionnaire to 45 government organizations that assess emerging threats across DOD, State, DHS, and ODNI, and had a 78-percent response rate. GAO conducted a content analysis of the responses to identify specific threats and develop broad threat categories. To supplement the data from the questionnaire, GAO reviewed national security strategies and agency documents provided by DOD, State, DHS, and ODNI, and interviewed key agency officials. This chapter is a public version of a classified report that GAO issued on September 28, 2018. Information that DOD deemed classified and sensitive has been omitted.

WHAT GAO FOUND

DOD, State, DHS, and ODNI independently identified various threats to the United States or its national security interests. In analyzing more than 210 individual threats identified by organizations across DOD, State, DHS, and ODNI, as well as its review of national security strategies and related documents, and interviews with key agency officials, GAO developed four broad categories for 26 long-range emerging threats that officials identified: Adversaries' Political and Military Advancements, Dual-Use Technologies, Weapons, and Events and Demographic Changes.

The figure below contains examples of the 26 threats in 4 categories—as identified by DOD, State, DHS, and ODNI—in response to GAO's questionnaire.

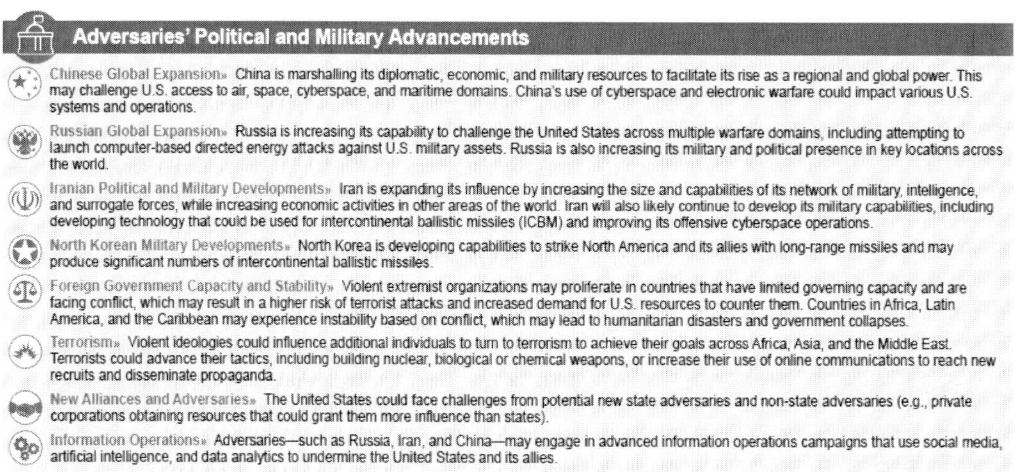

Emerging Threats As Identified by DOD, State, DHS, and ODNI. (Continued).

Dual-Use Technologies

Artificial Intelligence (AI)» Adversaries could gain increased access to AI through affordable designs used in the commercial industry, and could apply AI to areas such as weapons and technology.

Quantum Information Science» Quantum communications could enable adversaries to develop secure communications that U.S. personnel would not be able to intercept or decrypt. Quantum computing may allow adversaries to decrypt information, which could enable them to target U.S. personnel and military operations.

Internet of Things (IoT)» The United States may face difficulties protecting networks and data as IoT grows and traditional approaches for security (e.g., encryption) may no longer effectively protect information. Adversaries could also disrupt IoT-enabled critical infrastructure and devices.

Autonomous and Unmanned Systems» Adversaries are developing autonomous capabilities that could recognize faces, understand gestures, and match voices of U.S. personnel, which could compromise U.S. operations. Unmanned ground, underwater, air, and space vehicles may be used for combat and surveillance.

Biotechnology» Actors—which may include state or non-state entities such as violent extremist organizations and transnational criminal organizations—could alter genes or create DNA to modify plants, animals, and humans. Such biotechnologies could be used to enhance the performance of military personnel. The proliferation of synthetic biology—used to create genetic code that does not exist in nature—may increase the number of actors that can create chemical and biological weapons.

Other Emerging Technologies» Actors may gain access to new technologies previously limited to militaries, such as affordable and sophisticated encryption technologies, which would hinder U.S. efforts to monitor terrorist and criminal activities. Other emerging technologies—such as additive manufacturing (i.e., 3D printing)—may be vulnerable to cyber attacks or be used to manufacture restricted materials, such as weapons.

Weapons

Weapons of Mass Destruction» An increasing number of actors may gain access to these weapons. Adversaries could steal nuclear materials from existing facilities or develop new types of biological weapons using genetic engineering and synthetic biology.

Electronic Warfare» Adversaries are developing electronic attack weapons to target U.S. systems with sensitive electronic components, such as military sensors, communication, navigation, and information systems. These weapons are intended to degrade U.S. capabilities and could restrict situational awareness or may affect military operations.

Hypersonic Weapons» China and Russia are pursuing hypersonic weapons because their speed, altitude, and maneuverability may defeat most missile defense systems, and they may be used to improve long-range conventional and nuclear strike capabilities. There are no existing countermeasures.

Counterspace Weapons» China and Russia are developing anti-satellite weapons to threaten U.S. space operations. China is developing capabilities to conduct large-scale anti-satellite strikes using novel physical, cyber, and electronic warfare means.

Missiles» Adversaries are developing missile technology to attack the United States in novel ways and challenge U.S. missile defense, including conventional and nuclear ICBMs, sea-launched land-attack missiles, and space-based missiles that could orbit the earth.

Intelligence, Surveillance, Reconnaissance (ISR) Platforms» Future advances in AI, sensors, data analytics, and space-based platforms could create an environment of "ubiquitous ISR", where people and equipment could be tracked throughout the world in near-real time. China, Russia, Iran, and North Korea are developing multiple ISR platforms.

Aircraft» China and Russia are developing new aircraft, including stealth aircraft, which could fly faster, carry advanced weapons, and achieve greater ranges. Such aircraft could force U.S. aircraft to operate at farther distances and put more U.S. targets at risk.

Undersea Weapons» Russia has made significant advancements in submarine technology and tactics to escape detection by U.S. forces. China is developing underwater acoustic systems that could coordinate swarm attacks—the use of large quantities of simple and expendable assets to overwhelm opponents—among vehicles and provide greater undersea awareness. Adversaries could achieve breakthroughs in anti-submarine warfare—such as using AI to locate U.S. submarines—or attack U.S. undersea infrastructure, which could cripple communications.

Cyber Weapons» Adversaries, such as China, Russia, Iran, and North Korea, may launch cyber attacks against critical U.S. infrastructure (e.g., electric, oil and gas, and nuclear power systems) and military infrastructure (e.g., communications and ISR platforms). Adversaries could also launch cyber attacks on the U.S. health care system, threatening patient safety by disrupting access to medical care. Finally, adversaries are also developing tools to directly attack hardware and embedded components in aviation systems, which can manipulate or destroy data.

Events and Demographic Changes

Infectious Diseases» New and evolving diseases from the natural environment—exacerbated by changes in climate, the movement of people into cities, and global trade and travel—may become a pandemic. Drug-resistant forms of diseases previously considered treatable could become widespread again.

Climate Change» Extreme weather events—such as hurricanes and megadroughts—could intensify and affect food security, energy resources, and the health care sector. Diminishing permafrost could expand habitats for pathogens that cause disease. The loss of Arctic sea ice could open previously closed sea routes, potentially increasing Russian and Chinese access to the region and challenging the freedom of navigation that the United States currently has.

Internal and International Migration» Governments in megacities (i.e., over 10 million people) across Asia, Latin America, and Africa may not have the capacity to provide adequate resources and infrastructure, and may be vulnerable to natural or man-made disasters. Mass migration events may occur and threaten regional stability, undermine governments, and strain U.S. military and civilian responses.

Source: GAO analysis of DOD, State, DHS, and ODNI questionnaire responses, agency documents, and national security strategies. | GAO-19-204SP.

Emerging Threats As Identified by DOD, State, DHS, and ODNI.

* * *

December 13, 2018
Congressional Committees

The United States faces a complex array of threats to our national security, including our political, economic, military, and social systems. These threats will continue to evolve as new and resurgent adversaries develop politically and militarily, as weapons and technology advance, and as environmental and demographic changes occur. Our adversaries may include foreign governments, violent extremists, transnational criminal organizations, and megacorporations.[1] Threats may also come from events such as pandemics, human migration, regional conflict and instability, economic inequality, or the effects of climate change and environmental issues.

A variety of national intelligence and security organizations are responsible for national security, including identifying, analyzing, and countering emerging threats. Such organizations include: the Department of Defense (DOD), the Department of State (State), the Department of Homeland Security (DHS), and the Office of the Director of National Intelligence (ODNI).

For purposes of this chapter, we define "threat" as an actor with capability and intent, or an event with potential capability, to harm the United States or its national security interests. We define "emerging threat" as a threat that may be newly recognized; may have been recognized before but may potentially affect a new or different population, industry, or geographic area than previously affected; or may be an existing threat that has developed new attributes.

A House Committee report accompanying a bill for the National Defense Authorization Act for Fiscal Year 2018 included a provision for us to identify emerging threats of high national security consequence.[2] This chapter describes long-range emerging threats as identified by DOD, State, DHS, and ODNI.[3] For purposes of this chapter, we define long-range threats as threats that agency officials identified that may occur in approximately 5 or more years, or those threats that could occur in a future unknown time frame.[4]

This chapter is a public version of a classified report that we issued on September 28, 2018.[5] It omits classified and sensitive information about threats identified by executive branch agencies and described in 26 profiles in our classified report. It also omits classified and sensitive information in those profiles related to specific threats, the effects of those threats, specific warfare domains, and questions for oversight. Although the information provided in this chapter is more limited, the report addresses the same objectives as the classified report and uses the same methodology.

---

[1] Adversaries are potentially hostile or disruptive state or non-state actors. According to the 2018 National Defense Strategy, state actors and non-state actors, such as terrorists, transnational criminal organizations, and cyber hackers, have transformed the direction of global affairs with increased capabilities of mass disruption. Disruptive state actors include North Korea, Russia, China, and Iran. Non-state actors include violent extremist organizations such as al-Qaida and the Islamic State of Iraq and Syria. Transnational criminal organizations can participate in the sale of illegal drugs and counterfeit goods, human trafficking and smuggling, and other criminal activities. According to DOD officials, megacorporations are large companies that have the financial resources and a power base to exert influence on par with or exceeding non-state actors.

[2] H.R. Rep. No. 115-200, at 181 (2017).

[3] ODNI supports the Director of National Intelligence's role as head of the Intelligence Community. The Intelligence Community is comprised of 17 separate organizations such as the Central Intelligence Agency, the Defense Intelligence Agency, the Federal Bureau of Investigation, the National Security Agency, and intelligence components within agencies such as the Department of Homeland Security, Department of State, and the military services.

[4] We established this time frame because officials from DOD and ODNI stated that they consider threats occurring earlier than 5 years from today as near-term or mid-term threats, which receive greater attention and resources from defense and intelligence organizations than long-term threats.

[5] GAO, National Security: Long-Range Emerging Threats Facing the United States Identified by Federal Agencies, GAO-18-497SPC (Washington, D.C.: Sept. 28, 2018). (SECRET//NOFORN).

To identify long-range emerging threats, we administered a questionnaire to 45 selected organizations across DOD, State, DHS, and ODNI.[6] In the questionnaire, we asked respondents to identify and describe emerging threats that their organizations assess could occur in approximately 5 years or more from today, or those that have an unknown time frame. We received approximately 210 individual threats from 26 of these 45 organizations, which formed the basis of our threat profiles.[7] See appendix I for more details about the specific organizations that received the questionnaire. In addition, ODNI submitted a questionnaire but did not identify any threats on the questionnaire. Instead, ODNI officials referred us to their *Global Trends: Paradox of Progress* report and provided verbal input on long-range emerging threats.[8] We used this information to supplement questionnaire responses from DOD, State, and DHS organizations. In total, we received a 78-percent response rate (28 of 36) to our questionnaire.[9]

To supplement information from the questionnaire, we reviewed documents provided by DOD, State, DHS, and ODNI. For example, we reviewed the most recent national strategies that pertain to emerging threats and ODNI's 2017 *Global Trends: Paradox of Progress* report.[10] We also interviewed officials about long-range emerging threats from 22 organizations, including 11 DOD organizations, 6 State organizations, 4 DHS organizations, and ODNI. We selected these 22 organizations because they may have a role in identifying and assessing long-range emerging threats. This review did not assess any efforts to mitigate threats. We pretested the questionnaire instrument with officials from different agencies to confirm that it would be understood by respondents as intended, and determined that the data collected were sufficiently reliable for our purposes.

It is not possible to predict every potential long-range emerging threat. According to Intelligence Community officials, the further out in time predictions go, the more uncertain they become, because the future is a confluence of multiple trends with an infinite number of possible permutations. For example, adversaries may use emerging technologies together in novel and unpredicted ways to amplify their harm. Several DOD officials also noted that there will always be completely unpredictable events with no prior warning. Therefore, this chapter does not attempt to provide a comprehensive listing of all potential emerging threats to the United States that may arise over the next 5 or more years. Rather, it represents the assessments of agency experts who responded to our questionnaire, supplemented by

---

[6] We focused on DOD, State, DHS, and ODNI as among the federal agencies with primary responsibility for national security. We identified the 45 selected organizations within these agencies that assess long-range emerging threats through consultation with agency officials.

[7] Two additional organizations provided responses after the response period had ended. These responses were not used in the development of the threat profiles but were included in our response rate calculations.

[8] Office of the Director of National Intelligence, National Intelligence Council, Global Trends: Paradox of Progress, NIC 2017-001 (Washington, D.C.: January 2017). An ODNI official stated that the Global Trends: Paradox of Progress report lists some key threats over the next 5 to 20 years. In particular, ODNI officials emphasized economic threats such as U.S. debt and growing inequality; new technologies and ethical questions surrounding the use of those technologies; geopolitical conflict, including the spread of corruption to the developed world and the rise of China; and the spread of populism and nationalist identities around the world.

[9] Of the 45 organizations selected to receive our questionnaire, 9 organizations were excluded from our response rate calculations because 8 told us that they do not identify threats that meet our scope or definition, and 1 told us that a separate office within their organization had responded on their behalf. Of the remaining 36 organizations, 28 organizations provided responses (2 of which provided responses after the response period had ended, and were not used in the development of the threat profiles). In addition, 1 organization did not receive a questionnaire due to an administrative error and ODNI submitted an incomplete questionnaire that did not identify any threats. We did not receive responses from the remaining 6 organizations.

[10] NIC 2017-001.

information from national security strategies, related agency documents, and interviews with agency officials. Furthermore, many questionnaire responses focus on threats that originate outside the United States. For more information on our objective, scope, and methodology, see appendix I.

The performance audit upon which this chapter is based was conducted from July 2017 to September 2018 in accordance with generally accepted government auditing standards. Those standards require that we plan and perform the audit to obtain sufficient, appropriate evidence to provide a reasonable basis for our findings and conclusions based on our audit objectives. We believe that the evidence obtained provides a reasonable basis for our findings and conclusions based on our audit objective. We subsequently worked with DOD from September 2018 to December 2018 to prepare this public version of the original classified report for public release. This public version was also prepared in accordance with those standards.

BACKGROUND

Current Landscape of Emerging Threats

DOD officials noted that Western liberal democratic institutions around the world are being challenged in new and novel ways. Adversaries have had over 40 years to study the United States and Western institutions. As such, the nature of warfare has evolved to include "gray zone" conflict—defined as the area between war and peace—where weaker adversaries have learned how to seize territory and advance their agendas in ways not recognized as "war" by Western democracies. Also, these gray zone conflicts can offset superior U.S. economic and security structures. DOD officials added that adversaries around the world may erode democracies, often using democratic institutions, in the gray zone of conflict.[11] ODNI officials also noted that China and Russia are pursuing gray zone strategies to achieve their objectives without resorting to military conflict.

DOD officials provided a list of recent significant examples of adversary success in the gray zone of conflict, several of which have occurred without significant consequences, including:

- Russian and Chinese near-unrestricted thefts of U.S. intellectual property, Office of Personnel Management data theft, and penetrations of U.S. civil, utility, and military data and electoral voting systems;
- Russian seizure of Ukrainian territory, namely Crimea;
- Chinese seizure of the South China Seas and the building of military islands in defiance of international court rulings;
- China using bilateral economic deals to marginalize U.S. multilateral frameworks in Asia, Africa, Latin America, and the Pacific;

---

[11] Officials from the Defense Advanced Research Projects Agency noted that gray zone warfare is characterized by limited conflict that sits between normal state competition and what is traditionally thought of as war.

- Russia attempting to resurrect former Soviet client state relationships with Syria, Egypt, and Libya, and potentially with additional countries in the Middle East and North Africa;
- Iran realigning the Middle East by using proxy forces to create friendly governments including Syria, Iraq, and Yemen at the expense of U.S. leadership in the region;
- "Strongmen" in countries such as Venezuela, Egypt, and Turkey using democratic institutions to promote new paradigms independent of Western liberal norms; and
- The continued attraction of extremist groups, including the Islamic State and al-Qaida, as a preferable means to achieve Sunni Arab autonomy as a viable alternative to minority governance in countries with majorities that outnumber them (as in Syria and Iraq).

DOD officials said that, with current demographic trends, Western liberal democratic institutions will be tested in new ways as the nature of warfare changes. The challenge for the United States and its allies will be to develop responses faster than adversaries through a better understanding of the strategic environment. Officials added that this presents a challenge since the United States appears to be strategically surprised by an evolving world.

DOD officials also said that the United States must adapt to challenges from adversaries and better link security objectives and economic objectives, or risk further erosions of U.S. influence to adversaries such as China and Russia. Officials stated that China and Russia are more agile than the United States in creating relationships with other countries to degrade U.S. bilateral and multilateral frameworks. For example, China and Russia are working to define the United States as a "status quo" power trying to preserve the old world order in what is becoming a multipolar world. These officials added that the nature of conflict has changed, and so the United States must evolve.

Future Landscape of Emerging Threats

ODNI's January 2017 report *Global Trends: Paradox of Progress* describes future trends that will shape the direction of the world over the next 5 or more years. ODNI's report describes potential environments from which long-range threats may emerge, based on secen key global trends:

1. The rich population is shrinking, the poor population is not. Working-age populations are shrinking in wealthy countries and in China and Russia, and are growing in developing, poorer countries. This trend has the potential to increase economic, employment[12], urbanization and welfare pressures, and spur migration.[13]
2. The global economy is shifting. Weak economic growth will likely persist in the near term. Major economies will confront shrinking workforces and diminishing productivity gains while recovering from the 2008-2009 financial crises with high debt, weak demand, and doubts about globalization. Inequality and wealth

[12] NIC 2017-001.

[13] In its report, ODNI states this trend as "the rich are aging, the poor are not.

concentrations—combined with corruption and eroding trust in authorities—are driving a wave of political change.

3. Technology is accelerating progress but causing discontinuities. Rapid technological advancements will increase the pace of change and create new opportunities, but will aggravate divisions between winners and losers. Automation and artificial intelligence will threaten to change industries faster than economies can adjust, potentially displacing workers and limiting the usual route for poor countries to develop. Biotechnologies such as genome editing will revolutionize medicine and other fields, while sharpening moral differences.
4. Ideas and identities are driving a wave of exclusion. Growing global connectivity amid weak economic growth will increase tensions within and between societies. Populism will increase on the right and the left. Some leaders will use nationalism to shore up control. Religious influence will be increasingly consequential, and nearly all countries will see economic forces boost women's status and leadership roles, but backlash against this trend also will occur.
5. Governing is getting harder. The public will demand that governments deliver security and prosperity. However, flat revenues, distrust, polarization, and a growing list of emerging issues will hamper government performance. Technology will expand the range of players who can block or circumvent political action.
6. The nature of conflict is changing. The risk of conflict will increase due to diverging interests among major powers, an expanding terror threat, continued instability in weak states, and the spread of lethal, disruptive technologies. Disrupting societies will become more common, with long-range precision weapons, cyber, and robotic systems to target infrastructure from afar, and with more accessible technology to create weapons of mass destruction.
7. Climate change, environment, and health issues will demand attention. A range of global hazards pose imminent and longer-term threats that will require collective action to address—even as cooperation becomes harder. More extreme weather, water and soil stress, and food insecurity will disrupt societies. Sea-level rise, ocean acidification, glacial melt, and pollution will change living patterns. Tensions over climate change will grow.

The Global Trends report also points out that conflicts in the next 5 to 20 years will be more:

- *Diffuse*—referring to state, non-state, and sub-state entities having greater accessibility to means of warfare;
- *Diverse*—referring to the means of warfare varying across a wider spectrum, from nonmilitary capabilities to advanced conventional weapons and weapons of mass destruction; and
- *Disruptive*—referring to a greater emphasis by states and terror groups on targeting critical infrastructure, societal cohesion, and government functions, rather than defeating enemy forces on the battlefield through traditional military means.[14]

[14] See NIC 2017-001. [14]NIC 2017-001.

Roles and Responsibilities of Agencies That Identify and Mitigate Emerging Threats

DOD, State, DHS, and the Intelligence Community have key roles in identifying and mitigating longterm emerging threats. Specifically:

- DOD has a role in, among other things, defending the homeland from limited ballistic missile and cruise missile attack; large-scale terrorist attack; chemical, biological, radiological, or nuclear attack; and space, electromagnetic, or kinetic attacks against our critical infrastructure. DOD also works to prevent adversaries such as state and non-state actors from acquiring, proliferating, or using weapons of mass destruction, and is the lead agency to defend U.S. military and intelligence infrastructure from cyber attacks and conduct offensive cyber operations. DOD also works to rebuild the military strength and maximize the competitive advantage of the United States and its partners, while constraining the ability of our adversaries to achieve their military objectives. DOD efforts may include preventing terrorists from directing or supporting operations against the U.S. homeland and its partners, and bolstering its partners against coercion. Finally, DOD assists State and the U.S. Agency for International Development with natural disaster and conflict response around the world.
- State is the lead U.S. foreign affairs agency and the lead institution for conducting American diplomacy. State plays a role in protecting and advancing the interests of the United States by, in part, countering threats and adversaries, deepening U.S. security relationships and partnerships around the world, and strengthening our allies and alliances. State also engages in security and capacity building and other non-military assistance, such as border patrol, with other countries. In conjunction with DOD and the U.S. Agency for International Development, State also responds to natural disasters and conflict-induced crises around the world.
- DHS plays a role in preventing a variety of threats within the homeland, particularly terrorist attacks within the United States. DHS also seeks to reduce the vulnerability of the United States to terrorism, assisting in the recovery from terrorist attacks that do occur within the United States, and disrupting connections between illegal drug trafficking and terrorism, and for coordinating efforts to sever such connections. DHS officials added that DHS is also the lead agency for defense of civilian cyber infrastructure (such as .gov accounts) from cyber-attacks, and for aiding private-sector critical-infrastructure cyber security. DHS officials also said that DHS has primary responsibility for border and transportation security issues, including interdicting illicit smuggling of humans and contraband into the homeland, traveler security screening, and, via the U.S. Coast Guard, securing the maritime approaches to the homeland.
- ODNI supports the Director of National Intelligence in his role as the head of the Intelligence Community, acts as the principal advisor to the President, National Security Council, and the Homeland Security Council for intelligence matters related to national security, and oversees and directs the implementation of the National

Intelligence Program.[15] ODNI's activities include integrating intelligence analysis and collection, driving secure information sharing, setting strategic direction and priorities for national intelligence resources and capabilities, developing and implementing unifying intelligence strategies, and advancing capabilities to provide the United States with a global intelligence advantage.

DOD, STATE, DHS AND ODNI IDENTIFIED A VARIETY OF EMERGING THREATS TO U.S. NATIONAL SECURITY THAT MAY OCCUR OVER THE NEXT APPROXIMATELY 5 OR MORE YEARS

DOD, State, DHS, and ODNI independently identified various emerging threats to the United States or its national security interests. Our analysis of these threats led to 26 threat profiles that fell within four broad categories: 1) Adversaries' Political and Military Advancements, 2) Dual-Use Technologies, 3) Weapons, and 4) Events and Demographic Changes, as shown in figure 1.

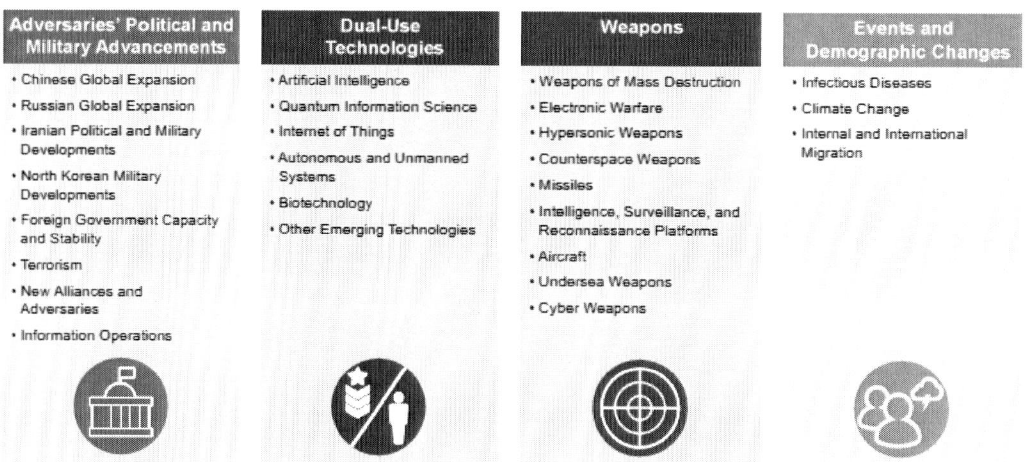
Adversaries' Political and Military Advancements
• Chinese Global Expansion
• Russian Global Expansion
• Iranian Political and Military Developments
• North Korean Military Developments
• Foreign Government Capacity and Stability
• Terrorism
• New Alliances and Adversaries
• Information Operations
Dual-Use Technologies
• Artificial Intelligence
• Quantum Information Science
• Internet of Things
• Autonomous and Unmanned Systems
• Biotechnology
• Other Emerging Technologies
Weapons
• Weapons of Mass Destruction
• Electronic Warfare
• Hypersonic Weapons
• Counterspace Weapons
• Missiles
• Intelligence, Surveillance, and Reconnaissance Platforms
• Aircraft
• Undersea Weapons
• Cyber Weapons
Events and Demographic Changes
• Infectious Diseases
• Climate Change
• Internal and International Migration

Source: GAO analysis of DOD, State, DHS, and ODNI questionnaire responses, agency documents, and national security strategies. | GAO-19-204SP.

Figure 1. GAO's Four Broad Categories for 26 Long-Range Emerging Threats Identified by DOD, State, DHS, and ODNI.

---

[15] The National Intelligence Program is intended to provide the resources to develop and maintain intelligence capabilities that support national priorities. Intelligence Reform and Terrorism Prevention Act of 2004, Pub. L. No. 108-458, § 1011 (2004). According to 50 U.S.C. § 3003 (6) "the term 'National Intelligence Program' refers to all programs, projects, and activities of the intelligence community, as well as any other programs of the intelligence community designated jointly by the Director of National Intelligence and the head of a United States department or agency or by the President. Such term does not include programs, projects, or activities of the military departments to acquire intelligence solely for the planning and conduct of tactical military operations by United States Armed Forces."

ADVERSARIES' POLITICAL AND MILITARY ADVANCEMENTS

Our adversaries are developing new political and military policies, strategies, doctrines, and tactics to advance their interests. These activities may or may not be intended to harm the United States and its national security interests. Agency officials identified examples such as Russia's integration of irregular warfare, influence operations, deception, and cyber attacks. Figure 2 shows the identified threats for this category.

Threat »	Description »	Examples »
Chinese Global Expansion	China is marshalling its diplomatic, economic, and military resources to facilitate its rise as a regional and global power. This may challenge U.S. access to air, space, cyberspace, and maritime domains. China's use of cyberspace and electronic warfare could impact various U.S. systems and operations.	• Expansion and Power Projection • Fusion of Military and Civilian Sectors and Control of Supply Chain • Cyber and Electronic Warfare
Russian Global Expansion	Russia is increasing its capability to challenge the United States across multiple warfare domains, including attempting to launch computer-based directed energy attacks against U.S. military assets. Russia is also increasing its military and political presence in key locations across the world.	• Military Capabilities across Warfare Domains • Global Military and Political Influence • Biotechnology Advancements
Iranian Political and Military Developments	Iran is expanding its influence by increasing the size and capabilities of its network of military, intelligence, and surrogate forces, while increasing economic activities in other areas of the world. Iran will also likely continue to develop its military capabilities, including developing technology that could be used for intercontinental ballistic missiles (ICBM) and improving its offensive cyberspace operations.	• Military and Economic Influence • Ballistic Missiles • Cyber Attacks
North Korean Military Developments	North Korea is developing capabilities to strike North America and its allies with long-range missiles and may produce significant numbers of intercontinental ballistic missiles.	• Nuclear Strike against the Continental United States • Numerical Overmatch of Ballistic Missile Systems
Foreign Government Capacity and Stability	Violent extremist organizations may proliferate in countries that have limited governing capacity and are facing conflict, which may result in a higher risk of terrorist attacks and increased demand for U.S. resources to counter them. Countries in Africa, Latin America, and the Caribbean may experience instability based on conflict, which may lead to humanitarian disasters and government collapses.	• Governments' Ability to Address Influences from Violent Extremist Organizations • Foreign Militaries' Reduced Military Readiness • Instability in Africa • Instability in Latin America and the Caribbean
Terrorism	Violent ideologies could influence additional individuals to turn to terrorism to achieve their goals across Africa, Asia, and the Middle East. Terrorists could advance their tactics, including building nuclear, biological or chemical weapons, or increase their use of online communications to reach new recruits and disseminate propaganda.	• Proliferation of Terrorism and Violent Ideologies • Terrorist Use of Chemical, Biological, and Nuclear Materials • New Tactics and Techniques
New Alliances and Adversaries	The United States could face challenges from potential new state adversaries and non-state adversaries (e.g., private corporations obtaining resources that could grant them more influence than states).	• Disrupted Alliances • Rise of New Nation-State and Non-State Adversaries • Foreign Nation-States' Influences on International Agreements and Standards
Information Operations	Adversaries—such as Russia, Iran, and China—may engage in advanced information operations campaigns that use social media, artificial intelligence, and data analytics to undermine the United States and its allies.	• Exploitation and Theft of U.S. Information • Weaponized Information

Source: GAO analysis of DOD, State, DHS, and ODNI questionnaire responses, agency documents, and national security strategies. | GAO-19-204SP.

Figure 2. Threats Identified under Adversaries' Political and Military Advancements.

DUAL-USE TECHNOLOGIES

These are technologies that may be developed by governments or the private sector for benign or beneficial purposes, but may have a dual-use application. For instance, in an adversary's hands, these technologies may pose a risk to the United States. Agency officials identified examples such as unmanned vehicles, artificial intelligence, and encryption technologies. Figure 3 shows the identified threats for this category.

Threat »	Description »	Examples »
Artificial Intelligence (AI)	Adversaries could gain increased access to AI through affordable designs used in the commercial industry, and could apply AI to areas such as weapons and technology.	• Nation-State and Non-State Development of AI • Intelligent Systems with General AI
Quantum Information Science	Quantum communications could enable adversaries to develop secure communications that U.S. personnel would not be able to intercept or decrypt. Quantum computing may allow adversaries to decrypt information, which could enable them to target U.S. personnel and military operations.	• Quantum Communications • Quantum Computing
Internet of Things (IoT)	The United States may face difficulties protecting networks and data as IoT grows and traditional approaches for security (e.g., encryption) may no longer effectively protect information. Adversaries could also disrupt IoT-enabled critical infrastructure and devices.	• Unsecure Networks and Data • Attacks on IoT-Enabled Infrastructure • Attacks on Commercial and Military Devices
Autonomous and Unmanned Systems	Adversaries are developing autonomous capabilities that could recognize faces, understand gestures, and match voices of U.S. personnel, which could compromise U.S. operations. Unmanned ground, underwater, air, and space vehicles may be used for combat and surveillance.	• Enhancement of Autonomous Systems • Weapons with Autonomous Navigation • Autonomous and Unmanned Vehicles
Biotechnology	Actors—which may include state or non-state entities such as violent extremist organizations and transnational criminal organizations—could alter genes or create DNA to modify plants, animals, and humans. Such biotechnologies could be used to enhance the performance of military personnel. The proliferation of synthetic biology—used to create genetic code that does not exist in nature—may increase the number of actors that can create chemical and biological weapons.	• Human Genetic Modification and Synthetic Biology • Plant and Animal Genetic Modification • Other Biotechnology Applications • Increase Access to Technology
Other Emerging Technologies	Actors may gain access to new technologies previously limited to militaries, such as affordable and sophisticated encryption technologies, which would hinder U.S. efforts to monitor terrorist and criminal activities. Other emerging technologies—such as additive manufacturing (i.e., 3D printing)—may be vulnerable to cyber attacks or be used to manufacture restricted materials, such as weapons.	• Expansion of Removable Media and Storage • Additive Manufacturing • New Materials • Development of Technologies that Address Electric Power Scarcity • Advancements in Camouflage Technology • Advanced Sensors

Source: GAO analysis of DOD, State, DHS, and ODNI questionnaire responses, agency documents, and national security strategies. | GAO-19-204SP.

Figure 3. Threats Identified under Dual-Use Technologies.

WEAPONS

These threats are inherently threatening military devices that may be used by our adversaries to inflict harm upon the United States or its national security interests. These weapons do not have potential beneficial or benign uses from the perspective of the United States. Agency officials identified examples such as hypersonic missiles, weaponized pathogens, or stealth aircraft. Figure 4 shows the identified threats for this category.

EVENTS AND DEMOGRAPHIC CHANGES

Events and demographic changes are occurrences with no adversary behind them and therefore no intent to harm the United States. Nevertheless, events and demographic changes may have the capability to harm the United States or its national security interests in the absence of mitigating factors. Agency officials identified examples such as influenza pandemic, climate change, food shortages, and the growth of megacities. Figure 4 shows the identified threats for this category.

Threat »	Description »	Examples »
Weapons of Mass Destruction	An increasing number of actors may gain access to these weapons. Adversaries could steal nuclear materials from existing facilities or develop new types of biological weapons using genetic engineering and synthetic biology.	• Global Proliferation of Weapons of Mass Destruction • Development and Use of Nonstrategic Nuclear Weapons • New Forms of Biological Weapons
Electronic Warfare	Adversaries are developing electronic attack weapons to target U.S. systems with sensitive electronic components, such as military sensors, communication, navigation, and information systems. These weapons are intended to degrade U.S. capabilities and could restrict situational awareness or may affect military operations.	• Electronic Attack Weapons • Attacks on Communications and Navigation Systems
Hypersonic Weapons	China and Russia are pursuing hypersonic weapons because their speed, altitude, and maneuverability may defeat most missile defense systems, and they may be used to improve long-range conventional and nuclear strike capabilities. There are no existing countermeasures.	• Hypersonic Weapons and Missile Defense • Hypersonic Ballistic and Cruise Missiles • Hypersonic Glide Vehicles • Future Development and Convergence
Counterspace Weapons	China and Russia are developing anti-satellite weapons to threaten U.S. space operations. China is developing capabilities to conduct large-scale anti-satellite strikes using novel physical, cyber, and electronic warfare means.	• Anti-Satellite Weapons • Increased Access to Space and Anti-Satellite Weapons
Missiles	Adversaries are developing missile technology to attack the United States in novel ways and challenge U.S. missile defense, including conventional and nuclear intercontinental ballistic missiles, sea-launched land-attack missiles, and space-based missiles that could orbit the earth.	• Advancements in Missile Technology • Adversary Plans for Intercontinental Ballistic Missiles • Orbital Missiles • Sea-to-Land Missiles • Adversary Missile Defense
Intelligence, Surveillance, Reconnaissance (ISR) Platforms	Future advances in artificial intelligence, sensors, data analytics, and space-based platforms could create an environment of "ubiquitous ISR", where people and equipment could be tracked throughout the world in near-real time. China, Russia, Iran, and North Korea are developing multiple ISR platforms.	• Worldwide and Ubiquitous Surveillance • Adversary Improvements in Radar and Surveillance Platforms
Aircraft	China and Russia are developing new aircraft, including stealth aircraft, which could fly faster, carry advanced weapons, and achieve greater ranges. Such aircraft could force U.S. aircraft to operate at farther distances and put more U.S. targets at risk.	• Russian Aircraft • Chinese Aircraft
Undersea Weapons	Russia has made significant advancements in submarine technology and tactics to escape detection by U.S. forces. China is developing underwater acoustic systems that could coordinate swarm attacks—the use of large quantities of simple and expendable assets to overwhelm opponents—among vehicles and provide greater undersea awareness. Adversaries could achieve breakthroughs in anti-submarine warfare—such as using artificial intelligence to locate U.S. submarines—or attack U.S. undersea infrastructure, which could cripple communications.	• Russian Improvements in Undersea Stealth • Unmanned Underwater Vehicles • Anti-Submarine Warfare • Attack on Undersea Cables
Cyber Weapons	Adversaries, such as China, Russia, Iran, and North Korea, may launch cyber attacks against critical U.S. infrastructure (e.g., electric, oil and gas, and nuclear power systems) and military infrastructure (e.g., communications and ISR platforms). Adversaries could also launch cyber attacks on the U.S. health care system, threatening patient safety by disrupting access to medical care. Finally, adversaries are also developing tools to directly attack hardware and embedded components in aviation systems, which can manipulate or destroy data.	• Attacks on Critical Infrastructure • Military Infrastructure • Cyber Attacks on Health Care • Malware and New Form of Attack

Source: GAO analysis of DOD, State, DHS, and ODNI questionnaire responses, agency documents, and national security strategies. | GAO-19-204SP.

Figure 4. Threats Identified under Weapons.

Threat »	Description »	Examples »
Infectious Diseases	New and evolving diseases from the natural environment—exacerbated by changes in climate, the movement of people into cities, and global trade and travel—may become a pandemic. Drug-resistant forms of diseases previously considered treatable could become widespread again.	• Pandemic Disease Event • Drug-Resistant Disease
Climate Change	Extreme weather events—such as hurricanes and megadroughts—could intensify and affect food security, energy resources, and the health care sector. Diminishing permafrost could expand habitats for pathogens that cause disease. The loss of Arctic sea ice could open previously closed sea routes, potentially increasing Russian and Chinese access to the region and challenging the freedom of navigation that the United States currently has.	• Extreme Weather Events • Loss of Arctic Sea Ice and Permafrost
Internal and International Migration	Governments in megacities (i.e., over 10 million people) across Asia, Latin America, and Africa may not have the capacity to provide adequate resources and infrastructure, and may be vulnerable to natural or man-made disasters. Mass migration events may occur and threaten regional stability, undermine governments, and strain U.S. military and civilian responses.	• Disasters in Megacities • A Mass Migration Event

Source: GAO analysis of DOD, State, DHS, and ODNI questionnaire responses, agency documents, and national security strategies. | GAO-19-204SP.

Figure 5. Threats Identified under Events and Demographic Changes.

Agency Comments and Our Evaluation

We provided a draft of the classified version of this chapter to the DOD, State, and DHS, as well as ODNI, for their review and comment. DOD concurred with our classified report and provided technical comments, which we addressed as appropriate. DOD's letter is included in appendix II. We also received technical comments from DHS and ODNI, which we addressed as appropriate. State did not provide comments.

We are sending copies of this chapter to the appropriate congressional committees, DOD, State, DHS, and ODNI.

Joseph W. Kirschbaum
Director
Defense Capabilities and Management

Brian M. Mazanec
Acting Director
International Affairs and Trade

List of Congressional Committees

The Honorable James M. Inhofe
Chairman

The Honorable Jack Reed
Ranking Member
Committee on Armed Services United States Senate

The Honorable Richard Shelby
Chairman

The Honorable Dick Durbin
Ranking Member
Subcommittee on Defense Committee on Appropriations
United States Senate

The Honorable Mac Thornberry
Chairman

The Honorable Adam Smith
Ranking Member
Committee on Armed Services House of Representatives

The Honorable Kay Granger
Chairwoman

The Honorable Pete Visclosky
Ranking Member
Subcommittee on Defense Committee on Appropriations
House of Representatives

APPENDIX I: OBJECTIVE, SCOPE, AND METHODOLOGY

This chapter is a public version of a classified report that we issued on September 28, 2018.[16] It omits classified and sensitive information about threats identified by executive branch agencies and described in 26 profiles in our classified report. It also omits classified and sensitive information in those profiles related to specific threats, the effects of those threats, specific warfare domains, and questions for oversight. Although the information provided in this chapter is more limited, the report addresses the same objectives as the classified report and uses the same methodology.

This chapter provides a summary of long-range emerging threats as identified by agencies that, among others, have primary responsibility for national security: the Department of Defense (DOD), Department of State (State), Department of Homeland Security (DHS), and the Office of the Director of National Intelligence (ODNI). We utilized questionnaires, national security strategies, agency documents, and interviews with agency officials to obtain information on these long-range emerging threats. For purposes of this chapter, we define long-range threats as threats that agency officials identified that may occur in approximately 5 or more years, or those threats that could occur in a future unknown time frame.

There is no standard definition of "emerging threat" within the federal government, and the use and definitions of the term vary among organizations. To develop a definition of emerging threat that generally reflected how multiple organizations use this term, we reviewed strategies and reports issued by federal government entities—such as the 2016 Joint Strategic Intelligence Estimate from the Joint Staff and Global Trends: Paradox of Progress from the National Intelligence Council—that describe issues, risks, threats, or events that could affect the national security interests of the United States and its allies. We also reviewed documents such as the DOD Dictionary of Military and Associated Terms and the Department of Homeland Security Risk Assessment Lexicon that define and standardize commonly-used terminology. We reviewed our past reports and publications by research institutions to understand how different organizations consider and utilize the concepts of "emergence" and "threat." We adapted the use of the term "emerging" from our prior work in

[16] GAO, National Security: Long-Range Emerging Threats Facing the United States Identified by Federal Agencies, GAO-18-497SPC (Washington, D.C.: Sept. 28, 2018). (SECRET//NOFORN)

emerging infectious diseases, and adapted the use of the term "threat" from the documents we reviewed.[17]

After developing a working definition of emerging threat, we solicited feedback on the definition through interviews with officials from DOD, State, and ODNI, including assessing whether the definition would be acceptable or understood within their respective organizations. We modified the definition based on their feedback. Furthermore, we limited the scope of emerging threats, as described in this chapter, to threats that may occur approximately 5 years or more from 2018, or those that have an unknown time frame. We established this time frame because officials from DOD and ODNI stated they consider threats occurring earlier than 5 years from today as near-term or mid-term threats, which receive greater attention and resources from defense and intelligence organizations than long-term threats.

As the primary mechanism for identifying emerging threats within our identified time frame, we developed a questionnaire that asked respondents to identify and describe emerging threats that their organizations assess could occur in approximately 5 years or more from today, or those that have an unknown time frame. To identify organizations within DOD, State, DHS, and the Intelligence Community to receive this questionnaire, we consulted with officials from DOD, State, DHS, and ODNI about the objective, scope, and methodology of our work. We then identified additional organizations through an iterative process whereby we contacted DOD, State, DHS and ODNI officials and solicited the names of additional organizations that assess emerging threats. We repeated this process until the referrals were mostly to organizations we had previously contacted.

Ultimately, we selected a total of 45 organizations to receive the questionnaire, comprised of 36 organizations identified through the iterative process described previously and the nine combatant commands.[18] We took several steps to ensure that the questionnaire would gather reliable information. The questionnaire was developed in collaboration with a survey specialist and was reviewed by a separate survey specialist. We requested and received comments from subject matter experts from DOD, State, and DHS. We also conducted six pretests of the questionnaire with potential recipients to assess how the questionnaire would be understood by the eventual recipients. The pretest participants included officials from each department requested to respond to the questionnaire (DOD, State, and DHS) who had not previously reviewed or provided comments on the questionnaire. We refined the questionnaire based on the results of each step. Additionally, we included an example to guide respondents to the type and length of content we wanted them to provide in their response. The final questionnaire was a Microsoft Word form that the respondents could return electronically.

---

[17] GAO, Emerging Infectious Diseases: Actions Needed to Address the Challenges of Responding to Zika Virus Disease Outbreaks, GAO-17-445 (Washington, D.C.: May 23, 2017)

[18] U.S. Cyber Command was elevated to a combatant command on May 5, 2018—after we sent the questionnaire. Therefore, U.S. Cyber Command was not included among the combatant commands that received a questionnaire.

Table 1. Organizations That Provided Completed Questionnaire Responses

Department of Defense	Department of State	Department of Homeland Security
Office of Assistant Secretary for Research and Engineering, Office of Net Technical Assessment	Bureau of Oceans and International Environment and Scientific Affairs	Countering Weapons of Mass Destruction Office
Office of Assistant Secretary for Research and Engineering, Deputy Assistant Secretary of Defense, Emerging Capabilities and Prototyping	Office of Medical Services, Directorate of Operational Medicine	Office of Science and Technology
Strategic Capabilities Office		Office of Intelligence and Analysis[a]
Office of Net Assessment		Federal Emergency Management Agency
Defense Advanced Research Projects Agency[a]		National Protection and Programs Directorate
Defense Intelligence Agency, Office for Space and Counterspace		
Defense Intelligence Agency, Defense Technology and Long Range Analysis		
Defense Intelligence Agency, National Center for Medical Intelligence		
National Security Agency		
U.S. Army, National Ground Intelligence Center		
U.S. Navy, Acquisition, Intelligence, and Requirements Office		
U.S. Air Force, National Air and Space Intelligence Center		
U.S. Marine Corps, Marine Corps Intelligence Activity		
U.S. Africa Command		
U.S. European Command		
U.S. Northern Command		
U.S. Indo-Pacific Command		
U.S. Southern Command		
U.S. Special Operations Command		
U.S. Strategic Command		
U.S. Transportation Command		

Source: GAO. | GAO-19-204SP.

[a] Defense Advanced Research Projects Agency and the Department of Homeland Security's Office of Intelligence and Analysis submitted completed questionnaires after our response period had ended. The information received in these questionnaires was not used in the development of the threat profiles.

Out of the 45 government organizations selected, 8 told us that they do not identify threats that meet our scope or definition, and 1 told us that a separate office within their organization had responded on their behalf, so these 9 organizations were excluded from our response rate calculations. Of the remaining 36 organizations, 26 provided responses by the end of the response period and 2 provided responses after the response period had ended so they were not used in the development of the threat profiles.[19] In addition, 1 organization did not receive a questionnaire due to an administrative error and ODNI submitted an incomplete questionnaire that did not identify any threats. Instead, ODNI referred us to their Global

[19] These responses were submitted more than 3 months after the submission deadline. Many of these responses were similar to previously submitted questionnaire responses, but some of the emerging threats were different.

Trends: Paradox of Progress report and provided verbal input on long-range emerging threats during two agency meetings.[20] We used this information to supplement questionnaire responses from DOD, State, and DHS organizations. We did not receive responses from the remaining six organizations. In total, we received a 78-percent response rate (28 of 36) of organizations that provided completed questionnaire responses. Table 1 lists the 28 organizations that provided completed responses to our questionnaire.

The 26 of 28 organizations that timely responded provided approximately 210 individual threats, 4 of which were later deemed outside of the scope of this review. The questionnaire responses are not generalizable to any other organizations.

We then conducted a content analysis of the questionnaire responses to categorize threats and to identify common themes across responding organizations. Two analysts independently reviewed and coded each threat described in the questionnaires according to the categorization framework. After all of the individual threats had been coded, the analysts met, discussed any differences, and reached agreement on the final coding for each individual threat. A third analyst adjudicated any unresolved differences between coders.

To consistently report on all emerging threats identified during this review, the analysts conducted a second phase of content analysis. Using primarily the list of descriptors and the threats coded to each descriptor, three analysts developed a list of 26 threats described in separate profiles in this chapter. In this process, some descriptors were combined into a single threat profile, while others were renamed to more accurately reflect the threats associated with the descriptor and threat profile. The analysts coded each of the approximately 210 individual threats into 1 of the 26 threat profiles. The analysts resolved any differences by discussion and consensus. We also reviewed documents provided by organizations that participated in this review to determine whether the documents identified emerging threats differently from those identified through the questionnaire responses and content analysis. We did not identify any additional emerging threats through this document review.

We also used information in related documents— such as a DOD risk assessment, DOD threat reports, GAO reports, a Defense Science Board report, National Academy of Sciences reports, and National Intelligence Council reports—to supplement the information gathered from the processes listed above.

To supplement the questionnaire responses and our review of the national security strategies and other documents, we interviewed officials from DOD, State, DHS, and ODNI. In total, we interviewed officials from 22 organizations, including 11 DOD organizations such as the Defense Intelligence Agency, several combatant commands, and the Joint Staff; 6 State organizations across 5 bureaus, including the Bureaus of Counterterrorism and Countering Violent Extremism, Intelligence and Research, and Oceans and International Environmental and Scientific Affairs; 4 DHS organizations, such as the Science and Technology Directorate and the Countering Weapons of Mass Destruction Office; and ODNI. We selected these 22 organizations because they may have a role in identifying and assessing long-range emerging threats. Additionally, we interviewed officials at the headquarters of the North Atlantic Treaty Organization, U.S. Africa Command, and U.S. European Command. We selected these sites

[20] An ODNI official stated that the *Global Trends: Paradox of Progress* report lists some key threats over the next 5 to 20 years. In particular, ODNI officials emphasized economic threats such as U.S. debt and growing inequality; new technologies and ethical questions surrounding the use of those technologies; geopolitical conflict, including the spread of corruption to the developed world and the rise of China; and the spread of populism and nationalist identities around the world.

because officials within DOD and State identified these organizations as representative military commands that identify and address emerging threats.

The performance audit upon which this chapter is based was conducted from July 2017 to September 2018 in accordance with generally accepted government auditing standards. Those standards require that we plan and perform the audit to obtain sufficient, appropriate evidence to provide a reasonable basis for our findings and conclusions based on our audit objectives. We believe that the evidence obtained provides a reasonable basis for our findings and conclusions based on our audit objectives. We subsequently worked with DOD from September 2018 to December 2018 to prepare this public version of the original classified report for public release. This public version was also prepared in accordance with those standards.

APPENDIX II: DOD COMMENTS

We received these comments on September 25, 2018. The draft report number for the classified version of this chapter, GAO-18-497C, was subsequently renumbered GAO-18-497SPC for the final classified report.

OFFICE OF THE UNDER SECRETARY OF DEFENSE
5000 DEFENSE PENTAGON
WASHINGTON, DC 20301-5000

INTELLIGENCE

MEMORANDUM FOR MR. JOSEPH KIRSCHBAUM, DIRECTOR, DEFENSE CAPABILITIES MANAGEMENT, U.S.GOVERNMENT ACCOUNTABILITY OFFICE

SUBJECT: Review of GAO Draft Report

Reference: GAO Draft Report, GAO-18-497C, "NATIONAL SECURITY: Long-Range Emerging Threats Facing the United States Identified by Federal Agencies, dated July 26, 2018 (GAO Code 102221)

This is the Department of Defense (DoD) response to the GAO Draft Report, GAO-18-497, "NATIONAL SECURITY: Long-Range Emerging Threats Facing the United States Identified by Federal Agencies, dated July 26, 2018 (GAO Code 102221). The Department appreciates the opportunity to review and comment on the draft report. We concur with the report as a whole with some recommendations.

The security review determined that the overall classification of the report must remain SECRET//NOFORN, except as indicated when separated from the report. Paragraphs have been portioned marked in accordance with security guidelines.

Overall, we find this GAO study of high quality while providing an accurate although sobering macro picture of how the US stands in the world against emerging threats.

Wendell C. Warner, DISES
Director, Geographic Combatant Command
Intelligence Support

In: Top 10 Reports and Testimonies in December 2018
Editor: Sarah J. Nygaard
ISBN: 978-1-53615-507-5

Chapter 7

NAVY AND MARINE CORPS: REBUILDING SHIP, SUBMARINE, AND AVIATION READINESS WILL REQUIRE TIME AND SUSTAINED MANAGEMENT ATTENTION*

John H. Pendleton

WHY GAO DID THIS STUDY

The 2018 National Defense Strategy emphasizes that restoring and retaining readiness is critical to success in the emerging security environment. The Navy and Marine Corps are working to rebuild the readiness of their forces while growing and modernizing their aging fleet of ships and aircraft. However, achieving readiness recovery goals will take years as both services continue to be challenged to rebuild readiness amid continued operational demands.

This statement provides information on current and future readiness challenges facing (1) the Navy ship and submarine fleet and (2) Navy and Marine Corps aviation. GAO also discusses prior recommendations on Navy and Marine Corps readiness and progress to address them.

This statement is based on previously published work since 2015 related to Navy and Marine Corps readiness challenges, including shipyard workforce and capital investment, ship crewing, weapon system sustainment, the fighter pilot workforce, and modernizing force structure. GAO conducted site visits to the Pacific fleet in November 2018 and analyzed updated data, as appropriate.

* This is an edited, reformatted and augmented version of United States Government Accountability Office; Testimony, Before the Subcommittees on Seapower and Readiness and Management Support, Committee on Armed Services, U.S. Senate, Publication No. GAO-19-225T dated December 12, 2018.

What GAO Recommends

GAO has made a total of 45 recommendations in the prior work described in this statement. The Department of Defense concurred with most of them, and has many actions underway, but has not yet fully implemented any. Attention to these recommendations can assist the Navy and the Marine Corps as they seek to rebuild the readiness of their forces.

What GAO Found

The Navy has taken steps to address training shortfalls in the surface fleet, but faces persistent maintenance and personnel challenges as it seeks to rebuild ship and submarine readiness. While the Navy has corrective actions underway, they will take years to implement. Following ship collisions in 2017, the Navy has taken steps to ensure its crews are trained to standards prior to deployment and made significant progress in those efforts. However, the Navy has struggled to complete ship maintenance—with only 30 percent of maintenance completed on time since fiscal year 2012—leading to thousands of days that ships were unavailable for training and operations (see Figure). Additionally, manning shortfalls and experience gaps continue to contribute to high sailor workload and are likely to continue through at least fiscal year 2021. The Navy has developed a plan to improve shipyards and is re-examining its ship manning, among other actions; however, these positive steps have not yet fully addressed GAO's recommendations. Looking to the future, the Navy has indicated that it wants to grow its fleet to meet demands. However, the costs of such growth are not yet known and would likely require resourcing well above currently planned levels.

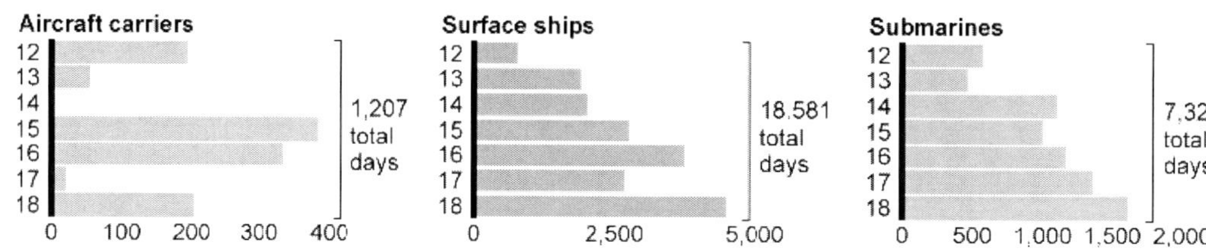

Source: GAO analysis of Navy data. | GAO-19-225T.

Days of Maintenance Delay by Type of Ship, Fiscal Years 2012 through 2018.

Navy and Marine Corps aircraft availability has been limited due to numerous challenges (see Figure). Specifically, the seven aircraft GAO reviewed have generally experienced decreasing availability since fiscal year 2011 and did not meet availability goals in fiscal years 2017 and 2018. The F-35—the future of naval aviation—also has not met availability goals due to part shortages and poor sustainment planning. In September 2018, the Department of Defense established aggressive targets for aircraft availability. While the Navy and Marine Corps are taking actions to improve aircraft availability, including addressing GAO's recommendations, aviation readiness will take many years to recover.

Aircraft	Aging aircraft		Maintenance		Supply support	
	Delays acquiring replacement aircraft	Unexpected replacement of parts and repairs	Delays in depot maintenance	Shortage of depot maintainer personnel	Parts obsolescence	Diminishing manufacturing source
AV-8B	✓	✓	✓	✓	✓	✓
C-2A		✓	✓	✓	✓	✓
E-2C		✓	✓	✓	✓	✓
E-2D			✓	✓	✓	✓
EA-18 G			✓	✓		✓
F/A-18 A-D	✓	✓	✓	✓	✓	✓
F/A-18 E-F		✓	✓	✓		✓

Source: GAO analysis of Navy data. | GAO-19-225T.

Sustainment Challenges Affecting Selected Navy and Marine Corps Aircraft.

Chairmen Wicker and Sullivan, Ranking Members Hirono and Kaine, and Members of the Subcommittees:

Thank you for the opportunity to be here today to discuss issues related to Navy and Marine Corps readiness.

In June 2017, we issued a report highlighting five key mission challenges facing the Department of Defense (DOD).[1] In that report, we noted that the United States faces an extremely challenging national security environment at the same time it is grappling with addressing an unsustainable fiscal situation in which DOD accounts for approximately half of the federal government's discretionary spending. Within this environment, DOD is working to both rebuild the readiness of its current forces and modernize to meet future threats. Since we issued that report, the department released a new National Defense Strategy in January 2018 that prioritizes the long-term challenges posed by highly capable adversaries and emphasizes the need to rebuild readiness. Additionally, Congress has passed appropriations to fund DOD's effort to restore readiness.

This statement provides information on current and future readiness challenges facing the (1) Navy ship and submarine fleet and (2) Navy and Marine Corps aviation. In appendix I, we also summarize our recommendations related to Navy and Marine Corps readiness that we have made in prior reports and we summarize any progress the Navy and Marine Corps have made to implement those recommendations.[2]

This statement is based on prior reports we issued from 2015 through 2018 examining Navy and Marine Corps readiness challenges, shipyard workforce and capital investment, ship crewing, weapon system sustainment, the fighter pilot workforce, and force structure.[3] To perform our prior work, we analyzed Navy and Marine Corps readiness, maintenance, personnel, and training data, and interviewed cognizant Navy and Marine Corps officials

[1] This report included a detailed discussion of our priority recommendations to DOD. Since August 2015, we have identified priority recommendations in letters to the Secretary of Defense—recommendations that we have made to DOD that we believe the department should give a high priority to addressing. See GAO, *Department of Defense: Actions Needed to Address Five Key Mission Challenges*, GAO-17-369 (Washington, D.C.: June 13, 2017). As of April 2018, 85 priority recommendations remained open.

[2] Appendix I does not include classified recommendations made in classified reports, reports without recommendations, and reports in which we directed recommendations exclusively to the Office of the Secretary of Defense or the Department of the Air Force.

[3] A list of related classified and unclassified GAO products is provided in the Related GAO Products pages at the end of this statement.

involved in operations. The reports cited throughout this statement contain more details on the scope of the work and the methodology used to carry it out. This statement also includes updates to information as of November 2018, as appropriate, based on Navy and Marine Corps documentation and discussions with senior Navy leadership, the Fleet Forces Command, the Pacific Fleet, and other officials. We also conducted 10 group discussions with officers and enlisted personnel aboard a cruiser and a destroyer based in Yokosuka, Japan in November 2018 to discuss crew workload, training, and ship manning.[4] We have also issued several classified reports since 2015 examining these issues and made recommendations to the Navy and the Marine Corps; however, this statement does not include that work.

We conducted the work on which this testimony is based in accordance with generally accepted government auditing standards. Those standards require that we plan and perform the audit to obtain sufficient, appropriate evidence to provide a reasonable basis for our findings and conclusions based on our audit objectives. We believe that the evidence obtained provides a reasonable basis for our findings and conclusions based on our audit objectives.

BACKGROUND

We testified before the Senate Committee on Armed Services in September 2017 after four significant mishaps at sea resulted in the loss of 17 sailors' lives and serious damage to Navy ships.5 We reported on some of the Navy's challenges, including the degraded condition and expired training certifications of ships homeported overseas, reductions to ship crews that contributed to sailor overwork and safety risks, and an inability to complete maintenance on time. Since that time, the Navy has completed two internal reviews to address these and other challenges, identifying 111 recommendations to improve surface fleet readiness. The Navy formed an executive group to guide and closely track the implementation of recommendations, and its reform efforts are ongoing. As of November 2018, the Navy reported that it had implemented 78 (i.e., 70 percent) of these recommendations. Navy officials recognize that full implementation will take significant time and management attention to address the fundamental readiness challenges identified. In Figure 1, we show photographs of two of the four Navy ships involved in significant mishaps that occurred in 2017. Both the USS Fitzgerald and the USS John S. McCain were involved in collisions that resulted in sailor fatalities.

DOD has reported that more than a decade of conflict, budget uncertainty, and reductions in force structure have degraded its readiness; in response, the department has made rebuilding readiness a priority. The 2018 National Defense Strategy emphasizes that restoring and retaining readiness across the entire spectrum of conflict is critical to success in the emerging security environment. Nevertheless, DOD reported that readiness of the total military force remains low and has remained so since 2013. Our work has shown that the Navy has experienced increasing maintenance challenges as a high pace of operations has continued and maintenance has been deferred.[6] Maintenance and personnel challenges also

---

[4] Discussions were held separately with Navy officers and enlisted personnel. The results of the discussions are not generalizable beyond the individuals we talked to.

[5] GAO, *Navy Readiness: Actions Needed to Address Persistent Maintenance, Training, and other Challenges Affecting the Fleet*, GAO-17-809T (Washington, D.C.: Sept. 19, 2017).

[6] GAO-17-369.

hinder readiness recovery of Navy aircraft. For the Marine Corps, our work has shown that ground force readiness has improved and remained stable in recent years, but acute readiness problems remain in aviation units.

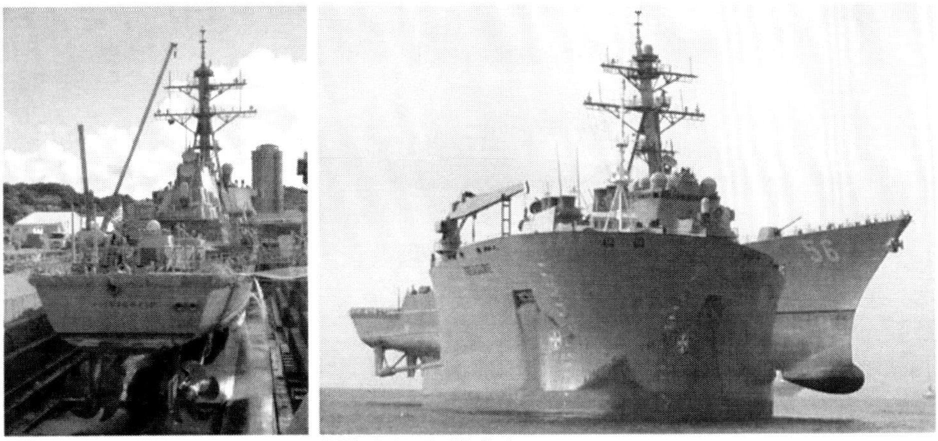

USS *Fitzgerald* **USS *John S. McCain***

Source: Defense Visual Information Distribution Service. | GAO-19-225T.

Figure 1. USS *Fitzgerald* Receiving Dry Dock Repairs and USS *John S. McCain* on Heavy Lift Transport after 2017 Collisions.

Over the past year, DOD has made department-wide progress in developing a plan to rebuild the readiness of the military force, with the military services providing regular input on the status of their readiness recovery efforts.[7] In August 2018, we reported that the Office of the Secretary of Defense has developed a Readiness Recovery Framework that the department is using to guide the services' efforts and plans to use to regularly assess, validate, and monitor readiness recovery.[8] The Office of the Secretary of Defense and the services have recently revised readiness goals and accompanying recovery strategies, metrics, and milestones to align with the 2018 National Defense Strategy and Defense Planning Guidance. We have ongoing work assessing DOD's progress in achieving its overall readiness goals.[9]

DOD's readiness rebuilding efforts are occurring in a challenging context that requires the department to make difficult decisions regarding how best to address continuing operational demands while preparing for future challenges. Our work has shown that an important aspect of this, across all of the services, is determining an appropriate balance between maintaining and upgrading legacy weapon systems currently in operational use and procuring new ones to overcome rapidly advancing future threats.

---

[7] In September 2016, we reviewed DOD and the military services' plans to rebuild readiness and reported that the efforts may be at risk without a department-wide plan for moving forward. We made five recommendations on implementing and overseeing readiness rebuilding efforts. See GAO, *Military Readiness: DOD's Readiness Rebuilding Efforts May Be at Risk without a Comprehensive Plan*, GAO-16-841 (Washington, D.C.: Sept. 7, 2016).

[8] GAO, *Military Readiness: Update on DOD's Progress in Developing a Readiness Rebuilding Plan*, GAO-18-441RC (Washington, D.C.: Aug. 10, 2018). The Readiness Recovery Framework identifies primary readiness issues that each of the military services face, actions to address identified issues, and milestones and metrics to assess progress in addressing identified issues.

[9] Section 333 of the John S. McCain National Defense Authorization Act for Fiscal Year 2019, Pub. L.No. 115-232 (2018), requires us to report annually until 2021 on the readiness of the armed forces to conduct full spectrum operations in the ground, sea, air, space, and cyber domains.

The Navy Fleet Faces Challenges in Rebuilding Readiness and the Costs Associated with Expanding the Fleet to Enhance Readiness in the Future Are Unknown

Based on updated information we received in November 2018, the Navy has taken steps to provide dedicated training time so its surface forces may meet existing Navy training standards and their training is certified when they deploy. However, the Navy continues to struggle with rebuilding the readiness of the existing fleet due to enduring maintenance and manning challenges. As the Navy seeks to expand its fleet by 25 percent, these challenges will likely be further exacerbated and the Navy will likely face additional affordability challenges.

Navy Has Taken Steps to Address Training Shortfalls in the Surface Fleet

After the collisions in 2017, the Navy focused on training surface ship crews to its existing standards. We testified in September 2017 that there were no dedicated training periods built into the operational schedules of the cruisers and destroyers based in Japan and 37 percent of training certifications for these surface ship crews had lapsed as of June 2017. Since that time, the Navy has worked to ensure surface ships are certified before they are deployed. For example, the Navy has established controls to limit waivers that allowed training lapses to worsen, now requiring multiple high-level approvals for ships to operate uncertified. Based on our analysis of updated data, the Navy has improved markedly in the percentage of cruisers and destroyers with lapsed certifications in Japan, from 41 percent of certifications expired in September 2017 to 9 percent as of November 2018, with less than 3 percent of certifications expired on ships in operational status.

While the Navy has demonstrated its commitment to ensuring that crews are certified prior to deploying, training for amphibious operations and higher-level collective training may not be fully implemented for several years. In September 2017, we reported that some Marine Corps units were limited in their ability to complete training to conduct an amphibious operation—a military operation that is launched from the sea to introduce a landing force ashore—by several factors, including a decline in the number of amphibious ships from 62 in 1990 to 32 as of November 2018, access to range space, and a high pace of deployments, among others. We recommended that the Navy and the Marine Corps develop an approach to mitigate their amphibious operations training shortfalls as the services await the arrival of additional amphibious ships into the fleet. Marine Corps officials told us that the Marine Corps and the Navy are working together to maximize amphibious training opportunities. Additionally, the Navy has plans to phase in high-level collective training into the operational schedules of its ships homeported in Japan over the next several years. Previously, advanced and integrated training involving multiple ships was conducted ad hoc if at all for ships homeported in Japan. Such collective training is important because the 2018 National Defense Strategy states that the department's principal priority is to prepare for threats from strategic competitors due to the magnitude of the threat they pose. However, in November 2018, officials from Fleet Forces Command told us that fully implementing its training approach to prepare for advanced adversaries would not be fully implemented across the fleet for several years.

The Fleet Faces Persistent Maintenance and Personnel Challenges as the Navy Seeks to Rebuild Readiness

We have reported that the Navy faces persistent challenges in completing maintenance on time and providing sufficient manning to its ships. Unless these challenges are addressed, the Navy will be hampered in its ability to rebuild readiness and prepare for the future.

Maintenance Delays for Ships and Submarines Reduce Time for Training and Operations

Our work has found that the Navy has been unable to complete ship and submarine maintenance on time, resulting in continuing schedule delays that reduce time for training and operations and create costly inefficiencies in a resource constrained environment. The Navy's readiness recovery is premised on the rigorous adherence to deployment, training, and maintenance schedules. However, we reported in May 2016 on the difficulty that both the public and private shipyards were having in completing maintenance on time.[10] We reported that, from 2011 through 2014, about 28 percent of scheduled maintenance for surface combatants was completed on time and 11 percent was completed on time for aircraft carriers. We updated these data as of November 2018 to include maintenance periods completed through the end of fiscal year 2018 and found that the Navy continues to struggle to complete maintenance on time. For fiscal years 2012-2018, our analysis for key portions of the Navy fleet shows that 30 percent of Navy maintenance was completed on time, leading to more than 27,000 days in which ships were delayed and unavailable for training and operations as shown in Figure 2 below.

In addition to affecting training and operations, maintenance delays are costly. In November 2018, we examined attack submarine maintenance delays and reported that the Navy was incurring significant operating and support costs to crew, maintain, and support attack submarines that are delayed getting into and out of shipyard maintenance periods. We estimated that over the past 10 years the Navy has spent $1.5 billion in fiscal year 2018 constant dollars to support attack submarines that provide no operational capability—those sitting idle no longer certified to conduct normal operations—while waiting to enter the shipyards, and those delayed in completing their maintenance at the shipyards (see Figure 3).[11] We recommended that the Navy analyze how it allocates its maintenance workload across public and private shipyards. DOD concurred with our recommendation, stating that it has taken the first steps to take a more holistic view of submarine maintenance requirements and impacts across both the public and private shipyards. In an update provided in November

---

[10] GAO, *Military Readiness: Progress and Challenges in Implementing the Navy's Optimized Fleet Response Plan*, GAO-16-466R (Washington, D.C.: May 2, 2016).

[11] While acknowledging the magnitude of these costs, Navy officials stated that there may be some benefits that could be realized from supporting these idle attack submarines since crews on idle attack submarines can conduct some limited training. GAO, *Navy Readiness: Actions Needed to Address Costly Maintenance Delays Facing the Attack Submarine Fleet*, GAO-19-229 (Washington, D.C.: Nov. 19, 2018).

2018, the Navy told us that they are developing a contracting strategy to conduct two additional depot maintenance periods at private shipyards in the future.

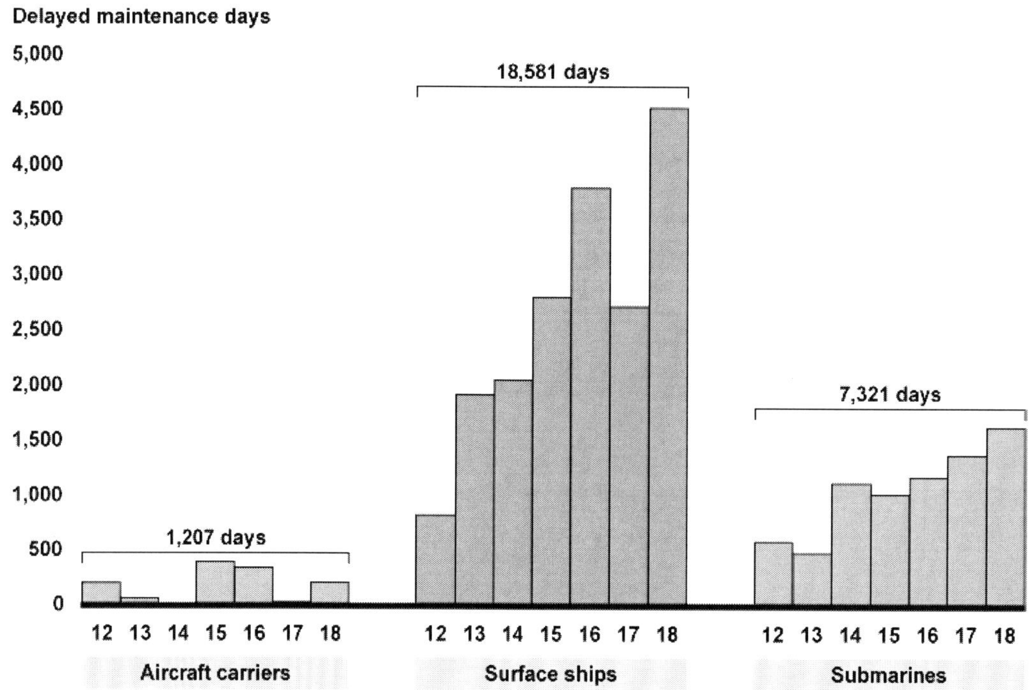

Source: GAO analysis of Navy data. | GAO-19-225T.

Note: In order to standardize the analysis across data for aircraft carriers, surface ships, and submarines, we calculated days of maintenance delay based on the difference between actual and planned completion dates. Additionally, these delayed maintenance days are arranged by the fiscal year in which they occurred. We included maintenance delays for converting decommissioned submarines to training ships because those conversions require shipyard resources and workers, and restrict the use of limited drydocks. Delayed maintenance days for aircraft carrier and submarine data for this analysis are limited to the Navy's public shipyards and do not include data from private shipyards. As we reported in November 2018, attack submarine maintenance performed at private shipyards also experienced delays in execution. Additionally, data are not captured in this analysis for aircraft carrier and submarine maintenance availabilities that began prior to fiscal year 2010, as well as surface ship maintenance availabilities that began prior to fiscal year 2012, that may have resulted in delays that occurred after fiscal year 2012. Data showing delayed maintenance days for aircraft carriers and submarines are as of November 2018; for surface ships the data are as of October 2018.

Figure 2. Aircraft Carrier, Surface Ship, and Submarine Days of Maintenance Delay, Fiscal Years 2012–2018.

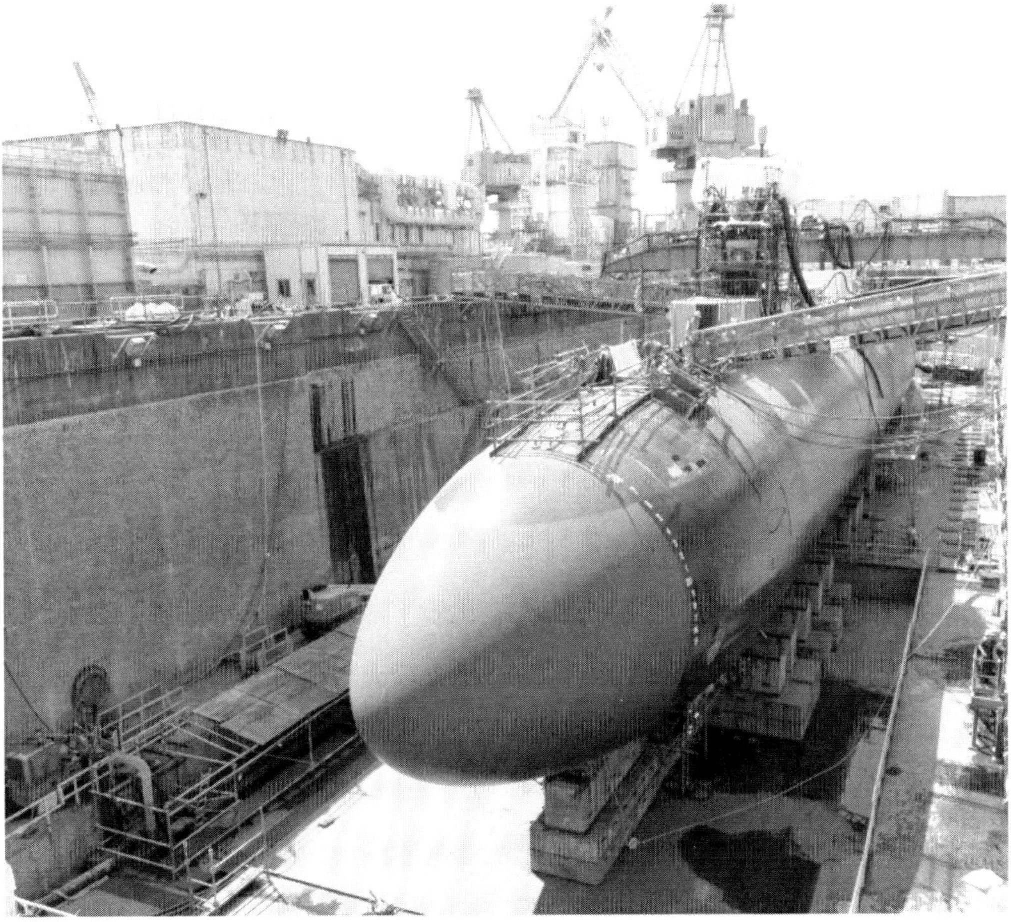

Source: U.S. Navy. | GAO-19-225T.

Figure 3. USS Albany Undergoing an Extended Maintenance Period at Norfolk Naval Shipyard.

Our prior work has shown that three primary factors at the naval shipyards contribute to maintenance delays:

- Poor conditions and aging equipment limit the ability of the shipyards to meet current and future demands. We reported in September 2017 that facility and equipment limitations at the shipyards contributed to maintenance delays for the aircraft carriers and submarines, hindering the shipyards' ability to support the Navy. Specifically, we found that the shipyards would be unable to support an estimated one-third of maintenance periods planned over the next 23 years.[12] We recommended that the Navy take steps to improve its management of shipyard investments; the Navy concurred with this recommendation and we are encouraged by its response.[13]

[12] This estimate did not factor in planned increases to the fleet that would make the shortfalls even greater.

[13] GAO, *Naval Shipyards: Actions Needed to Improve Poor Conditions that Affect Operations*, GAO-17-548 (Washington, D.C.: Sept. 12, 2017). Senate Report 115-130, accompanying a bill for the Military Construction, Veterans Affairs, and Related Agencies Appropriations 2018 and Senate Report 115-125, accompanying a bill for the National Defense Authorization Act for Fiscal Year 2018 directed the Secretary of

For example, the Navy has developed a plan for the optimal placement of facilities and major equipment at each public shipyard, which the Navy estimates can ultimately increase its maintenance efficiency by reducing personnel and materiel travel by an average of 65 percent. This equates to recovering about 328,000 man days per year—an amount roughly equal to that of an aircraft carrier maintenance period. However, the Navy's preliminary estimate —that this effort will require an estimated $21 billion and 20 years to address—is well beyond historical funding levels, and does not include some potentially significant costs (e.g., for utilities, roads, or environmental remediation).[14]

- Shipyard workforce gaps and inexperience are limiting factors. The Navy has reported a variety of workforce challenges at the Navy's four public shipyards such as hiring personnel in a timely manner and providing personnel with the training necessary to gain proficiency in critical skills.[15] The Navy has noted that some occupations require years of training before workers become proficient. According to Navy officials, a large portion of its workforce is inexperienced. For example, 45 percent of the Puget Sound and 30 percent of the Portsmouth Naval Shipyards' skilled workforce have fewer than 5 years of experience. According to DOD officials, workforce shortages and inexperience contribute to maintenance delays. For example, at Pearl Harbor Naval Shipyard, two submarines were delayed approximately 20 months, in part because of shortages in ship fitters and welders, among other skilled personnel. Most of DOD's depots, which include the naval shipyards, have taken actions to maintain critical skills through retention incentives, bonuses, and awards. We plan to issue a report examining DOD's depot skill gaps, including those at the naval shipyards, later this month.
- Depot supply support may not be cost-effective. In June 2016, we reported that the naval shipyards and other depots had not implemented actions that would likely improve the cost-effectiveness of their supply operations. Specifically, the Navy had not transferred certain functions to the Defense Logistics Agency (DLA) at the shipyards in the same manner as the Navy and Air Force did for their aviation depots.[16] The Navy and Air Force aviation depots that transferred these functions to

---

the Navy to submit a report providing an engineering master plan for the optimal placement of facilities and major equipment to support ship repair functions at each public shipyard, including an investment strategy to address the infrastructure requirements at each shipyard.

[14] Naval Sea Systems Command, *Report to Congress: Shipyard Infrastructure Optimization Plan, Report on the Navy's Strategic Plan for Addressing the Infrastructure Deficiencies at the Public Naval Shipyards* (Washington, D.C.: February 2018).

[15] The four public naval shipyards—Portsmouth Naval Shipyard, Norfolk Naval Shipyard, Puget Sound Naval Shipyard and Intermediate Maintenance Facility, and Pearl Harbor Naval Shipyard and Intermediate Maintenance Facility—provide depot-level maintenance, which the Navy describes as the most involved and time-consuming maintenance work (e.g., overhauls, alterations, refits, restorations, nuclear refueling, and deactivations). Two private shipyards—General Dynamics Electric Boat and Huntington Ingalls Industries-Newport News Shipbuilding—build the Navy's nuclear-powered ships and in some cases provide depot-level maintenance.

[16] The Navy's aviation depots are called Fleet Readiness Centers. The Navy operates three Fleet Readiness Centers at Cherry Point, North Carolina; Jacksonville, Florida; and North Island, California. The Air Force's aviation depots are referred to as Air Logistics Complexes and are located in Warner Robins, Georgia; Oklahoma City, Oklahoma; and Ogden, Utah.

DLA had reaped a number of efficiencies in their supply operations, including a 10-percent reduction in backorders over a 5-year period. We recommended that the Navy analyze whether such a transfer of functions is warranted at the shipyards and the Navy concurred with the recommendation.[17] However, as of October 2018, the Navy had not conducted a comprehensive analysis of transferring these functions and had provided no plans to do so.

Navy Processes for Determining Manning of Ships Do Not Account for All Ship Workload

In May 2017, we reported that the Navy's process for determining manpower requirements—the number and skill mix of sailors needed on the Navy's ships—did not fully account for all ship workload.[18] The Navy was using outdated standards to calculate the size of ship crews that may have been leading to overburdened crews working long hours. We recommended steps to help ensure the Navy's manpower requirements meet the needs of the existing and future surface fleet, and the Navy has been studying ship workload and revising its guidance. As of November 2018, the Navy was continuing to analyze the manpower requirements of its ship classes to better size and compose ship crews, and the Navy was also working to improve shipboard manning. However, these efforts are not yet complete and it is too early to assess their effectiveness. Until manpower requirements are reassessed across the fleet, the Navy risks that ship crews will continue to be undersized and sailors will be overworked with potential negative effects on readiness and safety.

Additionally, the Navy provided information in November 2018 that showed that it is taking steps to ensure that ships have a minimum percentage of crew assigned and with the appropriate skills. The Navy has prioritized manning its surface ships homeported overseas. The Navy established a minimum threshold of filling at least 95 percent of authorized billets in its ship crews with sailors (referred to as fill), with a minimum goal of 92 percent of those sailors having the right qualifications for the billet (known as fit). According to Navy officials, the Navy is for the most part meeting its fill goals Navy-wide, but has not consistently met its fit goals. However, during group discussions in November 2018 with ship crews and interviews with Navy officials in Japan, we learned that the Navy's methods for tracking fit and fill do not account for sailor experience and may be inaccurately capturing the actual presence of sailors onboard and available for duty on its ships. Moreover, sailors consistently told us that ship workload has not decreased, and it is still extremely challenging to complete all required workload while getting enough sleep. Navy officials told us that manning challenges will continue through at least fiscal year 2021 as the Navy increases its end strength and trains its new sailors to gain the proper mix of skills to operate and maintain the fleet.

[17] GAO, *Defense Inventory: Further Analysis and Enhanced Metrics Could Improve Service Supply and Depot Operations*, GAO-16-450 (Washington, D.C.: June 9, 2016).

[18] GAO, *Navy Force Structure: Actions Needed to Ensure Proper Size and Composition of Ship Crews*, GAO-17-413 (Washington, D.C.: May 18, 2017).

Navy Plans to Expand Its Fleet but Full Costs Are Unknown and Manning an Expanded Fleet Likely Will Be Challenging

To meet continued operational demands, the Navy is planning for the most significant fleet size increase in over 30 years. According to the Navy's fiscal year 2019 shipbuilding plan, the Navy plans to build and maintain a fleet of 355 battle force ships—an increase of about 25 percent above the Navy's current force of 287 ships.[19] To reach its goal, the Navy plans to buy 301 ships through 2048 and extend the service life of its 66 Arleigh Burke class destroyers and up to 7 attack submarines.[20] Together, the fiscal year 2019 shipbuilding plan and the service life extensions would allow the Navy to reach a 355-ship fleet by the 2030s.

Congressional Budget Office reporting and our past work have shown that the Navy has consistently and significantly underestimated the cost and timeframes for delivering new ships to the fleet. For example, the Navy estimates that buying the new ships specified in the fiscal year 2019 plan would cost $631 billion over 30 years while the Congressional Budget Office has estimated that those new ships would cost $801 billion—a difference of 27 percent.[21] We also reported in June 2018 that acquisition outcomes for ship classes built during the last 10 years have often not achieved cost, schedule, quality, or performance goals that were established.[22] Furthermore, we have reported that:

- all 8 of the lead ships delivered over the past decade that we reviewed were provided to the fleet behind schedule, and more than half of those ships were delayed by more than 2 years,[23] and
- six ships of different classes valued at $6.3 billion were delivered to the Navy with varying degrees of incomplete work and quality problems.[24]

As a result of past cost and schedule problems, our work has shown that the Navy has a less-capable and smaller fleet today than it planned over 10 years ago. The Navy has also received $24 billion more in funding than it originally planned in its 2007 long-range shipbuilding plan but has 50 fewer ships in its inventory today, as compared with the goals it first established. Therefore, we have reported that as the Navy moves forward in implementing its shipbuilding plan it will be paramount for the Navy to learn from and apply lessons learned from the past.

---

[19] Department of the Navy, *Report to Congress on the Annual Long-Range Plan for Construction of Naval Vessels for Fiscal Year 2019* (February 2018). This plan reflects the Navy's plan to meet its 2016 force structure assessment.

[20] Of the 301 ships, the Navy plans to purchase 245 combat ships and 56 combat logistics and support ships.

[21] Congressional Budget Office, *An Analysis of the Navy's Fiscal Year 2019 Shipbuilding Plan* (Washington, D.C.: October 2018). CBO's estimates are higher than the Navy's because CBO and the Navy made different assumptions about the design and capabilities of some future ships, used different estimating methods, and treated growth in shipbuilding labor and materials costs differently.

[22] GAO, *Navy Shipbuilding: Past Performance Provides Valuable Lessons for Future Investments,* GAO-18-238SP (Washington, D.C.: June 2018).

[23] GAO-18-238SP.

[24] GAO, *Navy Shipbuilding: Policy Changes Needed to Improve the Post-Delivery Process and Ship Quality*, GAO-17-418 (Washington, D.C.: July 13, 2017). According to Navy officials, incomplete work and quality problems in acquisition programs shifts repair costs from the shipbuilding accounts to the fleet's operations and maintenance accounts and contributes to a maintenance backlog from the first day the fleet is responsible for the ship.

In addition to the cost of buying the ships and submarines to expand fleet size, the Navy will likely face affordability challenges with regard to the manning of an expanded fleet with the right number of sailors with the right mix of skills. In May 2017, we reported that the personnel costs for surface ship classes in fiscal years 2000-2015 were the largest share of total operating and support costs and that careful planning will be needed as new ships are brought into the fleet.[25] We also reported that crew sizes on recently inducted ship classes grew from original projections as the Navy gained experience operating them. For example, the total crew size of Littoral Combat Ships has grown from 75 in 2003 to 98 personnel in 2016, a 31-percent increase. Navy officials told us that they plan to better articulate the personnel and resources needed for a larger fleet after fully accounting for workload and right-sizing ship crews. The Navy's end strength has since increased by over 11,000 personnel from fiscal year 2017 levels, which should help alleviate manning challenges as the fleet grows. In November 2018, officials from Fleet Forces Command provided us with projections of its manning shortfalls continuing through at least fiscal year 2021 and steps it was planning to take to mitigate them.

NAVY AND MARINE CORPS AGING AIRCRAFT AND F-35S FACE MAINTENANCE AND SUPPLY CHALLENGES THAT AFFECT READINESS REBUILDING NOW AND IN THE FUTURE

Our work has shown that Navy and Marine Corps aircraft availability has been limited by aging aircraft, delayed maintenance, and insufficient supply support. Pilot and maintenance personnel shortfalls further limit readiness recovery across legacy air platforms. The growing F-35 program, which is meant to replace many aging aircraft, has presented additional operational and sustainment challenges, which will likely persist into the future if not corrected. DOD, the Navy, and the Marine Corps have emphasized mission capability of critical aviation platforms— including the Navy and Marine Corps F/A-18s and F-35s—and are taking steps to improve availability, but these efforts will take time to realize results.

Aircraft Availability Has Been Limited by Aging Fleets with Maintenance and Supply Challenges

Navy and Marine Corps aircraft availability has been limited by challenges associated with aging aircraft fleets, depot maintenance, and supply support challenges that limit the services' ability to keep aviation units ready.[26] The Navy and Marine Corps spend billions of dollars each year on sustainment, such as for spare parts and depot maintenance, to meet aircraft availability goals.[27] However, aircraft availability rates have generally declined since

[25] GAO-17-413. According to DOD, operating and support costs—which include personnel and maintenance costs—have traditionally constituted about 70 percent of a ship's total life-cycle costs.

[26] GAO, *Weapon System Sustainment: Selected Air Force and Navy Aircraft Generally Have Not Met Availability Goals, and DOD and Navy Guidance Need to Be Clarified*, GAO-18-678 (Washington, D.C.: Sept. 10, 2018).

[27] Based on our analysis of the operating and support (O&S) costs in fiscal years 2011- 2016, maintenance cost generally is one of the largest portions—about 42 percent—of total O&S costs for the seven aircraft we reviewed. GAO-18-678.

fiscal year 2011. While specific aircraft availability data are considered sensitive by the Navy and the Marine Corps, and cannot be discussed in detail, we found in September 2018 that the Navy and the Marine Corps generally did not meet aircraft availability goals in fiscal years 2011-2016 for the seven aircraft we reviewed. In updating data in November 2018, we found that none of the aircraft met aircraft availability goals for fiscal years 2017 and 2018.

According to the Navy, the pace of operations has increased wear and tear on its aircraft and decreased the time available for maintenance and modernization—a necessity for an aging fleet. For example, the average age of a legacy F/A-18A-D Hornet is 26 years, of an AV-8B Harrier is 21 years, and of the C-2A Greyhound is 29 years. Both services expect these aircraft will continue to be used for the foreseeable future and in some cases into the 2030s.[28]

The Navy and the Marine Corps face delays in the arrival of the F-35 to replace their legacy F/A-18A-D Hornets and AV-8B Harriers.[29] To compensate for the delay, the Navy and the Marine Corps are planning to procure additional aircraft, such as the F/A-18E-F Super Hornet, and extend the service life and upgrade the capabilities of their legacy aircraft. However, these efforts and the sustainment of the Navy and Marine Corps legacy aircraft fleet face key challenges as shown in Figure 4.

Aircraft	Aging aircraft		Maintenance		Supply support	
	Delays in acquiring replacement aircraft	Unexpected replacement of parts and repairs	Delays in depot maintenance	Shortage of depot maintainer personnel	Parts obsolescence[a]	Diminishing manufacturing source[b]
AV-8B	✓	✓	✓	✓	✓	✓
C-2A		✓	✓	✓	✓	✓
E-2C		✓	✓	✓	✓	✓
E-2D			✓	✓	✓	✓
EA-18 G			✓	✓		✓
F/A-18 A-D	✓	✓	✓	✓	✓	✓
F/A-18 E-F		✓	✓	✓		✓

Source: GAO analysis of Navy data. | GAO-19-225T.

[a]Obsolescence is a lack of availability of a part due to its lack of usefulness or it is no longer current or available for production.

[b]Diminishing manufacturing source is a loss or impending loss of manufacturers or suppliers of items.

Figure 4. Sustainment Challenges Affecting Selected Navy and Marine Corps Aircraft.

Specifically, our prior work has shown that the Navy and the Marine Corps are confronted with two sets of challenges in sustaining their aircraft:

- Depot maintenance complexities for aging aircraft and spare parts availability. Depot maintenance on aging weapon systems, including Navy and Marine Corps aircraft, becomes less predictable as structural fatigue occurs and parts that were not expected

[28] GAO-18-678.

[29] GAO-18-678.

to be replaced begin to wear out.[30] While the Navy and the Marine Corps reported that sustainment funding accounts, such as those for depot maintenance and spare parts, have been funded at increased levels in fiscal years 2017 and 2018, efforts to improve spare parts availability take time to produce results due to long lead times for acquiring some items. In addition, Navy and Marine Corps aircraft face challenges associated with diminishing manufacturing sources and parts obsolescence. DOD has a program intended to manage these risks, but we reported in September 2017 that its implementation varied across DOD weapon system program offices.[31] We made recommendations to improve the program's management; DOD concurred and has initiated improvement efforts.

- Maintenance personnel inexperience and retention. The Navy has had difficulty attracting and retaining skilled maintainers, such as sheet metal workers and machinists at its aviation depots (i.e., Fleet Readiness Centers), which directly affects its ability to complete planned maintenance. Some of the depots experienced challenges attracting and retaining skilled personnel due to competition with nearby contractors that are able to offer higher pay, according to Navy depot officials. Similar to the shipyards, the aviation depots also lack experienced personnel, affecting the efficiency and quality of maintenance. For example, 41 percent of the skilled workers at Fleet Readiness Center Southwest have 2 years or fewer of experience. Workforce inexperience and attrition of skilled personnel were some of the reasons cited for machining defects detected in the landing gear for F/A-18, E-2, and C-2A aircraft by a recent Navy report.[32] All of the depots have undertaken retention efforts such as incentives, bonuses, and awards to address these issues.

Until the Navy and Marine Corps address maintenance and supply challenges it will be difficult to meet Secretary of Defense-established mission capability goals. Specifically, in September 2018, the Secretary of Defense issued a memorandum emphasizing that a key component of implementing the 2018 National Defense Strategy is ensuring critical aviation platforms meet their mission capability targets by the end of fiscal year 2019. The memorandum established a goal of achieving a minimum of 80-percent mission capable rates for various aircraft, including for the Navy's and Marine Corps' F/A-18 inventories, by the end of fiscal year 2019 while also reducing operating and maintenance costs. To accomplish this, the Navy and the Marine Corps developed the Return to Readiness strategy in November 2018 that includes a broad array of actions to improve the availability of spare parts and evaluate the application of best commercial practices to naval aviation sustainment, among other actions. Office of the Secretary of Defense and Navy program officials told us, and based on our prior work we agree, that this goal will be challenging to achieve by the end of fiscal year 2019.

---

[30] For additional information on this issue, see GAO, *Defense Inventory: Further Analysis and Enhanced Metrics Could Improve Service Supply and Depot Operations*, GAO-16-450 (Washington, D.C.: June 9, 2016).

[31] The Diminishing Manufacturing Sources and Material Shortages program is meant to address parts supply challenges. GAO, *Defense Supply Chain: DOD Needs Complete Information on Single Sources of Supply to Proactively Manage the Risks*, GAO-17-768 (Washington, D.C.: Sept. 28, 2017).

[32] Commander, *Fleet Readiness Centers: Fleet Readiness Southwest Landing and Arresting Gear Quality Escape Investigation Report*, May 11, 2017.

Pilot Shortages Have Worsened in Recent Years and Are Projected to Remain through 2023

We reported in April 2018 that fighter pilot shortages in the Navy and the Marine Corps have been worsening in recent years and shortfalls are projected to remain through at least fiscal year 2023.[33] Our analysis of Navy and Marine Corps data showed that the Navy's shortage of first operational tour fighter pilots more than doubled from 12 percent in fiscal year 2013 to 26 percent in fiscal year 2017.[34] Similarly, the Marine Corps' overall shortage of fighter pilots quadrupled from 6 percent in fiscal year 2006 to 24 percent in fiscal year 2017.

Also, as we reported in April 2018, service officials attributed the pilot shortages to reduced training opportunities and increased attrition due to career dissatisfaction, among other factors. Officials from both services stated at the time that they have ensured that deploying squadrons have been fully staffed with fighter pilots by using various approaches including using senior pilots to staff junior positions and having pilots deploy more frequently and for longer periods. However, we reported that squadron leaders and fighter pilots said that these approaches had a negative impact on the fighter pilot training and retention and ultimately may be exacerbating the situation.

Further compounding their pilot shortages, we also found that the services have not recently reevaluated squadron requirements to reflect an increased fighter pilot workload. As a result, the reported shortage actually could be greater. The services were taking actions, including increasing retention incentives for fighter pilots. To help determine the magnitude of the shortages and help target strategies to better meet their personnel needs, we recommended, and the Navy and Marine Corps agreed, to reevaluate fighter pilot squadron requirements.

New F-35 Aircraft Facing Sustainment and Operational Challenges

Sustainment challenges are not just an issue for older aircraft, but represent an enduring challenge for the F-35 Lightning II aircraft—a key component to the future of tactical aviation for the Navy and Marine Corps. The Navy and Marine Corps are both flying F-35s now as the program ramps up development, and they plan to procure nearly 700 aircraft over the coming decades. The sustainment costs of the F-35 fleet are projected to exceed $1 trillion over its 60-year life cycle. In October 2017, we reported that:

- F-35B aircraft (including Marine Corps aircraft) were *available* (i.e., the aircraft were safe to fly, available for use, and able to perform at least one tasked mission) about 52 percent of the time from March 2017 through June 2017, which fell short of the 65-percent goal established by the Marine Corps for non-deployed units and
- F-35B aircraft (including Marine Corps aircraft) were *fully mission capable* (i.e., the aircraft were capable of accomplishing all tasked missions) about 15 percent of the

[33] GAO, *Military Personnel: DOD Needs to Reevaluate Fighter Pilot Workforce Requirements,* GAO-18-113 (Washington, D.C.: Apr. 11, 2018).

[34] A fighter pilot's first operational tour at sea is completed between 3 and 6 years of service.

time from March 2017 through June 2017, which fell short of the 60-percent goal established by the Marine Corps for non-deployed units.[35]

We also reported on numerous sustainment challenges leading to less than desirable outcomes for F-35 warfighter readiness. For example, F-35 aircraft were unable to fly 22 percent of the time because of parts shortages from January 2017 through August 7, 2017. Additionally, DOD's capabilities to repair F-35 parts at military depots were 6 years behind schedule, which resulted in average part repair times that are twice that of the program's objective.

As DOD gains experience with the F-35, our work has shown that the department has encountered additional challenges. In 2017, the Marine Corps became the first military service to station F-35 aircraft overseas, transferring aircraft to Iwakuni, Japan. While in the Pacific, DOD expects to disperse its F-35s into smaller detachments to outmaneuver the enemy and counter regional threats. However, in April 2018, we reported that this approach posed logistics and supply challenges.[36] In June 2018, we reported that the F-35 program had not improved its reliability and maintainability over the past year and continued to fall short on half of its performance targets.[37] Furthermore, we found that the program may not meet its required targets before each variant of the F-35 is expected to demonstrate maturity—the point at which the aircraft has flown enough hours to predictably determine reliability and maintainability over its lifespan. This means that the Navy and the Marine Corps may have to decide whether they are willing to accept less reliable and maintainable aircraft than originally planned. Among other outcomes, this could result in higher maintenance costs and lower aircraft availability than anticipated which also could pose readiness challenges in the future. As we reported in October 2017, the poor reliability of certain parts is already contributing to shortages of F-35 spare parts.[38]

Challenges posed by the F-35 program are largely the result of sustainment plans that do not fully include or consider key requirements. Our work has shown that planning for sustainment and aligning its funding are critical if DOD wants to meet its aircraft availability goals and effectively deploy to support operations. To address the challenges associated with F-35 sustainment and operational deployment, we recommended that DOD revise its sustainment plans, align associated funding, and mitigate the risks associated with key supply chain-related challenges for deployed F-35s in the Pacific, among others.[39] DOD concurred with these recommendations and stated that it is taking steps to address them. Furthermore, as previously discussed, the Secretary of Defense has established an 80-percent mission capability goal for critical aviation assets, including the F-35. Due to current low availability and numerous sustainment issues, the F-35 fleet will be challenged in meeting the goal.

---

[35] GAO, *F-35 Aircraft Sustainment: DOD Needs to Address Challenges Affecting Readiness and Cost Transparency*, GAO-18-75 (Washington, D.C.: Oct. 26, 2017). At the time of our October 2017 report, the information presented here, including aircraft availability and mission capability rates, and the goals for those metrics, were not considered sensitive by the department. The Navy considers the current rates and goals to be sensitive.

[36] GAO, *Warfighter Support: DOD Needs to Share F-35 Operational Lessons Across the Military Services*, GAO-18-464R (Washington, D.C.: Apr. 25, 2018). This was a public version of a more detailed March 2018 classified report.

[37] GAO, *F-35 Joint Strike Fighter: Development Is Nearly Complete, but Deficiencies Found in Testing Need to Be Resolved*, GAO-18-321 (Washington, D.C.: June 5, 2018).

[38] GAO-18-75.

[39] GAO-18-75 and GAO-18-464R.

In sum, the Navy's and Marine Corps' significant readiness challenges have developed over more than a decade of conflict, budget uncertainty, and reductions in force structure. Both services have made encouraging progress identifying the causes of their readiness decline and have begun efforts to arrest and reverse it; however, our prior work shows that fully addressing the persistent readiness challenges will require years of sustained management attention. Our work cited today contains 25 specific recommendations to the Navy and the Marine Corps and an additional 20 recommendations to various other DOD components to assist these services in rebuilding the readiness of their forces and in modernizing for the future. Attention to these recommendations can assist the Navy and the Marine Corps as they seek to rebuild the readiness of their forces.

Chairmen Wicker and Sullivan, Ranking Members Hirono and Kaine, and Members of the Subcommittees, this concludes my prepared statement. I would be pleased to respond to any questions you may have at this time.

Appendix I: Implementation Status of Prior GAO Recommendations Related to Navy and Marine Corps Readiness

Over the past 4 years, we have issued a number of reports related to Navy and Marine Corps readiness and we used them to develop this statement. Table 1 summarizes the recommendations in these reports.[40] The Department of Defense (DOD) concurred with most of the 45 recommendations and has many actions underway. However, DOD has not fully implemented any of the recommendations to date. For each of the reports, the specific recommendations and any progress made in implementing them are summarized in Tables 2 through 16.

Table 1. Recommendations That GAO Has Made Since 2015 on Navy and Marine Corps Readiness Cited in This chapter

Product date	Product title and number	Number of open recommendations
Recommendations to Navy and Marine Corps		
November 19, 2018	*Navy Readiness: Actions Needed to Address Costly Maintenance Delays Facing the Attack Submarine Fleet* (GAO-19-229)	1[a]
September 10, 2018	*Weapon System Sustainment: Selected Air Force and Navy Aircraft Generally Have Not Met Availability Goals, and DOD and Navy Guidance Need to Be Clarified* (GAO-18-678)	1[b]
April 11, 2018	*Military Personnel: DOD Needs to Reevaluate Fighter Pilot Workforce Requirements* (GAO-18-113)	2[c]
March 28, 2018	*Military Aircraft: F-35 Brings Increased Capabilities, but the Marine Corps Needs to Assess Challenges Associated with Operating in the Pacific* (GAO-18-79C)	2[d]
September 26, 2017	*Navy and Marine Corps Training: Further Planning Needed for Amphibious Operations Training* (GAO-17-789)	3
September 12, 2017	*Naval Shipyards: Actions Needed to Improve Poor Conditions That Affect Operations* (GAO-17-548)	3

[40] This summary does not include classified recommendations made in classified reports, reports without recommendations, and reports in which we directed recommendations exclusively to the Office of the Secretary of Defense or the Department of the Air Force.

Product date	Product title and number	Number of open recommendations
July 13, 2017	*Navy Shipbuilding: Policy Changes Needed to Improve the Post-Delivery Process and Ship Quality* (GAO-17-418)	4
May 18, 2017	*Navy Force Structure: Actions Needed to Ensure Proper Size and Composition of Ship Crews* (GAO-17-413)	4
September 7, 2016	*Military Readiness: DOD's Readiness Rebuilding Efforts May Be at Risk without a Comprehensive Plan* (GAO-16-841)	3[e]
May 29, 2015	*Navy Force Structure: Sustainable Plan and Comprehensive Assessment Needed to Mitigate Long-Term Risks to Ships Assigned to Overseas Homeports* (GAO-15-329)	2
Subtotal		25
Recommendations to DOD components in coordination with Navy and Marine Corps		
June 5, 2018	*F-35 Joint Strike Fighter: Development Is Nearly Complete, but Deficiencies Found in Testing Need to Be Resolved* (GAO-18-321)	2
April 25, 2018	*Warfighter Support: DOD Needs to Share F-35 Operational Lessons Across the Military Services* (GAO-18-464R)	2[f]
October 26, 2017	*F-35 Aircraft Sustainment: DOD Needs to Address Challenges Affecting Readiness and Cost Transparency* (GAO-18-75)	4
September 28, 2017	*Defense Supply Chain: DOD Needs Complete Information on Single Sources of Supply to Proactively Manage the Risks* (GAO-17-768)	6
June 9, 2016	*Defense Inventory: Further Analysis and Enhanced Metrics Could Improve Service Supply and Depot Operations* (GAO-16-450)	6
Subtotal		20
Total		45

Source: GAO analysis.| GAO-19-225T.

Note: This table does not include classified recommendations made in classified reports, reports without recommendations, and reports in which we directed recommendations exclusively to the Office of the Secretary of Defense or the Department of the Air Force.

[a]GAO-19-229 is an unclassified version of a GAO-19-192C that included three additional classified recommendations to Navy leadership, that are not counted here.

[b]GAO-18-678 included a recommendation directed to the Office of the Secretary of Defense, that is not counted here.

[c]GAO-18-113 included a recommendation directed to the Secretary of the Air Force, that is not counted here.

[d]GAO-18-79C is a classified report that included four recommendations, all of which were deemed unclassified by DOD. Two recommendations were directed to the Commandant of the Marine Corps and are included here. The other two recommendations were directed to the F-35 Program Executive Officer and are included in GAO-18-464R.

[e]GAO-16-841 included two recommendations directed to the Office of the Secretary of Defense, and are not counted here.

[f]GAO-18-464R is an unclassified version of GAO-18-79C. Two recommendations were directed to the F-35 program office and are included here. The other two recommendations were directed to the Commandant of the Marine Corps and are included in GAO-18-79C.

Table 2. Status of Recommendations from Navy Readiness: Actions Needed to Address Costly Maintenance Delays Facing the Attack Submarine Fleet (GAO-19-229)

Recommendation #1:	
The Secretary of the Navy should ensure that the Chief of Naval Operations conducts a business case analysis to inform maintenance workload allocation across public and private shipyards; this analysis should include an assessment of private shipyard capacity to perform attack submarine maintenance, and should incorporate a complete accounting of both (a) the costs and risks associated with attack submarines sitting idle and (b) the qualitative benefits associated with having the potential to both mitigate risk in new submarine construction and provide additional availability to the combatant commanders.	**Status:** Open **Concurrence:** Yes **Comments:** In response to our report, DOD stated that it has taken the first steps to take a more holistic view of submarine maintenance requirements and impacts across both the public and private shipyards. In an update provided in November 2018, the Navy told us that they are developing a contracting strategy to conduct two additional depot maintenance periods at private shipyards in the future.

Source: GAO analysis. | GAO-19-225T.

Note: This table does not include three recommendations directed to Navy leadership that were deemed classified by DOD.

Table 3. Status of Recommendations from Weapon System Sustainment: Selected Air Force and Navy Aircraft Generally Have Not Met Availability Goals, and DOD and Navy Guidance Need to Be Clarified (GAO-18-678)

Recommendation #1:	
The Secretary of the Navy should update or issue new guidance clarifying the requirements for documenting sustainment strategies for legacy weapon systems, including for fixed-wing aircraft.	**Status:** Open **Concurrence:** Yes **Comments:** We will monitor DOD's efforts to address this recommendation.

Source: GAO analysis. | GAO-19-225T.
Note: This table does not include a recommendation that was directed to the Office of the Secretary of Defense.

Table 4. Status of Recommendations from Military Personnel: DOD Needs to Reevaluate Fighter Pilot Workforce Requirements (GAO-18-113)

Recommendation #1:	
The Secretary of the Navy should ensure that the Chief of Naval Operations reevaluate fighter pilot squadron requirements, to include updating current assumptions of fighter pilot workload and assessing the impact of future incorporation of Unmanned Aerial Systems platforms into combat aviation.	**Status:** Open **Concurrence:** Yes **Comments:** DOD noted that across the Navy, many organizations and offices including the resource sponsor (Naval Air Forces) will play integral roles in determining the future size and mix of manpower requirements for fighter pilot squadrons. We will continue to monitor DOD actions taken to address this recommendation.
Recommendation #2:	
The Secretary of the Navy should ensure that the Commandant of the Marine Corps and the Deputy Commandant for Aviation reevaluate fighter pilot squadron requirements.	**Status:** Open **Concurrence:** Yes **Comments:** DOD noted that across the Marine Corps, many organizations and offices in addition to the Deputy Commandant for Aviation play integral roles in the continuous evaluation and determination regarding current and future size and mix of manpower requirements for fighter and attack squadrons. We will continue to monitor DOD actions taken to address this recommendation.

Source: GAO analysis. | GAO-19-225T.
Note: This table does not include a recommendation that was directed to the Secretary of the Air Force.

Table 5. Status of Recommendations from Military Aircraft: F-35 Brings Increased Capabilities, but the Marine Corps Needs to Assess Challenges Associated with Operating in the Pacific (GAO-18-79C)

Recommendation #1:	
The Commandant of the Marine Corps should assess the risks associated with key supply chain-related challenges related to operating and sustaining the F-35 in the Pacific, and determine how to mitigate these risks.	**Status:** Open **Concurrence:** Yes **Comments:** According to DOD officials, as of July 2018, the Marine Corps was engaging in a number of risk mitigation efforts for key supply-chain-related challenges related to operating and sustaining the F-35 in the Pacific, working with key stakeholders, including the Joint Program Office, industry, and entities such as the Defense Logistics Agency and the U.S. Transportation Command. Current risk mitigation efforts already underway include a strategy to ensure that spare parts with a delivery time of greater than 2 years are placed on contract, as are plans to increase local repair capability to capitalize on resident skill already possessed by the local Marine Aviation Logistics Squadron. Other risk mitigation

Recommendation #1:	
	efforts currently under consideration include material lay-in investments to improve supplier capacity and performance, and assessment of the delivery times for off-station repair parts to mitigate future risks. The Marine Corps continues to assess supply-chain-related challenges in the Pacific and will continue to develop risk mitigation strategies in response to those challenges. We are encouraged by the Marine Corps' focus on the potential risks associated with key supply-chain- related challenges in the Pacific. However, until these assessments are complete and the Marine Corps has determined how to mitigate these risks, this recommendation will remain open.
Recommendation #2:	
The Commandant of the Marine Corps should determine the F-35's ability to support distributed operations through the use of exercises and/or analyses.	**Status:** Open **Concurrence:** Yes **Comments:** According to DOD officials, as of July 2018, the Marine Corps continued to assess the F-35's ability to support distributed operations through the Marine Corps' Training and Exercise Employment Plan in preparation for real world operations. These exercises include land-based and shipboard operations. The Marine Corps has also established Deployment Transfer Locations throughout the Pacific in order to support distributed operations. We are encouraged by the Marine Corps' continued focus on the F-35's ability to support distributed operations in the Pacific. However, until the Marine Corps determines its ability to support distributed operations through exercises and/or analyses, this recommendation will remain open.

Source: GAO analysis. | GAO-19-225T.

Note: This report is classified and included four recommendations, all of which were deemed unclassified by DOD. Two recommendations were directed to the Commandant of the Marine Corps and are included here. The other two recommendations were directed to the F-35 Program Executive Officer and are included in Table 13, which summarizes GAO-18-464R.

Table 6. Status of Recommendations from Navy and Marine Corps Training: Further Planning Needed for Amphibious Operations Training (GAO-17-789)

Recommendation #1:	
The Secretary of the Navy, in coordination with the Chief of Naval Operations and the Commandant of the Marine Corps, should develop an approach, such as building upon the Amphibious Operations Training Requirements review, to prioritize available training resources, systematically evaluate among training resource alternatives to achieve amphibious operations priorities, and monitor progress toward achieving them.	**Status:** Open **Concurrence:** Yes **Comments:** Marine Corps officials told us that as of August 2018, the Marine Corps has ongoing actions intended to address this recommendation. For example, the Marine Corps is developing an annual requirements order detailing the naval ship services required to execute amphibious operations training. Once issued, the order will be used to schedule naval ship training support to optimize amphibious training opportunities and to identify joint- and service-level exercises that may provide venues and resources for amphibious operations training. These officials stated that the Navy and Marine Corps are also developing joint amphibious training plans to support Marine Corps amphibious readiness standards. Completion of these actions should allow the Navy and Marine Corps to better mitigate amphibious operations training shortfalls.
Recommendation #2:	
The Secretary of the Navy, in coordination with the Chief of Naval Operations and the Commandant of the Marine Corps, should clarify the organizations responsible and time frames to define and articulate common	**Status:** Open **Concurrence:** Yes **Comments:** As of August 2018, the Department of the Navy had identified ongoing actions intended to address this recommendation. Specifically, the Navy is developing a joint Navy and Marine Corps

Table 6. (Continued)

Recommendation #2:	
outcomes for naval integration and use those outcomes to (1) develop a joint strategy; (2) more fully establish compatible policies, procedures, and systems; (3) better leverage training resources; and (4) establish mechanisms to monitor results.	strategy for naval integration with common outcomes. Additionally, the Navy is studying the feasibility of developing compatible Navy and Marine Corps scheduling systems to address amphibious training requirements. Completion of these actions should help align Navy and Marine Corps efforts to maximize training opportunities for amphibious operations.
Recommendation #3:	
The Commandant of the Marine Corps should develop guidance for the development and use of virtual training devices that includes (1) developing requirements for virtual training devices that consider and document training tasks and objectives, required proficiency, and available training time; (2) setting target usage rates and collecting usage data; and (3) conducting effectiveness analysis of virtual training devices that defines a consistent process for performing the analysis, including the selection of the devices to be evaluated, guidelines on conducting the analysis, and the data that should be collected and assessed.	**Status:** Open **Concurrence:** Yes **Comments:** As of August 2018, the Marine Corps had completed some actions intended to address the recommendation, and had additional actions ongoing. For example, in June 2017 the Marine Corps issued the Marine Corps Ground Training Simulations Implementation Plan. The plan provides a framework for the Marine Corps' use of current and future simulations technology and virtual training environments to align training efforts and resource requirements. According to Marine Corps officials, as part of the implementation plan, the Marine Corps is also developing an analysis of alternatives to inform its virtual training developmental efforts that considers training tasks, required proficiency, and available training time. Additionally, Marine Corps officials told us they are implementing the Ground Simulation Training Effectiveness Program, which provides guidelines on conducting effectiveness analysis, including selecting the devices to be evaluated and identifying the data that should be collected and assessed. Once fully implemented, these actions should help the Marine Corps more effectively and efficiently integrate virtual training devices into operational training.

Source: GAO analysis. | GAO-19-225T.

Table 7. Status of Recommendations from Naval Shipyards: Actions Needed to Improve Poor Conditions That Affect Operations (GAO-17-548)

Recommendation #1:	
The Secretary of the Navy should develop a comprehensive plan for shipyard capital investment that establishes (1) the desired goal for the shipyards' condition and capabilities; (2) an estimate of the full costs to implement the plan, addressing all relevant requirements, external risk factors, and associated planning costs; and (3) metrics for assessing progress toward meeting the goal that include measuring the effectiveness of capital investments.	**Status:** Open **Concurrence:** Yes **Comments:** As of October 2018, Naval Sea Systems Command had produced a Shipyard Optimization Report, a plan intended to guide the overhaul and improvement of the naval shipyards, which the Navy presented to Congress in February 2018. However, the plan did not include metrics for assessing progress. Navy officials have stated that the Navy intends to develop metrics to meet this element, but that this development will take place during a second phase that will be complete in fiscal year 2019.
Recommendation #2:	
The Secretary of the Navy should conduct regular management reviews that include all relevant stakeholders to oversee implementation of the plan; review metrics; assess the progress made toward the goal; and make adjustments, as necessary, to ensure that the goal is attained.	**Status:** Open **Concurrence:** Yes **Comments:** In June 2018, the Navy issued NAVSEA Notice 5450, which established a new program management office responsible for planning, developing, scheduling, budgeting, and sustaining the replacement of shipyard facilities and equipment. By creating this office, the Navy has taken a first step toward establishing a result-oriented management approach, but

Recommendation #2:	
	additional steps, such as identifying all relevant stakeholders, holding meetings, and reviewing oversight metrics are needed to fully address this recommendation.
Recommendation #3:	
The Secretary of the Navy should provide regular reporting to key decision makers and Congress on the progress the shipyards are making to meet the goal of the comprehensive plan, along with any challenges that hinder that progress, such as cost. This may include reporting on progress to reduce their facilities restoration and modernization backlogs, improve the condition and configuration of the shipyards, and recapitalize capital equipment.	**Status:** Open **Concurrence:** Yes **Comments:** DOD officials stated in October 2018 that the Naval Sea Systems Command's Shipyard Optimization Report, along with the creation of the Readiness Reform Oversight Council, address this recommendation. While the Readiness Reform Oversight Council does appear to involve some of the key stakeholders who should be receiving the regular reporting we recommended, regular reporting on progress cannot be achieved with only a single disclosure at the beginning of the effort. While it is possible that the newly created Shipyard Program Management Office will be able to provide such reporting, that organization is still being developed. We will continue to monitor DOD actions taken to address this recommendation.

Source: GAO analysis. | GAO-19-225T.

Table 8. Status of Recommendations from Navy Shipbuilding: Policy Changes Needed to Improve the Post-Delivery Process and Ship Quality (GAO-17-418)

Recommendation #1:	
The Secretary of the Navy should revise the Navy's ship delivery policy to clarify what types of deficiencies need to be corrected and what mission capability (including the levels of quality and capability) must be achieved at (1) delivery and (2) when the ship is provided to the fleet (at the obligation work limiting date). In doing so, the Navy should clearly define what constitutes a complete ship and when that should be achieved.	**Status:** Open **Concurrence:** No **Comments:** Navy acquisition officials confirmed that the ship delivery policy, OPNAVINST 4700.8K, is the primary policy governing the delivery and post-delivery process for ships. Additionally, we reviewed the other policies identified by DOD during the course of our audit and found that they were not focused on construction and the post-delivery period, and did not provide guidance on the level of quality and completeness expected when ships are provided to the fleet. As such, we maintain that the Navy's ship delivery policy is a key instruction for ensuring that complete, mission-capable ships are provided to the fleet. In line with our finding that the Navy's ship delivery policy has not ensured complete and mission-capable ships are being delivered to the fleet, Congress included a provision in the John S. McCain National Defense Authorization Act for Fiscal Year 2019 that stipulated that the Navy could no longer count ships toward its battle force at commissioning, which occurs shortly after delivery, and instead may only count ships in the battle force once they were both commissioned and capable of contributing to the Navy's missions. In continuing to not acknowledge the importance of its ship delivery policy and taking steps to clarify it, the Navy is missing important opportunities to improve the completeness and capability of its ships and remains at risk of providing ships to the fleet with significant quality problems. To fully implement this recommendation, the Navy should revise its ship delivery policy to clearly define what constitutes a complete and defect-free ship and by when that should be achieved.

Table 8. (Continued)

Recommendation #2:	
The Secretary of the Navy should reconcile policy with practice to support the Navy Board of Inspection and Survey's role in making a recommendation for fleet introduction. Accomplishing this may require a study of the current timing of ship trials, and the costs and benefits associated with adding a Navy Board of Inspection and Survey assessment prior to providing ships to the fleet.	**Status:** Open **Concurrence:** No **Comments:** DOD noted that the current timing of Navy Board of Inspection and Survey trials provides the Navy with an opportunity to ensure contractual obligations have been met and identify construction deficiencies for correction during the post-delivery period. DOD also stated that adding another Navy Board of Inspection and Survey trial at the end of the post-delivery period would not be cost-effective and could delay ship deployment schedules. However, we found that most of the significant construction deficiencies identified prior to delivery were not corrected until the post-delivery period, and that the Navy Board of Inspection and Survey generally did not have an opportunity to inspect these corrections before ships were provided to the fleet. Given this, we maintain that the Navy should re-assess the timing of its post-delivery trials in support of the Navy Board of Inspection and Survey's responsibility to make recommendations for fleet introduction. Until this occurs, the Navy will continue to be at risk of providing ships to the fleet with significant deficiencies.
Recommendation #3:	
The Secretary of the Navy should reflect additional ship milestones in Selected Acquisition Reports to Congress, including obligation work limiting dates and readiness to deploy.	**Status:** Open **Concurrence:** Partial **Comments:** DOD agreed to report obligation work limiting dates in its Selected Acquisition Reports to Congress and is in the process of making this change. DOD plans include obligation work limiting dates in the Navy's 2018 Selected Acquisition Reports and to fully implement this change by March 2019. However, DOD did not agree to report ready-to-deploy dates in the Selected Acquisition Reports to Congress, noting that operational factors outside of acquisition concerns can affect the timing of this milestone. While we agree that readiness to deploy is a fleet determination, we continue to believe that this date is important for congressional oversight, as it remains the best milestone for determining when a ship has achieved a sufficient level of completeness to operate under the Navy's current framework for ship delivery.
Recommendation #4:	
The Secretary of the Navy should, in Selected Acquisition Reports to Congress, ensure that the criteria used to declare initial operational capability aligns with DOD guidance, and reflect the definition of this milestone in the reports.	**Status:** Open **Concurrence:** Yes **Comments:** For shipbuilding programs that have not yet achieved initial operational capability, the Navy will include the initial operational capability definition in its 2018 Selected Acquisition Reports to Congress. DOD is in the process of making this change and plans to complete the effort by March 2019. However, to fully meet the intent of this recommendation, DOD should report the initial operational capability definition for all shipbuilding programs, not just those that have yet to reach this milestone. The department also needs to ensure that the criteria used to declare initial operational capability align with DOD guidance. Taking these additional steps would result in more meaningful and consistent information being provided to Congress.

Source: GAO analysis. I GAO-19-225T.

Table 9. Status of Recommendations from Navy Force Structure: Actions Needed to Ensure Proper Size and Composition of Ship Crews (GAO-17-413)

Recommendation #1:	
The Secretary of the Navy should have the Navy conduct a comprehensive reassessment of the Navy standard workweek and make any necessary adjustments.	**Status:** Open **Concurrence:** Yes **Comments:** As of November 2018, the Navy was in the process of conducting a study of afloat workload to establish accurate fleet manpower requirements and inform manning level changes, with a report on the study expected in November 2018. The results of the study are expected to be promulgated to cognizant stakeholders, and revisions will be made to the Navy Total Force Manpower Policies and Procedures Instruction (OPNAVINST 1000.16L) in February 2019.
Recommendation #2:	
The Secretary of the Navy should have the Navy update guidance to require examination of in-port workload and identify the manpower necessary to execute in-port workload for all surface ship classes.	**Status:** Open **Concurrence:** Yes **Comments:** As of November 2018, the Navy had completed two in-port workload studies, and had planned future studies for various ship classes. These studies are expected to inform an update to OPNAVINST 1000.16L in February 2019.
Recommendation #3:	
The Secretary of the Navy should have the Navy develop criteria and update guidance for reassessing the factors used to calculate manpower requirements periodically or when conditions change.	**Status:** Open **Concurrence:** Yes **Comments**: As of November 2018, the Navy Total Force Manpower Training and Education Requirements Division published a Manpower Guidance Memorandum on March 1, 2018, that outlines the requirement for reassessing the factors used to calculate manpower requirements. This is expected to inform the planned revision to OPNAVINST 1000.16L.
Recommendation #4:	
The Secretary of the Navy should have the Navy identify personnel needs and the costs associated with the planned larger Navy fleet size, including consideration of the updated manpower factors and requirements.	**Status:** Open **Concurrence:** Yes **Comments:** As of November 2018, Navy officials confirmed that this recommendation has an anticipated implementation date of February 2019, adding that total ownership costs that capture all facets of personnel needs and costs will be adjusted based upon the Navy's growth linked to the 30-year ship building plan and aviation master plan. The refinement of all manpower determination planning factors and assumptions, the ongoing data collection and analysis garnered from the in-port workload studies, and the outcome of the operational afloat workweek study are expected to inform all existing and future force structure manpower requirements.

Source: GAO analysis. | GAO-19-225T.

Table 10. Status of Recommendations from Military Readiness: DOD's Readiness Rebuilding Efforts May Be at Risk without a Comprehensive Plan (GAO-16-841)

Recommendation #1:	
The Secretaries of the Departments of the Army, the Navy, and the Air Force should establish comprehensive readiness rebuilding goals to guide readiness rebuilding efforts and a strategy for implementing identified goals, to include resources needed to implement the strategy.	**Status:** Open **Concurrence:** Partial **Comments:** The military services have defined their readiness rebuilding goals and, in some cases, extended these goals since we reported in 2016. Further, through the department's Readiness Recovery Framework, the military services have identified key readiness issues that their respective forces face and actions to

Table 10. (Continued)

Recommendation #1:	
	address these issues, as well as metrics by which to assess progress toward achieving overall readiness recovery goals. The Office of the Secretary of Defense continues to work with the military services to ensure that the services' actions and metrics clearly align with readiness recovery goals in an executable strategy. We will continue to monitor progress regarding DOD's Readiness Recovery Framework before closing this recommendation as implemented.
Recommendation #2:	
The Secretaries of the Departments of the Army, the Navy, and the Air Force should develop metrics for measuring interim progress at specific milestones against identified goals for all services.	**Status:** Open **Concurrence:** Partial **Comments:** The military services have taken steps to develop metrics for measuring interim progress at specific milestones against identified readiness recovery goals. Through the Readiness Recovery Framework process, the military services have identified key readiness issues that their respective forces face and actions to address these issues, as well as metrics to assess progress toward readiness recovery goals that include quantifiable deliverables at specific milestones. The Office of the Secretary of Defense continues to work with the military services to ensure that the services' metrics and milestones clearly align with readiness recovery goals. We will continue to monitor progress regarding DOD's Readiness Recovery Framework before closing this recommendation as implemented.
Recommendation #3:	
The Secretaries of the Departments of the Army, the Navy, and the Air Force should identify external factors that may impact readiness recovery plans, including how they influence the underlying assumptions, to ensure that readiness rebuilding goals are achievable within established time frames. This should include, but not be limited to, an evaluation of the impact of assumptions about budget, maintenance time frames, and training that underpin the services' readiness recovery plans.	**Status:** Open **Concurrence:** Partial **Comments:** DOD noted that the department would continue to work with the military services to refine their readiness recovery goals and identify the requisite resources needed to meet them. We will continue to monitor progress regarding DOD's Readiness Recovery Framework before closing this recommendation as implemented.

Table 11. Status of Recommendations from Navy Force Structure: Sustainable Plan and Comprehensive Assessment Needed to Mitigate Long-Term Risks to Ships Assigned to Overseas Homeports (GAO-15-329)

Recommendation #1:	
The Secretary of the Navy should fully implement the Navy's optimized fleet response plan and develop and implement a sustainable operational schedule for all ships home ported overseas.	**Status:** Open **Concurrence:** Yes **Comments:** In August 2015, the Navy reported that it had approved and implemented six different revised optimized fleet response plan schedules that covered all ships home ported overseas. We closed the recommendation as implemented in 2015. In 2017, the Navy suffered four significant mishaps at sea resulting in the loss of 17 sailors' lives and serious damage to its ships. Three of the four ships involved were homeported in Japan. The resulting Navy investigations revealed that due to heavy operational demands, the Navy had not fully implemented the revised operational schedules it developed in 2015 for ships based

Recommendation #1:	
	in Japan. In light of this information, we re-opened this recommendation. As of October 2018, the Navy had developed a change to the operational schedule for ships homeported in Japan, and is expecting to codify this revised schedule in November 2018. The Navy also established Commander, Naval Surface Group, Western Pacific to oversee surface ship maintenance, training, and certification for ships based in Japan. We will continue to monitor the Navy's adherence to these revised schedules before closing this recommendation as implemented.
Recommendation #2:	
The Secretary of the Navy should develop a comprehensive assessment of the long-term costs and risks to the Navy's surface and amphibious fleet associated with the Navy's increasing reliance on overseas homeporting to meet presence requirements, make any necessary adjustments to the Navy's overseas presence based on this assessment, and reassess these risks when making future overseas homeporting decisions and developing future strategic laydown plans.	**Status:** Open **Concurrence:** Yes **Comments:** As of November 2018, the Navy had tasked the Office of the Chief of Naval Operations Assessments Division to conduct an assessment of the long-term costs and risks to the Navy's fleet associated with the Navy's increasing reliance on overseas homeporting. The Office of the Chief of Naval Operations plans to complete the review by the end of 2018.

Source: GAO analysis. | GAO-19-225T.

Table 12. Status of Recommendations from F-35 Joint Strike Fighter: Development Is Nearly Complete, but Deficiencies Found in Testing Need to Be Resolved (GAO-18-321)

Recommendation #1:	
The F-35 program office should resolve all critical deficiencies before making a full-rate production decision.	**Status:** Open **Concurrence:** Yes **Comments:** DOD stated that critical deficiencies would be resolved before full-rate production, expected in October 2019. As of August 2018, DOD had not resolved these deficiencies.
Recommendation #2:	
The F-35 program office should identify what steps are needed to ensure the F-35 meets reliability and maintainability requirements before each variant reaches maturity, and update the Reliability and Maintainability Improvement Program with these steps.	**Status:** Open **Concurrence:** Yes **Comments:** As August 2018, DOD had not taken actions to implement this recommendation. We will monitor DOD's efforts to address this recommendation.

Source: GAO analysis. | GAO-19-225T.

Table 13. Status of Recommendations from Warfighter Support: DOD Needs to Share F-35 Operational Lessons across the Military Services (GAO-18-464R)

Recommendation #1:	
The F-35 Program Executive Officer should test operating the F-35 disconnected from its Autonomic Logistics Information System (ALIS) for extended periods of time in a variety of scenarios to assess the risks related to operating and sustaining the aircraft, and determine how to mitigate any identified risks.	**Status:** Open **Concurrence:** Yes **Comments:** According to DOD officials, as of July 2018, the Initial Operational Test and Evaluation test plan did not include an evaluation of continued disconnected operations. However, the military services are planning more limited operational tests in the near future. For example, the Marine Corps is planning a future deployment to demonstrate an ability to rapidly deploy with three to four aircraft, and operate for 2 to 3 days without connectivity back to the squadron kit. While this is not intended to replicate an extended 30-day disconnected operation, it may provide initial indications of

Table 13. (Continued)

Recommendation #1:	
	how extended disconnected operations may function. As the emerging ALIS strategy comes into focus, particularly in terms of the decentralized maintenance capability, it is expected that a robust test plan will be developed and implemented. We are encouraged that the department is aware of the issue and working toward, as necessary, potential mitigation strategies. However, until the F-35 is tested disconnected from ALIS for extended periods of time in a variety of scenarios to assess any risks related to operating and sustaining the aircraft, this recommendation will remain open.
Recommendation #2:	
The F-35 Program Executive Officer should formally share or make available, through a new or existing communications mechanism, F-35 operational lessons learned across the services.	**Status:** Open
	Concurrence: Yes
	Comments: According to DOD officials, as of July 2018, the Air Force, the Marine Corps, and the Navy all had robust systems for capturing and sharing F-35 operational lessons learned. However, although these systems are accessible by members of the other services, there is a general lack of awareness of how to access systems across the military services. The department is considering a number of possible solutions to facilitate cross-service sharing of lessons learned, with most of the solutions requiring action from the individual services. For example, there has been discussion of utilizing the already-established Joint Lessons Learned Information System website, and creating a specific repository for the F-35. We are encouraged that the department is aware of the importance of sharing operational lessons learned across the services and that a solution is likely on the horizon. However, until the department reaches a consensus and implements the optimal path forward, this recommendation will remain open.

Source: GAO analysis. I GAO-19-225T

Note: This chapter is an unclassified version of GAO-18-79C. Two of the four recommendations were directed to the F-35 program office and are included here. The remaining two recommendations were directed to the Commandant of the Marine Corps and are included in Table 5, which summarizes recommendations made in GAO-18-79C.

Table 14. Status of Recommendations from F-35 Aircraft Sustainment: DOD Needs to Address Challenges Affecting Readiness and Cost Transparency (GAO-18-75)

Recommendation #1:	
The Under Secretary of Defense for Acquisition, Technology and Logistics, in coordination with the F-35 Program Executive Officer, should revise sustainment plans to ensure that they include the key requirements and decision points needed to fully implement the F-35 sustainment strategy and align funding plans to meet those requirements.	**Status:** Open
	Concurrence: Yes
	Comments: Officials from the Office of the Under Secretary of Defense for Acquisition and Sustainment (USD (A&S)) said that as of October 2018, USD (A&S) and the F-35 Program Executive Officer (PEO) were focusing actions and resources toward achieving key production, development and sustainment objectives by 2025. For sustainment, the two primary objectives are to increase F-35 availability and reduce sustainment costs. According to these officials, the PEO, with industry- and department-level input, is updating sustainment plans to accelerate depot repair capacity, reduce spares demand and improve the stability, security, and mission capabilities of the Autonomic Logistics Information System. These efforts and others will inform the Fiscal Year 2020-2024 Program Budget decisions, to ensure that investments return the most in terms of increased availability and reduced cost. Officials said that these actions, strategy updates and investments will continue over the

Recommendation #1:	
	Future Year's Defense Plan. We will continue to monitor DOD's efforts to revise the department's sustainment plans and align the department's future budgets to support those plans, but it is too soon to determine the extent to which these efforts—when completed—will address the concerns that we identified our report.
Recommendation #2:	
	Status: Open
The Under Secretary of Defense for Acquisition, Technology and Logistics, in coordination with the F-35 Program Executive Officer, should re-examine the metrics that it will use to hold the contractor accountable under the fixed-price, performance-based contracts to ensure that such metrics are objectively measurable, are fully reflective of processes over which the contractor has control, and drive desired behaviors by all stakeholders.	**Concurrence:** Yes
	Comments: Officials from USD (A&S) said that as of October 2018, the F-35 PEO re-examines sustainment metrics every year, so that the department can objectively measure and hold the contractor accountable for delivering increased availability and reduced cost, and to align sustainment processes and deliverables to those that the contractor controls. In the fiscal year 2018 annual sustainment contract, the PEO established a fee structure to better motivate the contractor to deliver threshold performance values, established an improved metric compared with the 2017contract, and initiated a new fee for delivery of supply chain performance metrics directly under the contractor's control. Officials said that the PEO will continue to re-examine metrics annually to ensure that they align with government and industry interests, drive desired behavior, increase F-35 availability, and reduce cost. We recognize the department's progress related to this recommendation, but the key metrics being used by the F-35 program to incentivize the contractor remain a concern as they are not fully reflective of processes over which the contractor has control. This could make it difficult to hold the contractor accountable under performance based contracts, as we reported. We will continue to monitor DOD's efforts to re-examine metrics to ensure that they are objectively measureable, fully reflective of processes over which the contractor has control, and drive desired behaviors by all stakeholders.
Recommendation #3:	
	Status: Open
The Under Secretary of Defense for Acquisition, Technology and Logistics, in coordination with the F-35 Program Executive Officer, should, prior to entering into multi-year, fixed-price, performance-based contracts, ensure that DOD has sufficient knowledge of the actual costs of sustainment and technical characteristics of the aircraft after baseline development is complete and the system reaches maturity.	**Concurrence:** Yes
	Comments: Officials from USD (A&S) said that as of October 2018, the F-35 PEO is overseeing a Sustainment Actual Cost Working Group, made up of representatives from both the Office of the Secretary of Defense and the F-35 Joint Program Office. The working group is striving to improve DOD's insight into the actual cost of F-35 sustainment. According to these officials, to date, the working group has identified a number of gaps in the cost data that the department receives from prime and subcontractors and is now collaborating with the vendors and with contracting officials to find ways to improve the quality, granularity, and timeliness of the actual F-35 cost data that the department receives. In addition, the F-35 system has not yet completed key operational tests or reached system maturity. Until DOD has a full understanding of the actual costs of sustainment and technical characteristics of the aircraft at system maturity, DOD may not be well positioned to enter into a long-term, fixed-price, performance-based contract. We will continue to monitor DOD's efforts in this area.
Recommendation #4	
	Status: Open
The Under Secretary of Defense for Acquisition, Technology and Logistics, in coordination with the F-35 Program Executive Officer, should take steps to improve communication with the services and provide	**Concurrence:** Yes
	Comments: Officials from USD (A&S) said that as of October 2018, USD (A&S) was undertaking a study on F-35 Sustainment Affordability and Transparency, in response to the Senate Armed Services Committee report accompanying a bill for the National

Table 14. (Continued)

Recommendation #4	
more information about how the F-35 sustainment costs they are being charged relate to the capabilities received.	Defense Authorization Act for Fiscal Year 2018. According to these officials, the study examines affordability and transparency issues between the services and the F-35 Joint Program Office, which inhibit the services' visibility into expected F-35 costs versus budgets, what they are paying for in sustainment, and what they are getting for that money. Work on this study is ongoing. We will review DOD's report, once completed, to determine the extent to which DOD's efforts address our recommendation.

Source: GAO analysis. | GAO-19-225T.

Table 15. Status of Recommendations from Defense Supply Chain: DOD Needs Complete Information on Single Sources of Supply to Proactively Manage the Risks (GAO-17-768)

Recommendation #1:	
The Under Secretary of Defense for Acquisition, Technology and Logistics, in conjunction with the Defense Contract Management Agency and the military departments, should assess whether risk mitigation actions have been identified in the event of a loss of each task critical assets facility in the defense industrial base and, based	**Status:** Open **Concurrence:** Yes **Comments:** DOD officials stated that the department addressed this recommendation by issuing DOD Instruction 3020.45 in August 2018; however, DOD did not have an update on how the department will share this information with congressional decision makers.
on this assessment, develop risk mitigation actions with associated implementation plans and timelines and provide this information to congressional and DOD decision makers.	
Recommendation #2:	
The Under Secretary of Defense for Acquisition, Technology and Logistics, in conjunction with the Defense Contract Management Agency and the military departments, should provide congressional and DOD decision makers with information on the potential effects on defense capabilities in the event of a loss of each task critical assets facility in the defense industrial base.	**Status:** Open **Concurrence:** Yes Comments: DOD officials stated that as of August 2018, the department's efforts to address this recommendation were in progress and stated that the issuance of the mission assurance instruction furthered this progress. However, DOD did not provide information on its plan to develop a mechanism to share this information with Congress.
Recommendation #3:	
The Under Secretary of Defense for Acquisition, Technology and Logistics, in conjunction with the Defense Contract Management Agency and the military departments, should provide congressional and DOD decision makers with information on DOD's organic facilities that have been identified as task critical assets, similar to the information provided previously on commercial facilities. This information also should include (1) the potential effects on defense capabilities in the event of a loss of the facility and (2) risk mitigation actions and associated implementation plans with timelines.	**Status:** Open **Concurrence:** Yes **Comments:** DOD officials stated that as of August 2018, the department's efforts to address this recommendation were in progress and that the issuance of the mission assurance instruction furthered this progress. However, DOD did not provide information on its plan to develop a mechanism to share this information with Congress.

Recommendation #4:	
The Under Secretary of Defense for Acquisition, Technology and Logistics, in conjunction with the Defense Contract Management Agency and the military departments, should take steps to share information on risks identified through the annual Critical Asset Identification Process with relevant program managers or other designated service or program officials. At a minimum, relevant officials should receive information on the most critical facilities (such as task critical assets) that produce parts supporting their programs. This information-sharing could occur through service-specific channels of communication or another method of internal communication deemed appropriate by DOD.	**Status:** Open **Concurrence:** Yes **Comments:** DOD officials stated that as of August 2018, they were in the process of developing proactive steps to share information on risks identified through the annual Critical Asset Identification Process with relevant program managers, or with other designated service or program officials as necessary. They further stated that the issuance of the mission assurance instruction will assist with these efforts. We will assess this instruction and will continue to monitor DOD actions taken to address this recommendation.
Recommendation #5:	
The Under Secretary of Defense for Acquisition, Technology and Logistics, in conjunction with the military departments, should develop a mechanism to ensure that program offices obtain information from contractors on single source of supply risks.	**Status:** Open **Concurrence:** Yes **Comments:** DOD officials stated that as of August 2018, assessing the health of the defense industrial base and associated supply chains was the focus of an Executive Order issued in July 2017 and that the resulting interagency report will be released within the next year. DOD officials stated that the issuance of this report will provide significant information toward addressing this recommendation. We will assess this report upon issuance.
Recommendation #6:	
The Under Secretary of Defense for Acquisition, Technology and Logistics, in conjunction with the military departments, should issue a department-wide Diminishing Manufacturing Sources and Material Shortages policy, such as an instruction, that clearly defines requirements of Diminishing Manufacturing Sources and Material Shortages management and details responsibilities and procedures to be followed by program offices to implement the policy.	**Status:** Open **Concurrence:** Yes **Comments:** The DOD official that is the lead for the Diminishing Manufacturing Sources and Material Shortages program stated that as of August 2018, the department was in the process of addressing this recommendation. A working group lead by the official and comprising of all relevant offices developed a draft Diminishing Manufacturing Sources and Material Shortages instruction and accompanying manual that details program requirements, responsibilities, and procedures to be followed. The official expects the instruction and manual to be issued by December 2019.

Source: GAO analysis. | GAO-19-225T.

Table 16. Status of Recommendations from Defense Inventory: Further Analysis and Enhanced Metrics Could Improve Service Supply and Depot Operations (GAO-16-450)

Recommendation #1:	
The Assistant Secretary of Defense for Logistics and Materiel Readiness, in conjunction with the Director, Defense Logistics Agency, and the Secretaries of the Army and the Navy and the Commandant of the Marine Corps, to assess through a comprehensive business case analysis—drawing on lessons learned from previous efforts—the costs and benefits of the Defense Logistics Agency managing the retail supply, storage, and distribution functions at the Army and Marine Corps depots and Navy shipyards.	**Status:** Open **Concurrence:** Yes **Comments:** As of August 2018, the Department of Defense (DOD) had designated the transfer of these retail functions as an operating priority and identified it as a key reform effort within logistics in the department. The Marine Corps has conducted its analysis and decided to transition additional supply, storage, and distribution functions to the Defense Logistics Agency over a 4-year period, with all implementation activities scheduled to be complete by 2022. The Navy and Defense Logistics Agency are working on a strategic memorandum of understanding to guide decisions on the role of the Defense Logistics Agency at the Navy shipyards, according to a senior DOD official. Without the Navy finalizing its

Table 16. (Continued)

Recommendation #1:	
	business case analyses, decision makers will not be positioned to make cost-effective decisions regarding supply operations at military depots.
Recommendation #2:	
The Assistant Secretary of Defense for Logistics and Materiel Readiness, in conjunction with the Director, Defense Logistics Agency, and the Secretaries of the Army and the Navy and the Commandant of the Marine Corps to use the analysis to make a decision on the degree to which the Defense Logistics Agency should manage these functions at the Army and Marine Corps depots and Navy shipyards.	**Status:** Open **Concurrence:** Yes **Comments:** As of August 2018, DOD had designated the transfer of these retail functions as an operating priority and identified it as a key reform effort within logistics in the department. The Marine Corps has conducted its analysis and decided to transition additional supply, storage, and distribution functions to the Defense Logistics Agency over a 4-year period, with all implementation activities scheduled to be completed by 2022. However, the Navy has not made any decisions regarding the additional transfer of supply, storage and distribution functions to the Defense Logistics Agency. Without the Navy making decisions based on business case analyses on the degree to which additional supply, storage, and distribution functions will transfer to the Defense Logistics Agency, DOD will not be assured that it is operating its supply operations at military depots in a cost-effective manner.
Recommendation #3:	
The Assistant Secretary of Defense for Logistics and Materiel Readiness, in conjunction with the Director, Defense Logistics Agency, and the Secretaries of the Army, Navy, and Air Force and the Commandant of the Marine Corps to develop and implement metrics that measure the accuracy of planning factors, such as the schedule, bill of materials, and replacement factors used for depot maintenance.	**Status:** Open **Concurrence:** Yes **Comments:** As of August 2018, DOD has begun to identify metrics that measure the accuracy of planning factors used for depot maintenance. However, these metrics are not scheduled to be fully implemented until December 2018.
Recommendation #4:	
The Assistant Secretary of Defense for Logistics and Materiel Readiness, in conjunction with the Director, Defense Logistics Agency, and the Secretaries of the Army, the Navy, and the Air Force and the Commandant of the Marine Corps to take action, as appropriate and necessary, to resolve any issues identified through measuring the accuracy of planning inputs in an effort to improve supply and depot maintenance operations.	**Status:** Open **Concurrence:** Yes **Comments:** As of August 2018, DOD had begun to identify metrics that measure the accuracy of planning factors used for depot maintenance. However, these metrics are not scheduled to be fully implemented until December 2018. Thus, no actions have been taken to resolve any identified issues based on the results of the metrics.
Recommendation #5:	
The Assistant Secretary of Defense for Logistics and Materiel Readiness, in conjunction with the Director, Defense Logistics Agency, the Secretaries of the Army, the Navy, and the Air Force, and the Commandant of the Marine Corps to take steps to develop and implement metrics, to the extent feasible, to measure and track disruption costs created by the lack of parts at depot maintenance industrial sites by, for example, establishing a team of supply and depot maintenance experts from the Defense Logistics Agency and the services to assess potential data sources, approaches, and methods.	**Status:** Open **Concurrence:** Yes **Comments:** As of September 2018, DOD had begun examining potential methods for measuring and tracking disruption costs created by the lack of parts at depot maintenance industrial sites. However, DOD and the services have identified a number of data challenges in being able to compute such costs and are in the process of working through those issues so that they can begin measuring and tracking disruption costs.

Recommendation #6:	
The Assistant Secretary of Defense for Logistics and Materiel Readiness, in conjunction with the Director, Defense Logistics Agency, the Secretaries of the Army, the Navy, and the Air Force, and the Commandant of the Marine Corps to take action as appropriate to address any inefficiencies identified by the disruption cost metrics in supply and depot maintenance operations.	**Status:** Open **Concurrence:** Yes **Comments:** As of August 2018, DOD had begun to develop metrics that measure and track disruption costs created by the lack of parts at depot maintenance industrial sites. However, these metrics are not scheduled to be implemented until October 2018. Thus, no actions have been taken to resolve any identified issues based on the results of the metrics.

Source: GAO analysis. | GAO-19-225T.

In: Top 10 Reports and Testimonies in December 2018 ISBN: 978-1-53615-507-5
Editor: Sarah J. Nygaard

Chapter 8

STATE AND LOCAL GOVERNMENTS' FISCAL OUTLOOK: 2018 UPDATE*

United States Government Accountability Office

ABBREVIATIONS

BEA	Bureau of Economic Analysis
CBO	Congressional Budget Office
CHIP	Children's Health Insurance Program
CMS	Centers for Medicare & Medicaid Services
CPI	Consumer Price Index
GDP	Gross Domestic Product
HHS	Health & Human Services
NIPA	National Income and Product Accounts
OASDI Trustees	the Board of Trustees of the Federal Old-Age and Survivors Insurance and Federal Disability Insurance Trust Funds
PPACA	Patient Protection and Affordable Care Act
SALT	State and Local Tax
TCJA	Tax Cuts and Jobs Act

WHY GAO DID THIS STUDY

Fiscal sustainability presents a national challenge shared by all levels of government. Since 2007, GAO has published simulations of long-term fiscal trends in the state and local government sector, which have consistently shown that the sector faces long-term fiscal pressures. While most states have requirements related to balancing their budgets, deficits can

* This is an edited, reformatted and augmented version of United States Government Accountability Office; Report to the Congress, Publication No. GAO-19-208SP, dated December 2018.

arise because the planned annual revenues are not generated at the expected rate, demand for services exceeds planned expenditures, or both, resulting in a near-term operating deficit.

This chapter updates GAO's state and local fiscal model to simulate the fiscal outlook for the state and local government sector. This includes identifying the components of state and local expenditures likely to contribute to the sector's fiscal pressures. In addition, this chapter identifies considerations related to federal policy and other factors that could contribute to uncertainties in the state and local government sector's long-term fiscal outlook.

GAO's model uses the Bureau of Economic Analysis's National Income and Product Accounts as the primary data source and presents the results in the aggregate for the state and local sector as a whole. The model shows the level of receipts and expenditures for the sector until 2067, based on current and historical spending and revenue patterns. In addition, the model assumes that the current set of policies in place across state and local government remains constant to show a simulated long-term outlook.

What GAO Found

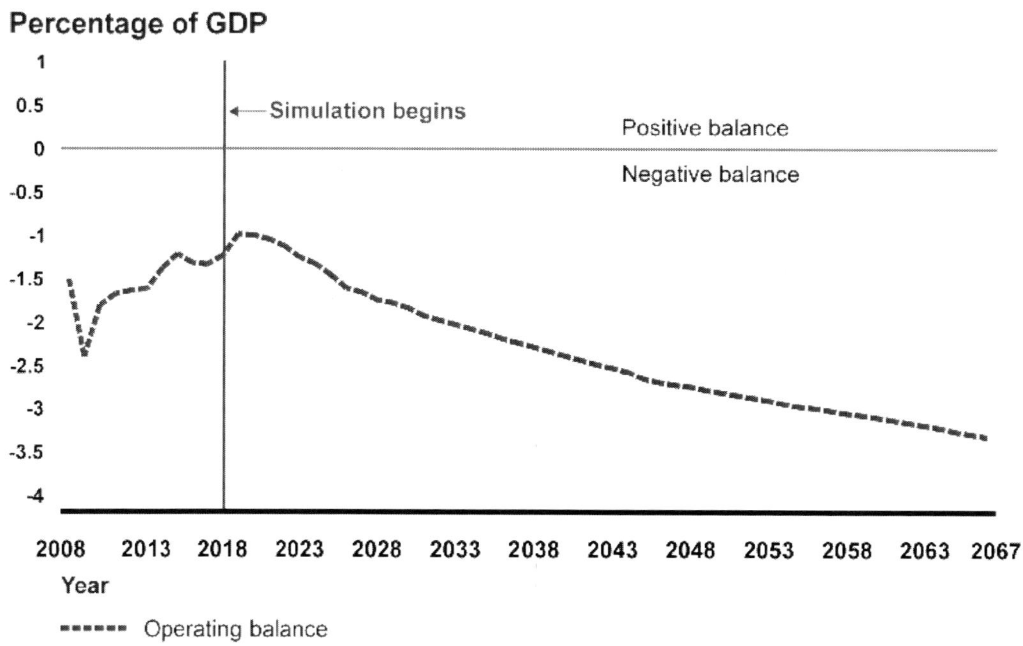

Source: GAO analysis of data from the Agency for Healthcare Research and Quality, Bloomberg, the Board of Governors of the Federal Reserve System, the Board of Trustees of the Federal Old-Age and Survivors Insurance and Federal Disability Insurance Trust Funds, the Bureau of Economic Analysis, the Bureau of Labor Statistics, the Census Bureau, the Centers for Medicare & Medicaid Services, the Congressional Budget Office, and the Federal Reserve Bank of St Louis. | GAO-19-208SP.

State and Local Government Sector Operating Balance as a Percentage of Gross Domestic Product (GDP), 2008 through 2067.

GAO's simulations suggest that the state and local government sector will likely face an increasing difference between revenues and expenditures during the next 50 years as reflected by the operating balance—a measure of the sector's ability to cover its current expenditures out of its current receipts. While both expenditures and revenues are projected to increase as a percentage of gross domestic product (GDP), a difference between the two is projected to persist because expenditures are expected to grow faster than revenues throughout the simulation period.

GAO's simulations also suggest that growth in the sector's overall spending is largely driven by health care expenditures—in particular, Medicaid spending and spending on health benefits for state and local government employees and retirees. These expenditures are projected to grow as a share of GDP during the simulation period. GAO's simulations also suggest that revenues from personal income taxes and federal grants to states and localities will increase during the simulation period. However, revenues will grow more slowly than expenditures such that the sector faces a declining fiscal outlook.

GAO also identified federal policy changes that could affect the state and local government sector's fiscal outlook. For example, the effects of the recently-enacted Tax Cuts and Jobs Act will likely depend on how states incorporate the Act into their state income tax rules. In addition, other factors, such as economic growth and rates of return on pension assets, could shift future fiscal outcomes for the sector.

December 13, 2018
Report to the Congress

Fiscal sustainability presents a national challenge shared by all levels of government. The federal government and state and local governments share responsibility in fulfilling important national goals and providing essential services to citizens. State and local governments provide primary and secondary education, health care, libraries, police and fire protection services, social programs, roads and other infrastructure, public colleges and universities, and more. These subnational governments rely on the federal government for significant portions of their revenue. Given the nature of the partnership among levels of government in providing services, understanding potential future fiscal conditions of the state and local government sector is important for federal policymaking.

To provide Congress and the public with this broader context, we developed a fiscal model of the state and local government sector, which we first reported on in 2007 and have regularly updated since.[1] This chapter updates our state and local fiscal model to simulate the fiscal outlook for the state and local government sector. This includes identifying the components of state and local expenditures that are likely to contribute to the sector's fiscal pressures. This chapter also identifies considerations related to federal policy and other factors that could contribute to uncertainties in the state and local government sector's fiscal outlook.

To develop simulations of the fiscal outlook for the state and local government sector, we use the Department of Commerce's Bureau of Economic Analysis's (BEA) National Income and Product Accounts (NIPA) as the primary data source and project the level of receipts and expenditures for the sector until 2067, based on current and historical spending and revenue patterns. Our model assumes that historical relationships between taxes and their tax bases persist, that the federal government continues to provide services to people at a level consistent with current policies, and that other current policies and relationships affecting

[1] See appendix III for a list of reports related to this work.

revenues do not change. Our model also assumes that the state and local government sector continues to provide levels of services to each resident consistent with current government policies. The model presents results in the aggregate for the state and local government sector as a whole, consistent with the nature of the NIPA source data. Because of this, the fiscal outlook for individual states and localities cannot be identified.

As part of our simulations, we also assess potential fiscal outcomes for the sector using an indicator of fiscal balance called the operating balance. The state and local government sector's operating balance is a measure of its ability to cover expenditures in a given year using revenues collected in the same year. Because subnational governments are generally required to balance or nearly balance their operating budgets, the design of our operating balance measure reflects this characteristic of subnational governments' operating budgets.[2] For additional information on the model's key assumptions, see appendix I.

To identify considerations related to federal policy that could contribute to uncertainties in the sector's fiscal outlook, we reviewed recent legislation, relevant legal precedents, economic literature, our prior reports, and reports from selected think tanks that analyze aspects of fiscal federalism. These think tanks include the Nelson A. Rockefeller Institute of Government, the Pew Charitable Trusts, the Tax Foundation Center for Federal Tax Policy, and the Urban Institute and Brookings Institution Tax Policy Center. We also conducted semistructured interviews on federal and intergovernmental policy issues and related data with associations representing state government officials, including the National Association of State Budget Officers, the National Conference of State Legislatures, the National Association of State Auditors, Comptrollers and Treasurers; specialists from credit rating agencies and their research divisions, such as Moody's Analytics and Standard & Poor's Global Ratings; and senior officials from the Federal Reserve Bank of Chicago, BEA, and the Congressional Budget Office (CBO). We selected these organizations and related reports based on a literature review and our prior work on state and local government fiscal issues. These interviews primarily focused on tax- and health-related federal policies because of their relevance to our simulation results. Specifically, our simulations have continually suggested that trends in tax revenues and health care spending have contributed to large and recurring fiscal challenges for the sector. The policy considerations we identified are not exhaustive. That is, we did not fully analyze every federal tax- and health-related policy that could create uncertainties for the state and local government sectors' fiscal outlook.

Further, to identify other factors that could contribute to uncertainties in the sector's fiscal outlook, we developed simulations using alternative assumptions of the growth of key model variables to describe how the operating balance measure would respond to changes in the growth projections of key variables over the simulation period. For additional information on our methodology for developing these simulations, see appendix II.

---

[2] Most states have some sort of requirement to balance operating budgets. To address fiscal pressures and comply with balanced budget requirements, state and local governments may offset increased costs in one program by making cuts to other programs. However, they may have less flexibility to adjust certain types of spending. For example, state and local government employee pension benefits are often defined in state law or local ordinances or charters, and, in that sense, pension benefits for current retirees are largely protected from states' or localities' responses to fiscal pressures. On the other hand, retiree health benefits for those employees may not have the same level of legal protection. Spending on programs such as street paving may have no legal protection, but instead be an implicit commitment grounded in the public's expectations for the provision of government services. Flexibility to adjust revenues may also be constrained explicitly (e.g., caps on tax increases) or implicitly (e.g., tax increases can be politically unpopular).

We conducted our work for this model update from February 2018 to December 2018 in accordance with all sections of our Quality Assurance Framework that are relevant to our objectives. The framework requires that we plan and perform the engagement to obtain sufficient and appropriate evidence to meet our stated objectives, and to discuss any limitations in our work. We believe that the information and data obtained, and the analysis conducted, provide a reasonable basis for any findings and conclusions in this product.

STATE AND LOCAL GOVERNMENTS WILL NEED TO MAKE POLICY CHANGES TO MAINTAIN LONG-TERM FISCAL BALANCE

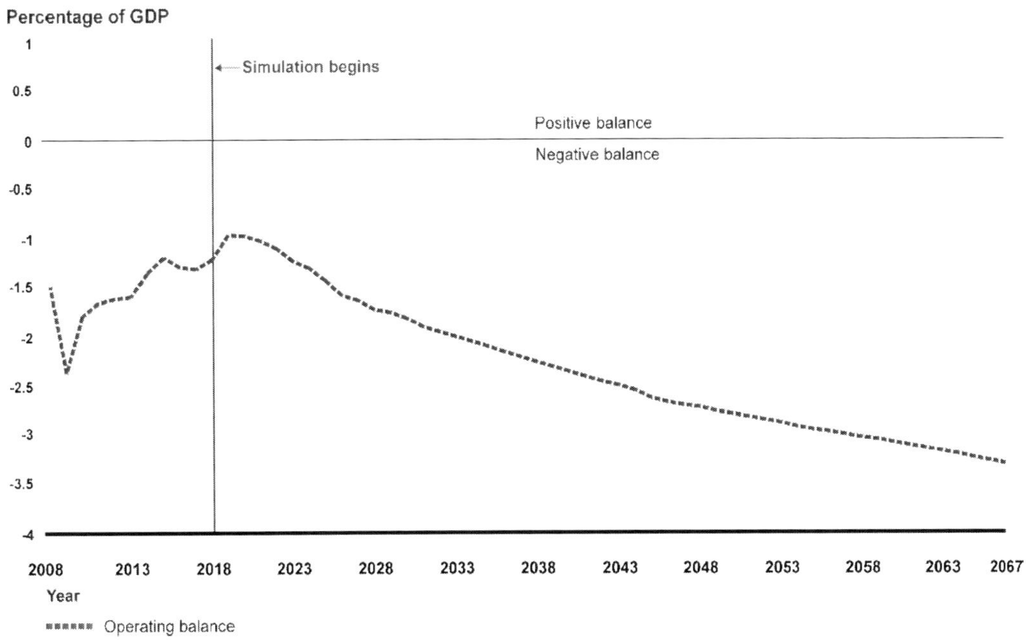

Source: GAO analysis of data from the Agency for Healthcare Research and Quality, Bloomberg, the Board of Governors of the Federal Reserve System, the Board of Trustees of the Federal Old-Age and Survivors Insurance and Federal Disability Insurance Trust Funds, the Bureau of Economic Analysis, the Bureau of Labor Statistics, the Census Bureau, the Centers for Medicare & Medicaid Services, the Congressional Budget Office, and the Federal Reserve Bank of St Louis. | GAO-19-208SP.

Note: The operating balance is defined as total receipts minus (1) capital outlays not financed by medium- and long-term debt issuance, (2) total current expenditures less depreciation, (3) current surplus of state and local government enterprises, and (4) net social insurance fund balance.

Figure 1. State and Local Government Sector Operating Balance as a Percentage of Gross Domestic Product (GDP), 2008 through 2067.

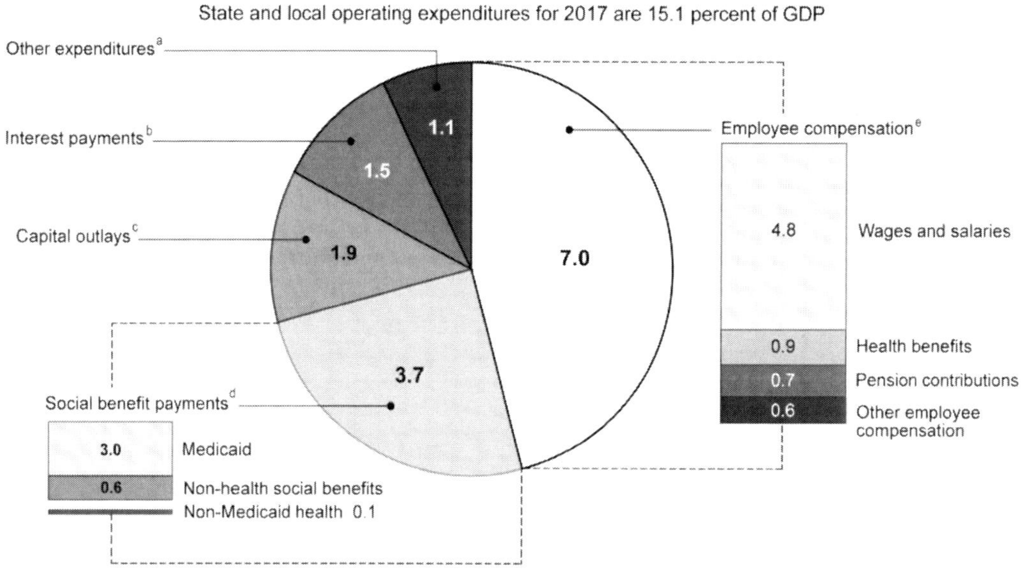

Source: GAO analysis of data from the Agency for Healthcare Research and Quality, Bloomberg, the Board of Governors of the Federal Reserve System, the Board of Trustees of the Federal Old-Age and Survivors Insurance and Federal Disability Insurance Trust Funds, the Bureau of Economic Analysis, the Bureau of Labor Statistics, the Census Bureau, the Centers for Medicare & Medicaid Services, the Congressional Budget Office, and the Federal Reserve Bank of St Louis. | GAO-19-208SP.

Notes: Operating expenditures are comprised of the spending components of the operating balance and include employee compensation, social benefit payments, capital outlays, interest payments, and other types of spending. State and local government sector operating expenditures were 15.1 percent of GDP in 2017. Percentages may not add to 15.1 due to rounding.

[a]Other expenditures include subsidy payments to railroads, purchases of intermediate goods, and the net balance of social insurance funds.

[b]Interest payments are payments on actual and imputed interest on outstanding debt.

[c]Capital outlays include spending on structures (i.e., residential and commercial buildings, highways and streets and sewer and water systems), equipment, intellectual property, and net purchases of land, excluding payments to states for long-term rights to extract oil.

[d]Social benefit payments are amounts paid to individuals to provide for needs arising from circumstances such as sickness, unemployment, retirement, and poverty. These payments include Medicaid and other general medical assistance, temporary disability insurance, education assistance, and a variety of other needs.

[e]Employee compensation includes wages and salaries, health benefits for employees and retirees, contributions to employee defined benefit pension funds, and other types of compensation, such as life insurance and workers compensation contributions.

Figure 2. State and Local Government Sector Operating Expenditures as a Percentage of Gross Domestic Product (GDP) in 2017.

Our simulations suggest that the sector will likely continue to face a difference between revenue and spending during the next 50 years. This long-term outlook is measured by the operating balance—a measure of the sector's ability to cover its current expenditures out of current receipts.[3] While both expenditures and revenues are projected to increase as a percentage of gross domestic product (GDP) during the simulation period, a difference between the two is projected to persist because expenditures are generally expected to grow at a faster rate than revenues.[4] (see Figure 1). Absent any policy changes by state and local governments, revenues are likely to be insufficient to maintain the sector's capacity to provide services at levels consistent with current policies during the next 50 years. Our simulations suggest that state and local governments will need to make policy changes to avoid fiscal imbalances before then and assure that revenues are at least equal to expenditures.

We simulated the state and local government sector's operating balance (the difference between the sector's operating revenues and operating expenditures) in order to understand the sector's long-term fiscal outlook. The sector's operating expenditures were 15.1 percent of GDP in 2017. As shown in Figure 2, these state and local government sector operating expenditures are comprised of employee compensation, social benefit payments, interest payments, capital outlays, and other expenditures. The sector's operating revenues were 13.8 percent of GDP in 2017. As shown in Figure 3, these state and local government sector operating revenues are comprised of taxes, transfer receipts, and other types of revenues.

One way of measuring the long-term fiscal challenges faced by the state and local government sector is through an indicator known as the "fiscal gap." The fiscal gap is an estimate of actions—such as revenue increases or expenditure reductions—that must be taken today and maintained for each year going forward to achieve fiscal balance during the simulation period. While we measured the gap as the amount of reductions in expenditures needed to prevent negative operating balances, increases in revenues, reductions in expenditures, or a combination of the two of sufficient magnitude would allow the sector to close the fiscal gap.

Our simulations suggest that the fiscal gap is about 14.7 percent of total expenditures or about 2.4 percent of GDP. That is, assuming no change in projected total revenues, eliminating the difference between the sector's expenditures and revenues during the 50-year simulation period would likely require action to be taken today, and maintained for each year equivalent to a 14.7 percent reduction in the sector's total expenditures (see Figure 4).[5] Alternatively, assuming no change in projected total expenditures, closing the fiscal gap by increasing revenue would also likely require actions of similar magnitude. More likely,

---

[3] The operating balance measure includes all receipts, excluding funds used for long-term investments, less current expenditures. To develop this measure, we subtract funds used to finance longer-term projects—such as investments in buildings and roads—from receipts since these funds would be unavailable to cover current expenses. Similarly, we exclude capital-related expenditures from spending. While most states have requirements related to balancing their budgets, deficits can arise because of unanticipated events such as recessions. These deficits can occur because the planned annual revenues are not generated at the expected rate, demand for services exceeds planned expenditures, or both, resulting in a near-term operating deficit. States have tapped fiscal reserves to cope with revenue shortfalls during recessions, as indicated by their reported total balances, which are composed of general fund ending balances and amounts in state budget stabilization "rainy day" funds. Figure 1 depicts the state and local simulated operating balance only, and does not include fiscal reserves or other budget measures used to cope with revenue shortfalls.

[4] Throughout this report we use GDP to refer to the U.S. GDP.

[5] Based on data from BEA, GDP totaled about $19.5 trillion in 2017.

eliminating the difference between expenditures and revenues would involve some combination of spending reductions and revenue increases.[6]

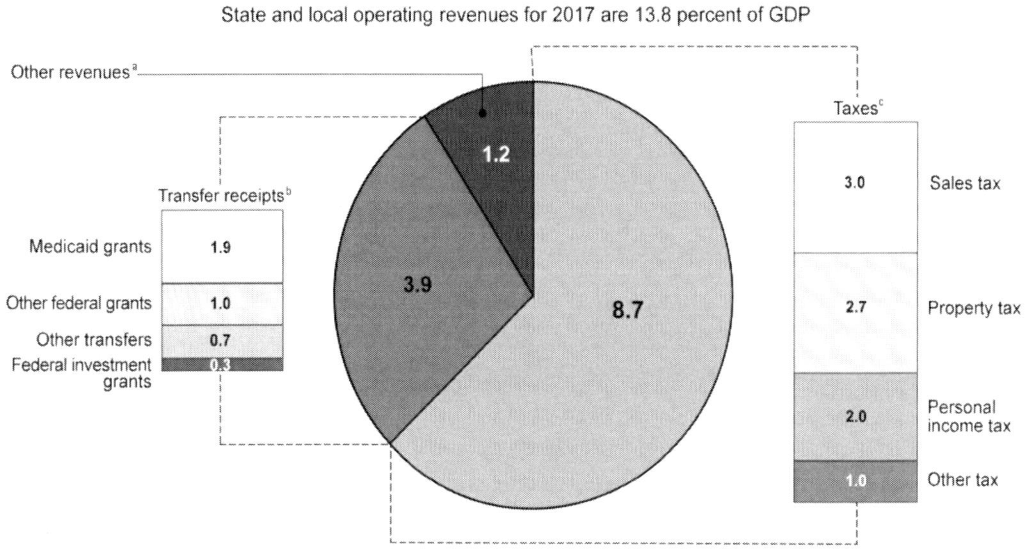

Source: GAO analysis of data from the Agency for Healthcare Research and Quality, Bloomberg, the Board of Governors of the Federal Reserve System, the Board of Trustees of the Federal Old-Age and Survivors Insurance and Federal Disability Insurance Trust Funds, the Bureau of Economic Analysis, the Bureau of Labor Statistics, the Census Bureau, the Centers for Medicare & Medicaid Services, the Congressional Budget Office, and the Federal Reserve Bank of St Louis. | GAO-19-208SP.

Notes: Operating revenues are comprised of the revenue components of the operating balance and include taxes, transfer receipts, and other types of revenues. State and local operating revenues were 13.8 percent of GDP in 2017.

[a]Other revenues include the issuance of medium- and long-term debt, interest earned and income from other assets including dividends, rents, and royalties on financial assets; and social insurance contributions (i.e., payments received for items such as disability insurance and workers compensation).

[b]Transfer receipts are receipts for which state and local governments provide nothing in return. Transfer receipts include Medicaid grants, other federal grants excluding Medicaid grants, other transfers (i.e., fines, fees, donations, and tobacco settlements), and federal investment grants (i.e., grants intended to finance capital infrastructure investments).

[c]Tax revenues include receipts from sales tax, property tax, personal income tax and other types of taxes (i.e., estate and gift tax, other personal tax, corporate income tax, and other production and import tax).

Figure 3. State and Local Government Sector Operating Revenues as a Percentage of Gross Domestic Product (GDP) in 2017.

[6] The "maintain balance" spending path shown in Figure 4 is illustrative. Our model assumes no economic effects from closing the state and local fiscal gap. Because abrupt spending declines or tax increases would likely have negative effects on both state and local governments, and the economy as a whole, the adjustments needed to achieve fiscal balance would likely need to be adopted gradually.

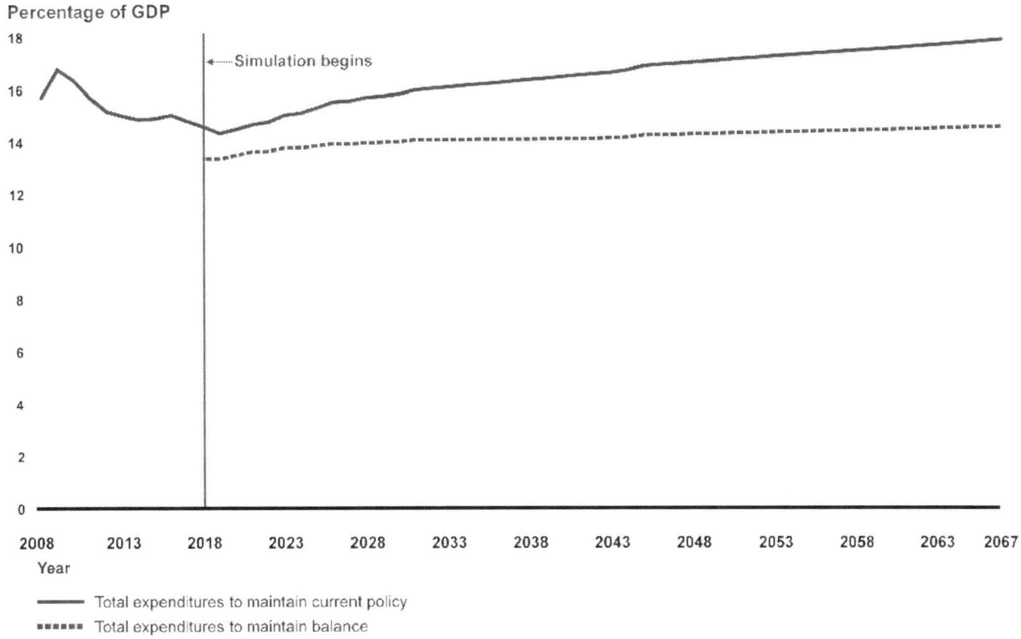

Source: GAO analysis of data from the Agency for Healthcare Research and Quality, Bloomberg, the Board of Governors of the Federal Reserve System, the Board of Trustees of the Federal Old-Age and Survivors Insurance and Federal Disability Insurance Trust Funds, the Bureau of Economic Analysis, the Bureau of Labor Statistics, the Census Bureau, the Centers for Medicare & Medicaid Services, the Congressional Budget Office, and the Federal Reserve Bank of St Louis. | GAO-19-208SP.

Figure 4. State and Local Government Action Required to Maintain Balance (Expenditure Reductions as a Percentage of Gross Domestic Product (GDP)), 2008 through 2067.

HEALTH CARE COST GROWTH AND OTHER FACTORS CONTRIBUTE TO THE STATE AND LOCAL SECTOR'S FISCAL IMBALANCE

Medicaid and Employee Health Benefits Are Key Drivers of Long-Term Spending

Our simulations suggest that growth in the sector's overall spending is largely driven by health care expenditures. As shown in Figure 5, these expenditures are projected to increase from about 4.1 percent of GDP in 2018 to 6.3 percent of GDP in 2067. Two types of health care expenditures—Medicaid spending and spending on health benefits for state and local government employees and retirees—will likely constitute a growing expenditure for state and local governments during the simulation period. Medicaid expenditures are expected to rise, on average, by 1 percentage point more than GDP each year.

According to CBO, growth in Medicaid spending reflects growth in both the number of people receiving Medicaid benefits and the cost of Medicaid benefits each person receives. Specifically, CBO reported that between 2019 and 2028, Medicaid spending is projected to grow at an average rate of 5.5 percent per year—nearly 5 percentage points of this growth is due to an increase in per capita costs and about 1 percentage point of this growth is due to an increase in enrollment. Data from CBO and the Centers for Medicare & Medicaid Services (CMS) also suggest that growth in Medicaid spending per capita is generally expected to outpace GDP growth in the future—referred to as excess cost growth.[7] Our estimates of Medicaid excess cost growth using CMS data suggest that Medicaid spending per capita will grow, on average, about 0.5 percent faster than GDP per capita for the period from 2018 through 2067.

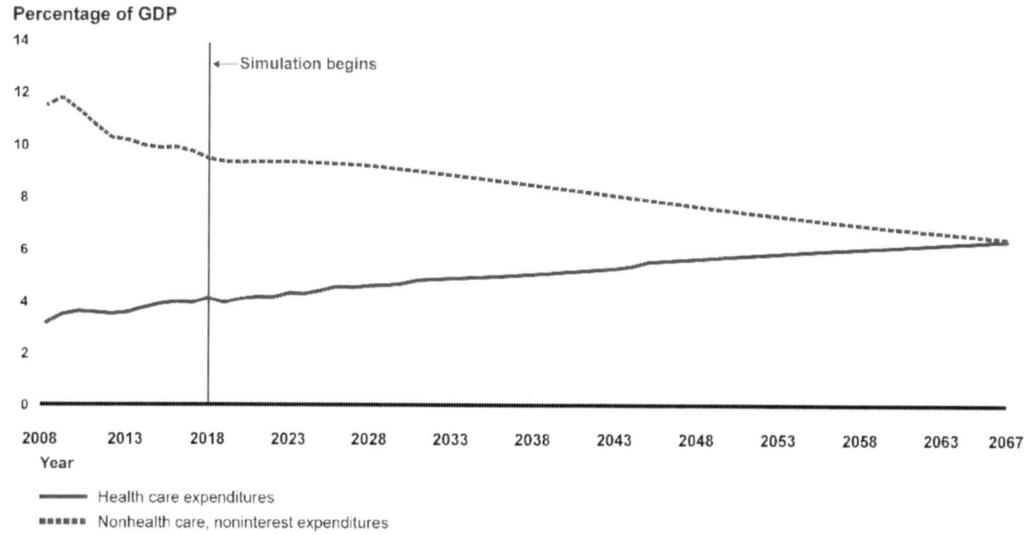

Source: GAO analysis of data from the Agency for Healthcare Research and Quality, Bloomberg, the Board of Governors of the Federal Reserve System, the Board of Trustees of the Federal Old-Age and Survivors Insurance and Federal Disability Insurance Trust Funds, the Bureau of Economic Analysis, the Bureau of Labor Statistics, the Census Bureau, the Centers for Medicare & Medicaid Services, the Congressional Budget Office, and the Federal Reserve Bank of St Louis. | GAO-19-208SP.

Note: Health expenditures include Medicaid social benefit payments, other social benefit payments for health care, and health benefits for state and local government employees and retirees. Nonhealth, noninterest expenditures include all other operating expenditures other than interest payments.

Figure 5. Health and Nonhealth, Noninterest Expenditures of State and Local Governments as a Percentage of Gross Domestic Product (GDP), 2008 through 2067.

Our simulations also suggest that health benefits for state and local government employees and retirees—a type of employee compensation spending—are likely to rise, on average, by 0.9 percentage points more than GDP each year. Growth in these health benefits also reflects growth in the projected number of employees and retirees and growth in the projected amount of health benefits for each employee and retiree. Growth in spending by states and local governments on health care per capita, which includes spending on employee and retiree health benefits, is generally expected to outpace GDP per capita. Data from CMS suggest that national health expenditures per capita are likely to grow on average about 0.8 percent faster than GDP per capita each year during the simulation period from 2018 through

[7] CBO's long-term projections of federal Medicaid spending incorporate average excess cost growth of about 1.5 percent annually from 2019 through 2028.

2067.[8] If employee and retiree health benefits follow trends in overall national health spending, they will likely make up an increasingly large share of total employee compensation going forward (see Figure 6).

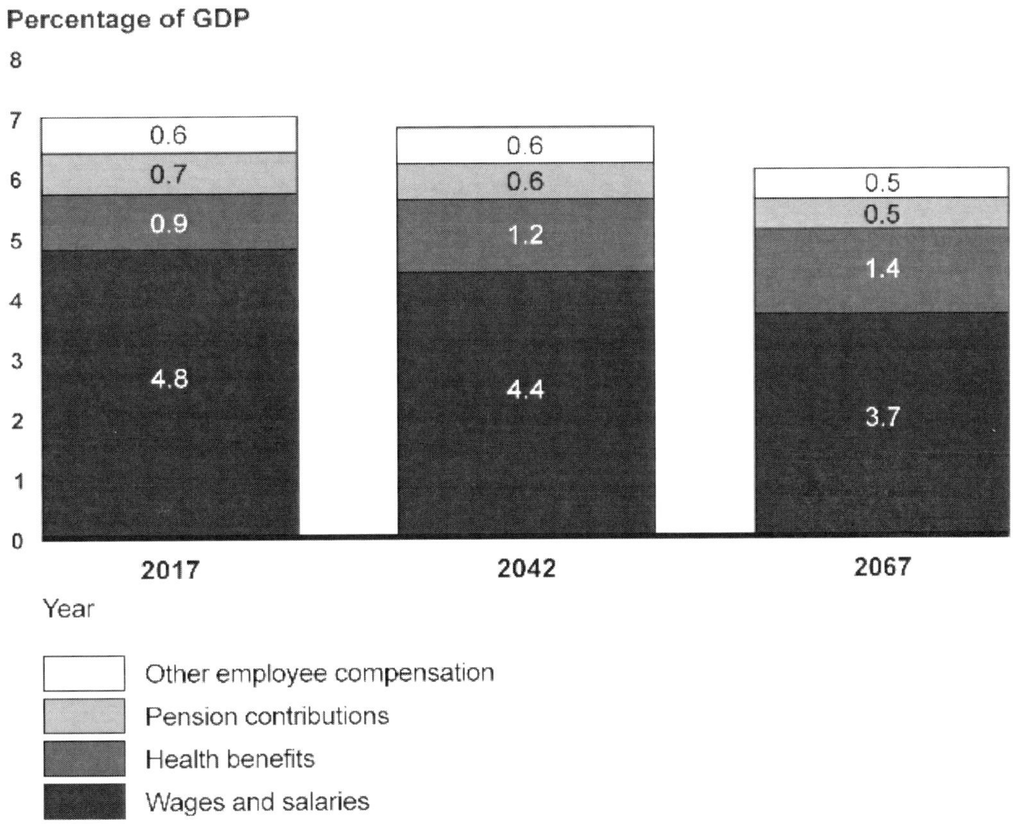

Source: GAO analysis of data from the Agency for Healthcare Research and Quality, Bloomberg, the Board of Governors of the Federal Reserve System, the Board of Trustees of the Federal Old-Age and Survivors Insurance and Federal Disability Insurance Trust Funds, the Bureau of Economic Analysis, the Bureau of Labor Statistics, the Census Bureau, the Centers for Medicare & Medicaid Services, the Congressional Budget Office, and the Federal Reserve Bank of St Louis. | GAO-19-208SP.

Note: State and local government spending on employee compensation includes compensation for general government employees only. Health benefits include health benefits for both active employees and for retirees. Other employee compensation includes benefits, such as life insurance and workers compensation contributions.

Figure 6. State and Local Government Sector Employee Compensation as a Percentage of Gross Domestic Product (GDP), 2017 through 2067.

---

[8] CMS measures national health expenditures as annual health spending in the United States for types of goods or services delivered (hospital care, physician and clinical services, retail prescription drugs, etc.) for sources of funding (private health insurance, Medicare, Medicaid, out-of-pocket spending, etc.) and for businesses, households, and governments.

While state and local government contributions to employee pension plans—another type of employee compensation spending—will likely decline as a percentage of GDP, as shown in Figure 6, our simulations nonetheless suggest that state and local governments may need to take steps to manage their pension obligations in the future. From 1998 through 2007, state and local governments' pension contributions amounted to about 8 percent of wages and salaries on average. In addition, for the period from 2008 through 2017, pension contributions amounted to about 12.3 percent of wages and salaries on average. Our simulations suggest that those pension contributions will need to be about 12.9 percent of wages and salaries for state and local governments to meet their long-term pension obligations.[9] This is the case even though pension asset values have increased in recent years, from about $2.4 trillion in 2008 to about $4.2 trillion in 2017 (adjusted for inflation and measured in 2012 dollars).[10] This suggests that state and local governments may need to take additional steps to manage their pension obligations by reducing benefits or increasing employees' contributions.

Along with pension contributions, other types of state and local government expenditures are projected to grow more slowly than GDP. For example, in 2017, wages and salaries of state and local government employees constituted a large expenditure for the sector. However, these expenditures are projected to decline as a percentage of GDP during the simulation period. Our simulations also suggest that state and local governments' capital outlays—which include spending on infrastructure, such as buildings, highways and streets, sewer systems, and water systems, as well as equipment and land— will grow more slowly than GDP if state and local governments continue to provide current levels of capital per resident.[11]

Growth in Medicaid Grants and Personal Income Taxes Drive Revenues

Our simulations suggest that federal grants overall will increase as a share of GDP, while Medicaid grants will likely grow more quickly than other types of federal grants (see Figure 7). Thus, Medicaid grants will likely make up an increasing share of revenues in the future. Since Medicaid is a matching formula grant program, the projected increase in federal Medicaid grants, therefore, reflects expected increased Medicaid expenditures that will be shared by state governments. Our simulations also suggest that federal investment grants (i.e., grants intended to finance capital infrastructure investments) and other federal grants

---

[9] Our model predicts future growth in the number of state and local government retirees based on the growth of the state and local government sector's workforce in earlier years.

[10] Our simulations are consistent with our past work, in which we have reported that while most state and local government pension plans have assets sufficient to cover benefit payments to retirees for a decade or more, plans have experienced a growing gap between assets and liabilities over the longer term. For additional information, see GAO, *The Nation's Retirement System: A Comprehensive Re-evaluation Is Needed to Better Promote Future Retirement Security*, GAO-18-111SP (Washington, D.C.: Oct. 18, 2017) and *State and Local Government Pension Plans: Economic Downturn Spurs Efforts to Address Costs and Sustainability*, GAO-12-322, (Washington, D.C.: Mar. 2, 2012).

[11] Some evidence suggests that maintaining current levels of capital per resident could become increasingly costly, at least for some types of capital. For example, according to CBO, nominal public spending on transportation and water infrastructure increased between 2003 and 2014. However, after adjusting for increases in the price of materials and other inputs during this period, spending actually decreased. For additional information see CBO, *Public Spending on Transportation and Water Infrastructure*, 1956 to 2014 (Washington, D.C.: March 2015).

unrelated to Medicaid (i.e., grants intended to finance education, social services, housing, and community investment) are likely to decline as a share of GDP.

Further, our simulations suggest that if historical relationships between state and local governments' tax revenues and tax bases persist, total tax revenues for the state and local government sector will increase from 8.8 percent of GDP in 2018 to 9.4 percent of GDP by the end of the simulation period. This increase is driven largely by the growth in personal income taxes, as shown in Figure 8. Specifically, our simulations suggest that personal income tax revenues will increase as a share of GDP by about 1 percentage point during the simulation period. Sales taxes and property taxes, on the other hand, are projected to remain relatively constant as a share of GDP during the simulation period through 2067.

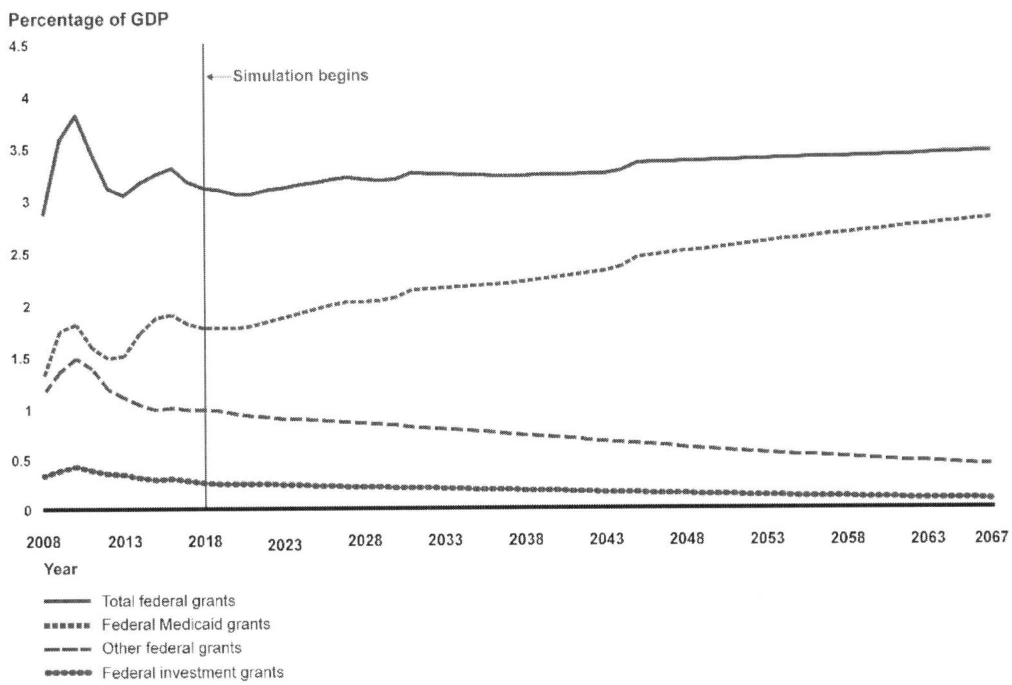

Source: GAO analysis of data from the Agency for Healthcare Research and Quality, Bloomberg, the Board of Governors of the Federal Reserve System, the Board of Trustees of the Federal Old-Age and Survivors Insurance and Federal Disability Insurance Trust Funds, the Bureau of Economic Analysis, the Bureau of Labor Statistics, the Census Bureau, the Centers for Medicare & Medicaid Services, the Congressional Budget Office, and the Federal Reserve Bank of St Louis. | GAO-19-208SP.

Note: Total federal grants to state and local governments are the sum of federal investment grants, federal Medicaid grants, and all other federal grants. Federal investment grants include grants that are intended to finance capital infrastructure investments.

Figure 7. Federal Grants to State and Local Governments as a Percentage of Gross Domestic Product (GDP), 2008 through 2067.

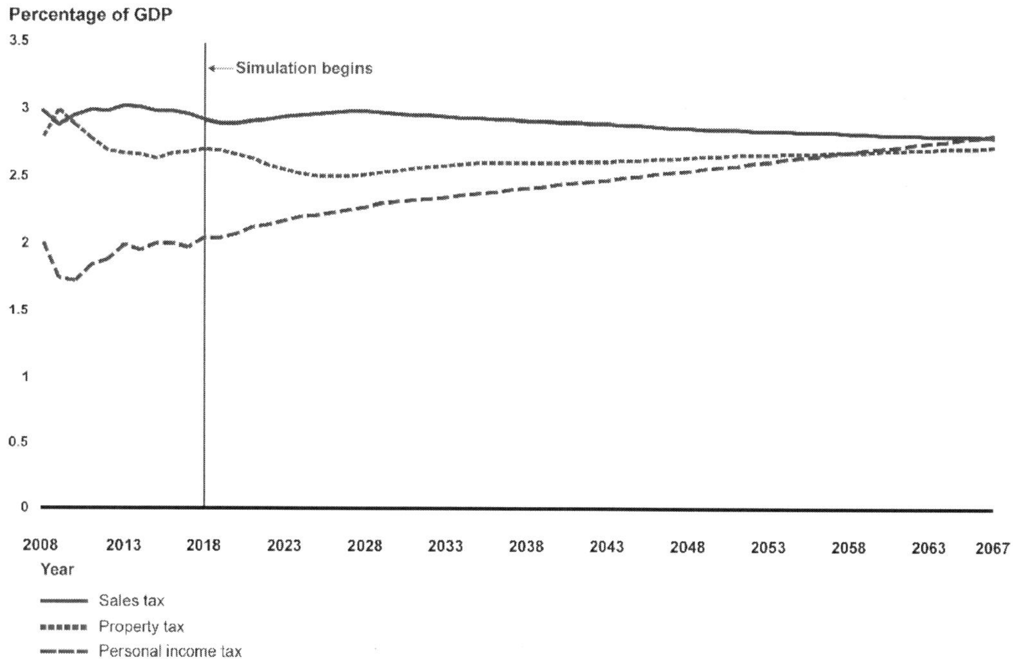

Source: GAO analysis of data from the Agency for Healthcare Research and Quality, Bloomberg, the Board of Governors of the Federal Reserve System, the Board of Trustees of the Federal Old-Age and Survivors Insurance and Federal Disability Insurance Trust Funds, the Bureau of Economic Analysis, the Bureau of Labor Statistics, the Census Bureau, the Centers for Medicare & Medicaid Services, the Congressional Budget Office, and the Federal Reserve Bank of St Louis. | GAO-19-208SP.

Note: Sales tax revenue is the sum of general sales tax revenue and excise tax revenue.

Figure 8. State and Local Government Tax Revenues as a Percentage of Gross Domestic Product (GDP), 2008 through 2067.

Policy Changes and Other Considerations Could Affect the State and Local Government Sector's Fiscal Outlook

While our long-term simulations do not account for pending or future federal policy changes that will result in changes to expenditures and revenues, an understanding of several recent federal policy changes related to taxes and health care are important to note because they present sources of uncertainty for the state and local government sector's long-term fiscal outlook. In addition, as is the case in any model that is reliant on historical data to simulate a long-term outlook, other considerations, such as economic growth and rates of return on pension assets, could shift future fiscal outcomes. These policy changes and uncertainties are discussed below and may help federal policy makers and state and local governments consider how these changes could affect the long-term outlook.

Tax-and Health-Related Policies Could Affect the Sector's Long-Term Fiscal Outlook

Tax Policies

Recently enacted legislation, such as Public Law 115-97, commonly referred to by the President and administrative documents as the Tax Cuts and Jobs Act (TCJA), could affect the sector's revenues over the long-term.[12] Enacted in December 2017, TCJA included significant changes to corporate and individual tax law, with implications for state and local government tax collections. In particular, for individual taxpayers, for tax years 2018 through 2025, tax rates were lowered for nearly all income levels, some deductions from taxable income were changed (personal exemptions were eliminated, while the standard deduction was increased), and certain credits, such as the child tax credit, were expanded.

The effect of TCJA on the long-term state and local fiscal outlook is still evolving, and will likely depend on how states incorporate the law's changes into their state income tax rules. That is, because some states link their state income taxes to federal income tax rules, states must decide whether to let the changes from TCJA flow through to their state income tax systems, or establish new state income tax rules. For example, some states have adopted the federal definition of taxable income as a starting point for state tax calculations, while other states use the federal definition of adjusted gross income as a starting point. The choices states make to continue to link to these definitions could have long-term implications for their state tax revenues. In addition, under TCJA, the amount of the federal itemized deductions allowed for all state and local income, sales, and property taxes (commonly referred to as the state and local tax (SALT) deduction) is now capped at $10,000 for tax years 2018 to 2025.[13] The magnitude or net effect of these changes is uncertain in that states are still working to understand the impact of the tax laws on their revenues. It remains to be seen whether and how states will see changes in their revenues in the future.

Moreover, a recent U.S. Supreme Court decision involving state sales taxes could have implications for states' ability to collect revenue. Specifically, the court's ruling in June 2018 in *South Dakota v. Wayfair, Inc.* held that states could require out-of-state sellers to collect and remit sales taxes on purchases made from those out-of-state sellers, even if the seller does not have a substantial physical presence in the taxing state.[14] Prior to this ruling, a seller that did not have a substantial physical presence in a state could not be required to collect and remit a sales tax on goods sold into the state. Instead, a purchaser may have been required to pay a use tax (i.e., a tax levied on the consumer for the privilege of use, ownership, or possession of taxable goods and services) in the same amount to his or her state government.[15] In 2017, we reported that states could realize between an estimated $8.5 billion and $13.4 billion in additional state sales tax revenue across all states if all sellers were required to collect taxes on all remote sales at current rates.[16] The extent to which states

---

[12] To provide for reconciliation pursuant to titles II and V of the concurrent resolution on the budget for fiscal year 2018, Pub. L. No. 115-97, 131 Stat. 2054 (2017) (hereinafter TCJA).

[13] 26 U.S.C. 164(b)(6).

[14] *South Dakota v. Wayfair, Inc.*, 138 S. Ct. 2080 (2018).

[15] However, we reported in 2017 that consumer compliance rates for use tax remittance are estimated to be very low. See GAO, *Sales Taxes: States Could Gain Revenue from Expanded Authority, but Businesses Are Likely to Experience Compliance Costs*, GAO-18-114 (Washington, D.C.: Nov. 16, 2017).

[16] GAO-18-114.

realize changes in sales tax revenue will likely depend on how they revise their state laws and enforcement efforts in response to this June 2018 ruling.

Health Care Policies

Enacted health care legislation could also affect the long-term fiscal position of state and local governments.[17] As we have reported in prior work, the effect of the Patient Protection and Affordable Care Act (PPACA) on the long-term state and local fiscal outlook could depend on how states implement PPACA, and on future rates of health care cost growth.[18] For example, consider the states that have opted, under PPACA, to expand Medicaid program coverage to millions of lower income adults. While the federal government is expected to cover a large share of the costs of the Medicaid expansion, these states are ultimately expected to bear some of the costs. Specifically, the federal government reimbursed 100 percent of the costs of the expanded population beginning in 2014.[19] This reimbursement rate will decline from the 2018 reimbursement rate of 94 percent to 90 percent by 2020. As such, the reduced federal reimbursement rate may affect those states that expanded their Medicaid populations in recent years.

As discussed earlier in this chapter, our simulations suggest that Medicaid spending will make up an increasing share of the state and local government sector's operating expenditures in the future. A weakening of the economy could add to the fiscal pressures states face in funding these Medicaid obligations. As our prior work has shown, past recessions in 2001 and 2007 hampered states' ability to fund increased Medicaid enrollment and maintain their existing services. Specifically, Medicaid enrollment increased during these recessions, in part due to increased unemployment, which led more individuals to become eligible for the program.[20]

We have also reported on the use of Medicaid demonstrations, which allow states to test new approaches to coverage to improve quality and access, or generate savings or efficiencies.[21] Specifically, CMS may waive certain Medicaid requirements and approve new types of expenditures that would not otherwise be eligible for federal Medicaid matching

---

[17] For additional information on Medicaid expansion, see GAO, *Medicaid: CMS Needs to Better Target Risks to Improve Oversight of Expenditures,* GAO-18-564, (Washington, D.C.: Aug. 6, 2018), *The Nation's Fiscal Health: Action Is Needed to Address the Federal Government's Fiscal Future,* GAO-18-299SP (Washington, D.C.: June 21, 2018), *Medicaid: Key Policy and Data Considerations for Designing a Per Capita Cap on Federal Funding,* GAO-16-726 (Washington, D.C.: Aug.10, 2016), *Medicaid: Changes to Funding Formula Could Improve Allocation of Funds to States,* GAO-16-377T (Washington, D.C.: Feb.10, 2016), and *Medicaid: Additional Efforts Needed to Ensure that State Spending is Appropriately Matched with Federal Funds,* GAO-16-53 (Washington, D.C.: Oct. 16, 2015).

[18] See for example, GAO, *State and Local Governments' Fiscal Outlook: 2016 Update*, GAO-17-213SP (Washington, D.C.: Dec. 8, 2016).

[19] Under PPACA, starting in 2014, states may opt to expand their Medicaid programs by covering nearly all adults with incomes at or below 133 percent of the federal poverty level. As of December 2017, 31 states and the District of Columbia expanded eligibility for their Medicaid programs under PPACA. This increased the number of people receiving Medicaid benefits.

[20] GAO, *Medicaid: Improving Responsiveness of Federal Assistance to States during Economic Downturns*, GAO-11-395 (Washington, D.C.: Mar. 31, 2011).

[21] For additional information on the use of Medicaid demonstrations, see GAO, *Medicaid: CMS Has Taken Steps to Address Program Risks but Further Actions Needed to Strengthen Program Integrity,* GAO-18-687T (Washington, D.C.: Aug. 21, 2018) and *Medicaid Demonstrations: Evaluations Yielded Limited Results, Underscoring Need for Changes to Federal Policies and Procedures,* GAO-18-220 (Washington D.C.: Jan. 19, 2018).

funds.[22] For example, under demonstrations, states have extended coverage to certain populations, provided services not otherwise eligible for Medicaid, and made payments to providers to incentivize delivery system improvements. We previously reported that, as of November 2016, nearly three-quarters of states have CMS-approved demonstrations. In fiscal year 2015, federal spending under demonstrations represented a third of all Medicaid spending nationwide.[23] We also reported that in 10 states, federal spending on demonstrations represented 75 percent or more of all federal spending on Medicaid.[24] Joint financing of Medicaid is a fixture of this federal-state partnership. Demonstration waivers hold the potential for changing state Medicaid spending. However, as we have reported, these demonstrations are required, under HHS policy, to achieve budget neutrality and not raise costs for the federal government.[25]

Economic Growth and Other Factors Could Affect the Sector's Fiscal Outlook

In addition to federal tax- and health-related policy changes, a number of other factors could affect the state and local government sector's long-term fiscal outlook. Specifically, we developed simulations using alternative assumptions of the growth of key model variables—which include economic growth, health care excess cost growth, and the rate of return on pension assets. We determined that changes in the growth projections of these key variables could affect the operating balance of state and local governments, thereby shifting future fiscal outcomes for the sector.[26]

Economic Growth

Future trends in GDP growth could affect the state and local government sector's fiscal outlook. Data from CBO and the Board of Trustees of the Federal Old-Age and Survivors Insurance and Federal Disability Insurance Trust Funds (OASDI Trustees) project real GDP to grow by 1.9 percent per year on average from 2018 through 2028, and by 2.1 percent per year on average after 2028, respectively.[27] Using these projections, our simulations suggest that maintaining current policies would cause the sector's expenditures to exceed its revenues and that the difference between revenues and expenditures would become increasingly

[22] Under section 1115 of the Social Security Act, the Secretary of Health & Human Services (HHS) may waive certain Medicaid requirements and approve new types of expenditures that would not otherwise be eligible for federal Medicaid matching funds for experimental, pilot, or demonstration projects that, in the Secretary's judgment, are likely to promote Medicaid objectives. See 42 U.S.C. § 1315(a). The Secretary has delegated the approval and administration of Medicaid section 1115 demonstrations to CMS, which requires that such demonstrations be budget neutral to the federal government; that is, the federal government should spend no more for Medicaid under a state's demonstration than it would have spent without the demonstration. There are also other types of waivers that states can apply for and use, including those approved under section 1915(c) of the Social Security Act, which authorizes the Secretary of HHS to waive requirements that states provide home and community based services that they would otherwise need to meet in the absence of the waiver.

[23] GAO-18-220.

[24] GAO-18-220.

[25] GAO-18-687T.

[26] For additional information on these simulations, see appendix II.

[27] Real GDP is a measure of the value of all the goods and services produced in the economy in a given year, adjusted for changes in the price level.

negative during the next several decades. However, simulations we developed using the OASDI Trustees' alternative projections of real GDP growth suggest that the difference between revenues and expenditures would expand before narrowing toward the end of the simulation period if real GDP were to grow at a faster rate—2.8 percent per year on average—as shown in Figure 9. Our simulations also show that if GDP were to grow at a slower rate—1.5 percent per year on average—the difference between revenues and expenditures would expand. This would result in an increasingly negative operating balance during the simulation period.

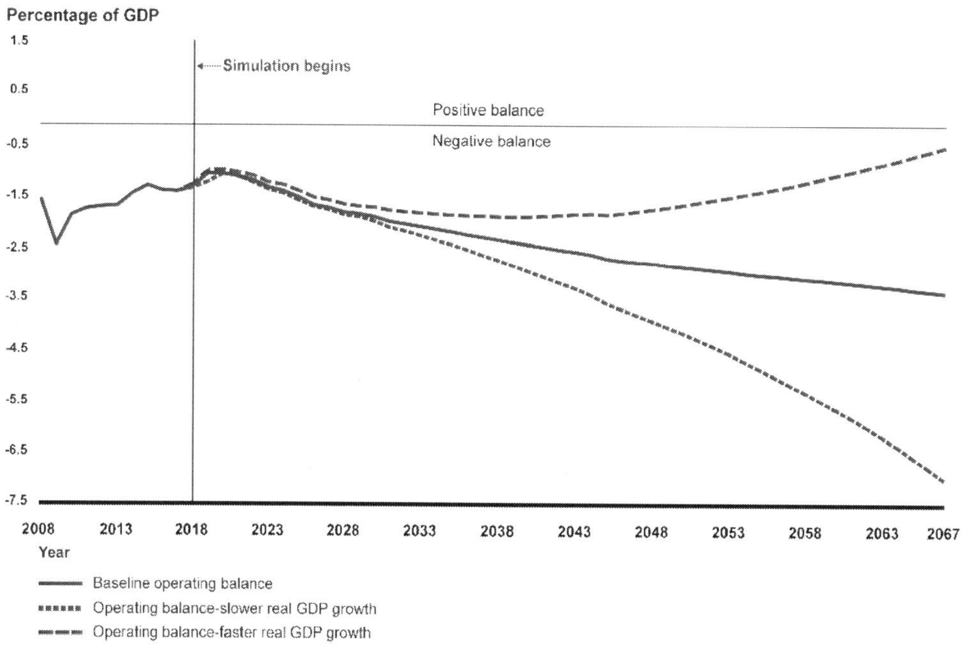

Source: GAO analysis of data from the Agency for Healthcare Research and Quality, Bloomberg, the Board of Governors of the Federal Reserve System, the Board of Trustees of the Federal Old-Age and Survivors Insurance and Federal Disability Insurance Trust Funds, the Bureau of Economic Analysis, the Bureau of Labor Statistics, the Census Bureau, the Centers for Medicare & Medicaid Services, the Congressional Budget Office, and the Federal Reserve Bank of St Louis. | GAO-19-208SP.

Note: The operating balance is defined as total receipts minus (1) capital outlays not financed by medium- and long-term debt issuance, (2) total current expenditures less depreciation, (3) current surplus of state and local government enterprises, and (4) net social insurance fund balance. For our baseline simulations, we used Congressional Budget Office projections of real GDP for the period from 2018 through 2028 and OASDI Trustees' intermediate projections of real GDP growth for the remainder of the simulation period. For our alternative simulations reflecting slower and faster real GDP growth, we used the OASDI Trustees' high- and low-cost projections of real GDP growth for the entire simulation period.

Figure 9. State and Local Government Sector Operating Balance under Alternative Gross Domestic Product (GDP) Growth Paths, 2008 through 2067.

Excess Cost Growth

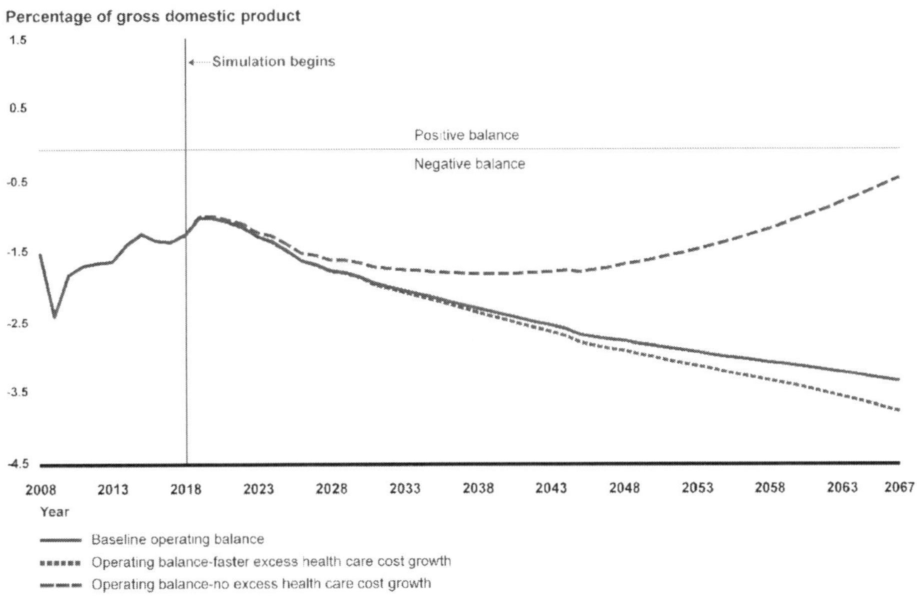

Source: GAO analysis of data from the Agency for Healthcare Research and Quality, Bloomberg, the Board of Governors of the Federal Reserve System, the Board of Trustees of the Federal Old-Age and Survivors Insurance and Federal Disability Insurance Trust Funds, the Bureau of Economic Analysis, the Bureau of Labor Statistics, the Census Bureau, the Centers for Medicare & Medicaid Services, the Congressional Budget Office, and the Federal Reserve Bank of St Louis. | GAO-19-208SP.

Note: The operating balance is defined as total receipts minus (1) capital outlays not financed by medium- and long-term debt issuance, (2) total current expenditures less depreciation, (3) current surplus of state and local government enterprises, and (4) net social insurance fund balance. For our baseline simulations, we used Medicaid cost growth derived from CMS's baseline projections for the period from 2029 through 2092, and we used CMS's baseline projections of national health care excess cost growth for the entire simulation period. For our alternative simulations reflecting higher excess cost growth, we used Medicaid cost growth derived from CMS's alternative projections for the period from 2029 through 2092, as well as CMS's alternative projections of national health expenditures excess cost growth. For our alternative simulations reflecting lower excess cost growth, we assumed that Medicaid excess cost growth is zero after 2028 and that national health expenditures excess cost growth is zero for the entire simulation period. For the period from 2018 through 2028, our simulations of variables related to Medicaid relied on CBO projections of two variables—federal spending on Medicaid, Children's Health Insurance Program, and exchange subsidies as a fraction of U.S. GDP and federal Medicaid grants to state and local governments—that already incorporate excess cost growth, so we could not apply alternative projections of Medicaid excess cost growth for these years.

Figure 10. State and Local Government Sector Operating Balance under Alternative Health Care Excess Cost Growth Paths, 2008 through 2067.

As discussed earlier in this chapter, excess cost growth in health care is another key determinant of the sector's fiscal balance. Data from CBO project Medicaid spending per capita to grow about 1.5 percent faster than GDP per capita on average for the period from 2019 through 2028. Data from CMS project Medicaid spending per capita to grow about 0.6

percent faster on average for the period from 2029 through 2067. Data from CMS also project national health expenditures per capita to grow about 0.8 percent faster than GDP per capita for the period from 2018 through 2067. Using these projections, our simulations suggest that maintaining current policies will cause the sector's expenditures to exceed its revenues, and that the difference between revenues and expenditures will become increasingly negative during the next several decades. However, simulations developed using alternative projections of excess cost growth in Medicaid and national health expenditures suggest that the difference between revenues and expenditures may be reduced but not eliminated within the simulation period if excess cost growth in health care is zero. In the scenario where excess cost growth rises faster—0.7 percent on average for Medicaid for the period from 2029 through 2067 and 1 percent for national health expenditures for the period from 2018 through 2067—our simulations show that the difference between revenues and expenditures will persist for the remainder of the simulation period (see Figure 10).

Rate of Return on Pension Assets

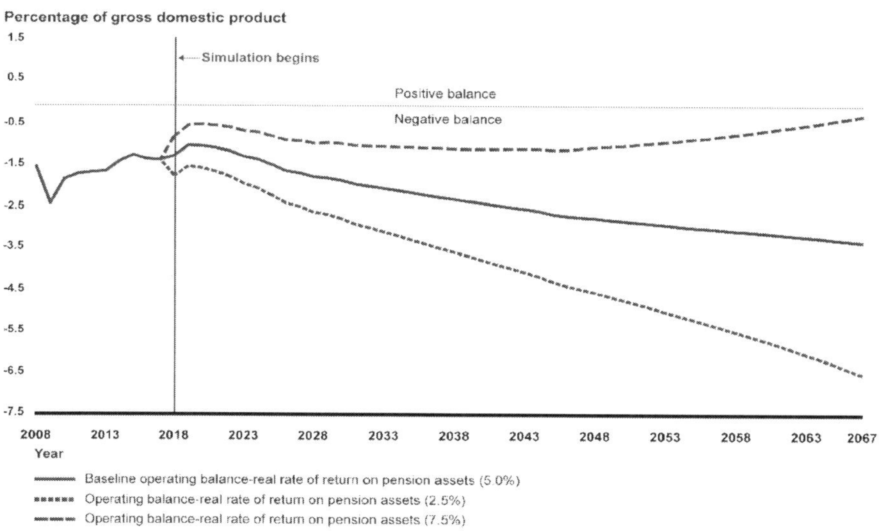

Source: GAO analysis of data from the Agency for Healthcare Research and Quality, Bloomberg, the Board of Governors of the Federal Reserve System, the Board of Trustees of the Federal Old-Age and Survivors Insurance and Federal Disability Insurance Trust Funds, the Bureau of Economic Analysis, the Bureau of Labor Statistics, the Census Bureau, the Centers for Medicare & Medicaid Services, the Congressional Budget Office, and the Federal Reserve Bank of St Louis. | GAO-19-208SP.

Note: The operating balance is defined as total receipts minus (1) capital outlays not financed by medium- and long-term debt issuance, (2) total current expenditures less depreciation, (3) current surplus of state and local government enterprises, and (4) net social insurance fund balance. The real rate of return on pension assets measures the return on pension assets after adjusting for changes in the price level. For our baseline simulations, we assumed that the real rate of return on pension assets is 5 percent throughout the simulation period, consistent with our prior work. For our alternative simulations reflecting higher and lower real rates of return on pension assets, we used real rates of return of 7.5 percent and 2.5 percent.

Figure 11. State and Local Government Sector Operating Balance under Alternative Assumptions for the Real Rate of Return on Pension Assets, 2008 through 2067.

The rate of return on pension assets could also affect the state and local government sector's fiscal outlook. Based on an inflation-adjusted rate of return on pension assets of 5 percent, our simulations suggest that state and local governments will need to make pension contributions equivalent to about 12.9 percent of their wages and salaries to meet their long-term pension obligations. However, this estimate is sensitive to the rate of return on state and local governments' pension assets. Simulations we developed using a higher rate of return—7.5 percent—suggest that pension contributions needed to meet pension obligations would be about 3 percent of state and local government employees' wages and salaries. In addition, under this scenario, our simulations suggest that the difference between revenues and expenditures will be reduced, but not eliminated within the simulation period. Alternatively, we estimated that if the rate of return on pension assets is relatively low—at 2.5 percent—required pension contributions would need to be about 23 percent of state and local government employees' wages and salaries during the simulation period. Under this scenario, our simulations show that the sector's negative operating balance will continue to grow larger throughout the simulation period. It follows therefore, that high rates of return on pension assets are associated with an improved outlook for state and local governments, and vice versa (see Figure 11).[28]

APPENDIX I: STATE AND LOCAL GOVERNMENT FISCAL MODEL SIMULATION METHODOLOGY

Data

To simulate measures of fiscal balance for the state and local government sector for the long term, we used aggregate data on the state and local government sector and national data on other variables from the following sources:

- Agency for Healthcare Research and Quality;
- Bloomberg;
- Board of Governors of the Federal Reserve System;
- Board of Trustees of the Federal Old-Age and Survivors Insurance and Federal Disability Insurance Trust Funds (OASDI Trustees);
- Bureau of Economic Analysis (BEA);
- Bureau of Labor Statistics;
- Census Bureau;
- Centers for Medicare & Medicaid Services (CMS);
- Congressional Budget Office (CBO); and
- Federal Reserve Bank of St. Louis.

[28] We do not consider the possibility of altered benefit promises here because we treat these as policy changes, which we hold fixed throughout in the model.

Model Specification

Overview

Our approach generally follows the approach used in GAO-08-317 and in subsequent updates of that report. Specifically, we developed a model that projects the levels of receipts and expenditures of the state and local government sector (henceforth, the sector) in future years based on current and historical spending and revenue patterns. We use Table 3.3 of the National Income and Product Accounts (NIPA)—State and Local Government Current Receipts and Expenditures—prepared by BEA at the U.S. Department of Commerce as an organizing framework for developing our model of the sector's revenues and expenditures (see Table 1). In this table, current revenues are grouped in five main categories.

- Current tax receipts. These receipts are tax payments made by persons or businesses to state and local governments. They include income taxes, general sales taxes, property taxes, and excise taxes. Current taxes also include fees for motor vehicle licenses, drivers' licenses, and business licenses.
- Social insurance contributions. These contributions finance the provision of certain social benefits to qualified persons, and include contributions from employers and employees for temporary disability insurance, worker's compensation insurance, and other programs.
- Income receipts from government assets. These receipts include interest, dividends, and rental income, such as royalties paid on drilling on the outer continental shelf. Also, state and local governments earn interest and dividend income on financial assets.
- Current transfer receipts. Transfer receipts are receipts for which state and local governments provide nothing of value in return. Current transfer receipts include federal grants, fines, fees, donations, and tobacco settlements. Also included are net insurance settlements, certain penalty taxes, court fees, and other miscellaneous transfers.
- Current surplus of government enterprises. This surplus is a profit-type measure for state and local government enterprises, such as water, sewer, gas, and electricity providers; toll providers; liquor stores; air and water terminals; public transit; and state lotteries. Some types of enterprises, such as state lotteries, consistently earn surpluses which are used to fund general government activities. In contrast, many enterprises run deficits, which, in turn, reduce receipts.

State and local governments also receive income from the sale of goods and services, such as school tuition. In the NIPAs, this income is treated as an offset against expenditures, not revenue. This income comes from voluntary purchases that might have been made from a private sector provider of such services.

In addition to current receipts, state and local governments receive capital transfer receipts. These receipts include estate and gift taxes, and federal government investment grants for capital such as highways, transit, air transportation, and water treatment plants.

Table 1. State and Local Government Receipts and Expenditures in National Income and Product Accounts (NIPA), 2017 (dollars in billions)

Description	Amount
Current receipts	2,484.2
Current tax receipts	1,689.9
Personal current taxes	421.2
Income taxes	386.7
Other	34.5
Taxes on production and imports	1,215.7
General sales taxes	395.7
Excise taxes	190.7
Property taxes	532.2
Other	97.1
Taxes on corporate income	52.9
Contributions for government social insurance	20.6
Income receipts on assets	86.0
Interest receipts	68.8
Dividends	5.9
Rents and royalties	11.3
Current transfer receipts	690.7
Federal grants	559.3
From business (net)	51.5
From persons	80.0
Current surplus of government enterprises	-2.9
Current expenditures	2,743.3
Consumption expenditures	1,744.5
Current transfer payments	712.3
Government social benefit payments to persons	712.3
Interest payments	286.0
To persons and business	282.8
To the rest of the world	3.2
Subsidies	0.6
Net state and local government saving	-259.1
Social insurance funds	4.0
Other	-263.1
Addenda:	
Total receipts	**2,558.3**
Current receipts	2,484.2
Capital transfer receipts	74.0
Total expenditures	**2,857.3**
Current expenditures	2,743.3
Gross government investment	364.8
Capital transfer payments	1.2
Net purchases of nonproduced assets	13.5
Less: Consumption of fixed capital (depreciation)	265.6
Net lending or net borrowing (-)	-299.0

Source: NIPA, Table 3.3. | GAO-19-208SP.

Note: Totals may not add due to rounding.

State and local government current expenditures are grouped into four main categories.

- Consumption expenditures. Generally, spending for which some value is provided in return. State and local government consumption spending is the sum of inputs used to provide goods and services, including compensation of general government employees, consumption of general government fixed capital (depreciation), and intermediate goods and services purchased, less sales to other sectors and own-account investment.
- Current transfer payments. Payments for which nothing of value is provided in return. For state and local governments, current transfer payments consist primarily of social benefits, which are payments to persons to provide for needs that arise from circumstances such as sickness, unemployment, retirement, and poverty. There are two kinds of social benefits—benefits from social insurance funds, such as temporary disability insurance and workers' compensation, and other social benefits, such as medical benefits from Medicaid and the state Children's Health Insurance Program (CHIP), family assistance from Temporary Assistance to Needy Families, education assistance, and other public assistance programs. While NIPA Table 3.3 also includes other current transfer payments to the rest of the world as part of current transfer payments, these amounts are generally equal to zero.
- Interest payments. These include actual and imputed interest and represent the cost of borrowing by state and local governments to finance their capital and operational costs.
- Subsidies. State and local government subsidies are largely payments to railroads.

State and local government spending also includes gross investment, capital transfer payments, and net purchases of nonproduced assets. Gross investment is spending on capital goods like structures, equipment, and intellectual property—items that are called fixed assets or capital because of their repeated or continuous use in providing government services for more than 1 year. Structures include residential and commercial buildings, highways and streets, sewer systems, and water systems. State and local government capital transfer payments include disaster-related insurance benefits paid to the U.S. territories and the Commonwealths of Puerto Rico and Northern Mariana Islands. Net purchases of nonproduced assets are composed of net purchases of land less oil bonuses (payments to states for the long-term rights to extract oil).

Our main indicator of the sector's fiscal balance is its operating balance net of funds for capital expenditures (henceforth, operating balance), which is a measure of the sector's ability to cover its current expenditures out of current revenues. The operating balance is defined as total receipts minus (1) capital outlays not financed by medium- and long-term debt issuance, (2) total current expenditures less depreciation, (3) current surplus of state and local government enterprises, and (4) net social insurance fund balance.[29]

[29] We refer to the sum of state and local government gross investment, net purchases of nonproduced assets, and capital transfer payments as capital outlays.

Alternative indicators of fiscal balance include net saving and net lending or borrowing.

- Net saving is the difference between current receipts and current expenditures. Since current expenditures exclude capital investment but include a depreciation measure, net saving can be thought of as a measure of the extent to which governments are covering their current operations from current receipts.
- Net lending or borrowing is the difference between total receipts and total expenditures, and is analogous to the federal unified surplus or deficit. Total receipts differ from current receipts because they include capital transfer receipts. Total expenditures differ from current expenditures because they include capital investment, capital transfer payments, and net purchases of nonproduced assets. However, they exclude fixed capital consumption. The former three categories are cash expenditures, while the latter is a noncash charge. Net lending or net borrowing represents the governments' cash surplus or borrowing requirement. This measure is normally negative because governments borrow to finance their capital investment (and sometimes to finance current operations as well).

The following equations describe how we simulated state and local government receipts and expenditures, as well as the intermediate variables used in those simulations. For this update, we started with historical data for 2017, or the most recent year available, and then simulated each variable for each year from 2018 through 2092 (the simulation period).

National Demographic, Macroeconomic, and Health Care Variables

To simulate state and local government receipts and expenditures, we use simulations of various national-level demographic, macroeconomic, and health care variables derived from projections produced by CBO, CMS, and the OASDI Trustees, and otherwise derived using our own assumptions (see Table 2). This approach is similar to the approach we have used in prior model updates.

State and Local Government Defined Benefit Pension Contribution Rate

To simulate state and local government spending on defined benefit pensions, we first estimate the contribution rate (as a fraction of state and local government general government wages and salaries) that state and local governments would need to make each year going forward to ensure that their pension systems are fully funded on an ongoing basis. Our goal is to estimate the financial commitments to employees that have been and are likely to continue to be made by the state and local sector to better understand the full fiscal outlook for the sector. As such, our analysis projects the liabilities that the sector is likely to continue to incur in the future based on simulations of future numbers of retirees receiving pension benefits and their benefit amounts; future numbers of employees, their wages and salaries, and their pension contributions; and assets in state and local government defined benefit pension funds. Although we are only interested in applying contribution rates over the simulation time frame, we actually have to derive the contribution rate for a longer time frame in order to find the steady-state level of necessary contributions.[30]

---

[30] We used a 400-year period to estimate the steady-state pension contribution rate.

Table 2. Simulation Approach for National Demographic, Macroeconomic, Health Care, and Other Key Variables

	Simulation approach for...	
Variable	**... 2018 through 2028**	**... 2029 through 2092**
Real U.S. gross domestic product (GDP)	Grows at the same rate as Congressional Budget Office (CBO) projection	Grows at the same rate as the Board of Trustees of the Federal Old-Age and Survivors Insurance and Federal Disability Insurance Trust Funds (OASDI Trustees) intermediate projection
U.S. GDP price index	Grows at the same rate as CBO projection	Grows at the same rate as prior year
U.S. consumer price index	Grows at the same rate as CBO projection	Grows at the same rate as prior year
U.S. private sector employment cost index	Grows at the same rate as CBO projection	Grows at the same rate as prior year
U.S. GDP	Grows at the same rate as CBO projection	Grows at the same rate as real U.S. GDP multiplied by the U.S. GDP price index
U.S. total wages and salaries	Grows at the same rate as CBO projection	Grows at the same rate as real U.S. GDP multiplied by the U.S. GDP price index
U.S. personal income	Grows at the same rate as CBO projection	Grows at the same rate as real U.S. GDP multiplied by the U.S. GDP price index
U.S. domestic corporate profits	Grows at the same rate as CBO projection	Grows at the same rate as real U.S. GDP multiplied by the U.S. GDP price index
3-month Treasury rate	Equals CBO projection	Remains constant at last value of CBO projection
10-year Treasury rate	Equals CBO projection	Remains constant at last value of CBO projection
Federal government spending on Medicaid, Children's Health Insurance Program, and exchange subsidies as a fraction of GDP	Equals CBO projection (which incorporates excess cost growth)	Equals CBO projection through 2047 (which assumes zero excess cost growth), then remains constant at 2047 value
U.S. population	Equals OASDI Trustees' intermediate projection	
National health expenditures excess cost growth multiplier	Equals Centers for Medicare & Medicaid Services (CMS) baseline projection	
Medicaid excess cost growth multiplier	Equals growth rate of national health expenditures less Medicare spending as a fraction of age and gender-adjusted U.S. GDP based on CMS baseline projections	
Federal government share of total Medicaid spending	Minimum of CBO's projected range of federal government share of Medicaid spending	
State and local government employment cost index	Grows at the same rate as U.S. private sector employment cost index	
Spread between 20-year and 1-year Treasury rates	Equal to its last historical value	
U.S. personal consumption expenditures less food and services	Two-step process that first simulates real personal consumption expenditures based on its elasticity with respect to real wages and salaries, and then adjusts for inflation using the U.S. GDP price index; see Table 8 and the "Estimated Historical Relationships" section below for details.	
U.S. market value of real estate	Two-step process that first simulates the real market value of real estate based on its elasticity with respect to real U.S. GDP and then adjusts for inflation using the U.S. GDP price index; see Table 8 and the "Estimated Historical Relationships" section below for details.	

Source: GAO. | GAO-19-208SP.

This longer time frame is required because the estimated contribution rate increases as the projection horizon increases and eventually converges to a steady state. If the projection period is of insufficient length, the steady-state level of contribution is not attained, and the necessary contribution rate is understated. We simulated variables used to estimate the pension contribution rate using the approach summarized in Table 3. This approach is similar to the approach we have used in prior model updates.

State and Local Government Defined Benefit Pension Contribution Rate

To simulate state and local government spending on defined benefit pensions, we first estimate the contribution rate (as a fraction of state and local government general government wages and salaries) that state and local governments would need to make each year going forward to ensure that their pension systems are fully funded on an ongoing basis. Our goal is to estimate the financial commitments to employees that have been and are likely to continue to be made by the state and local sector to better understand the full fiscal outlook for the sector. As such, our analysis projects the liabilities that the sector is likely to continue to incur in the future based on simulations of future numbers of retirees receiving pension benefits and their benefit amounts; future numbers of employees, their wages and salaries, and their pension contributions; and assets in state and local government defined benefit pension funds.

Table 3. Simulation Approach for Variables Used to Estimate State and Local Government Defined Benefit Pension Contribution Rate

Variable	Simulation approach
Real rate of return on state and local government pension assets	5 percent
Number of state and local government general government and government enterprise employees	Grows at the same rate as U.S. population
Number of state and local government retirees	Growth rate equals the weighted average of the growth rates of past general government and government enterprise employment
Wages and salaries for state and local government general government and government enterprise employees	Grows at the same rate as U.S. population times the private sector employment cost index
Mortality rate for retired state and local government employees receiving periodic benefit payments	Remains constant at the 2017 value of the mortality rate for Federal Old-Age, Survivors, and Disability Insurance Program beneficiaries
Employment cost index for state and local government retirees	Weighted average of past values of the state and local government employment cost index
Pension benefits paid for state and local government retirees	Grows at the same rate as the number of state and local government retirees times the employment cost index for state and local government retirees times the Consumer Price Index
State and local government employee pension contributions	Grows at the same rate as wages and salaries for state and local government employees

Source: GAO. | GAO-19-208SP.

Although we are only interested in applying contribution rates over the simulation time frame, we actually have to derive the contribution rate for a longer time frame in order to find the steady-state level of necessary contributions.[31] This longer time frame is required because the estimated contribution rate increases as the projection horizon increases and eventually

[31] We used a 400-year period to estimate the steady-state pension contribution rate.

converges to a steady state. If the projection period is of insufficient length, the steady-state level of contribution is not attained, and the necessary contribution rate is understated. We simulated variables used to estimate the pension contribution rate using the approach summarized in Table 3. This approach is similar to the approach we have used in prior model updates.

Future growth in the number of state and local government retirees— many of whom will be entitled to pension and health care benefits—is largely driven by the size of the workforce in earlier years. We simulated the number of state and local government retirees by assuming that the growth rate in the number of retirees is a weighted average of the growth rates in lagged general government and government enterprise employment. We estimated the weights using a regression of the percent change in the number of retirees on the percent change in employment 1, 6, 11, 16, 21, 26, 31, 36, and 41 years in the past. The coefficients on the past percentage changes in employment were constrained to be non-negative and to sum to 1. For this regression, we removed cyclical swings in employment using the Hodrick-Prescott filter.

Similarly, future changes in the real amount of pension benefits will be a function of past changes in real wages and salaries. As indicated in Table 3, we used a weighted average of past values of the state and local government employment cost index to simulate the employment cost index for state and local government retirees. We chose the weights to reflect changes in the share and average real benefit level of three subsets of the retiree population over time: (1) new retirees entering the beneficiary pool, (2) deceased retirees leaving the pool, and (3) continuing retirees from the previous year.

- We simulated the weight for new retirees in a year as the number of retirees less the number of continuing retirees divided by the number of retirees.
- We simulated the weight for deceased retirees as the mortality rate multiplied by last year's retirees divided by this year's retirees.
- We simulated the weight for continuing retirees as last year's retirees divided by this year's retirees.

Finally, we simulated the employment cost index for state and local government retirees as the sum of the weight on new retirees multiplied by the state and local government employment cost index and the weight on continuing retirees multiplied by the state and local government employment cost index 8 years prior, less the weight on deceased retirees multiplied by the state and local government employment cost index 21 years prior.

As discussed above, we started with historical data for 2017, or the most recent year available, simulated all of the variables in Table 3 over the long run, and then used the consumer price index (CPI) and the real return on pension assets to calculate the total present value of wages and salaries for state and local government general government and government enterprise employees, the total present value of real pension benefits paid to state and local government retirees, and the total present value of state and local government employees' pension contributions.[32] Then, we calculated the total present value of state and local governments' pension liabilities as the total present value of real pension benefits paid to state and local government retirees less the total present value of state and local

[32] We used the 400-year period from 2018 to 2417 to estimate the steady-state pension contribution rate.

government employees' pension contributions, and the value of assets in state and local government defined benefit pension funds in 2017. Finally, we estimated state and local governments' pension contribution rate as the ratio of the total present value of their pension liabilities to the total present value of wages and salaries for state and local government employees.

Interest Rates on State and Local Government Financial Assets and Liabilities

Table 4. Simulation Approach for Interest Rates on State and Local Government Financial Assets and Liabilities

Variable	Simulation approach
Effective interest rate on state and local government financial assets	Based on the historical relationship between the effective interest rate on state and local government financial assets and the 3-month Treasury rate; see Table 8 and the "Estimated Historical Relationships" section below for details
State and local government bond yields	Based on the historical relationship between state and local government bond yields and 10-year Treasury rates; see Table 8 and the "Estimated Historical Relationships" section below for details
Effective interest rate on medium-and long-term debt and federal government loans	Based on the historical relationship between the effective interest rate on medium-and long-term debt and federal government loans and state and local government bond yields; see Table 8 and the "Estimated Historical Relationships" section below for details

Source: GAO. | GAO-19-208SP.

Table 4 summarizes the approach we used to simulate interest rates on state and local government financial assets and liabilities. This approach is similar to the approach we have used in prior model updates.

State and Local Government Receipts

Table 5 summarizes our approach to simulating state and local government receipts. This approach is similar to the approach we have used in prior model updates.

These variables track state and local government receipts in Table 1 below as follows:

- State and local government personal income tax revenue is the sum of state personal income tax revenue and local personal income tax revenue;
- State and local government personal tax revenue is the sum of personal income tax revenue and other personal tax revenue;
- State and local government revenue from taxes on production and imports is the sum of general sales tax revenue, excise tax revenue, property tax revenue, and revenue from other taxes on production and imports;
- State and local government current tax revenue is the sum of personal tax revenue, revenue from taxes on production and imports, and corporate income tax revenue;
- State and local government current transfer receipts are equal to federal Medicaid grants minus Medicare Part D payments to the federal government, plus other federal grants (excluding investment grants), transfer receipts from businesses, and transfer receipts from persons;

Table 5. Simulation Approach for State and Local Government Receipts

	Simulation approach	
Variable	...for 2018 through 2028	...for 2029 through 2092
Federal investment grants to state and local governments	Grows at the same rate as Congressional Budget Office (CBO) projections of federal capital transfers	Grows at the same rate as U.S. population times the U.S. gross domestic product (GDP) price index
Federal Medicaid grants to state and local governments	Grows at the same rate as CBO projection (which incorporates Medicaid excess cost growth)	Grows at the same rate as federal spending on Medicaid, Children's Health Insurance Program, and exchange subsidies, multiplied by Medicaid excess cost growth
Medicare Part D payments from state and local governments to the federal government	Grows at the same rate as CBO projection	Grows at the same rate as federal Medicaid grants to state and local governments
Other federal non-Medicaid, non-investment grants to state and local governments	Equals difference between (1) total federal non-investment grants and (2) federal Medicaid grants to state and local governments net of Medicare Part D payments to the federal government	Grows at the same rate as U.S. population times the U.S. GDP price index
Estate and gift tax revenue for state and local governments	Equal to prior year's value times 1 plus the 10-year Treasury rate	
State government personal income tax revenue	Two-step process that first simulates real state personal income tax revenues based on their historical elasticity with respect to real taxable personal income, and then adjusts for inflation using the U.S. GDP price index; see Table 9 and the "Estimated Historical Relationships" section below for details	
Local government personal income tax revenue	Grows at the same rate as personal income	
Other personal tax revenue for state and local governments	Grows at the same rate as personal income	
General sales tax revenue for state and local governments	Grows at the same rate as personal consumption expenditures less food and services	
Excise tax revenue for state and local governments	Two-step process that first simulates real state and local government excise tax revenue based on its historical elasticity with respect to real wages and salaries and then adjusts for inflation using the U.S. GDP price index; see Table 9 and the "Estimated Historical Relationships" section below for details.	
Property tax revenue for state and local governments	Grows at the same rate as the U.S. market value of real estate	
Revenue from other taxes on production and imports for state and local governments	Grows at the same rate as U.S. GDP	
Corporate income tax revenue for state and local governments	Grows at the same rate as domestic corporate profits	
Social insurance contributions for state and local governments	Grow at the same rate as wages and salaries	
Income from state and local government financial assets	Equals the effective interest rate on financial assets times assets outstanding in prior year	
Transfers from businesses to state and local governments	Grow at the same rate as U.S. GDP	
Transfers from people to state and local governments	Grow at the same rate as U.S. GDP	
Surplus of state and local government enterprises	Equal to zero	

Source: GAO. | GAO-19-208SP.

These variables track state and local government receipts in Table 1 above as follows:

- State and local government personal income tax revenue is the sum of state personal income tax revenue and local personal income tax revenue;
- State and local government personal tax revenue is the sum of personal income tax revenue and other personal tax revenue;
- State and local government revenue from taxes on production and imports is the sum of general sales tax revenue, excise tax revenue, property tax revenue, and revenue from other taxes on production and imports;
- State and local government current tax revenue is the sum of personal tax revenue, revenue from taxes on production and imports, and corporate income tax revenue;
- State and local government current transfer receipts are equal to federal Medicaid grants minus Medicare Part D payments to the federal government, plus other federal grants (excluding investment grants), transfer receipts from businesses, and transfer receipts from persons;
- State and local government current receipts are the sum of current tax revenue, current transfer receipts, income on assets, social insurance contributions, and government enterprise surplus;
- State and local government capital transfer receipts are the sum of federal investment grants and estate and gift tax revenue; and
- State and local government total receipts are the sum of current receipts and capital transfer receipts.

State and Local Government Expenditures

Our general approach to simulating state and local government expenditures is to assume that state and local governments maintain the current level of public goods and services provision per capita (see Table 6). Thus, we generally assume that expenditures keep up with U.S. population growth and some measure of inflation, where the relevant rate of inflation varies depending on the specific type of expenditure. However, we use alternative approaches—described below—to simulate depreciation, interest payments, and social benefits for health care. This approach is similar to the approach we have used in prior model updates.

These variables correspond to state and local government expenditures in Table 1 as follows:

- Employee compensation is the sum of wages and salaries, pension contributions, health benefits for current employees, health benefits for retirees, and other compensation, for state and local government general government employees.
- Consumption expenditures are the sum of employee compensation, general government fixed capital consumption, and other general government consumption expenditures.
- Social benefit payments are the sum of Medicaid benefits, non-Medicaid health benefits, and non-health social benefits.
- Current expenditures are the sum of consumption expenditures, social benefit payments, interest payments, and subsidy payments.

- Total expenditures are the sum of current expenditures, gross investment, capital transfer payments, and purchases of nonproduced assets, minus general government and government enterprise fixed capital consumption.

Table 6. Simulation Approach for State and Local Government Expenditures

Variable	Simulation approach
Wages and salaries for state and local government general government employees	Grows at the same rate as U.S. population times the private sector employment cost index
Contributions to defined benefit pension funds for general government employees	Equal to wages and salaries for state and local government general government employees times the pension contribution rate
Health benefits for current state and local government employees	Grows at the same rate as U.S. gross domestic product (GDP), multiplied by national health expenditures excess cost growth
Health benefits for state and local government retirees	Grows at the same rate as the number of retirees times U.S. GDP per capita, multiplied by national health expenditures excess cost growth
Other state and local government employee compensation	Grows at the same rate as U.S. population times the U.S. employment cost index for private wages and salaries
State and local government purchases of nonproduced assets	Grows at the same rate as U.S. population times the U.S. GDP price index
Capital transfer payments from state and local governments	Equal to zero
Gross investment by state and local governments	Grows at the same rate as U.S. population times the U.S. GDP price index
Depreciation rate of state and local government capital	Equal to the last historical value of the 5-year moving average of the depreciation rate
Real state and local government capital stock	Equal to prior year capital stock less depreciation, plus gross investment adjusted for inflation using the U.S. GDP price index
Consumption of general government and government enterprise fixed capital	Equals the depreciation rate times the real capital stock in the prior year times the U.S. GDP price index
Consumption of state and local government general government fixed capital	Grows at the same rate as consumption of general government and government enterprise fixed capital
Other state and local government consumption spending	Grows at the same rate as U.S. population times the U.S. GDP price index
Medicaid social benefit payments from state and local governments	Equal to federal Medicaid grants divided by the federal government share of total Medicaid spending
Non-Medicaid social benefit payments for health care from state and local governments	Grow at the same rate as federal spending on Medicaid, Children's Health Insurance Program, and exchange subsidies (which incorporates Congressional Budget Office projections of excess cost growth for 2018 through 2028), multiplied by Medicaid excess cost growth for 2029 through 2092
Non-health social benefit payments from state and local governments	Grow at the same rate as U.S. population times the U.S. GDP price index
State and local government interest payments	Equal to the sum of (1) the amount of medium-and long-term debt and federal government loans outstanding in the prior year times the effective interest rate on medium- and long-term debt and federal government loans and (2) the amount of short-term debt outstanding in the prior year times the difference between the interest rate on medium- and long-term debt and federal government loans and the spread between long-term and short-term debt
State and local government subsidy payments	Grow at the same rate as U.S. population times the U.S. GDP price index
State and local government net social insurance fund balance	Grows at the same rate as wages and salaries

Source: GAO. | GAO-19-208SP.

State and Local Government Financial Assets and Liabilities

Table 7 summarizes our approach for simulating state and local government financial assets and liabilities. This approach is similar to the approach we have used in prior model updates.

Table 7. Simulation Approach for State and Local Government Financial Assets and Liabilities

Variable	Simulation approach
State and local government financial assets	Grow at the same rate as U.S. gross domestic product (GDP)
Medium-and long-term state and local government debt outstanding	Based on the historical relationship between (1) medium-and long-term debt issuance as a fraction of gross investment and nonproduced asset purchases in excess of federal investment grants and (2) the change in state and local government bond yields; see Table 9 and the "Estimated Historical Relationships" section below for details.
Federal government loans to state and local governments outstanding	Based on the historical relationship between real federal government lending to state and local governments and real U.S. GDP; see Table 9 and the "Estimated Historical Relationships" section below for details.
State and local government trade payables outstanding	Grow at the same rate as other consumption spending
Short-term state and local government debt outstanding	Equal to short-term debt outstanding in the prior year plus the change in financial assets minus (1) medium- and long-term debt issuance, (2) the change in trade payables, (3) borrowing from the federal government, and (4) net lending or borrowing

Source: GAO. | GAO-19-208SP.

Our method for simulating the sectors' short-term debt outstanding leverages the fact that for any entity, there is a direct relationship between budget outcomes and changes in financial position. Specifically, if expenditures exceed receipts, the gap needs to be financed by some combination of changes in financial assets and changes in financial liabilities. If governments spend more than they take in, they must pay for it by issuing debt, cashing in assets, or some combination of the two. Conversely, if receipts exceed expenditures and the sector is a net lender, its net financial investment (the net change in financial assets minus the net change in financial liabilities) must equal the budget surplus. The relationship between budget outcomes and the sector's financial position is shown in the following accounting identity:

total receipts – total expenditures = change in financial assets – change in financial liabilities.

The sector's financial liabilities include short-, medium-, and long-term debt; trade payables; and loans from the federal government, so the accounting identity can be rewritten as follows:

total receipts – total expenditures = change in financial assets – change in medium- and long-term debt – change in trade payables – change in federal government loans – change in short term debt.

For a given difference between total receipts and total expenditures, various combinations of changes in financial assets and changes in financial liabilities can satisfy this identity.

However, we assumed that financial assets grow at the same rate as U.S. GDP, that medium- and long-term debt outstanding is determined using the historical relationship described in Table 7, that federal government loans to state and local governments are determined using the historical relationship described in Table 7, and that trade payables grow at the same rate as other state and local government consumption spending. If the first four terms on the right hand side of the identity are already determined, then only the fifth term— the change in short-term debt—is free to satisfy this identity.

State and Local Government Fiscal Balance

As discussed above, our indicators of fiscal balance are operating balance, net saving, and net lending or borrowing. This approach is similar to the approach we have used in prior model updates. Recall that we defined operating balance as follows:

> operating balance = total receipts – (gross investment + capital transfer payments + net purchases of nonproduced assets – medium- and long-term debt issuance) – (current expenditures – consumption of general government fixed assets) – current surplus of state and local government enterprises – net social insurance fund balance.

By substituting for total receipts and current expenditures using the relationships described above and rearranging terms, we can also calculate operating balance using a formula that more easily identifies its revenue components—the items in the first set of parentheses—and expenditure components—the items in the second set of parentheses:

> operating balance = (current tax revenues + estate and gift tax revenues + social insurance fund contributions + income receipts from assets + current transfers + federal investment grants + medium- and long-term debt issuance) – (compensation of general government employees + social benefit payments + interest payments + gross investment + capital transfer payments + net purchases of nonproduced assets + other general government consumption expenditures + subsidy payments + net social insurance fund balance).

Estimated Historical Relationships

Some of our simulations are based on estimated historical relationships between pairs of variables:

- Elasticity of real personal consumption expenditures less food and services with respect to real wages and salaries;
- Elasticity of the real U.S. market value of real estate with respect to real U.S. GDP;
- Relationship between effective interest rates on financial assets and 3-month Treasury rates;
- Relationship between state and local government bond yields and 10- year Treasury rates;
- Relationship between effective interest rates on long-term state and local government debt and federal government loans and state and local government bond yields;

- Elasticity of real state personal income tax revenue with respect to real personal income;
- Elasticity of real state and local government excise tax revenue with respect to real wages and salaries;
- Relationship between long-term debt issuance as a fraction of gross investment and nonproduced asset purchases in excess of federal investment grants and the change in state and local government bond yields; and
- Relationship between real federal government lending to state and local governments and real U.S. GDP.

To estimate each of these historical relationships, we used the following approach: first, we assessed the order of integration of both variables using unit root tests of the levels and the first differences, where a variable is integrated of order 0 (I(0) or stationary) if we rejected the null hypothesis of a unit root in the levels at standard significance levels, and is integrated of order 1 (I(1) or first-order nonstationary) if we could not reject the null hypothesis of a unit root in the levels but we could do so for the first differences. For relationships between variables that were both stationary, we estimated an autoregressive distributed lag model,

$$y_t = \alpha_0 + \sum_{i=1}^{p} \alpha_i y_{t-i} + \sum_{j=0}^{q} \beta_j x_{t-j} + \varepsilon_t,$$

where y is the dependent variable, x is the independent variable, and ε is an independent, identically distributed error term. The long-run impact on y of a one unit change in x is given by $\sum_{j=0}^{q} \beta_j / (1 - \sum_{i=1}^{p} \alpha_i)$

We initially chose the number of lags based on the Bayesian Information Criteria and then added additional lags of the dependent variable, if needed, until the residuals were consistent with a white noise process at standard significance levels. For relationships between variables that were both first-order nonstationary, we used the same approach but also used the Pesaran, Shin, and Smith bounds test for the existence of a cointegrating (long-run equilibrium) relationship.[33] We concluded that the variables were cointegrated if we rejected the null hypothesis of no relationship at standard significance levels. Tables 8 and 9 summarize the estimated regression models as well as the results of the unit root, white noise, and cointegration tests.

Indicators of Fiscal Balance for the State and Local Government Sector

We simulated the model for the 75-year period from 2018 through 2092, and we used the results to calculate the operating balance for the state and local government sector as a percentage of U.S. GDP. Our results suggest that if the sector maintains current policy and continues to provide current per capita levels of public goods and services, then its operating

[33] Pesaran, M. Hashem, Yongcheol Shin, and Richard J. Smith, 2001, "Bounds Testing Approaches to the Analysis of Level Relationships," *Journal of Applied Econometrics* 16, 289-326.

balance will decline from about -1 percent of U.S. GDP to about -3 percent of U.S. GDP over the next 50 years.

Table 8. Estimated Regression Models Used in Simulations—Macroeconomic Variables and Interest Rates

Dependent variable	Natural log of real personal consumption expenditures less food and services	Natural log of real market value of real estate	Effective interest rates on financial assets	State and local government bond yields	Effective interest rates on medium-and long-term state and local government debt and federal government loans
Lagged by …					
…1 year	1.03[a]	1.56[a]	0.97[a]	0.81[a]	1.10[a]
	(0.09)	(0.08)	(0.10)	(0.13)	(0.13)
…2 years	-0.31[a]	-0.72[a]	-0.22[b]	-0.20[a]	-0.38[a]
	(0.09)	(0.08)	(0.08)	(0.06)	(0.12)
…0 years	0.54[a]	0.75[a]	0.20[a]	0.64[a]	0.26[a]
	(0.09)	(0.16)	(0.02)	(0.06)	(0.08)
…1 year	-0.70[a]	-0.93[a]		-0.39[a]	
	(0.14)	(0.23)		(0.11)	
…2 years	0.43[a]	0.35[b]			
	(0.09)	(0.17)			
Constant	-0.03	0.02	0.01[a]	0.01[a]	0.01[b]
	(0.04)	(0.06)	(0.00)	(0.00)	(0.01)
Estimated long-run change in dependent variable associated with a 1-unit change in independent variable	0.93[a] (0.02)	1.07[a] (0.04)	0.78[a] (0.06)	0.65[a] (0.04)	0.93[a] (0.21)
Dependent variable order of integration	I(1)	I(1)	I(1)	I(1)	I(1)
Independent variable order of integration	I(1)	I(1)	I(1)	I(1)	I(1)
Time period	1933-2017	1950-2017	1950-2017	1980-2016	1965-2016
White noise residuals	Yes	Yes	Yes	Yes	Yes
Cointegrated	Yes	Yes	Yes	Yes	Yes

Legend: a = $p<0.01$; b = $p<0.05$. Source: GAO. | GAO-19-208SP. Notes: Standard errors are in parentheses.

To shed light on how maintaining the operating balance at or above zero would affect the state and local government sector, we used the model to simulate the level of total expenditures that would keep the operating balance greater than or equal to zero. We then calculated the difference between the present value of total expenditures simulated assuming the sector maintains balance, and the present value of total expenditures simulated assuming the sector maintains current policies, both as a percentage of the present value of total expenditures assuming the sector maintains current policies, and as a percentage of the present value of U.S. GDP. We calculated all of the present values for the 50-year period from 2018 through 2067, and we used a discount rate equal to the average of the 3-month

Treasury rate and the 10-year Treasury rate for each year. Our results suggest that the difference between the present value of total expenditures that maintain balance and the present value of total expenditures that maintain current policies is about -14.7 percent of the present value of total expenditures that maintain current policies, or about -2.4 percent of the present value of U.S. GDP. That is, our simulations suggest that maintaining balance would require the sector to spend about 14.7 percent less than it would spend each year to maintain current policies. We note that a similar exercise based on simulating total revenues required to maintain the operating balance at or above zero would generate a similar result.

Table 9. Estimated Regression Models Used in Simulations— Tax Revenues and Financial Liabilities

Dependent variable	**Natural log of real state personal income tax revenue**	**Natural log of real state and local government excise tax revenue**	**Medium-and long-term debt issuance as a fraction of gross investment and nonproduced asset purchases in excess of federal investment grants**	**Real federal government lending to state and local governments**
Lagged by ...				
...1 year	0.64[a]	1.44[a]	0.26[b]	0.09
	(0.12)	(0.11)	(0.14)	(0.12)
...2 years	-0.11	-0.56[a]		
	(0.16)	(0.11)		
...3 years	0.25b			
	(0.15)			
...4 years	-0.20			
	(0.14)			
...5 years	0.14			
	(0.09)			
...0 years	1.76[a]	0.37[a]	-10.00	1.54
	(0.25)	(0.13)	(11.22)	(1.29)
...1 year	-1.41[a]	-0.98[a]		
	(0.26)	(0.19)		
... 2 years		0.71[a]		
		(0.12)		
Constant	-1.71[a]	-0.33[a]	0.35[a]	-0.03
	(0.52)	(0.12)	(0.11)	(0.05)
Estimated long-run change in dependent variable associated with a 1-unit change in independent variable	1.27[a] (0.08)	0.91[a] (0.07)	-13.58 (15.16)	1.70 (1.44)
Dependent variable order of integration	I(1)	I(1)	I(0)	I(0)
Independent variable order of integration	I(1)	I(1)	I(0)	I(0)
Time period	1970-2016	1970-2017	1966-2016	1950-2017
White noise residuals	Yes	Yes	Yes	Yes
Cointegrated	Yes	Yes	Not applicable	Not applicable

Notes: Standard errors are in parentheses.

Caveats and Limitations

Our approach has a number of limitations and the results should be interpreted with caution:

- The state and local government fiscal model is not designed for certain types of analyses. The simulations are not intended to provide precise predictions. Even though we know that these governments regularly make changes to tax laws and expenditures, the model essentially holds current policy in place and analyzes the fiscal future for the sector as if those policies were maintained because it would be highly speculative to make any assumptions about future policy adjustments.
- Fiscal outcomes, as related to the state and local government sector's financial position and solvency, may not reflect all aspects of the sector's fiscal health. Other indicators include economic indicators that go beyond the sector's financial position to include economic growth, income, or distributional equity, as well as indicators of the quality of services provided by the sector, including education, health care, infrastructure, and other public goods and services.
- Our unit of analysis is the state and local government sector as a whole, so our results provide an assessment of the sector's fiscal outlook. However, individual state and local governments likely exhibit significant heterogeneity in their expenditure and revenue patterns, so their fiscal outlooks will likely differ from that for the sector. Nevertheless, it is informative to assess the overall fiscal outlook of the sector because doing so reveals the outlook for the average state or local government. In addition, aggregate data on the sector are available on a more timely basis than data for individual state and local governments. This allows for a better assessment of the sector's current fiscal outlook. Our results for the sector also provide a baseline from which to view the experiences of individual state and local governments. Finally, assessing the fiscal outlook of the sector as a whole can help mitigate the tendency to extrapolate from the most visible, but potentially not representative, experiences of individual states or localities.

APPENDIX II: STATE AND LOCAL GOVERNMENT FISCAL MODEL ALTERNATIVE SIMULATIONS

Our baseline approach to simulating the fiscal outlook for the state and local government sector is described in appendix I. As part of our simulation approach, we used five variables with values for the simulation period—the period from 2018 through 2092—that are projected outside the model and that do not rely on maintaining historical relationships: U.S. population, real U.S. gross domestic product (GDP) growth, national health care excess cost growth, Medicaid excess cost growth, and the real rate of return on pension assets.

- U.S. population. For our baseline simulations, we used the Board of Trustees of the Federal Old-Age and Survivors Insurance and Federal Disability Insurance Trust Funds' (OASDI Trustees) intermediate population projections.

- Real U.S. GDP. For our baseline simulations, we projected real U.S. GDP to grow at the same rate as Congressional Budget Office (CBO) projections for the period from 2018 through 2028 and to grow at the same rate as the OASDI Trustees' intermediate projections of real U.S. GDP growth for the period from 2029 through 2092.
- National health expenditures excess cost growth. For our baseline simulations, we used Centers for Medicare & Medicaid Services' (CMS) baseline projection of national health expenditures excess cost growth.
- Medicaid excess cost growth. For our baseline simulations, for the period from 2029 through 2092, we used Medicaid excess cost growth derived from MCS's baseline projections.[34]
- Real rate of return on state and local government pension assets. For our baseline simulations, we assumed a 5 percent real rate of return on state and local government pension assets.

To assess the sensitivity of our results to changes in these baseline projections, we selected two alternative projections of each of these variables, one associated with a faster growth rate or rate of return and one associated with a slower growth rate or rate of return.

- U.S. population. For our alternative simulations, we used the OASDI Trustees' high cost and low cost population projections.
- Real U.S. GDP. For our alternative simulations, we used the OASDI Trustees' high cost and low cost projections of real U.S. GDP growth.
- National health expenditures excess cost growth. For our alternative simulations, we used CMS's alternative projection of national health expenditures excess cost growth. As another alternative, we simulated the model assuming excess cost growth for national health expenditures is zero.
- Medicaid excess cost growth. For our alternative simulations, for the period from 2029 through 2092, we used Medicaid excess cost growth derived from CMS's alternative projections for the period from 2029 through 2092. As another alternative, we simulated the model assuming Medicaid excess cost growth is zero for the period from 2029 through 2092.[35]
- Real rate of return on state and local government pension assets. For our sensitivity analysis, we used real rates of return of 2.5 percent and 7.5 percent.

Table 10 shows the average annual growth rate or rate of return associated with the baseline and alternative projections of each variable for the simulation period.

---

[34] For the period from 2018 through 2028, our simulations of variables related to Medicaid relied on CBO projections of two variables—federal spending on Medicaid, Children's Health Insurance Program, and exchange subsidies as a fraction of U.S. GDP and federal Medicaid grants to state and local governments—that already incorporate excess cost growth.

[35] For the period from 2018 through 2028, our simulations of variables related to Medicaid relied on CBO projections of two variables—federal spending on Medicaid, Children's Health Insurance Program, and exchange subsidies as a fraction of U.S. GDP and federal Medicaid grants to state and local governments—that already incorporate excess cost growth. Thus, we could not use alternative projections of Medicaid excess cost growth for these years.

Table 10. Average Annual Baseline and Alternative Projections of Key Exogenous Variables for the Period from 2018 through 2092 (percentage)

	Average annual U.S. population growth	Average annual growth of real U.S. gross domestic product	Average annual national health expenditures excess cost growth	Average annual Medicaid excess cost growth	Average annual real rate of return on state and local government pension fund assets
Baseline assumption	0.5	2.1	0.73	0.57	5.00
Slower alternative	0.3	1.4	0	0	2.50
Faster alternative	0.8	2.8	0.89	0.61	7.50

Source: GAO analysis of data from the Board of Trustees of the Federal Old-Age and Survivors Insurance and Federal Disability Insurance Trust Funds, the Centers for Medicare & Medicaid Services, the Congressional Budget Office, and GAO. | GAO-19-208SP.

Note: Average annual Medicaid excess cost growth is for the period from 2029 through 2092.

For our simulations based on alternative assumptions about U.S. population growth and real U.S. GDP growth, as well as simulations based on alternative assumptions about real pension asset returns, we simulated the model changing one variable at a time and leaving the others fixed at their baseline values. For example, for one simulation we used the slower assumption for real U.S. GDP growth and the baseline assumptions for all other variables. For our simulations based on alternative assumptions about excess cost growth for national health expenditures and for Medicaid, we changed both variables in the same direction and left the others fixed at their baseline values. For example, for one simulation we used zero excess cost growth for both national health expenditures and for Medicaid, and made the baseline assumption for the other variables. Thus, our sensitivity analysis is in the spirit of a partial equilibrium comparative statics analysis that sheds light on how each of the individual variables may affect the state and local government sector's fiscal outlook. However, these variables are likely to be correlated so future changes in one would likely be associated with changes in others.

In: Top 10 Reports and Testimonies in December 2018
Editor: Sarah J. Nygaard
ISBN: 978-1-53615-507-5

Chapter 9

VA HEALTH CARE: IMPROVEMENTS NEEDED IN SUICIDE PREVENTION MEDIA OUTREACH CAMPAIGN OVERSIGHT AND EVALUATION*

United States Government Accountability Office

ABBREVIATIONS

CDC	Centers for Disease Control and Prevention
OMHSP	Office of Mental Health and Suicide Prevention
PSA	Public Service Announcement
REACH VET	Recovery Engagement and Coordination for
Health	Veterans Enhanced Treatment
VA	Department of Veterans Affairs
VCL	Veterans Crisis Line
VHA	Veterans Health Administration

WHY GAO DID THIS STUDY

Veterans suffer a disproportionately higher rate of suicide than the civilian population. VA has estimated that an average of 20 veterans die by suicide per day, and in 2018, VA identified suicide prevention as its highest clinical priority. VHA's suicide prevention media outreach campaign—its collective suicide prevention outreach activities—helps raise awareness among veterans and others in the community about suicide prevention resources. VHA has contracted with an outside vendor to develop suicide prevention media outreach content.

* This is an edited, reformatted and augmented version of United States Government Accountability Office; Report to the Ranking Member Committee on Veterans' Affairs, House of Representatives, Publication No. GAO-19-66, dated November 2018.

GAO was asked to examine VHA's suicide prevention media outreach campaign. This chapter examines the extent to which VHA (1) conducts activities for its suicide prevention media outreach campaign, and (2) evaluates the effectiveness of its campaign. GAO reviewed relevant VHA documents and data on the amount, type, and cost of suicide prevention outreach activities since fiscal year 2013. GAO also reviewed VHA's contract for developing suicide prevention outreach content and interviewed VA and VHA officials.

What GAO Recommends

VHA should (1) establish an approach to oversee its suicide prevention media outreach campaign that includes clear delineation of roles and responsibilities, and (2) establish targets for its metrics to improve evaluation efforts. VA concurred with GAO's recommendations and described steps it will take to implement them.

What GAO Found

The Department of Veterans Affairs' (VA) Veterans Health Administration (VHA) conducts national suicide prevention media outreach on various platforms to raise awareness about VHA's suicide prevention resources. The primary focus of this campaign since 2010 has been to raise awareness of the Veterans Crisis Line (VCL), VHA's national hotline established in 2007 to provide support to veterans in emotional crisis. GAO found that VHA's suicide prevention media outreach activities declined in recent years due to leadership turnover and reorganization. For example, the amount of suicide prevention content developed by VHA's contractor for social media decreased in fiscal years 2017 and the first 10 months of 2018 after increasing in each of the 4 prior years.

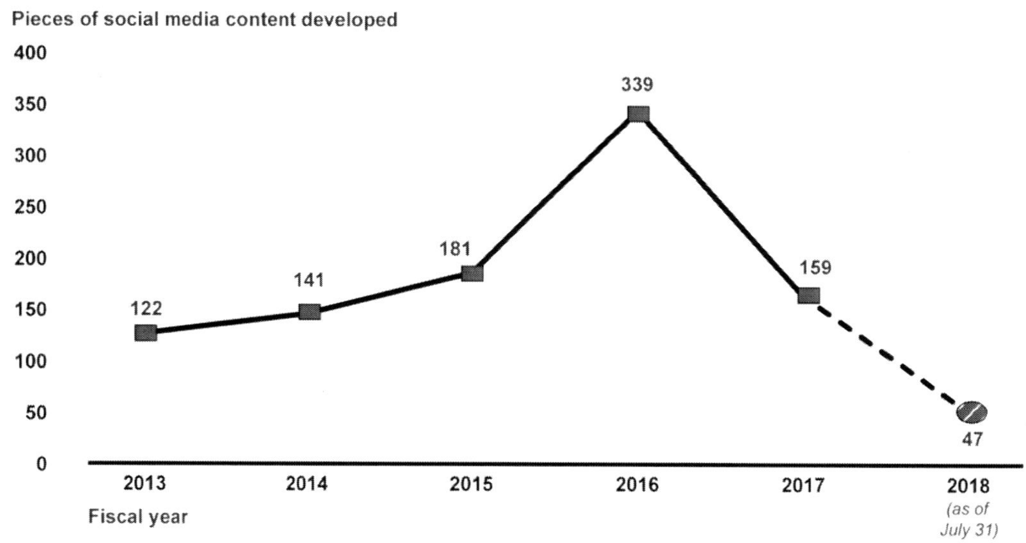

Source: Veterans Health Administration. | GAO-19-66.

Suicide Prevention Outreach Content for Social Media, since Fiscal Year 2013.

VHA officials reported not having leadership available for a period of time to make decisions about the suicide prevention media outreach campaign. GAO found that VHA did not assign key leadership responsibilities or establish clear lines of reporting, and as a result, its ability to oversee the outreach campaign was hindered. Consequently, VHA may not be maximizing its reach with suicide prevention media content to veterans, especially those who are at-risk.

VHA evaluates the effectiveness of its suicide prevention media outreach campaign by collecting data on metrics, such as the number of people that visit the VCL website. However, VHA has not established targets for the majority of these metrics. Officials said they have not established targets because, apart from one industry-wide target they use, they lack meaningful targets for evaluating the campaign. However, VHA could use information about how its metrics performed in the past to develop reasonable and meaningful targets for future performance. Without established targets for its metrics, VHA is missing an opportunity to better evaluate the effectiveness of its suicide prevention media outreach campaign.

November 15, 2018

The Honorable Tim Walz
Ranking Member
Committee on Veterans' Affairs
House of Representatives

Dear Mr. Walz:

Suicide is a public health problem facing all populations, particularly veterans. After military service, veterans suffer a disproportionately higher rate of suicide than the civilian population. According to the Department of Veterans Affairs (VA), veterans accounted for 14.3 percent of all deaths by suicide among United States adults in 2015, despite constituting only 8.3 percent of the adult population. VA reported in June 2018 that an average of 20 veterans died by suicide each day in 2015, and that an average of 6 of these 20 veterans (30 percent) were recent users of VA's Veterans Health Administration's (VHA) health care services.[1] Suicide is not unique to veterans; the Centers for Disease Control and Prevention (CDC) reports that suicide was the tenth leading cause of death in the United States in 2015.[2] However, according to VA, the rate of suicide is higher for veterans than non-veterans (see Figure 1).

VHA conducts national outreach to veterans and others in the community to raise awareness about suicide prevention and services available through VA, as one of several VHA initiatives to help reduce suicides in the veteran community.

[1] See Department of Veterans Affairs, *VA National Suicide Data Report* (Washington, D.C.: June 2018). VA's June 2018 report is based on 2015 data, the most recent year of data available. Recent users of VHA health care services is defined as those who received VHA care in 2015 or 2014.

[2] See Centers for Disease Control and Prevention, *Preventing Suicide: A Technical Package of Policy, Programs, and Practices* (Atlanta, Ga.: 2017).

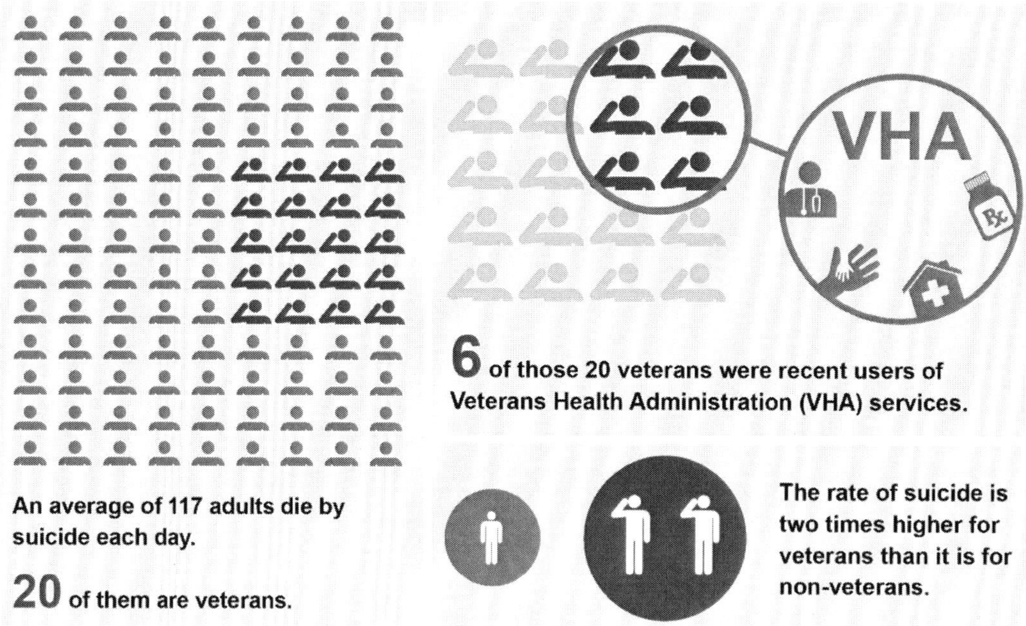

Source: Department of Veterans Affairs (VA). | GAO-19-66.

Note: See Department of Veterans Affairs, *VA National Suicide Data Report* (Washington, D.C.: June 2018). The report includes data from 2015, the most recent year of complete data available. In its agency comments, VA indicated that the rate of suicide is now one and a half times higher for veterans than it is for non-veterans, based on its September 2018 report, which includes data through 2016. See VA, *VA National Suicide Data Report* (Washington, D.C.: September 2018).

Figure 1. Veteran Suicide Rates Compared to Non-Veterans, 2015.

Since 2010, VHA has awarded multiple contracts to the same vendor to develop content for suicide prevention media outreach.[3] Questions have been raised about the effectiveness of VHA's collective suicide prevention media outreach activities, also referred to as its suicide prevention media outreach campaign. You asked us to review VHA's suicide prevention media outreach activities and related oversight. In this chapter, we examine:

1) the extent to which VHA conducts activities for its suicide prevention media outreach campaign; and
2) the extent to which VHA evaluates the effectiveness of its suicide prevention media outreach campaign.

To examine the extent to which VHA conducts activities for its suicide prevention media outreach campaign, we reviewed VHA's contract to develop suicide prevention outreach content from fiscal years 2013 through 2016 and its contract to develop suicide prevention and mental health outreach content in fiscal years 2017 and 2018.[4] VHA's first such contract began in 2010; however, the Federal Acquisition Regulation only requires federal agencies to

[3] Outreach "content" refers to materials for communicating with the public, such as flyers, and billboards, and social media posts. VHA's suicide prevention content typically includes images and information about its suicide prevention services and resources.

[4] Both contracts are with the same vendor, which we will refer to hereafter as VHA's "contractor."

maintain contract documentation for a period of 6 years after the last payment. Therefore, we did not include the initial contract or associated outreach in our review due to the lack of available documentation. We also requested and reviewed data on the amount and type of outreach content that VHA's contractor developed from fiscal year 2013 through fiscal year 2018.[5] We interviewed VHA officials responsible for implementation and oversight of the contract about the data. We also obtained written responses from the contractor about the steps it took to compile and ensure the accuracy of the data. On the basis of these actions, we found these data to be sufficiently reliable for the purpose of our reporting objective.

We also reviewed documentation and interviewed VHA officials who worked on the campaign about VHA's suicide prevention media outreach campaign, outreach activities, and VHA leadership officials' involvement in the campaign, and plans moving forward.[6] We compared VHA's outreach campaign and related activities with federal internal control standards related to control environment and monitoring.[7] We also interviewed relevant other VHA and VA officials who played a role in the suicide prevention media outreach campaign, including officials in VA's Office of Acquisitions, Logistics, and Construction and VHA's Office of Communications.

To examine the extent to which VHA evaluates the effectiveness of its suicide prevention media outreach campaign, we reviewed documentation of VHA's evaluation efforts, including monthly monitoring reports, to identify any performance metrics VHA monitors and any targets established for those metrics. We also reviewed the 2016 contract to identify any requirements for the contractor to monitor and report on the effectiveness of the campaign. Additionally, we interviewed VHA officials responsible for monitoring and evaluating the campaign and reviewed supporting documentation. Specifically, we asked officials about the extent to which they had evaluated the campaign's effectiveness since fiscal year 2013, their evaluation processes and tools, and any plans for completing future evaluations. We then compared VHA's evaluation efforts to criteria we developed in previous bodies of work for designing program evaluations, as well as to federal internal control standards for monitoring.[8]

We conducted this performance audit from December 2017 to November 2018 in accordance with generally accepted government auditing standards. Those standards require that we plan and perform the audit to obtain sufficient, appropriate evidence to provide a reasonable basis for our findings and conclusions based on our audit objectives. We believe

---

[5] In order to expedite this data request, VHA enlisted the assistance of the contractor to provide the data in the format and time frames required for this review. We requested the data on a subset of the types of content the contractor develops in order to focus on those types of media outreach most relevant to our work. For example, we did not focus on promotional items, such as magnets and keychains, and data on website maintenance. For fiscal year 2018, we obtained data through July 2018, the first 10 months of the fiscal year.

[6] Officials that worked on the campaign include the contracting officer's representative (the primary VHA official responsible for oversight of the contract) and other officials within VHA that worked directly on the campaign.

[7] GAO, *Standards for Internal Control in the Federal Government*, GAO-14-704G (Washington, D.C.: Sept. 10, 2014) and *Standards for Internal Control in the Federal Government*, GAO/AIMD-00-21.3.1 (Washington, D.C.: Nov. 1, 1999). Internal control is a process effected by an entity's management, oversight body, and other personnel that provides reasonable assurance that the objectives of an entity will be achieved.

[8] GAO, *Tax Administration: IRS Needs to Further Refine Its Tax Filing Season Performance Measures*, GAO-03-143 (Washington, D.C.: Nov. 22, 2002). Our prior work states that clearly articulating a program's strategy and performance expectations aids the selection of appropriate performance measures and data sources. For example, a well- articulated program logic model can help evaluate agency efforts. See also GAO, *Designing Evaluations: 2012 Revision,* GAO-12-208G (Washington, D.C.: Jan. 31, 2012), GAO-14-704G, and GAO/AIMD-00-21.3.1.

that the evidence obtained provides a reasonable basis for our findings and conclusions based on our audit objectives.

BACKGROUND

VA Suicide Prevention

VA has undertaken a number of initiatives to help prevent veteran suicide, including identifying suicide prevention as VA's highest clinical priority in its strategic plan for fiscal years 2018 through 2024 (see Figure 2).[9]

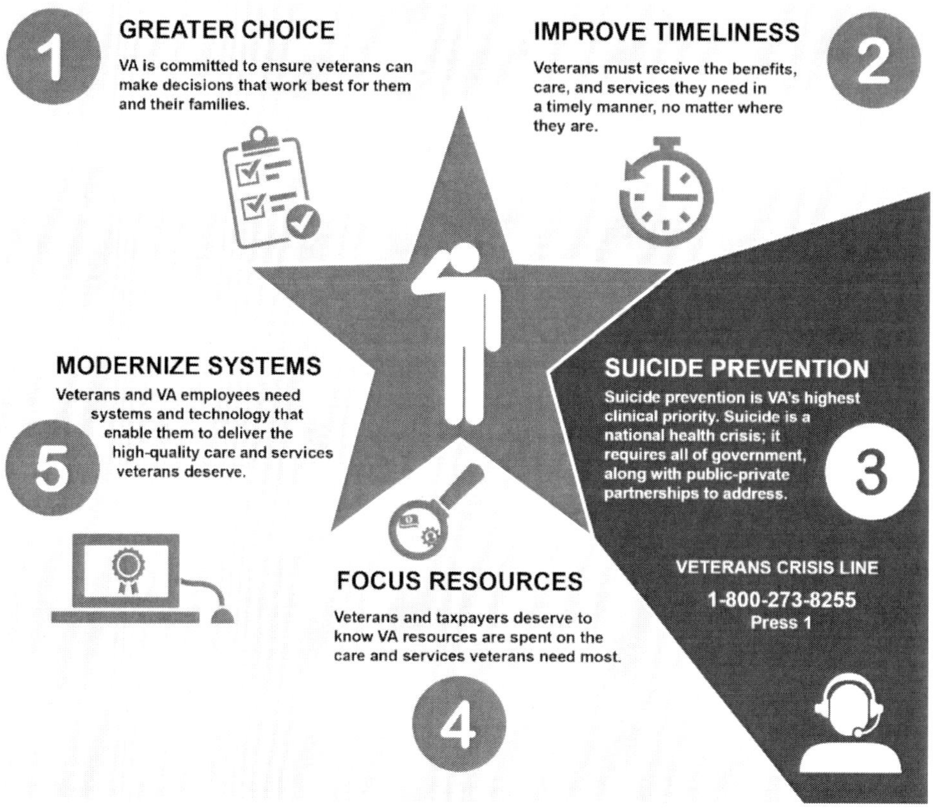

Source: VA (information); GAO (illustration). | GAO-19-66.

Figure 2. Top Five Priorities in the Department of Veterans Affairs' (VA) Strategic Plan for Fiscal Years 2018 – 2024.

VA uses CDC's research on risk factors and prevention techniques to inform its approach to suicide prevention in the veteran community. There is no single determining cause for suicide; instead, suicide occurs in response to biological, psychological, interpersonal, environmental, and societal influences, according to the CDC. Specifically, suicide is

[9] See Department of Veterans Affairs, *Department of Veterans Affairs Fiscal Years 2018-2024 Strategic Plan* (Washington, D.C.: Feb. 12, 2018).

associated with risk factors that exist at the individual level (such as a history of mental illness or substance abuse, or stressful life events, such as divorce or the death of a loved one), community level (such as barriers to health care), or societal level (such as the way suicide is portrayed in the media and stigma associated with seeking help for mental illness). According to VA, veterans may possess risk factors related to their military service, such as a service-related injury or a difficult transition to civilian life. CDC reports that protective factors—influences that help protect against the risk for suicide—include effective coping and problem- solving skills, strong and supportive relationships with friends and family, availability of health care, and connectedness to social institutions such as school and community.

VA's 2018 National Strategy for Suicide Prevention identifies four focus areas: (1) healthy and empowered veterans, families, and communities; (2) clinical and community preventative services; (3) treatment and support services; and (4) surveillance, research, and evaluation.[10]

Collectively, these four areas encompass 14 goals for preventing veteran suicide, one of which is implementing communication designed to prevent veteran suicide by changing knowledge, attitude, and behaviors.

VHA's suicide prevention media outreach campaign is just one of its initiatives intended to reduce veteran suicide. For example, in 2007, VHA established the Veteran's Crisis Line (VCL), a national toll-free hotline that supports veterans in emotional crisis.11 Veterans, as well as their family and friends, can access the VCL by calling a national toll-free number—1-800-273-8255—and pressing "1" to be connected with a VCL responder, regardless of whether these veterans receive health care through VHA. VHA added the option to communicate with VCL responders via online chat in 2009, followed by text messaging in 2011. Another VHA suicide prevention initiative is the Recovery Engagement and Coordination for Health – Veterans Enhanced Treatment initiative, or REACH VET. Established in 2016, REACH VET uses predictive modeling to analyze existing data from veterans' health records to identify veterans at increased risk for adverse outcomes, such as suicide, hospitalization, or illness.[12]

VHA's Suicide Prevention Media Outreach Campaign

Suicide prevention officials within VHA's Office of Mental Health and Suicide Prevention (OMHSP) are responsible for implementing the suicide prevention media outreach campaign. Since 2010, VHA has used a contractor to develop suicide prevention media outreach content and monitor its effectiveness. In September 2016, VHA awarded a new

---

[10] Department of Veterans Affairs, *National Strategy for Preventing Veteran Suicide 2018-2028* (Washington, D.C.: June 29, 2018).

[11] We have previously reported on the VCL and made recommendations for improving the timeliness and quality of VA's VCL responses. VA concurred with our recommendations and in July 2016, developed and implemented procedures to regularly test the VCL system. In addition, in July 2017, VA updated its VCL quality assurance plan to document measurable targets and time frames for key performance indicators needed to assess the VCL's performance. See GAO, *Veterans Crisis Line: Additional Testing, Monitoring, and Information Needed to Ensure Better Quality Service,* GAO-16-373 (Washington, D.C.: May 26, 2016).

[12] After being identified by REACH VET, veterans are contacted by VA health care providers to determine whether additional care or services are needed.

contract to the same contractor to provide both suicide prevention and mental health media outreach. Under the 2016 contract, the suicide prevention and mental health outreach campaigns remain separate and are overseen by separate suicide prevention and mental health officials, both within OMHSP.[13] VHA officials told us that beginning in fiscal year 2019, VHA will separate the contract for suicide prevention and mental health media outreach. Specifically, VHA will utilize an existing agreement with a different contractor for suicide prevention media outreach while the existing contractor will continue to provide mental health media outreach.[14]

According to VHA, the purpose of its suicide prevention media outreach campaign is to raise awareness among veterans, their families and friends, and the general public about VHA resources that are available to veterans who may be at risk for suicide. The primary focus of the outreach campaign since 2010 has been to raise awareness of the services available through the VCL.[15]

VHA's suicide prevention media outreach falls into two main categories: unpaid and paid. Unpaid media outreach content is typically displayed on platforms owned by VA or VHA, or is disseminated by external organizations or individuals that share VHA suicide prevention content at no cost, as discussed below (see Figure 3).[16]

- Social media. VA and VHA each maintain national social media accounts on platforms such as Facebook, Twitter, and Instagram, and post content, including suicide prevention content developed by VHA's contractor.[17] VHA also works with other federal agencies, non-governmental organizations, and individuals that post its suicide prevention content periodically.
- Public service announcements (PSA). VHA's contractor typically develops two PSAs per year, which various local and national media networks display at no cost to VHA.
- Website. VHA's contractor maintains the content displayed on the VCL website (veteranscrisisline.net), including much of the content it develops for other platforms, such as PSAs and social media content. Visitors to the website can both view the content on the website and share it on their own platforms.

Paid media outreach includes outreach on media platforms for which VHA must pay a fee to display its content (see Figure 4). Paid media falls into two categories, as discussed below.

---

[13] VHA officials said OMHSP was established in May 2017. Before May 2017, the suicide prevention program and the mental health program were organizationally located under different offices within VHA. In addition to these two programs, OMHSP also includes the VCL program, among others.

[14] Specifically, VHA said it will utilize an existing blanket purchase agreement through a GSA schedule contract. A blanket purchase agreement is a simplified method of filling anticipated repetitive needs for supplies or services that functions as a charge account, with terms and conditions agreed upon when the blanket purchase agreement is established. Federal Acquisition Regulation §§ 8.405-3, 13.303-1(a).

[15] See GAO-16-373.

[16] VHA also conducts unpaid outreach in the form of attending conferences and seminars, as well as developing materials to hand out to veterans and the community at these and other events. However, this type of outreach was not the focus of our report because it is not a national, media-based outreach effort.

[17] VHA has a VCL Facebook page, but officials told us that they intentionally do not populate it with suicide prevention content because it would not be an appropriate resource for providing timely support to veterans in emotional crisis.

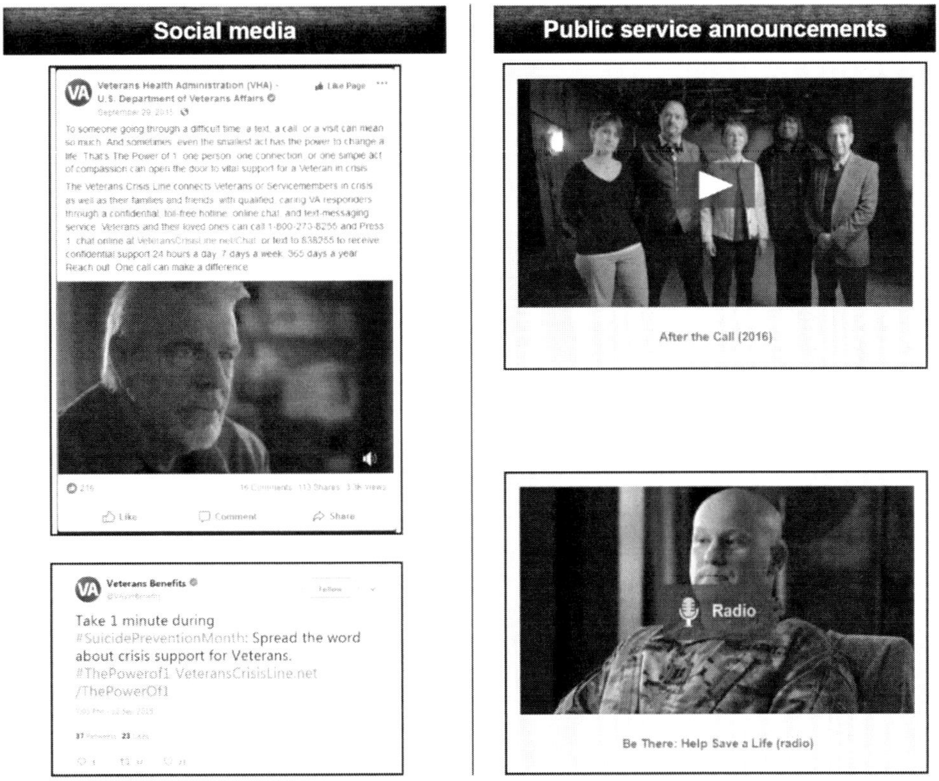

Source: © J. R. Reingold & Associates, Inc. | GAO-19-66.

Note: Unpaid media refers to outreach content that is displayed on platforms owned by the Department of Veterans Affairs, or is disseminated by external organizations or individuals that share VHA suicide prevention content at no cost.

Figure 3. Examples of the Veterans Health Administration's (VHA) Unpaid Suicide Prevention Media Outreach Content.

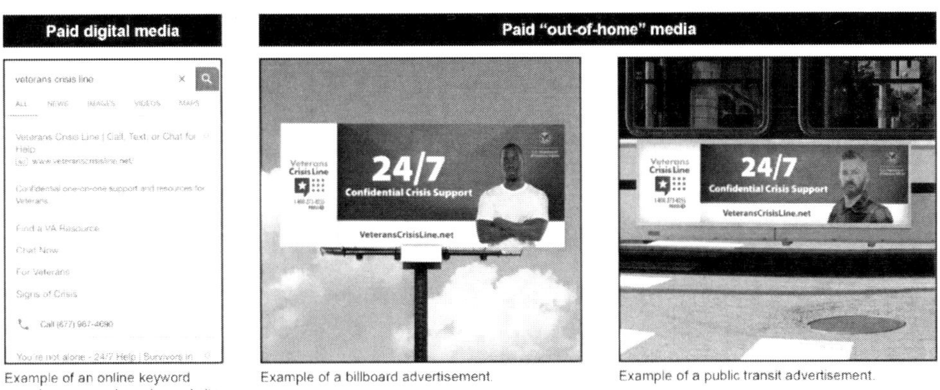
Paid digital media
Paid "out-of-home" media
veterans crisis line
24/7
Confidential Crisis Support
VeteransCrisisLine.net
Example of an online keyword search on a search engine website.
Example of a billboard advertisement.
Example of a public transit advertisement.

Source: © J. R. Reingold & Associates, Inc. | GAO-19-66.

Figure 4. Examples of the Veterans Health Administration's Paid Suicide Prevention Media Outreach Content.

- Paid digital media. An example of paid digital media includes online keyword searches, in which VHA pays a search engine a fee for its website to appear as a top result in response to selected keywords, such as "veterans crisis line" or "veteran suicide." Paid digital media also includes social media posts for which VHA pays a fee to display its content to a widespread audience, such as users with a military affiliation.
- Paid "out-of-home" media: "Out-of-home" refers to the locations where this type of content is typically displayed. Examples include billboards, bus and transit advertisements, and local and national radio commercials.

VHA recognizes September as Suicide Prevention Month each year. During this month, VHA establishes a theme and increases its outreach activities, including a combination of both paid and unpaid media outreach. According to VHA, it typically incorporates additional outreach techniques during this month, such as enlisting the support of celebrities or hosting live chat sessions on social media platforms, including Facebook and Twitter.

VHA's Suicide Prevention Media Outreach Activities Declined in Recent Years Due to Leadership Turnover and Reorganization

VHA's Suicide Prevention Media Outreach Activities Declined in Fiscal Years 2017 and 2018

VHA's suicide prevention media outreach activities declined in fiscal years 2017 and 2018 compared to earlier years of the campaign. We identified declines in social media postings, PSAs, paid media, and suicide prevention month activities, as discussed below.

- Social media. The amount of social media content developed by VHA's contractor decreased in 2017 and 2018, after increasing in each of the prior four years. Specifically, VHA reported that its contractor developed 339 pieces of social media content in fiscal year 2016, compared with 159 in fiscal year 2017, and 47 during the first 10 months of fiscal year 2018 (see Figure 5).[18]
- PSAs. VHA's contractor is required to develop two suicide prevention PSAs in each fiscal year. VHA officials said that the development of the two PSAs was delayed in fiscal year 2018. Specifically, as of August 2018, VHA reported that one PSA was completed, but had not yet aired, and another PSA was in development.[19] As a result of this delay, VHA had not aired a suicide prevention PSA on television or radio in

[18] The data includes the amount of content that was developed, not the number of times it was posted or displayed. This is because the outreach content developed by VHA's contractor is often disseminated on platforms that are not owned by VHA or its contractor.

[19] VHA released a PSA on suicide prevention in October 2017. However, VHA officials said this PSA was not developed by the contractor, but through a partnership with an outside organization, and it was developed for online dissemination, as opposed to television or radio.

over a year; this is the first time there has been a gap of more than a month since June 2012.

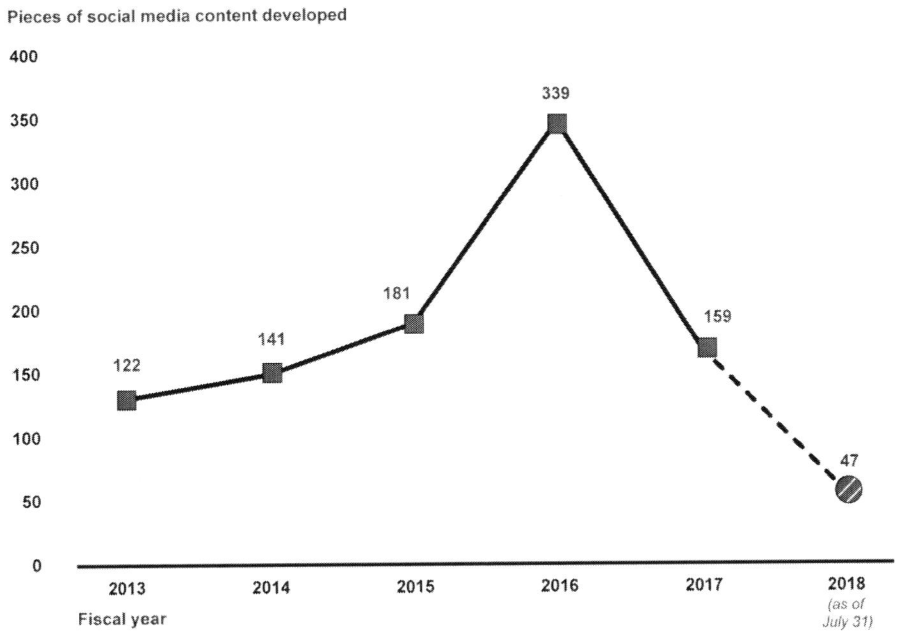

Source: Veterans Health Administration. | GAO-19-66.

Note: The table includes the amount of social media content developed, not the number of times it was posted on social media platforms or displayed in other locations.

Figure 5. Suicide Prevention Outreach Social Media Content Developed for the Veterans Health Administration, October 2012 through July 2018.

- Paid media. VHA had a total budget of $17.7 million for its suicide prevention and mental health media outreach for fiscal year 2018, of which $6.2 million was obligated for suicide prevention paid media. As of September 2018, VHA said it had spent $57,000 of its $6.2 million paid media budget.[20] VHA officials estimated that they would spend a total of $1.5 million on suicide prevention paid media for fiscal year 2018 and indicated that the remaining funds would be de-obligated from the contract at the end of the fiscal year and not used for suicide prevention media outreach. VHA officials indicated that the reason they did not spend the remaining funds on suicide prevention paid media in fiscal year 2018 was that the approval of the paid media plan was delayed due to changes in leadership and organizational realignment of the suicide prevention program. As a result, VHA officials said they limited the paid media outreach in fiscal year 2018 to activities that were already in place, including 25 keyword search advertisements, and 20 billboards and 8 radio advertisements in selected cities across the United States.

  In prior fiscal years, VHA conducted a variety of digital and out-of- home suicide prevention paid media. For example, in fiscal year 2015, with a suicide prevention

[20] VHA officials told us that because paid media is very effective, the amount of approved funds would be the biggest factor in determining the amount and type of paid media to conduct each year.

paid media budget of more than $4 million, VHA reported that it ran 58 advertisements on Google, Bing, and Facebook, and ran 30 billboards, 180 bus advertisements, more than 19,000 radio advertisements, 252 print advertisements, and 39 movie theatre placements in selected cities across the United States.[21] VHA ran similar types of paid media in fiscal years 2013, 2014, and 2016 with variation in quantities based on the approved budget in each of these years. In fiscal year 2017, VHA had a budget of approximately $1.7 million to spend on paid media for both the suicide prevention and mental health outreach campaigns. However, VHA spent less than 10 percent of the funds (approximately $136,000) to run paid advertisements on Google and Bing for suicide prevention in fiscal year 2017; the remainder was spent on mental health outreach.

- Suicide Prevention Month. VHA documentation indicated that Suicide Prevention Month 2017 was a limited effort. VHA officials said that this was because they did not begin preparing early enough. In May 2018, VHA officials indicated that they were similarly behind schedule for planning Suicide Prevention Month 2018, though they told us in August 2018 that they had caught up.

VHA Leadership Turnover and Reorganization Resulted in the Decline in Suicide Prevention Media Outreach Activities

VHA officials told us that the decrease in suicide prevention media outreach activities was due to leadership turnover and reorganization since 2017. For example, VHA officials said the National Director for Suicide Prevention position was vacant from July 2017 through April 2018. VHA filled the role temporarily with a 6-month detail from another agency from October 2017 through March 2018 and then hired this individual as the permanent director on April 30, 2018. VHA officials that worked on the campaign told us they did not have leadership available to make decisions about the suicide prevention campaign during this time. For example, VHA officials said they did not have a kick-off meeting between VHA leadership and VHA's contractor at the beginning of fiscal year 2018—a requirement of the contract—because there was no leadership available to participate in this meeting.[22]

The officials also reported that suicide prevention leadership was not available for weekly meetings to discuss suicide prevention outreach activities, even after the suicide prevention program obtained an acting director on detail from another agency. VHA staff said that at that time, they focused their suicide prevention media outreach efforts on areas that did not require leadership input, such as updating the VCL website. The absence of leadership available to provide direction and make decisions on the suicide prevention media outreach campaign is inconsistent with federal internal control standards for control environment, which require agencies to assign responsibilities to achieve its objectives.[23] If a key role is

[21] In fiscal years 2014, 2015, and 2016, VHA paid movie theatres to show suicide prevention PSAs during the previews.

[22] During kick-off meetings, VHA and its contractor typically discuss lessons learned from the prior year's campaign and the approach for the coming year, such as target audiences, outreach platforms, paid media, and new initiatives.

[23] GAO-14-704G and GAO/AIMD-00-21.3.1.

vacant, management needs to determine by whom and how those responsibilities will be fulfilled in order to meet its objectives.

Officials that worked on the campaign told us they shifted their focus away from the suicide prevention media outreach campaign toward the mental health outreach campaign due to reorganization of the offices responsible for suicide prevention activities in 2017. Specifically, under the new organization, and in the absence of suicide prevention program leadership, the officials began reporting directly to mental health program leadership and became more focused on the mental health outreach aspects of the contract.[24] Following the reorganization, officials that worked on the campaign did not have a clear line of reporting to the suicide prevention program. This is also inconsistent with federal internal control standards for control environment, which require agencies to establish an organizational structure and assign responsibilities, such as establishing lines of reporting necessary information to management.[25]

VHA officials told us that one of the highest priorities for the suicide prevention program since the beginning of fiscal year 2018 was to establish a national strategy for preventing veteran suicides. The national strategy, issued in June 2018, includes suicide prevention outreach as one of the strategy's 14 goals.[26] The national strategy also emphasizes VHA's plans to shift to a public health approach to suicide prevention outreach. The public health approach focuses less on raising awareness of the VCL and more on reaching veterans before the point of crisis.[27] VHA officials told us they have been trying to shift to a public health approach since 2016. Some of the campaign themes and messages have reflected this shift; for example, the "Be There" campaign theme that was adopted in fiscal year 2016—and has remained the theme since— emphasizes the message that everyone has a role in helping veterans in crisis feel less alone and connecting them to resources. However, VHA officials told us in May 2018 that they were just beginning to conceptualize what the suicide prevention outreach campaign should look like moving forward. Leadership officials also said that while they were developing the national strategy, they delegated the responsibility for implementing the suicide prevention outreach campaign to other officials working on the campaign.

The decline in VHA's suicide prevention media outreach activities over the past 2 fiscal years is inconsistent with VA's strategic goals, which identify suicide prevention as the agency's top clinical priority for fiscal years 2018 through 2024.[28] Further, VHA has continued to obligate millions of dollars to its suicide prevention media outreach campaign each year. Since fiscal year 2017, VHA has obligated $24.6 million to the contract for media outreach related to both suicide prevention and mental health.[29]

---

[24] VHA officials said that they had planned to appoint new staff to work specifically on the suicide prevention outreach campaign, but they had difficulty doing so until March 2018.

[25] GAO-14-704G and GAO/AIMD-00-21.3.1.

[26] VA, *National Strategy for Preventing Veteran Suicide 2018-2028.*

[27] Some VHA officials indicated that the shift away from raising awareness of the VCL was driven in part by reports that the VCL volume had exceeded its capacity for a period of time. However, VHA leadership officials, including the Director of the VCL, said that raising awareness of the VCL continues to be a priority.

[28] VA, *Department of Veterans Affairs Fiscal Years 2018- 2024 Strategic Plan.*

[29] Some of the deliverables in the fiscal year 2017 contract apply only to one campaign, while other deliverables are divided evenly between the two campaigns. Between fiscal years 2013 and 2016, VHA obligated over $16.8 million to the contract specifically for suicide prevention media outreach. These amounts include the cost of paid and unpaid media outreach, as well as indirect costs.

By not assigning key leadership responsibilities and clear lines of reporting, VHA's ability to oversee the suicide prevention media outreach activities was hindered and these outreach activities decreased. As a result, VHA may not have exposed as many people in the community, such as veterans at risk for suicide, or their families and friends, to its suicide prevention outreach content. Additionally, without establishing responsibility and clear lines of reporting, VHA lacks assurance that it will have continuous oversight of its suicide prevention media outreach activities in the event of additional turnover and reorganization in the future, particularly as VHA begins implementing the suicide prevention media outreach campaign under its new agreement that begins in fiscal year 2019.

VHA Monitors Metrics for Its Suicide Prevention Media Outreach Campaign, but Has Not Established Targets against Which to Evaluate the Campaign's Effectiveness

VHA Monitors Metrics for Its Suicide Prevention Media Outreach Campaign

VHA works with its contractor to create and monitor metrics to help gauge the effectiveness of its suicide prevention media outreach campaign in raising awareness among veterans and others about VHA services, such as the VCL. The metrics primarily focus on the number of individuals who were exposed to or interacted with VHA's suicide prevention content across various forms of outreach, including social media, PSAs, and websites.[30] According to VHA, the metrics are intended to help VHA ensure that its media outreach activities achieve intended results, such as increasing awareness and use of the resources identified on the VCL website.[31] Examples of metrics monitored by VHA and its contractor include those related to (1) social media, such as the number of times a piece of outreach content is displayed on social media; (2) PSAs, such as the total number of markets and television stations airing a PSA; and (3) the VCL website, such as the total traffic to the website, as well as the average amount of time spent on a page and average number of pages viewed per visit.

VHA's contractor is required to monitor the metrics and report results on a monthly basis. Specifically, the contractor provides monthly monitoring reports to VHA that summarize how outreach is performing, such as the number of visits to the VCL website that were driven from paid media sources. Officials noted these reports are key sources of

---

[30] Specifically, for its suicide prevention media outreach, VHA tracks reach, impressions and engagement. For the purposes of this report, "reach" refers to the number of unique people who may have seen a piece of outreach content, while "impressions" typically estimate the total number of times a piece of outreach content was displayed to people. For example, if VHA posts two tweets and 100 people see both of them, the reach is 100 while the impressions are 200. Meanwhile, "engagement" typically measures the number of times the audience interacted with a piece of outreach content, including click-through rates (the percentage of people exposed to an advertisement who click on it to access the advertised website) and social media "likes." These metrics can help VHA gauge the extent to which its outreach is raising awareness of the VCL and other VHA services through its outreach.

[31] VHA officials acknowledged that some metric outcomes can be affected by events or factors outside of VHA's control. For example, certain public events can raise awareness of suicide risk and increase calls to the VCL or visits to the VCL website.

information for VHA on the results of its outreach. VHA officials also told us they informally discuss certain metrics during weekly meetings with VHA's contractor. In addition, VHA works with its contractor to conduct a more in-depth analysis of outreach efforts during and after Suicide Prevention Month each year.

VHA Lacks Metric Targets to Evaluate the Effectiveness of Its Suicide Prevention Media Outreach Campaign

VHA has not established targets for the majority of the metrics it uses to help gauge the effectiveness of its suicide prevention media outreach campaign. As a result, VHA does not have the information it needs to fully evaluate the campaign's effectiveness in raising awareness of VHA's suicide prevention resources among veterans, including the VCL.[32] For example, we found that VHA's contractor's monitoring reports—a summary of key metrics that VHA uses to routinely monitor information regarding the campaign—generally focused on outreach "highlights" and positive results. The reports did not set expectations based on past outreach or targets for new outreach, and lacked more comprehensive information on whether outreach performed against these expectations. For example:

- A monitoring report from 2018 showed that during one month, there were 21,000 social media mentions of keywords specific to VA suicide prevention, such as "VCL" or "veteran suicide," across social media platforms. These mentions earned 120 million impressions; however, there was no indication of the number of keyword mentions or impressions that VHA expected based on its media outreach activities. In addition, the report did not indicate the proportion of mentions that VHA believed were specifically driven by its outreach activities, and there also was no indication of whether these mentions were positive or negative, or what actions to take based on this information.[33]
- Another monitoring report from January 2017 showed that paid advertising drove 39 percent of overall website traffic during one month, while unpaid sources drove the remaining 61 percent. However, there was no information indicating the amounts of paid advertising that VHA conducted during this monitoring period, and whether this amount of website traffic from paid advertising met expectations.
- VHA's 2016 Suicide Prevention Month summary report showed that there were 194,536 visits to the VCL website, roughly an 8 percent increase from the Suicide Prevention Month in 2015. However, the report did not indicate whether this increase from the prior year met expectations, or a different result was expected.

---

[32] While VHA has not established targets for the majority of its metrics, we found that VHA had established one specific target for its suicide prevention PSAs. Specifically, VHA officials told us their goal for each PSA is to rank in the top 10 percent of the Nielsen ratings; VHA's contractor tracks these metrics and provides feedback to VHA through PSA monitoring reports. Nielsen ratings are a tool used to measure audience television viewership and are produced by The Nielsen Company (U.S.), LLC, a data analytics company.

[33] The social media mentions metric can capture negative publicity about VHA or the VCL. For example, it could include Instagram or Facebook posts about unsatisfactory experiences with the VCL, such as long wait times.

VHA officials told us that they have not established targets for most of the suicide prevention media outreach campaign because they lack meaningful targets for the metrics to help evaluate the campaign. VHA officials said that the only target they have established is for each PSA to rank in the top 10 percent of the Nielsen ratings because this is the only meaningful target available that is accepted industry-wide.[34] VHA officials stated that using any other targets would be arbitrary. For the remaining metrics, VHA officials told us they assess the outcomes of their campaign by comparing data from year to year, and examining any changes in the outcomes over time.[35] However, VHA could set targets that capture the number of people who viewed or interacted with its outreach content, similar to its Nielsen target set for television viewership. Doing so would help VHA evaluate whether the campaign has been effective in raising awareness of VHA's suicide prevention resources. Further, creating targets for these additional metrics need not be arbitrary, because VHA could use information about how its metrics performed in the past to develop reasonable and meaningful targets for future performance. VHA could also adjust the targets over time to reflect changes in its metrics or approach to the campaign, such as changes to its paid media budget each year.

Federal internal control standards for monitoring require agencies to assess the quality of its performance by evaluating the results of activities. Agencies can then use these evaluations to determine the effectiveness of its programs or need for any corrective actions.[36] Further, VA's June 2018 National Strategy for Preventing Veteran Suicide also emphasizes the importance of the agency evaluating the effectiveness of its outreach.[37] The absence of established targets leaves VHA without a framework to effectively evaluate its campaign. Our prior work has shown that establishing targets allows agencies to track their progress toward specific goals. In particular, we have developed several key attributes of performance goals and measures including, when appropriate, the development of quantifiable, numerical targets

---

[34] Apart from noting the lack of meaningful targets for their metrics, officials also noted that it is generally difficult to determine whether behavioral shifts have occurred in veterans as a result of VA's outreach efforts and that they have struggled to study these types of outcomes. For example, in 2017, OMHSP proposed collaborating with VA's Center of Excellence for Suicide Prevention, whose mission is in part to use research to inform the implementation of effective veteran suicide prevention strategies, to (1) examine the metrics for the suicide prevention media outreach campaign, and (2) obtain veterans perspectives on the campaign. However, officials said that this effort did not commence due to the lack of senior leadership during and after this time. Officials indicated they would like to continue with their evaluation efforts in the future. VA's Center of Excellence has completed other studies that have examined the effects of VA's suicide prevention campaign. For example, one study that examined associations between VA's suicide prevention campaign and the use of crisis support services found that there were significant increases in call volume to the VCL to both targeted and broad resources during the campaign. See Elizabeth Karras, Naiji Lus, Guoxin Zuo, Xin M. Tu, Brady Stephens, John Draper, Caitlin Thompson, and Robert M. Bossarte, "Measuring Associations of the Department of Veterans Affairs' Suicide Prevention Campaign on the Use of Crisis Support Services," *Suicide and Life-Threatening Behavior,* 46 (4) August 2016: 447-456.

[35] VHA officials shared that their general approach has been to improve their suicide prevention media outreach activities each year by increasing the number of materials issued and website visits because, officials said, this means more people are being reached. They said that the indirect result of reaching more people is that the number of VCL calls are increasing, meaning more people are aware of VA's outreach activities. However, officials also recognized the number of visits to the website will likely reach a maximum after a certain point, and their goal might shift to maintaining the number of website visits rather than increasing it.

[36] GAO-14-704G and GAO/AIMD-00-21.3.1.

[37] VA, *National Strategy for Preventing Veteran Suicide 2012-2018.*

for performance goals and measures.[38] Such targets can facilitate future evaluations of whether overall goals and objectives were achieved by allowing for comparisons between projected performance and actual results. Further, establishing targets for its outreach metrics will enable VHA officials to determine whether outreach performed as expected and raised awareness of VHA resources such as the VCL, including identifying outreach efforts that worked particularly well and those that did not. In doing so, VHA officials will have the opportunity to make better informed decisions in their suicide prevention media outreach campaign to support VA's overall goal of reducing veteran suicides.

Conclusion

VA has stated that preventing veteran suicide is its top clinical priority; yet VHA's lack of leadership attention to its suicide prevention media outreach campaign in recent years has resulted in less outreach to veterans. While VHA identifies the campaign as its primary method of raising suicide prevention awareness, it has not established an effective oversight approach to ensure outreach continuity. This became particularly evident during a recent period of turnover and reorganization in the office responsible for the suicide prevention outreach campaign. Moving forward, VHA has an opportunity to improve its oversight to ensure that its outreach content reaches veterans and others in the community to raise awareness of VHA's suicide prevention services, particularly as VHA begins working with a new contractor beginning in fiscal year 2019.

VHA is responsible for evaluating the effectiveness of its suicide prevention media outreach campaign in raising awareness about VHA services that are available to veterans who may be at risk for suicide. To do so, VHA collects and monitors data on campaign metrics to help gauge the effectiveness of its suicide prevention media outreach campaign in raising such awareness, but has not established targets for the majority of these metrics because officials reported that there are no meaningful, industry-wide targets for them. We disagree with VHA's assertion that other targets would not be meaningful; VHA collects data on its metrics that it can use to develop reasonable and meaningful targets for future performance. In the absence of established targets, VHA cannot evaluate the effectiveness of the campaign, and make informed decisions about which activities should be continued to support VA's overall goal of reducing veteran suicides.

Recommendations for Executive Action

We are making the following two recommendations to VA:

1) The Under Secretary for Health should establish an approach for overseeing its suicide prevention media outreach efforts that includes clear delineation of roles and

---

[38] GAO-03-143 and GAO-12-208G.

responsibilities for those in leadership and contract oversight roles, including during periods of staff turnover or program changes. (Recommendation 1)

2) The Under Secretary for Health should require officials within the Office of Suicide Prevention and Mental Health to establish targets for the metrics the office uses to evaluate the effectiveness of its suicide prevention media outreach campaign. (Recommendation 2)

Agency Comments and Our Evaluation

We provided a draft of this chapter to VA for review and comment. In its written comments, summarized below and reprinted in Appendix I, VA concurred with our recommendations. VA described ongoing and planned actions and provided a timeline for addressing our recommendations. VA also provided technical comments, which we incorporated as appropriate.

In response to our first recommendation, to establish an oversight approach that includes delineation of roles and responsibilities, VA acknowledged that organizational transitions and realignments within OMHSP contributed to unclear roles and responsibilities in 2017 and 2018. VA said that OMHSP has made organizational improvements, including hiring a permanent Director for Suicide Prevention and establishing a new organizational structure. In its comments, VA requested closure of the first recommendation based on these actions.

However, to fully implement this recommendation, VA will need to provide evidence that it has established an oversight approach for the suicide prevention media outreach campaign. This would include providing information about the roles and responsibilities, as well as reporting requirements, for contract and leadership officials involved in the suicide prevention media outreach campaign under the new organizational structure and the new contract. VA will also need to demonstrate that it has a plan in place to ensure continued oversight of the suicide prevention media campaign in the event of staff turnover or program changes.

In response to our second recommendation, to establish targets against which to evaluate suicide prevention metrics, VA said it has plans to work with communications experts to develop metrics, targets, and an evaluation strategy to improve its evaluation of its suicide prevention program efforts, including outreach. VA expects to complete these actions by April 2019.

As agreed with your office, unless you publicly announce the contents of this chapter earlier, we plan no further distribution until 30 days from the report date. At that time, we will send copies to the appropriate congressional committees and the Secretary of Veterans Affairs.

Sincerely yours, Debra A. Draper
Director, Health Care

Appendix I: Comments from the Department of Veterans Affairs

THE SECRETARY OF VETERANS AFFAIRS
WASHINGTON

October 31, 2018

Ms. Debra A. Draper
Director
Health Care
U.S. Government Accountability Office
441 G Street, NW
Washington, DC 20548

Dear Ms. Draper:

The Department of Veterans Affairs (VA) has reviewed the Government Accountability Office (GAO) draft report: ***"VA HEALTH CARE: Improvements Needed in Suicide Prevention Media Outreach Oversight and Evaluation"*** (GAO-19-66).

The enclosure contains technical comments and sets forth the actions to be taken to address the draft report recommendations.

VA appreciates the opportunity to comment on your draft report.

Sincerely,

Robert L. Wilkie

Department of Veterans Affairs (VA) Comments to
Government Accountability Office (GAO) Draft Report
"VA HEALTH CARE: Improvements Needed in Suicide Prevention Media Outreach Campaign Oversight and Evaluation"
(GAO-19-66)

GAO Recommendation 1: The Under Secretary for Health should establish an approach for overseeing its suicide prevention media outreach efforts that includes delineation of roles and responsibilities for those in leadership and contract oversight roles, including during periods of staff turnover or program changes.

VA Comment: Concur. Suicide prevention is the Department of Veterans Affairs' (VA) highest priority. Every death by suicide is a tragedy, and we will not relent in our efforts to connect Veterans in need with life-saving support. VA's goal is to reduce suicide among Veterans. We can save lives.

VA's published National Strategy for Preventing Veteran Suicide provides the framework for identifying priorities, organizing efforts, and contributing to a national focus on Veteran suicide prevention over the next decade. The strategy aligns with the 2012 National Strategy for Suicide Prevention, consists of 4 strategic directions, 14 goals, 43 objectives, leverages the public health approach to suicide prevention, and focuses on the importance of collaboration and urgency.

The four strategic directions are:

1. Healthy and Empowered Veterans, Families, and Communities
   Work with community partners and policymakers to promote resources for Veterans and to promote mental health awareness and treatment.

2. Clinical and Community Preventive Services
   Share resources, training opportunities, interventions, and lethal means safety resources with providers outside VA and with clergy, first responders, law enforcement officials, and community partners.

3. Treatment, Recovery, and Support Services
   Work with local emergency departments and hospitals to promote Veteran suicide prevention resources and to ensure continuity of care for all Veterans admitted to an inpatient mental health unit.

4. Surveillance, Research, and Evaluation
   Share the VA National Suicide Data Report and National Strategy for Preventing Veteran Suicide with community partners.

VA has a comprehensive approach to suicide prevention. Here are just a few of our substantial efforts:

1. Expanding the Veterans Crisis Line that connects Veterans in crisis and their families and friends with qualified, caring VA responders through a confidential toll-free hotline, online chat, or text. Veterans and their loved ones can call **1-800-273-8255 and Press 1**, chat online, or send a text message to 838255 to receive confidential support 24 hours a day, 7 days a week, 365 days a year. More information is available at https://www.veteranscrisisline.net/.

2. Creating new cross-sector partnerships across various disciplines: faith communities, employers, schools, and health care organizations to name a few. Together we can reach more people.

3. Implementing the Joint Action Plan for Supporting Veterans During Their Transition From Uniformed Service to Civilian Life

4. Launching S.A.V.E. online suicide prevention training that educates yourself or your employees about how to recognize suicide risk factors and warning signs.

5. Implementing the Mayor's Challenge, which equips communities to build coalitions to prevent Veteran suicide. This partnership between VA and the Department of Health and Human Service Substance Abuse and Mental Health Services Administration (SAMHSA) helps local leaders in city governments work together to prevent suicide among Veterans. We have 27 Mayors now and we want more.

6. #BeThere prevention initiative teaches members of the community how simple acts can help save a Veteran in crisis. More information is available at https://www.veteranscrisisline.net/BeThere.aspx.

7. Make the Connection campaign is an online resource that connects Veterans, their family members and friends, and other supporters with information and solutions to issues affecting their lives. More information is available at https://maketheconnection.net/.

8. Coaching into Care (1-888-823-7458) is a national telephone service of VA. Coaching into Care aims to educate, support, and empower family members and friends who are seeking care or services for a Veteran. More information is available at https://www.mirecc.va.gov/coaching/.

9. Recovery Engagement and Coordination for Health – Veterans Enhanced Treatment Program (REACH VET) is an innovative program that applies principles of predictive medicine to prevent suicide.

10. About Face videos feature the real stories of Veterans who have experienced post-traumatic stress disorder with additional perspectives from their family members and VA clinicians. https://www.ptsd.va.gov/apps/AboutFace/.

11. How to Talk to a Child About a Suicide Attempt in Your Family: If there has been a recent suicide attempt in your family, this may be one of the toughest experiences you and your children may ever face. It is important to take care of yourself, so that you are better able to care for your child.

12. Paid media outreach such as advertisements on digital and social media.

VA's suicide prevention efforts are successful:

- Over 16,000 American citizens have downloaded VA's S.A.V.E. training to prevent suicides. Annual S.A.V.E. training is mandatory for VA employees, and in September 2018 alone over 52,000 VA employees completed it.
- The number of Veterans receiving mental health care in VA doubled over the past 10 years, now we are helping over 1.7 million Veterans with their mental health concerns.
- VA repeatedly meets our goals for being in the top 10 percent Nielsen ranking for our suicide prevention public service announcements.
- The Veterans Crisis Line serves about 2000 callers a day. Over the past 10 years, the Veterans Crisis Line has answered over 3 million calls, more than 363,000 online chats, and more than 83,000 text messages.
- Last year, VA's suicide prevention coordinators did 18,836 community outreach events and reached approximately 1,932,902 people.
- Over 102,000 people visited our #BeThere campaign page last year.
- Twenty-seven mayors are taking the challenge to reduce Veteran suicide in their cities. VA wants every city to take action to prevent suicide.
- During Suicide Prevention Month (September 2018) VA saw a lot of success with #BeThere messaging:
    - 50+ million #BeThere Twitter Chat impressions
    - 18 million+ social media reach (over past 7 days)
    - 2.6 million Thunderclap social media reach
    - 1,800+ registrants for Action Alliance's Messaging Webinar
    - 100+ private and public sector partners

In 2018, VA partnered with Johnson & Johnson on a broadly promoted public service announcement featuring Tom Hanks speaking that GAO did not include in the draft report. YouTube alone had over 30,000 views. VA showcased it as part of the #BeThere campaign. This outreach effort was supported through a non-monetary Memorandum of Agreement with Johnson & Johnson, at no cost to the Veterans Health Administration (VHA).

Regarding Paid Media spending, VHA estimates that the total amount spent in fiscal year (FY) 2018 will be about $1.5M. This will include money spent in September 2018 for Suicide Prevention Month paid media. VHA will not have final invoices for an exact total until sometime after October 2018. As indicated above, paid media is only one component of VHA's comprehensive suicide prevention effort, and it is a small portion of VHA's annual expenditures for suicide prevention.

VHA acknowledges that organizational transitions and realignments within Office of Mental Health and Suicide Prevention (OMHSP) contributed to unclear roles and responsibilities from mid-2017 to mid-2018. OMHSP has made significant organizational structure improvements to clearly delineate roles and responsibilities for those in leadership and contract oversight roles since that time. Organizational improvements within the Executive Leadership team and the Suicide Prevention team also ensure continuity during periods of staff turnover and program changes. OMHSP has hired a permanent Director for Suicide Prevention, and established and received approval for a permanent organizational structure which creates a clear chain of command within OMHSP and to VHA. With this new robust organizational structure in place, the Director for Suicide Prevention oversees communications and outreach activities in a more organized and deliberate manner. Similarly, contractual tasks related to these outreach activities fall within the Deputy Director for Partnerships' portfolio.

VHA has completed work on this recommendation and requests GAO close this recommendation as implemented. In support of our closure request, VHA has submitted the final, signed OMHSP organizational chart to GAO. Completion Date: July 2018

Recommendation 2: The Under Secretary for Health should require officials within the Office of Suicide Prevention and Mental Health to establish targets for the metrics the office uses to evaluate the effectiveness of its suicide prevention media outreach campaign.

VA Comment: Concur. GAO recognized that OMHSP has a robust monitoring process in place to track both reach and engagement of our suicide prevention outreach campaigns. Beyond quantitative data, OMHSP also tracks qualitative measures of success such as establishing partnerships with prominent organizations or securing promotion of our resources from high-profile public figures.

VHA has looked at broad indicators of impact for its suicide prevention outreach efforts for some time. VHA's current Agency Priority Goal is to provide core recommended interventions to Veterans targeted through its predictive risk modeling algorithms and to reduce Veteran suicide through a "Mayor's Challenge" partnership program. The growth in demand for services at the Veterans Crisis Line (VCL) has grown year over year and has been supported through ongoing outreach. In particular over FY 2018, the demand for chat and text services at VCL increased by over 25 percent and nearly 30 percent, respectively. Local outreach activities have also been part of national strategy including annual Community Mental Health Summits at VHA facilities. In 2018 there were 149 Summits with over 13,500 participants, and 83 percent of participants reported gaining a better understanding of suicide prevention resources and services through VHA and in their community.

VHA accepts GAO's recommendation to do more. OMHSP has begun to leverage VA expertise in health communication and evaluation to determine additional measures of effectiveness. These measures will be benchmarked against similar national program metrics. This effort is part of a larger initiative that is underway to determine program measures of effectiveness for the entire suicide prevention program. After receiving results from communications experts, OMHSP will finalize metrics, targets and the subsequent evaluation strategy. Target Completion Date: April 2019.

In: Top 10 Reports and Testimonies in December 2018
Editor: Sarah J. Nygaard
ISBN: 978-1-53615-507-5

Chapter 10

WORKING CHILDREN: FEDERAL INJURY DATA AND COMPLIANCE STRATEGIES COULD BE STRENGTHENED*

United States Government Accountability Office

ABBREVIATIONS

ASEC	Annual Social and Economic Supplement
BLS	Bureau of Labor Statistics
CAIS	Childhood Agricultural Injury Survey
CFOI	Census of Fatal Occupational Injuries
CPS	Current Population Survey
DOL	U.S. Department of Labor
ETA	Employment and Training Administration
FLSA	Fair Labor Standards Act of 1938, as amended
NASS	National Agricultural Statistics Service
NAWS	National Agricultural Workers Survey
NEISS-Work	National Electronic Injury Surveillance System-Occupational Supplement
NIOSH	National Institute for Occupational Safety and Health
OSHA	Occupational Safety and Health Administration
OSH Act	Occupational Safety and Health Act of 1970, as amended
SOII	Survey of Occupational Injuries and Illnesses
USDA	U.S. Department of Agriculture
WHD	Wage and Hour Division
WHISARD	Wage and Hour Investigative Support and Reporting

* This is an edited, reformatted and augmented version of United States Government Accountability Office; Report to Congressional Requesters, Publication No. GAO-19-26, dated November 2018.

WHY GAO DID THIS STUDY

Children aged 17 and under in the United States work for various reasons: some are encouraged to work to develop independence and responsibility; others work because of financial need. At the same time, research suggests working children are at risk for work-related injuries and fatalities. GAO was asked to update its 2002 child labor report to discuss the current status of working children in the United States, including those working in agriculture.

This chapter examines (1) children working in the United States since 2003, (2) work-related fatalities and injuries to such children for the period, and (3) how DOL oversees compliance with the child labor provisions of the Fair Labor Standards Act. GAO analyzed federal data from several sources, including DOL and other agencies; reviewed relevant federal laws and regulations; and interviewed officials from DOL, including staff in six WHD district offices that were selected based on factors such as investigations with at least one child labor violation, and all five regional offices. GAO also spoke with stakeholders knowledgeable about child labor, such as employer and employee labor groups.

WHAT GAO RECOMMENDS

GAO is making four recommendations to DOL, including that DOL should evaluate the feasibility of measuring injuries and illnesses to certain worker populations, and establish metrics for child labor-related outreach in agriculture. DOL generally agreed with all four recommendations.

WHAT GAO FOUND

The number of working children has fluctuated with the economy since 2003. An estimated 3.3 million children aged 15 to 17 worked in the summer months of 2003, and the number of working children reached a low of 1.9 million by 2011. It then increased to 2.5 million by 2017, but has not returned to its pre-recession level, as shown below. GAO's analysis of the U.S. Department of Commerce and the Department of Labor's (DOL) Current Population Survey data found that non-agricultural industries employed an estimated 2.5 million working children aged 15 to 17 in the summer months of 2017. Further, GAO found that the leisure and hospitality industry employed the largest number of children.

Since 2003, the majority of work-related child fatalities were in agriculture, and while available data are incomplete, they indicate that work-related injuries have declined. Although agriculture employs a small percentage of working children, DOL data indicate that from 2003 to 2016, the year for which the most recent data are available, over half of the 452 work-related fatalities among children were in agriculture. Also, according to DOL estimates, the number of work- related injuries and illnesses to children has declined, but these estimates do not include certain populations. While DOL is conducting a pilot study to enhance its work-related injury and illness data, this pilot does not include children, including those 14 or under. DOL has not evaluated the feasibility of measuring this population. As a result, DOL is missing opportunities to more accurately quantify injuries to children, which could better inform its compliance and enforcement efforts.

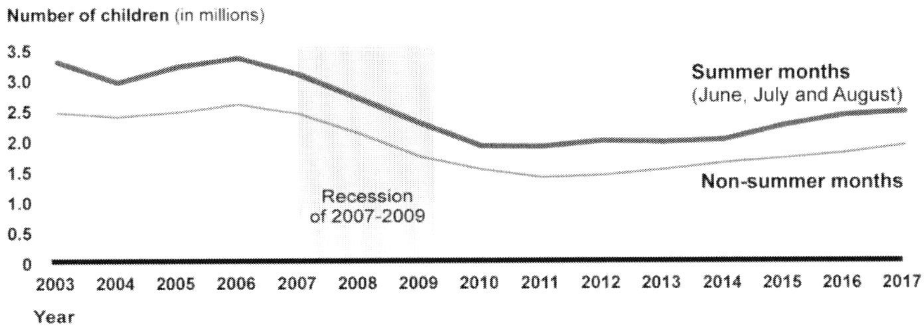

Source: GAO analysis of Current Population Survey (CPS) data. | GAO-19-26.

Estimated Number of Working Children Aged 15 to 17 in the United States, 2003 to 2017.

DOL's Wage and Hour Division (WHD) uses a strategic enforcement approach to oversee compliance with the child labor provisions of the Fair Labor Standards Act and collaborates within DOL to exchange information on potential violations. WHD officials told GAO that their enforcement and compliance efforts include outreach to industries with vulnerable workers, including children. However, WHD has not developed metrics for child labor-related outreach in agriculture. Federal internal control standards state that management should define objectives clearly to enable the identification of risks, such as by defining objectives in measurable terms. Without such metrics, WHD may not be effectively addressing the risks faced by children working in agriculture.

November 2, 2018

The Honorable Rosa DeLauro
Ranking Member
Subcommittee on Labor, Health and Human Services, Education, and
Related Agencies Committee on Appropriations
House of Representatives

The Honorable Lucille Roybal-Allard
House of Representatives

Children in the United States are often encouraged to work because early work experiences are thought to develop independence and responsibility; some children may also work because of financial need. At the same time, federal research suggests that working children are at risk for work-related injuries or fatalities.[1] Working children (aged 17 and under) are afforded certain protections, such as prohibitions on working in certain hazardous

[1] Department of Health and Human Services, Centers for Disease Control and Prevention, National Institute for Occupational Safety and Health, *Young Worker Injury Deaths: A Historical Summary of Surveillance and Investigative Findings*, Publication No. 2017-168 (Morgantown, WV: July 2017).

occupations,[2] under the child labor provisions of the Fair Labor Standards Act of 1938, as amended (FLSA) and regulations issued by the Department of Labor (DOL)[3]—the federal agency generally responsible for enforcing the FLSA.[4] In 2002, we reported that DOL could strengthen its efforts to protect children who work across all industries— particularly those with high rates of injuries—and strengthen its data collection for enforcement planning.[5]

You asked us to update our 2002 report to describe the current status of working children in the United States, including those working in agricultural occupations, and to report on the enforcement of the FLSA and associated regulations. For this chapter, we use the term "working children" to describe individuals aged 17 and under, in paid employment, unless otherwise noted. This chapter examines (1) what is known about children working in the United States, including those working in agriculture; (2) what is known about work-related fatalities and injuries to children working in the United States, including those working in agriculture; and (3) how DOL oversees compliance with the child labor provisions of the FLSA, including any efforts to collaborate within DOL.

To address the first two objectives, we analyzed national federal data from several sources.[6] Specifically, for the first objective, we analyzed employment and demographic characteristics data from DOL's Bureau of Labor Statistics' (BLS) Current Population Survey (CPS) from 2003 to 2017,[7] as well as employment and poverty data from the 2017 Annual Social and Economic Supplement data to produce estimates of child worker populations and demographic trends.[8] For additional information on children working in agricultural occupations, we also analyzed employment and demographic characteristics data from DOL's National Agricultural Worker Survey from fiscal years 2003 to 2016, the Department of Health and Human Services' National Institute for Occupational Safety and Health's (NIOSH) Childhood Agricultural Injury Survey for the years the data were collected during

---

[2] These protections include age-based limitations on the number of hours and times of day children can work and minimum ages below which children cannot work. Minimum ages for working children vary, as discussed later in the report. Agricultural employers are subject to separate child labor provisions under the Fair Labor Standards Act of 1938, as amended, including different age limits and occupational restrictions.

[3] Pub. L. No. 75-718, 52 Stat. 1060 (codified as amended at 29 U.S.C. §§ 201-219); 29 C.F.R. pt. 570. In addition to the child labor provisions, the FLSA also requires covered employers to comply with certain minimum wage and overtime requirements.

[4] Other federal laws, administered by other agencies, may also apply to working children. For example, under the Federal Insecticide, Fungicide, and Rodenticide Act, the Environmental Protection Agency has implemented measures to protect workers from pesticide exposure through its Worker Protection Standard, which, among other things, establishes a minimum age of 18 for workers engaged in certain pesticide-related tasks. For purposes of this report, we focus on the child labor provisions under the FLSA and its implementing regulations, and exclude from our scope any requirements under other laws and regulations.

[5] GAO, *Child Labor: Labor Can Strengthen Its Efforts to Protect Children Who Work,* GAO-02-880 (Washington D.C.: Sept. 27, 2002).

[6] None of the analyses in this report are intended to assess compliance with the FLSA, because the definitions of terms used in these data sets may not be the same as the definitions in the FLSA and DOL's regulations, among other reasons.

[7] Our 2002 report provided information from 1990 to 2001. In 2002, the CPS variables used to identify the race and ethnicity of working children, as well as the industries and occupations they may be employed in, significantly shifted. Accordingly, we chose to begin our analysis with 2003.

[8] We generally refer to these data as CPS data throughout this report. The CPS and its Annual and Social Economic Supplement are sponsored jointly by the Census Bureau and the Department of Labor's Bureau of Labor Statistics. To produce our estimates, we analyzed monthly CPS data from 2003 to 2017 and data from the March 2017 CPS Annual and Social Economic Supplement, which contains data for calendar year 2016.

the same time period,[9] as well as overall agricultural workforce data from the U.S. Department of Agriculture's 2012 Census of Agriculture.[10]

To address the second objective, we analyzed data on work-related child fatalities from BLS's Census of Fatal Occupational Injuries and data on work-related child injuries and illnesses from its Survey of Occupational Injuries and Illnesses for 2003 to 2016.[11] For additional information on work-related injuries to children, we also analyzed injury and illness data from NIOSH's National Electronic Injury Surveillance System from 2003 to 2016 and the Childhood Agricultural Injury Survey (CAIS) for the years the data was collected.[12] Given that each data set has its own strengths and limitations and that analysis across data sets can compound such limitations, we sent our analyses to the appropriate officials to ensure we accurately characterized the data and that our analyses across data sets appropriately accounted for data limitations. See appendix I for a detailed list of the data sources we analyzed for these objectives.

To address the third objective regarding how DOL oversees compliance with the child labor provisions of the FLSA, we analyzed data from DOL's Wage and Hour Division's (WHD) Wage and Hour Investigative Support and Reporting Database (WHISARD) from fiscal years 2010 to 2016, which tracks investigations, violations, and penalties assessed.[13] We also interviewed WHD officials at the five regional offices and six selected district offices to obtain information on WHD's enforcement of the child labor provisions of the FLSA.[14] Specifically, in each WHD region we interviewed the regional Child Labor Coordinator, and in each district office we interviewed a WHD investigator, Community Outreach Resource and Planning specialist, and district director. We selected WHD district offices to include different concentrations of investigations with at least one child labor violation, obtain geographic diversity, and ensure representation across agricultural and non-agricultural sectors. The findings from our interviews with regional and district WHD staff are not generalizable but provide examples of WHD's enforcement and compliance assistance efforts with regard to the child labor provisions of the FLSA.

To inform all of our objectives, we interviewed DOL staff in the national office, including WHD and Occupational Safety and Health Administration (OSHA) officials, and additional stakeholders, such as employer and employee labor groups, to learn about overall child labor trends in agricultural and non-agricultural sectors.[15] We also reviewed relevant federal laws, regulations, and guidance pertaining to child labor.[16]

---

[9] The CAIS was conducted in 2001, 2004, 2006, 2009, 2012, and 2014. We analyzed CAIS data from 2004, 2006, 2009, 2012, and 2014, as this report's scope begins with 2003.

[10] The 2012 Census of Agriculture was the most recent Census for which data are available.

[11] 2016 is the most recent year for which data are available from these data sets.

[12] We analyzed CAIS data from the same selected years for all analyses (i.e., 2004, 2006, 2009, 2012, and 2014). NIOSH combined 2 years of CAIS injury data to produce estimates of work-related injuries to children with less than 33 percent relative standard error, and thus within NIOSH's standards for reporting.

[13] Data for fiscal year 2016 was the most current data available at the time of our audit work. Throughout this report, investigations—and any violations found and resulting penalties—are counted in the fiscal year in which they concluded, although the investigations work may have been done in a prior fiscal year.

[14] WHD has five regional offices—Atlanta, Chicago, Dallas, Philadelphia, and San Francisco—and 54 district offices nationwide.

[15] We conducted 11 stakeholder interviews with a range of organizations, including those focused on employers, occupational health and safety, or working children.

[16] States may also have laws protecting working children, such as state child welfare laws and state child labor laws; however, a review of state laws was outside the scope of this report. Additionally, as noted previously, other

To assess the reliability of all of the data sets used in our study, we reviewed documentation, interviewed or obtained information from officials responsible for the data, and tested the data for inaccuracies. We determined that the data fields we used are sufficiently reliable for the purposes of our reporting objectives. See appendix I for more detailed information about our scope and methodology.

We conducted this performance audit from March 2017 to November 2018 in accordance with generally accepted government auditing standards. Those standards require that we plan and perform the audit to obtain sufficient, appropriate evidence to provide a reasonable basis for our findings and conclusions based on our audit objectives. We believe that the evidence obtained provides a reasonable basis for our findings and conclusions based on our audit objectives.

BACKGROUND

Fair Labor Standards Act and Federal Enforcement

The child labor requirements under the FLSA and its implementing regulations vary, depending on the age of the child and whether or not the child works in agriculture. With respect to non-agricultural employment, children aged 16 and 17 may work in any occupation other than those declared by the Secretary of Labor to be particularly hazardous for such individuals or detrimental to their health or well-being,[17] and there are no limits on the number of hours or times of day they may work.[18] The non- agricultural employment of children aged 14 and 15 is limited to occupations and time periods that DOL has determined will not interfere with their schooling and to conditions which will not interfere with their health and well-being. Accordingly, DOL has issued regulations that limit the types of jobs, number of hours, and times of day that these children may work.[19] For example, among other things, children aged 14 and 15 may engage in work such as office or clerical work, certain types of food service, and the dispensation of gasoline, outside of school hours, subject to maximum daily and weekly limits. In general, children aged 13 and under may not be employed in non-agricultural work other than work that is not covered by the FLSA, such as casual babysitting, and work that is exempt from the child labor provisions, such as delivering newspapers.[20]

More details about child labor provisions for non-agricultural employment are in Table 1.

---

federal laws such as the Federal Insecticide, Fungicide, and Rodenticide Act that may apply to working children are outside the scope of this report.

[17] See 29 U.S.C. § 203(l) and 29 C.F.R. §§ 570.50-570.68 (DOL's "hazardous occupations orders" for non-agricultural occupations). See table 2 for a list of these orders.

[18] However, working children may still be subject to the FLSA minimum wage and overtime provisions. Unless otherwise exempt, a child working in non-agricultural employment is generally entitled to receive the same minimum wage and overtime protections as adult workers.

[19] See generally 29 U.S.C. § 203(l) and 29 C.F.R. §§ 570.31-570.39. Employment that is not specifically permitted is prohibited.

[20] See 29 U.S.C. § 213(d). In addition, children under 16 (including those 13 and under) may be employed by their parent, or a person standing in place of a parent, in any occupation other than manufacturing, mining, or an occupation declared to be hazardous by DOL for children aged 16 and 17. 29 U.S.C. § 203(l), 29 C.F.R. § 570.2(a)(2).

Table 1. Child Labor Provisions for Non-Agricultural Employment

Age	Occupations allowed	Hours allowed	Times of day	Other conditions
13 or under[a]	Employment generally prohibited.	Not applicable.	Not applicable.	Not applicable.
14 and 15[a]	Limited to those occupations and time periods that DOL has determined will not interfere with their schooling and to conditions that will not interfere with their health and well-being, such as office and clerical work, among others.[b] Mining, manufacturing, and occupations declared to be hazardous by DOL for children aged 16 and 17 are expressly prohibited.	Only outside of school hours.[c] Daily limits: No more than 3 hours per day on days when school is in session; no more than 8 hours per day on days when school is not in session. Weekly limits: No more than 18 hours per week during weeks when school is in session; no more than 40 hours per week during weeks when school is not in session.	Between Labor Day and June 1: Between 7 am and 7 pm June 1 through Labor Day: Between 7 am and 9 pm	Certain exceptions apply for children participating in an approved Work Experience and Career Exploration Program, children participating in an approved Work Study program, and children who are employed as professional sports attendants, among others.[d]
16 and 17	Any occupations other than those declared by the Secretary of Labor to be particularly hazardous for the employment of children aged 16 and 17, or detrimental to their health or well-being.[e]	No specific restrictions for allowable work.[c]	No restrictions for allowable work.	Certain exceptions may apply; for example, some of the hazardous occupations orders contain limited exemptions for eligible apprentices and student-learners.

Source: GAO review of the Fair Labor Standards Act of 1938, as amended, applicable regulations, and Department of Labor guidance. | GAO-19-26.

[a]Children under age 16, including those aged 13 and under, may engage in work that is not covered by the FLSA, such as casual babysitting; and work that is exempt from the child labor provisions, such as acting or performing in motion pictures, theatrical productions, or radio or television productions, or delivering newspapers. In addition, if they are employed by their parent, or a person standing in place of a parent, children under age 16 may work in any occupation other than mining, manufacturing, or an occupation declared to be hazardous by DOL for children aged 16 and 17. There are no specific restrictions on the number of hours or times of day for these types of permissible work, although minimum wage and overtime requirements may apply.

[b]Other examples include, but are not limited to, doing errand and delivery work by foot, bicycle, and public transportation; lifeguarding (15-year-olds only); dispensing gasoline and oil; and car cleaning, washing, and polishing by hand. See 29 C.F.R. § 570.34.

[c]Minimum wage and overtime requirements may also apply.

[d]For example, children aged 14 and 15 participating in a Work Experience and Career Exploration Program that meets certain requirements may be employed for up to 23 hours per week and up to 3 hours per day when school is in session, including during school hours. 29 C.F.R. § 570.36. According to DOL guidance, the program is designed to provide a work experience and career exploration program for students who can benefit from a career-oriented education.

[e]DOL has established 17 "hazardous occupations orders," declaring certain non-agricultural occupations to be particularly hazardous for the employment of children between the ages of 16 and 18 years, or detrimental to their health or well-being (referred to in this table as "occupations declared to be hazardous by DOL for children aged 16 and 17"). See 29 C.F.R. §§ 570.50-570.68.

Further, children under age 18 are generally prohibited from working in the 17 non-agricultural hazardous occupations that DOL has established by regulation, subject to limited exemptions (see Table 2). These orders apply either on an occupational basis, irrespective of the industry, or on an industry basis, specifying the occupations in the industry that are not permitted. For example, one of the orders generally prohibits all occupations in connection with mining, other than coal, but allows work in offices, in a warehouse or supply house, in a laboratory, and in repair or maintenance shops not located underground, among other exceptions.[21]

Table 2. Non-Agricultural Hazardous Occupations Orders

Hazardous occupations order number	Hazardous occupations order title
1	Occupations in or about plants or establishments manufacturing or storing explosives or articles containing explosive components
2	Occupations of motor-vehicle driver and outside helper
3	Coal mine occupations
4	Forest fire fighting and forest fire prevention occupations, timber tract occupations, forestry service occupations, logging occupations, and occupations in the operation of any sawmill, lath mill, shingle mill, or cooperage stock mill
5	Occupations involved in the operation of power-driven woodworking machines
6	Exposure to radioactive substances and to ionizing radiations
7	Occupations involved in the operation of power-driven hoisting apparatus
8	Occupations involved in the operation of power-driven metal forming, punching, and shearing machines
9	Occupations in connection with mining, other than coal
10	Occupations in the operation of power-driven meat-processing machines and occupations involving slaughtering, meat and poultry packing, processing, or rendering
11	Occupations involved in the operation of bakery machines
12	Occupations involved in the operation of balers, compactors, and paper-products machines
13	Occupations involved in the manufacture of brick, tile, and kindred products
14	Occupations involving the operation of circular saws, band saws, guillotine shears, chain saws, reciprocating saws, wood chippers, and abrasive cutting discs
15	Occupations involved in wrecking, demolition, and ship-breaking operations
16	Occupations in roofing operations and on or about a roof
17	Occupations in excavation operations

Source: 29 C.F.R. §§ 570.50-570.68. | GAO-19-26.

Notes: Although referred to as hazardous occupations orders, the Department of Labor (DOL) has issued these orders by regulation. Each order describes specific work activities, including definitions and exceptions, that DOL has declared to be particularly hazardous for minors between the ages of 16 and 18, or detrimental to their health or well-being. In addition, the Fair Labor Standards Act of 1938, as amended, and DOL regulations prohibit children aged 14 and 15 from performing any work proscribed by these orders. This table includes only the titles of each order, not the specific work activities, definitions, and exemptions.

Under the FLSA, different child labor requirements apply to agricultural occupations.[22] For example, there are no occupational restrictions for children aged 16 and 17 working in

[21] 29 C.F.R. § 570.60(a).

[22] For purposes of the FLSA, "agriculture" includes "farming in all its branches and among other things includes the cultivation and tillage of the soil, dairying, the production, cultivation, growing, and harvesting of any agricultural or horticultural commodities, the raising of livestock, bees, fur-bearing animals, or poultry, and any practices (including any forestry, or lumbering operations) performed by a farmer or on a farm as an incident to or in conjunction with such farming operations, including preparation for market, delivery to storage or to market or to carriers for transportation to market." 29 U.S.C. § 203(f). Migrant and seasonal agricultural employees, regardless of their age and whether hired directly by the farmer or provided by a farm labor contractor—when covered by the FLSA—are entitled to the same protections under the FLSA as other farm workers, according to WHD guidance.

agriculture.[23] In accordance with the FLSA, DOL has issued 11 hazardous occupations orders for agricultural occupations, declaring certain occupations to be particularly hazardous for children under age 16 (see Table 3).[24]

Table 3. Agricultural Hazardous Occupations Orders

Hazardous occupations order number	Hazardous occupations
1	Operating a tractor of over 20 power-take-off horsepower, or connecting or disconnecting an implement or any of its parts to or from such a tractor.
2	Operating or assisting to operate[a] any of the following machines: (1) corn picker, cotton picker, grain combine, hay mower, forage harvester, hay baler, potato digger, or mobile pea viner; (2) feed grinder, crop dryer, forage blower, auger conveyor, or the unloading mechanism of a nongravity-type self-unloading wagon or trailer; or (3) power post-hole digger, power post driver, or nonwalking type rotary tiller.
3	Operating or assisting to operate[a] any of the following machines: trencher or earthmoving equipment, fork lift, potato combine; or power- driven circular, band, or chain saw.
4	Working on a farm in a yard, pen, or stall occupied by a bull, boar, or stud horse maintained for breeding purposes; or a sow with suckling pigs or cow with newborn calf (with umbilical cord present).
5	Felling, bucking, skidding, loading or unloading timber with butt diameter of more than 6 inches.
6	Working from a ladder or scaffold (painting, repairing, or building structures, pruning trees, picking fruit, etc.) at a height of over 20 feet.
7	Driving a bus, truck, or automobile when transporting passengers, or riding on a tractor as a passenger or helper.
8	Working inside a fruit, forage, or grain storage designed to retain an oxygen deficient or toxic atmosphere; an upright silo within 2 weeks after silage has been added or when a top unloading device is in operating position; a manure pit; or a horizontal silo while operating a tractor for packing purposes.
9	Handling or applying (including cleaning or decontaminating equipment, disposal or return of empty containers, or serving as a flagman for aircraft applying) agricultural chemicals classified under the Federal Insecticide, Fungicide, and Rodenticide Act as Category I of toxicity, identified by the word "poison" and the "skull and crossbones" on the label; or Category II of toxicity, identified by the word "warning" on the label.
10	Handling or using a blasting agent, including but not limited to, dynamite, black powder, sensitized ammonium nitrate, blasting caps and primer cord.
11	Transporting, transferring, or applying anhydrous ammonia.

Source: 29 C.F.R. § 570.71 | GAO-19-26.

Notes: Although referred to as hazardous occupations orders, the Department of Labor (DOL) has issued these orders via regulation. Each agricultural occupation listed in this table has been declared by the DOL to be particularly hazardous for the employment of children under the age of 16. These orders do not apply to children employed by a parent or a person standing in place of a parent on a farm owned or operated by such parent or person.

[a] "Operating or assisting to operate" includes starting, stopping, adjusting, feeding, or any other activity involving physical contact associated with the operation.

---

[23] Minimum wage requirements may apply; however, agricultural employees are generally not subject to the overtime provisions of the FLSA. See 29 U.S.C. § 213(b)(12).

[24] See 29 U.S.C. § 213(c)(2); 29 C.F.R. §§ 570.70-570.72 (DOL's hazardous occupations orders for agricultural employment).

Table 4. Child Labor Provisions for Agricultural Employment

Age	Allowable occupations	Allowable hours	Other conditions
Under 12[a, b]	Non-hazardous (agricultural).[c]	Only outside of school hours.	Children must be employed with the consent of their parent (or a person standing in place of a parent) on a farm where all employees are exempt from the minimum wage requirements due to its size.[d]
12 and 13[a]	Non-hazardous (agricultural).[c]	Only outside of school hours.	Children must be employed either with the written consent of their parent (or a person standing in place of a parent); or on the same farm where such parent or person is employed.
14 and 15[a]	Non-hazardous (agricultural).[c]	Only outside ofschool hours.[e]	Exceptions: Student-learners in a vocational agricultural program may work in specified hazardous (agricultural) occupations under certain conditions.[f] Children aged 14 to 15 who have successfully completed the tractor operation or machine operation training program under 4-H (or a similar program) or a program of the U.S. Office of Education Vocational Agriculture Training Program may work inthe hazardous (agricultural) occupations for which they have been trained. Certain conditions of employment apply for children working under these exemptions.[g]
16 and 17	All	Any (no hour restrictions).	Not applicable.

Source: GAO review of the Fair Labor Standards Act of 1938 (FLSA), as amended, applicable regulations, and Department of Labor guidance. | GAO-19-26.

[a]Children of any age may be employed in any agricultural occupation if employed by their parent (or a person standing in place of a parent) on a farm owned or operated by that parent, and there are no hour restrictions for children so employed.

[b]The FLSA provides that employers may apply for waivers from the Department of Labor (DOL) to permit local children aged 10 and 11 to be employed outside of school hours in the hand harvesting of short season crops under certain conditions. DOL issued regulations in 1978 setting forth the procedures for implementing this waiver provision. See 29 U.S.C. § 213(c)(4), 29 C.F.R. pt. 575. However, DOL was enjoined from issuing such waivers by a 1980 court decision resulting from a legal challenge to these regulations. See National Ass'n of Farmworkers Organizations v. Marshall, 628 F.2d 604 (D.C. Cir. 1980). According to officials, DOL does not have any record that it has issued a waiver under this authority since 1980.

[c]The FLSA provides a minimum age of 16-years-old for any agricultural occupations which DOL finds and declares to be particularly hazardous for persons under the age of 16. 29 U.S.C. § 213(c)(2). DOL has issued 11 hazardous occupations orders for agricultural employment. See 29 C.F.R. §§ 570.70–570.72. In this table we refer to occupations covered by these orders as "hazardous (agricultural)" and occupations not covered by these orders as "non-hazardous (agricultural)."

[d]The FLSA minimum wage and overtime provisions do not apply with respect to an agricultural employer who did not, during any calendar quarter in the preceding calendar year, use more than 500 "man-days" of agriculture labor.

[e]For children who have graduated from high school, the entire year would be considered outside of school hours and, therefore, their employment in agriculture would be permitted at any time.

[f]For example, the child must be employed under a written agreement that provides that the work shall be incidental to the training.

[g]For example, the employer is subject to certain supervision requirements, and must keep the child's certificate of completion on file, among other things.

Children younger than 16 may generally only work in agricultural occupations other than the ones covered by these orders, and only outside of school hours (see Table 4).[25] Additional

[25] 29 U.S.C. § 213(c)(1), (c)(2). Exceptions may apply to eligible student-learners in a vocational agricultural program, and children who have completed certain training in tractor or machine operation. See 29 C.F.R. §§ 570.71-570.72.

restrictions apply to children under the age of 14.[26] Children of any age may be employed in any agricultural occupation at any time, if they are employed by their parent (or a person standing in place of a parent) on a farm owned or operated by that parent or person.[27] Unlike some of the requirements for non-agricultural occupations, the FLSA does not limit the number of hours per day or week that children may work in agriculture, nor does it place limits on when that work may occur outside of school hours.

The child labor provisions of the FLSA do not cover all children. In addition to the exemptions and exceptions already discussed, some employers may not meet the criteria for FLSA coverage.[28] Children may also be covered under a state's child labor laws, which may provide more stringent child labor protections than the federal law.[29]

DOL's Role in Enforcing the Child Labor Provisions of the Fair Labor Standards Act

DOL, through its WHD, is the federal agency responsible for enforcing the FLSA, including the child labor provisions and associated regulations.[30]

According to DOL regulations, the child labor provisions seek to protect the safety, health, well-being, and opportunities for schooling of youthful workers.[31] DOL also oversees workplace safety and health through OSHA, which is responsible for setting and enforcing workplace safety and health standards under the Occupational Safety and Health Act of 1970, as amended (OSH Act).[32] Employers must follow applicable workplace safety and health standards, which generally require them to take steps to prevent workers, including those aged 17 and under, from being injured or becoming ill on the job. To carry out their respective responsibilities, WHD and OSHA conduct inspections, investigate complaints, and offer compliance assistance programs and training, among other efforts.

To enforce the FLSA, WHD's national office establishes annual performance measures for enforcement and compliance activities, including those related to the child labor provisions of the FLSA. WHD's national office also establishes the planning framework used

---

[26] For example, children aged 12 and 13 must be employed either with the written consent of their parent (or a person standing in place of a parent); or on the same farm where their parent is employed. 29 C.F.R. § 570.2(b). See table 4 for more information on the specific restrictions for children under age 14.

[27] 29 U.S.C. § 213(c)(2); 29 C.F.R. §§ 570.2(b), 570.70(b).

[28] The FLSA generally covers all employees of businesses that are engaged in interstate commerce and that have an annual gross volume of sales or business of $500,000 or more (referred to as "enterprise coverage"). Even when there is no enterprise coverage, employees may be covered by the FLSA's protections if they are individually engaged in interstate commerce or in the production of goods for interstate commerce. The FLSA's "hot goods" provision, in section 12(a), permits DOL to seek a court order to prevent the interstate shipment of goods that were produced in or about an establishment where a child labor violation occurred in the past 30 days. According to DOL officials, application of the hot goods provision does not require that the child who was employed in violation of FLSA's child labor provisions was personally engaged in the production of those goods. See 29 U.S.C. § 212(a).

[29] A review of state laws was outside the scope of this report.

[30] WHD is also responsible for enforcing several other statutes, including the Davis-Bacon Act and related acts, the Migrant and Seasonal Agricultural Worker Protection Act, and the Family and Medical Leave Act, among others.

[31] 29 C.F.R. § 570.101(a).

[32] Pub. L. No. 91-596, 84 Stat. 1590 (codified as amended at 29 U.S.C. §§ 553, 651-78). Under the OSH Act, states may choose to operate their own occupational safety and health programs in accordance with state plans approved by OSHA.

by WHD's 5 regional and 54 district offices to develop regional and local initiatives, which can include both enforcement and outreach activities. In addition, WHD's national office is responsible for providing guidance and training to its field offices and for assessing the results of their child labor compliance efforts. The field offices have discretion to organize their work to meet performance targets, and to create and implement these initiative plans each fiscal year.[33] WHD has also developed a Community Outreach Resource and Planning Specialist position for its district offices, whose primary duties include outreach and enforcement planning for WHD district offices.[34] In 2010, WHD's national office began emphasizing the use of data to develop its strategy for enforcement and compliance assistance activities, including the creation of a priority industry list, which would help the agency plan where to focus its enforcement activities.

Since 2010, WHD has addressed child labor as a component of its FLSA outreach and enforcement activities. WHD outreach efforts include presentations to stakeholder groups and employers. WHD's enforcement actions include on-site investigations of employers and other activities designed to bring employers into compliance with the law. When WHD determines, as a result of an investigation, that an employer has violated the child labor provisions of the FLSA, WHD may assess penalties or take other enforcement actions.[35] The penalties for child labor violations depend on the size of the business and the gravity of the violations, including any history of prior violations, evidence of willfulness or failure to take reasonable precautions, and whether any children were killed or injured as a result.

In 2011, WHD proposed some revisions to the FLSA agricultural child labor regulations. According to the proposed rule, these revisions were intended to implement specific recommendations made by NIOSH, increase parity between the agricultural and nonagricultural child labor provisions, and address other WHD-identified areas for improvement.[36]

After reviewing public comments, WHD withdrew the proposed rule in 2012.[37] In the notice withdrawing the proposed rule, WHD stated that it would instead pursue a non-regulatory approach to address the safety and health of children working in agriculture, such as collaborating with farming organizations to develop educational programs on hazardous agricultural work practices and conditions.[38]

---

[33] In addition to the national office, WHD operates offices at the regional, district, area, and field levels. For the purposes of this report, we generally refer to all WHD offices outside of the national office as "field offices," unless otherwise noted.

[34] As of June 2018, WHD had a Community Outreach and Resource Planning Specialist staff person in the majority of WHD's 54 district offices nationwide.

[35] 29 U.S.C. § 216(e); 29 C.F.R. pts. 579, 580. In addition to civil money penalties, the FLSA also authorizes DOL to seek injunctions to halt the interstate shipment of goods produced in violation of the child labor provisions, 29 U.S.C. § 212(a), to seek injunctions against violators of the child labor provisions to compel their compliance with the law, 29 U.S.C. § 217, and for willful violations, to seek criminal penalties including a fine of not more than $10,000 and/or imprisonment of not more than 6 months, 29 U.S.C. § 216(a).

[36] Child Labor Regulations, Orders and Statements of Interpretation; Child Labor Violations—Civil Money Penalties, 76 Fed. Reg. 54,836 (Sept. 2, 2011).

[37] WHD held a public hearing and received written comments on the proposed rule through December 2011. After consideration of the public comments, WHD announced its decision to pursue a non-regulatory approach to address the safety and health of children employed in agriculture rather than amending the existing child labor rules.

[38] Child Labor Regulations, Orders and Statements of Interpretation; Child Labor Violations—Civil Money Penalties, 77 Fed. Reg. 31,549 (May 29, 2012).

Data Sources

Several key federal sources provide information on the number and characteristics of working children aged 17 and under in the United States. The CPS, compiled monthly by DOL's BLS, is the primary source of labor force statistics, including for children aged 15 to 17.[39] The CPS is a survey of U.S. households and provides nationally representative information on the number of working children in the United States, as well as how many hours they worked and the industries in which they worked.[40] This survey includes data regarding children aged 15 to 17 who work in agriculture, including children on U.S. farms who were members of the household working for 15 or more hours per week (with or without pay) and children working on farms employing 10 or fewer workers.[41] The CPS and its Annual Social and Economic Supplement also provide demographic information on working children, such as age, race, ethnicity, and family income.

Agricultural Employers: U.S. Farm Characteristics and Family Farms

Agricultural production has shifted to much larger farming operations over the last 3 decades, even as the number of small farms has grown, according to the U.S. Department of Agriculture's Economic Research Service. Overall, larger farms —those with at least $1 million in sales—account for an increasing share of production, with 51 percent of the value of U.S. farm production coming from large farms in 2015, compared to 31 percent in 1991.

A "family farm" is any of the nation's approximately 2 million farms where the majority of the business is owned by the principal operator. The U.S. Department of Agriculture's Economic Research Service defines large-scale family farms as those with gross income of $1 million or more, and small family farms as those with a gross income of less than $350,000. Ninety percent of U.S. farms are classified as small, and these farms accounted for 51 percent of the land operated by farms in 2016, according to the Economic Research Service.

Source: GAO analysis of U.S. Department of Agriculture information. | GAO-19-26.

[39] CPS is a joint survey sponsored by the Census Bureau and BLS. CPS estimates contained in this report are estimated standard errors and are presented along with an approximate margin of error at the 95 percent confidence level or relative standard errors. We express our confidence in the precision of a particular sample's estimates with a confidence interval. By adding and subtracting the margin of error from the estimate, we construct a confidence interval that would contain the actual population value for 95 percent of the samples that CPS could have drawn. All margins of error for CPS estimates presented in this report are approximations. We calculated the approximate margins of error following CPS guidance and technical documentation. In order to estimate the margin of error for estimates of our subgroups of interest, a number of approximations were required. As a result, the margins of error provide a general order of magnitude. A relative standard error is equal to the standard error of a survey estimate divided by the survey estimate.

[40] The CPS includes all people residing in the United States, including those who are foreign born—people who were not U.S. citizens at birth—which include legally-admitted immigrants, refugees, temporary residents such as students and temporary workers, and undocumented immigrants. The CPS data, however, do not separately identify the number of people in these categories.

[41] BLS's CPS does not count unpaid family workers, on farms or in other family businesses, who work less than 15 hours per week. According to BLS officials, the CPS collects information on workers on farms, including those that employ 10 or fewer workers. BLS officials also stated that its research indicates some concerns with the data quality of the CPS variable used on firm size. BLS officials stated they believe that firm size can be better determined through surveys of establishments rather than surveys of households (such as the CPS).

In addition to CPS data, the Department of Health and Human Services' NIOSH and DOL also collect data specific to children aged 17 and under working in agriculture:

- NIOSH's Childhood Agricultural Injury Survey (CAIS) is conducted in selected years by surveying a random sample of 50,000 U.S. farms.[42] This survey collects data on children working in both crop and livestock agriculture, as well as working children on farms employing 10 or fewer workers, and children working on U.S. farms who are members of the household, referred to as "household children," regardless of their pay status or household status.[43]
- DOL's National Agricultural Workers Survey (NAWS) is an employment-based, annual survey of demographic, employment, and health characteristics of workers in crop agriculture, including those on crop farms employing 10 or fewer workers.[44] This survey does not include data on livestock agricultural workers or unpaid household workers.[45]

The primary sources of data on children who are injured or killed as a result of work-related incidents come from BLS and NIOSH. BLS reports on fatalities through its Census of Fatal Occupational Injuries, which collects data on fatalities through multiple sources such as death certificates, workers' compensation reports, and federal and state agency administrative reports. BLS collects data on the number of nonfatal work- related injuries and illnesses in its Survey of Occupational Injuries and Illnesses from a sample of the work-related injury and illness records that employers in private industry are required to maintain. NIOSH collects data on work-related injuries in its National Electronic Injury Surveillance System, which collects information from a nationally representative sample of hospital emergency departments to produce its annual estimate. NIOSH, in collaboration with the U.S. Department of Agriculture's National Agricultural Statistics Service, has also collected data on work-related injuries to children in agriculture through the CAIS.

[42] CAIS data were collected in 2001, 2004, 2006, 2009, 2012, and 2014. From 2001 through 2012, CAIS was based on a sample of 50,000 U.S. farm operations from the Census of Agriculture. In 2014, the CAIS sample was increased to 75,000 farming operations.

[43] For the purposes of this report, working household children are those who live and work without pay on a farm owned by their parents. CAIS collects data on hired labor (those working for pay), household labor (those living on the farm where they are working), and visitors (a visiting relative to the farm operation or a non-relative visitor). Working household children are those who live and work on a farm owned by their parents.

[44] NAWS surveys hired farm workers, including crop workers, workers at nurseries, workers at packing houses, and workers brought to farms by labor contractors. Approximately 1,500 of these workers each round are randomly selected for an in-person interview, and NAWS conducts three rounds of interviews per year, to account for the seasonality of agricultural production and employment. We note that a farm employing 10 or fewer workers may represent a large operation.

[45] Migrant child workers are within the scope of NAWS and CAIS, as these surveys are conducted at the job site and such workers are not excluded from the survey. According to DOL, migrant child workers are child farm workers who generally travel to the job site such that the farm worker is not reasonably able to return to his or her permanent residence within the same day. According to agency officials, workers in the United States on a H-2A visa—a temporary work visa for foreign agricultural workers with a job offer for temporary or seasonal agricultural work in the United States—are excluded in the NAWS survey, but are generally included in the CPS and CAIS.

Status of 2002 GAO Recommendations on Child Labor

In our 2002 report on child labor, we made seven recommendations related to the report's findings on limitations to DOL's compliance efforts regarding the child labor provisions of the FLSA.[46] DOL disagreed with many of the conclusions and recommendations in the report but has implemented all but one of these recommendations.[47] We recommended that DOL:

- provide additional guidance to staff,
- consider enhancing the CPS data collected on working children,
- routinely obtain and review data from its internal investigations database and use this data to ensure effective resource use for child labor compliance,
- use existing BLS and NIOSH data to better target compliance efforts,
- develop methods of measuring WHD's child labor compliance efforts,
- develop additional specific, measurable goals for improving compliance in industries in which children face the greatest risk of being injured or killed, and
- provide training to all WHD staff on how to obtain information from the internal investigations database.

For the CPS specifically, we recommended that BLS enhance data collection on working children by expanding the CPS to include 14-year- olds or beginning a new cohort of another survey of children, the National Longitudinal Study of Youth. DOL generally agreed with this recommendation, and the agency conducted an assessment of the feasibility of expanding the CPS.

THE NUMBER OF WORKING CHILDREN GENERALLY FLUCTUATED WITH THE ECONOMY

The Number of Working Children Declined until about 2011 and Has Since Increased, and Most Working Children Are Employed in Non-Agricultural Industries

According to our analysis of CPS data, the estimated number of working children aged 15 to 17 has generally fluctuated with the economy; however, this number has not reached pre-recession levels. Specifically, the number of children aged 15 to 17 who worked during summer months—June through August—was an estimated 3.3 million in 2003, and then reached a low of 1.9 million in 2011. By 2017, an estimated 2.5 million children worked during summer months, which remains below pre- recession levels. Fewer children worked

[46] GAO-02-880.

[47] DOL did not implement the recommendation to use existing BLS and NIOSH data to better target WHD's child labor compliance efforts, citing concerns that doing so would require disaggregating the data at a level that would jeopardize participants' confidentiality. We disagreed that such disaggregation would be required.

during non-summer months— September through May—however, they followed a similar trend (see Figure 1).[48]

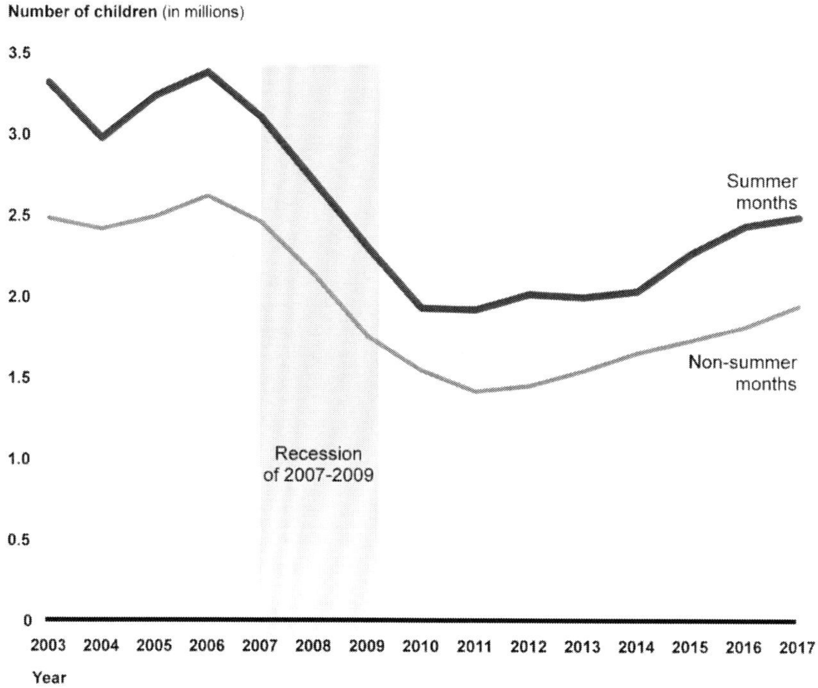

Source: GAO analysis of Current Population Survey (CPS) data. | GAO-19-26.

Notes: We defined "summer months" as June through August, and "non-summer months" as January through May and September through December during a calendar year. These definitions are not intended to align with how summer is defined in the Fair Labor Standards Act child labor regulations. These estimates have relative standard errors of 10 percent or less. For more details, see appendix II.

Figure 1. Estimated Number of Working Children Aged 15 to 17 in the United States, 2003 to 2017.

More children work in summer months and children generally work more hours in the summer than they do in non-summer months, according to the CPS data. For more details, see appendix II.

We conducted some additional analyses focusing on hours worked by 15- year-olds, because they are subject to different requirements than children aged 16 and 17.[49]

---

[48] More specifically, we define "non-summer months" as January through May and September through December during a calendar year. Our definitions of summer and non- summer months are not intended to align with how summer is defined in the FLSA child labor regulations. We used our definition of summer and non-summer months in our analysis as we found this categorization to be the most workable given the arrangement and content of the CPS data set. These estimates have relative standard errors of 10 percent or less.

[49] Our analysis does not show whether this work complied with the FLSA, due in part to differences between the data and definitions used in our analysis and the applicable FLSA requirements. As previously discussed, under the FLSA and DOL regulations, children aged 14 and 15 engaged in non-agricultural occupations may generally work up to 18 hours per week during weeks when school is in session, and up to 40 hours per week during weeks when school is not in session. School is generally considered to be in session for any week the local public school district where the child resides while employed is in session, and in which students are required to attend for at least one day or partial day. However, various exceptions may apply; for example, there are no hour restrictions for children employed by their parents. The data we used for our analysis do not

Specifically, we analyzed the number of hours children aged 15 worked in summer (June, July, and August) and non- summer months—which do not necessarily correspond to any given school year.[50] From 2003 through 2017 the percentage of working 15- year-olds we estimated that worked 40 or more hours per week in non- agricultural industries in summer months ranged from a low of 8 percent in 2004 to a high of 19 percent in 2014.[51] The percentage we estimated that worked 19 or more hours per week in non-agricultural industries in non-summer months ranged from a low of 14 percent in 2004 to a high of 31 percent in 2015 (see app. II for more details).[52]

We also analyzed the demographic characteristics of working children. Our analysis of demographic characteristics of working children in CPS found that working females aged 15 to 17 comprised about 52 percent of the working child population in 2017 summer months; and the percentage of white-only working children decreased from 2003 to 2017, while the percentage of working children of other races and ethnicities—black only, Hispanic, and other races combined—increased during the time period,[53] irrespective of industry or occupation. Our analysis of demographic characteristics of working children in CPS's Annual Social and Economic Supplement (ASEC) also found that while 27 percent of the children who did not work were low-income, only 15 percent of the children who worked were in that category.[54] Children in low-income families were less likely to work than their higher income counterparts. About 11 percent of children in low-income families worked in 2016 compared to 21 percent of children in higher income families. For the results of our analyses of these demographic characteristics, see appendix III.

Our analysis of CPS Annual Social and Economic Supplement data also shows that, in 2016, the vast majority of working children aged 15 to 17 worked in non-agricultural industries,[55] such as leisure and hospitality or wholesale and retail. As shown in Figure 2, we estimated the leisure and hospitality industry employed over 1.1 million children aged 15 to 17, wholesale and retail employed about 440,000, and more than 60,000 children aged 15 to 17 worked in the construction and mining industry.[56]

---

allow us to determine whether school was in session, or whether an exception applies, for the reported hours worked by 15-year-olds.

[50] We were unable to tabulate the extent to which 14-year-olds worked because, according to BLS, such data are not collected in the CPS or in other BLS surveys.

[51] These estimates for summer months are for 2004 and 2014 and have relative standard errors of 24 percent and 20 percent, respectively. The 2009 summer estimate is the only estimate from 2003 to 2017 that has a relative standard error higher than or equal to 30 percent (is 30 percent), and should be interpreted with caution.

[52] These estimates for non-summer months are from 2004 and 2015 and have relative standard errors of 19 percent and 17 percent, respectively.

[53] The CPS treats ethnicity separately from race. As a result, a child can be identified in the CPS as both white and Hispanic, or as both black and Hispanic, among other designations. For the purposes of our report, we categorized any respondent identifying as Hispanic, irrespective of their reported race, as Hispanic. We further categorized respondents who identified as being non bi- or multiracial white or black as being white only and black only. We counted the following respondents as other races: respondents of two or more races, Asians, and other races such as Native American or Pacific Islander.

[54] In this report, we defined low-income as having income below 150 percent of the poverty threshold. Poverty thresholds are set by the U.S. Census Bureau and take into account family size and composition to determine who is in poverty.

[55] Industry worked is determined based on industry of longest job worked in 2016.

[56] The estimates for these industries have margins of error of +/-96,000, +/-64,500, and +/-24,600, respectively.

We conducted an additional analysis of the children working in the construction and mining industry and found that an estimated 40,000 (+/-19,600) worked in construction and extraction occupations. In addition, according to the data, an estimated 12,000 (+/-8,800) worked in office and administrative support occupations.[57] We recognize our analysis does not show whether this work complied with FLSA requirements, in part because we could not identify the specific work activities performed by the children employed in these industries. Many activities in the construction and mining industry, such as roofing operations or activities about coal mines are prohibited, and some activities, such as office work, may be permissible, depending on the circumstances.[58]

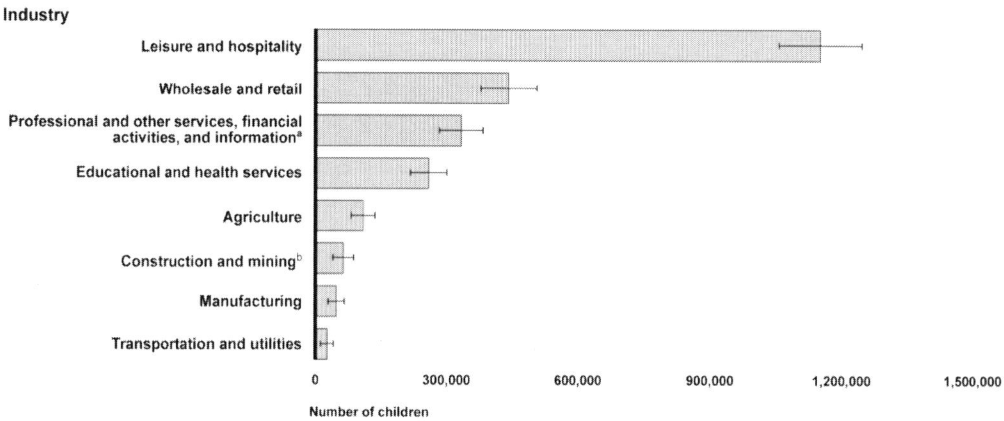

Source: GAO analysis of Current Population Survey (CPS) 2017 Annual Social and Economic Supplement data, which reports calendar year 2016 data. | GAO-19-26.

Notes: Our analysis does not show whether this work complied with the Fair Labor Standards Act (FLSA) and federal child labor regulations, due in part to a lack of precision in the data compared with the applicable FLSA requirements. Margins of error for estimates at the 95 percent confidence level are shown by chart whiskers.

[a]Professional and other services, financial activities, and information include legal, accounting, and other professional, scientific, and technical services, among others.

[b]Construction and mining industry also includes quarrying, and oil and gas extraction.

Figure 2. Industries in Which Children Aged 15 to 17 Worked, 2016.

Children aged 15 to 17 worked in a variety of occupations in 2016.[59] The top three occupations were cashiers (an estimated 375,000 working children), waiters and waitresses (141,000), and athletics-related occupations (103,000).[60] See appendix IV for detailed results.

[57] The relative standard error was greater than 30 percent (35 percent) and the estimate should be interpreted with caution.

[58] See, for example, 29 C.F.R. §§ 570.53, 570.60, 570.67 (hazardous occupations order numbers 3, 9, and 16). As described in tables 1 and 2, the FLSA's occupational restrictions vary depending on the age of the child, his or her specific occupation, and whether any exceptions apply. The data we used for our analysis do not allow us to determine the specific work activities performed, or whether an exception applies, among other things.

[59] We analyzed 2017 CPS Annual Social and Economic Supplement data, which contains information regarding annual work experience for 2016.

[60] These estimates have margins of error of +/-52,000, +/-36,000, and +/-27,000, respectively. Detailed occupation information is presented in appendix IV.

Federal Agencies Collect Some Information on Children Working in Agriculture

Federal data sets collect some information on children working in agriculture, but two we analyzed differ regarding which children they include.[61] For example, the data sets differ in the age range of children included in the data sets and the extent to which they include household workers, which may comprise a substantial percentage of children working in agriculture, as shown below. Our analysis of the CPS and CAIS data indicates the following:[62]

- CPS. According to our CPS analysis, an estimated 3.1 percent of children aged 15 to 17 worked in agriculture during summer months in 2003, and 2.9 percent worked in agriculture in summer months in 2017.[63] However, because the CPS does not measure certain groups of children, this is an undercount of children working in agriculture.[64]
- CAIS. Our analysis of CAIS data suggests higher numbers of children working on U.S. farms than do CPS data but capture a similar trend. Specifically, CAIS data indicate the number of children working in agriculture declined from an estimated 790,000 in 2004 to 524,000 in 2014 (see Figure 3).[65] The CAIS also collects information on children aged 17 and under working on U.S. farms who were members of the household ("working household children"). Our analysis of CAIS data indicate a substantial proportion of children working in agriculture are household children, which is a group that BLS officials stated is not fully represented in the CPS.[66] Our analysis indicates the number of working household children decreased from more than 590,000 in 2004 to 375,000 in 2014, the most recent year for which these data are available.[67] Further, about two-thirds of these working

---

[61] These two data sets are CPS, which is sponsored jointly by the Census Bureau and the Department of Labor's Bureau of Labor Statistics, as well as CAIS, which is NIOSH's collaborative effort with the U.S. Department of Agriculture's National Agricultural Statistics Service (NASS).

[62] We also analyzed data from the National Agricultural Worker Survey (NAWS), which is specific to hired workers in crop agriculture. See appendix V for our analyses of this data set.

[63] These estimates have a relative standard error of 21 percent and 25 percent, respectively. For non-summer months, we estimate 2.4 percent of working children aged 15 to 17 worked in agriculture in 2003, and 2.6 percent in 2017. These estimates have a relative standard error of 23 and 25 percent, respectively. See appendix II for additional results on our estimates of children working in agricultural industries from 2003 to 2017.

[64] CPS does not count as employed those children working less than 15 hours without pay for a family business. Further, because the CPS does not include workers aged 14 or under, it is not capturing the full population of children working in agriculture. BLS officials stated that CPS is not able to adequately identify the extent to which children are working in agriculture.

[65] These estimates have margins of error of 54,000 and 42,000, at the 95 percent confidence level, respectively.

[66] Our analysis of CAIS data indicates that in 2014, for example, more than 70 percent of working children aged 17 and under were working household youth. CAIS uses a different definition of household children from CPS. CPS counts as employed any child aged 15 or older who works 15 or more hours per week. For purposes of the CAIS, working household children are those who live and work on a farm owned by their parents, regardless of hours worked. CAIS collects data on hired labor (those working for pay), household labor (those living on the farm where they are working), and visitors (a visiting relative to the farm operation or a non-relative visitor).

[67] These estimates have margins of error at the 95 percent confidence level of 19,500 and 15,000, respectively. Our analyses of CAIS data also show that the proportion of working household children to hired children working on U.S. farms has remained relatively stable. For example, working household children comprised

household children—an estimated 246,000—were aged 14 and under in 2014. See appendix VI for detailed information regarding the characteristics of children working on U.S. farms.

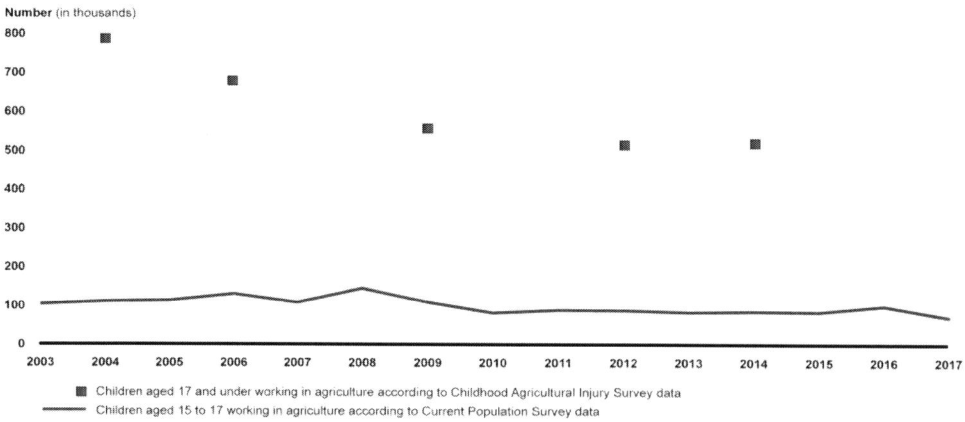

Source: GAO analysis of Childhood Agriculture Injury Survey and Current Population Survey data. | GAO-19-26.

Notes: The Childhood Agricultural Injury Survey was conducted in certain noncontiguous years and its estimates include information on children aged 17 and under who work in agriculture, including both hired workers and household workers (those living on the farm where they are working) or visitors (a visiting relative to the farm operation or a non-relative visitor) regardless of their pay status or household status. The Current Population Survey is an ongoing monthly survey and its estimates include children aged 15 to 17 working in agriculture and do not capture unpaid household workers working fewer than 15 hours per week. The estimates for CPS in the figure represent working children in summer months, which we defined as June, July, and August. CPS estimates have relative standard errors of 27 percent or less. The estimates for CAIS have relative standard errors of 10 percent or less.

Figure 3. Selected Federal Data on Children Working in Agriculture.

CHILDREN WORKING IN AGRICULTURE COMPRISED THE MAJORITY OF WORK- RELATED CHILD FATALITIES, AND DATA ON WORK-RELATED INJURIES ARE INCOMPLETE

BLS Data Indicate Work- Related Child Fatalities Have Generally Declined, and Agricultural Occupations Account for the Largest Percentage of Fatalities

According to BLS's Census of Fatal Occupational Injuries data, the annual number of work-related child fatalities has declined overall since 2003. More specifically, BLS data show a decline from 53 fatalities among children aged 17 and under in 2003 to 14 fatalities in 2013, and then an increase to 30 fatalities in 2016, the most recent year of available data. This

approximately 75 percent of all children working on farms in 2004, compared to approximately 71 percent in 2014.

trend was also similar to the trend in the number of working children (as presented in Figure 1) and the number of hours worked by children aged 15 to 17 during the same time period (see Figure 4).

Our analysis of Census of Fatal Occupational Injuries data found that certain groups of working children sustained disproportionately high percentages of work-related fatalities from 2003 to 2016. For example, while we estimated fewer than 5.5 percent of working children worked in agriculture in any year from 2003 to 2017,[68] this population sustained more than 50 percent of all work-related child fatalities from 2003 to 2016. According to available BLS data, fatalities were also disproportionately high among children aged 15 and under, children working in a family business, and among children working for an employer with 10 or fewer workers (see Table 5).

Table 5. Percentage of Work-Related Child Fatalities from 2003 to 2016 Compared to Estimated Percentage of Children Working in Selected Categories, 2017 (Categories Are Not Mutually Exclusive)

	Number of work-related child fatalities, 2003 to 2016	Percentage of that category of work-related fatalities to total fatalities	Estimated child workforce percentage, 2017
Children working in agriculture	237[a]	52	3[b]
Children aged 15 and under	197	44	7[b]
Children working in a family business	192	42	3[c]
Children working for employer with 10 or fewer workers	259[d]	76	Not available[e]

Source: GAO analysis of Census of Fatal Occupational Injuries and Current Population Survey (CPS) data. | GAO-19-26.

Notes: Estimates for children working in agriculture, children aged 15 and under, children working in a family business in the "Estimated child workforce percentage, 2017" column are for summer months—which we defined as June, July and August—and have relative standard errors of 25, 9, and 18 percent, respectively. For 2017 non-summer months, our estimates of working youth aged 15 to 17 indicate 3 percent of children worked in agriculture, 4 percent were 15-year-olds, and 3 percent were children working in a family business. These estimates have relative standard errors of 25, 8, and 15 percent, respectively.

[a]This data point is for children aged 17 and under. For children aged 15 to 17 working in agriculture, there were 125 work-related fatalities from 2003 to 2016. Accordingly, fatalities to children working in agriculture accounted for 40 percent of all fatalities to children aged 15 to 17 during the time period.

[b]CPS data do not include information on children aged 14 or younger. Thus, the estimate for children working in agriculture is for working children aged 15 to 17, and the estimate for working children aged 15 and under is for working 15-year-olds.

[c]This estimate is for unpaid children aged 15 to 17 working in a family business and self-employed children. According to BLS, self-employed workers consist of individuals who are family members working in a family business, as well as those who are self-employed, self-employed contractors, and partners or owners of an unincorporated business, professional practice, or farm. BLS's estimate for work-related child fatalities working in a family business includes paid and unpaid youth.

[d]Employer size was unknown for 25 percent of child fatalities.

[e]We analyzed CPS Annual Social and Economic Supplement data and found that, of working children, an estimated 474,000 out of 2.4 million (or about 20 percent of) employed 15 to 17-year-olds work at firms employing 9 or fewer workers, and an estimated 604,000 out of 2.4 million (or 25 percent of) working 15 to 17-year-olds worked at firms employing 10 to 49 workers in 2016. These estimates have margins of error of about 58,000 and 71,000, respectively. We were unable to estimate the percentage that worked at firms employing 10 or fewer workers because the Annual Social and Economic Supplement survey does not collect or capture that specific data point.

---

[68] The relative standard errors for all years during the period were less than 25 percent.

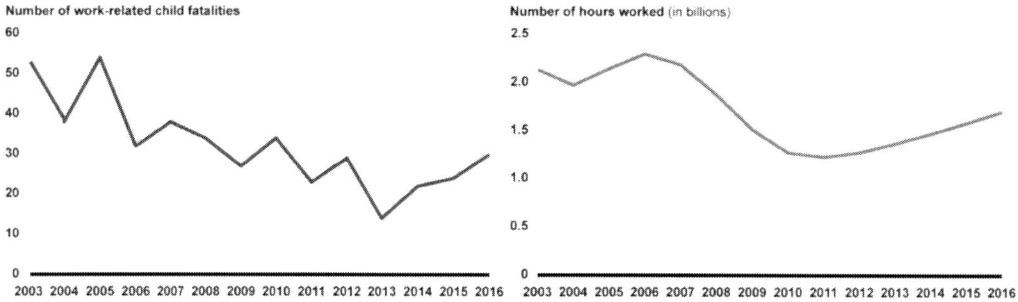

Source: GAO analysis of Census of Fatal Occupational Injuries data (facilities data) and Current Population Survey data (hours worked data). | GAO-19-26.

Notes: The number of annual hours worked is for children aged 15 to 17 because the Current Population Survey does not collect information for working children aged 14 or under. BLS officials stated the agency does not have research regarding standard errors for estimated total hours worked for 15- to 17-year-olds, and did not provide guidance on how to calculate such standard errors. GAO did not calculate the standard errors for the number of annual hours worked.

Figure 4. Number of Work-Related Fatalities to Children Aged 17 and Under and Estimated Number of Hours Worked by Children Aged 15 to 17, 2003 to 2016.

Children Working in Agriculture

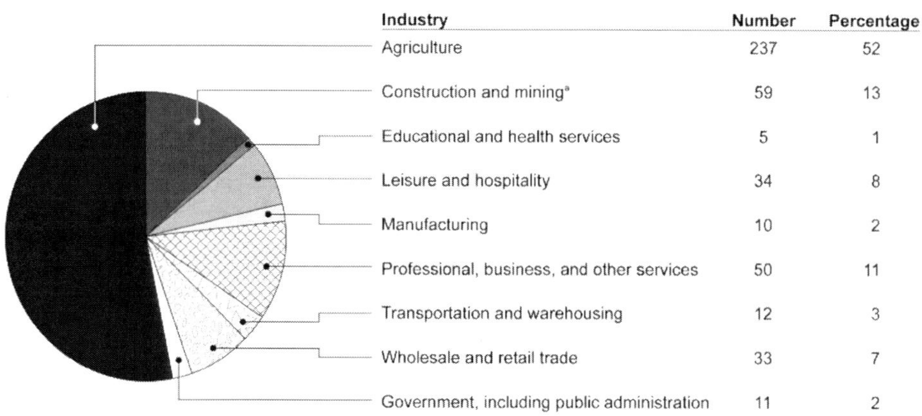

Source: GAO analysis of Census of Fatal Occupational Injuries data. | GAO-19-26.

Notes: The total number of fatalities to children aged 17 and under from 2003 to 2016 was 452. The sum of individual categories totals 451. According to Bureau of Labor Statistics officials, categories may not sum to totals due to the exclusion of unpublishable data. Percentages of major categories do not total 100 due to rounding and the exclusion of unpublishable data. The professional, business, and other services category includes information, professional and business services, and other services except public administration. The government category includes federal government, local government, and public administration.

[a]Construction and mining industry also includes quarrying, and oil and gas extraction.

Figure 5. Work-Related Child Fatalities, by Industry, 2003 to 2016.

Although children working in agriculture make up a small proportion of working children,[69] we found that from 2003 to 2016, 52 percent of work- related fatalities among children aged 17 and under were in agriculture,[70] with 32 percent in crop agriculture specifically. The construction, mining, quarrying, and oil and gas extraction industries accounted for 13 percent of child fatalities, as shown in Figure 5. For detailed information on work- related child fatalities by industry, see appendix VII.

Children Aged 15 and under

As shown in Table 6, children aged 15 and under comprised 44 percent of the work-related child fatalities from 2003 to 2016, and those aged 14 and under comprised 31 percent of fatalities during the same period. We estimated that children aged 15 comprised 7 percent of the child workforce (aged 15 to 17) during summer months, and 4 percent during non-summer months in 2017.[71]

Table 6. Number and Percentage of Work-Related Child Fatalities, by Age, 2003 to 2016

Age	Number of fatalities	Percentage of work-related child fatalities	Cumulative percentage
12 and under	73	16	16
13	25	6	22
14	44	10	31
15	55	12	44
16	110	24	68
17	145	32	100
Total	452	100	

Source: GAO analysis Census of Fatal Occupational Injuries (CFOI) data. | GAO-19-26.

Notes: The cumulative percentage for children aged 14 and under is more precisely 31.4 percent. Summing the individually rounded percent fatalities to children aged 12 and under, 13 and under, and 14 and under would total 32 percent, but we are presenting the cumulative percentage for work-related fatalities to children aged 14 and under as 31, based on the original, non-rounded data.

Children Working in a Family Business

Children working in a family business accounted for about 3 percent of all working children, but they represented about 42 percent of all work- related fatalities to children aged 17 and under.[72]

---

[69] In 2017, children aged 15 to 17 comprised an estimated 2.9 percent of the working child population in summer months, and an estimated 2.6 percent in non-summer months, according to our analysis. Both of these estimates have relative standard errors of 25 percent. BLS does not provide information on children aged 14 or under who are working, and thus might be employed in agriculture.

[70] Agriculture, as classified in the North American Industry Classification System which is used by the CFOI, includes non-crop agriculture, for example the raising of livestock, fish, or other activities such as logging; it also includes crop agriculture, for example the planting and harvesting of fruits, vegetables, and other foods. See appendix VII for more detailed information regarding work-related child fatalities by sub-industry.

[71] These estimates have relative standard errors of 9 percent and 8 percent, respectively. Further, children employed in agriculture comprised 74 percent of work-related fatalities involving children aged 15 and under, according to BLS data.

[72] This estimate is for unpaid children aged 15 to 17 working in a family business and self- employed children. According to BLS, self-employed workers consist of individuals who are family members working in a family business, as well as those who are self-employed, self-employed contractors, and partners or owners of an unincorporated business, professional practice, or farm. BLS's estimate for work-related child fatalities working in a family business includes paid and unpaid children.

Children Working for Employers with 10 or Fewer Workers

This group accounted for 76 percent of the work-related child fatalities for which employer size was reported from 2003 to 2016, according to BLS data. According to BLS officials, in 25 percent (113 out of 452) of BLS's reported work-related child fatalities, the size of establishment is unknown. Using CPS Annual Social and Economic Supplement data, we estimated that in 2016, 20 percent of working children aged 15 to 17 were working at firms employing 9 or fewer workers and an estimated 25 percent worked at firms employing 10 to 49 workers.[73]

We also analyzed the demographic characteristics of working children aged 17 and under who incurred work-related fatalities from 2003 to 2016. Our analysis of BLS data indicated that boys incurred 87 percent of these fatalities.[74] In addition, of those work-related fatalities that were reportable by race and ethnicity,[75] Hispanic children incurred 20 percent of them, and white only children incurred 75 percent. Further, transportation incidents, such as a work-related collision on or off a roadway with a motorized vehicle, were the cause of the highest number of work-related fatalities to children aged 17 and under. See appendix VIII for detailed results of these demographic analyses.

The Estimated Number of Work-Related Injuries and Illnesses to Children Has Declined, but Data Have Limitations

The two primary sources of nationwide data on child work-related injuries and illnesses indicate similar trends in the number of injuries and illnesses since 2003, yet these sources differ substantially in the magnitude of their estimates and methodologies for determining the number of working children incurring such injuries or illnesses each year.[76] For example, our analysis of both BLS's Survey of Occupational Injuries and Illnesses and NIOSH's National Electronic Injury Surveillance System—Occupational Supplement data sets indicates a decrease in the number of work-related injuries and illnesses that children incurred from 2006 to about 2010. BLS's estimates continue to decrease in 2011, and then rise from 2012 through 2016. In contrast, NIOSH estimates do not have a discernable increase from 2011 through 2016. However, as shown in Figure 6, NIOSH's estimates of the number of work-related childhood injuries and illnesses are generally more than 5 times higher than BLS's estimates.[77]

---

[73] We were unable to estimate the percentage that worked at firms employing 10 or fewer workers because the ASEC survey does not collect or capture that specific data point. BLS officials stated that there may be some quality concerns with the employer size variable in the Annual Social and Economic Supplement—which is a household survey— and that information regarding employer size would be better captured in a survey of employers.

[74] Because some data do not meet publication criteria, BLS reported gender information for 451 of the 452 work-related fatalities to children from 2003 to 2016.

[75] Because some data do not meet publication criteria, BLS reported race and ethnic information for 451 of the 452 work-related fatalities to children aged 17 and under from 2003 to 2016.

[76] The two primary sources of data for child work-related injuries and illnesses, as detailed in appendix I, are the Survey of Occupational Illness and Injuries, for which BLS collects information from a sample of employer records to estimate incidence rates and counts of workplace injuries and illnesses, and the National Electronic Injury Surveillance System- Occupational Supplement, for which NIOSH collects data from a sample of U.S. hospital emergency departments on civilian workers who were injured on the job.

[77] NIOSH's National Electronic Injury Surveillance System-Occupational Supplement estimated the number of work-related injuries to children aged 17 and under in 2016 to be 26,300, with an associated margin of error at

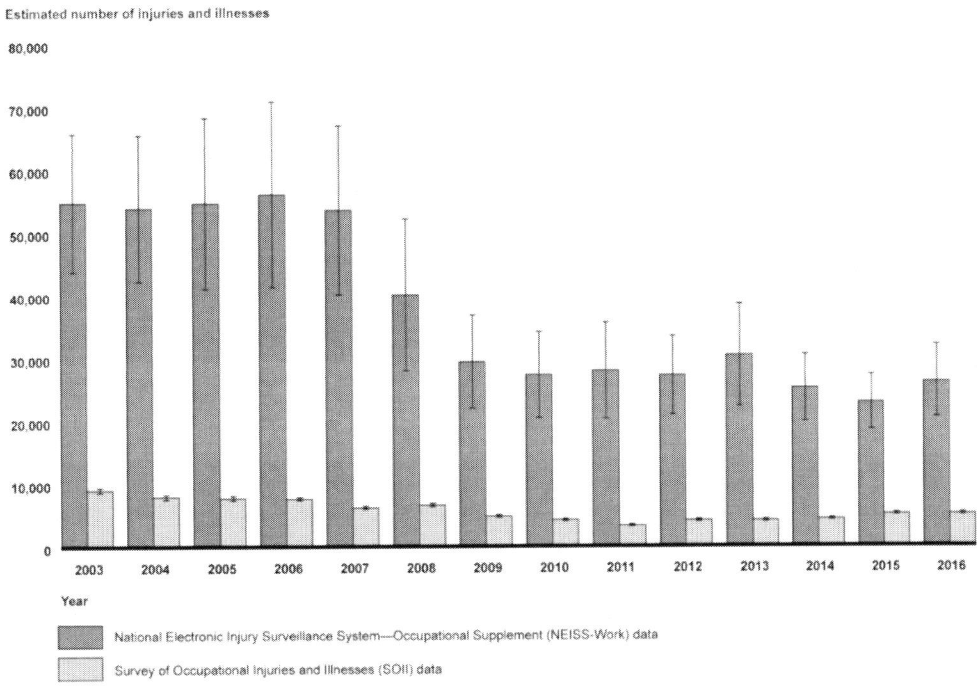

Source: GAO analysis of Department of Health and Human Services' National Institute for Occupational Safety and Health (NIOSH) National Electronic Injury Surveillance System – Occupational Supplement (NEISS-Work) data and Bureau of Labor Statistics (BLS) Survey of Occupational Injuries and Illnesses (SOII). | GAO-19-26.

Notes: BLS's SOII data set is more specifically for children aged 15 to 17. BLS's Survey of Occupational Injuries and Illnesses data presented here includes injuries or illnesses that resulted in one day of missed work. As shown in appendix IX, BLS also provided estimates for work-related injuries and illnesses to children aged 15 and under, which ranged from a low of 90, or 0.01 percent of all work-related injuries and illnesses resulting in a day way from work, to a high of 420, or 0.04 percent of all work related injuries and illnesses to children resulting in a day away from work. NIOSH's National Electronic Injury Surveillance System-Occupational Supplement (NEISS-Work) data set counts injuries to workers who sought treatment in one of the NEISS-Work sampled emergency departments for an occupational injury or illness. BLS officials stated that about 5 percent of its estimated injuries and illnesses to adults and children in private industry, and local and state government in 2016 were illnesses. NIOSH technical information notes that NEISS-Work data from 2003 to 2014 include illnesses such as those that began at work (heart attacks or stroke), chronic conditions, and exacerbated long-term injuries; it estimates 5 to 10 percent of all cases were such illnesses. NEISS-Work data from 2015 on do not capture most illnesses. Margins of error for estimates at the 95 percent confidence level are shown by chart whiskers. For more details, see appendix IX.

Figure 6. Estimated Number of Work-Related Injuries and Illnesses to Children Aged 17 and Under (National Institute for Occupational Safety and Health) and Aged 15 to 17 (Bureau of Labor Statistics), 2003 to 2016.

---

the 95 percent confidence level of +/-5,800. The margin of error of the 2010 estimate at the 95 percent confidence level (27,300 mean estimate) is +/-6,900.

Some of the differences in the estimates may be related to how the agencies collect the data. Specifically, BLS relies on surveyed employer records to collect its data—including detailed demographic data, such as the injured person's age—for individual cases serious enough to cause workers to miss at least one day of work.[78] It provides annual estimates for the number of work-related injuries and illnesses to children aged 17 and under, and separately for children aged 15 and under.[79] NIOSH estimates, based on emergency room records, include estimates for work-related injuries and illnesses to children aged 17 and under, and separately for children aged 14 and under. See appendix IX for annual BLS and NIOSH estimates of work-related injuries and illnesses to children.

BLS data indicate that the median number of days that children missed work due to work-related injuries and illnesses remained relatively constant from 2003 to 2016. According to BLS estimates, 42 percent of the work-related injuries and illnesses to children aged 17 and under in 2016 required them to miss 1 or 2 days of work, and about 10 percent of the injuries during this period required them to miss 31 or more days. Unlike fatalities data, BLS injury and illnesses data show that in 2016, the industry that employed the most children aged 15 to 17—leisure and hospitality—had the most work-related injuries and illnesses to children aged 17 and under. For more detailed results, see appendix X.

Injuries to Children Working in Agriculture

NIOSH Childhood Agricultural Injury Survey (CAIS) data estimated that there were 4,774 work-related injuries to children aged 17 or under on U.S. farms, based on a combined estimate of its 2012 and 2014 data.[80]

CAIS data—which include both working household children aged 17 or under and children on farms employing 10 or fewer workers—also indicate that about half of the work-related injuries to children on U.S. farms are to those aged 14 and under (see Table 7).

Further, CAIS data indicate that a substantial portion of work-related injuries to children on U.S. farms are incurred by children working in the farm owner's household, rather than children hired or visiting the farm.[81]

---

[78] BLS also collects information regarding a broad array of work-related injuries or illnesses from surveyed employers. It does not capture detailed case and demographic information regarding individual cases, such as the injured person's age, gender, and race, unless the individual case is one that is serious enough to cause a worker to miss at least one day of work.

[79] BLS published some estimates for work-related injuries to 14-year-olds in certain years; for more information, see appendix IX. In October 2009, GAO found that disincentives for workers to report and for employers to record injuries affect the accuracy of BLS's injury and illness data. See GAO, *Workplace Safety and Health: Enhancing OSHA's Records Audit Process Could Improve the Accuracy of Worker Injury and Illness Data*, GAO-10-10 (Washington, D.C.: Oct. 15, 2009).

[80] CAIS defines an injury as being any nonfatal traumatic event occurring on the farm operation resulting in at least 4 hours of restricted activity, or requiring professional medical treatment. CAIS defines a work injury as being any injury that occurred while performing work or chores on the farm that was associated with the farm business, regardless of whether the work was performed for pay. NIOSH combined 2 years of CAIS data to produce an estimate with less than 33 percent relative standard error, and thus within NIOSH's standards for reporting.

[81] CAIS defines a household worker as a member of a farm operator's household (farm operator, his/her spouse, child/step child); a visitor as a visiting relative to the farm operation or a non-relative visitor; and a hired worker as being a paid worker or laborer hired directly by a farm operator. NIOSH officials we interviewed stated that they did not plan to conduct another CAIS and that compiling a sample large enough to meet statistical reporting thresholds as they have done in the past would result in a prohibitive cost.

Table 7. National Estimates of Work-Related Injuries to Children Aged 17 and under on U.S. Farms, by Age Group

	2004 and 2006 combined data on injuries (margin of error)	2012 and 2014combined data on injuries (margin of error)
Aged 10 and under	2,400 (+/-1,085)	742a (+/-458)
Aged 14 and under	5,385 (+/-1,611)	2,420 (+/-940)
Aged 15 to 17	5,067 (+/-1,346)	2,353 (+/-823)
Aged 17 and under	10,452 (+/-1,999)	4,774b(+/-1,191)

Source: Source: GAO analysis of Childhood Agricultural Injury Survey (CAIS) data for 2004, 2006, 2012, and 2014. | GAO-19-26.

Notes: CAIS defines an injury as being any nonfatal traumatic event occurring on the farm operation resulting in at least 4 hours of restricted activity, or requiring professional medical treatment. CAIS defines a work injury as being any injury that occurred while performing work or chores on the farm (associated with the farm business), regardless of whether the work was performed for pay. NIOSH combined 2 years of CAIS data to produce an estimate with less than 33 percent relative standard error, and thus within NIOSH's standards for reporting.

[a]Estimate should be interpreted with caution because it has relative standard error of 32 percent.

[b]Number does not total to sum of estimated number of children aged 14 and under and 15 to 17 due to rounding.

Table 8 provides further details.

Table 8. National Estimates of Work-Related Injuries to Household and Non-Household Children Aged 17 or under on U.S. Farms

	2004 and 2006 combined data injuries (margin of error)	2012 and 2014 combined data injuries (margin of error)
Household children aged 17 or under	4,722 (+/-1427)	3,258 (+/-1013)
Non-household children aged 17 or under	1,022 (+/-531)	1,516 (+/-706)

Source: GAO analysis of Childhood Agricultural Injury Survey (CAIS) data for 2004, 2006, 2012, and 2014. | GAO-19-26.

Notes: While the estimated number of household children aged 17 or under incurring work-related injuries appears to decrease, and the estimated number of non-household children aged 17 or under incurring work-related injuries appears to increase from the 2004-2006 to 2012-2014 reporting periods, we cannot with confidence state that the trends are statistically reliable and instead note that there are no discernible trends. NIOSH combined 2 years of CAIS data to produce an estimate with less than 33 percent relative standard error, and thus within NIOSH's standards for reporting. CAIS defines a household worker as a member of a farm operator's household (farm operator, his/her spouse, child/step child).

In contrast to NIOSH's Childhood Agricultural Injury Survey, BLS's Survey of Occupational Illnesses and Injuries does not include data on two substantial groups of children working in agriculture: household children aged 17 or under and children working on farms employing 10 or fewer workers.[82]

BLS's estimates of the proportion of work-related injuries and illnesses incurred by children working in agriculture are lower than the proportion of work-related child fatalities incurred by children working in agriculture. For example, BLS estimated that in 2016, children working in agriculture incurred about 1 percent of the estimated 4,760 injuries and illnesses to children in the workplace across all industries—while 52 percent of all work-

[82] According to the U.S. Department of Agriculture's Census of Agriculture, as of 2012, farms employing 10 or fewer hired workers employed about half of all agricultural workers.

related fatalities occurred among children working in agriculture (from 2003 to 2016).[83] BLS officials told us that they did not have a definitive explanation for this difference, but noted that unlike its fatalities data set, many children working in agriculture were outside the scope of the agency's injury and illness data set—such as those working for agricultural employers with 10 or fewer workers or household workers.[84]

BLS officials also stated that the nature of work-related injuries causing fatalities may be different than those resulting in nonfatal injuries; however, they said they did not know of any research examining this issue.

BLS officials said the agency has begun exploring ways to enhance the measurement and counting of work-related injuries and illnesses in its Survey of Occupational Injuries and Illnesses data and is conducting a pilot Household Survey of Occupational Injuries and Illnesses for 2017 and 2018, which surveys members of a household rather than employers. They expect results to be available at the conclusion of fiscal year 2019. The current pilot survey is aimed at determining the feasibility of fielding a statistically reliable sample of households with workers who may have experienced work-related injuries and illnesses. The pilot's scope includes all workers in the United States 18 years and older who worked for pay or profit in the previous year. However, the pilot does not measure injuries and illnesses to children aged 17 and under, including household children and working children on farms employing 10 or fewer workers.[85]

BLS, within DOL, is the principal federal agency responsible for measuring labor conditions.[86] Its mission is to collect, analyze, and disseminate essential economic information to support private and public decision making. BLS is responsible for producing accurate and statistically valid estimates of work-related injuries and illnesses at U.S. workplaces.[87] BLS injury and illness data collected via its Survey of Occupational Injuries and Illnesses are used by federal agencies and others to understand trends in worker health and safety. Federal standards for internal control state that agencies should use quality information to achieve agency objectives.[88] These standards define quality information as appropriate, current, complete, accurate, accessible, and provided on a timely basis. BLS injury and illness data are not complete because they do not measure certain worker populations, including child household workers and those employed on farms with 10 or fewer workers. Without evaluating the feasibility of measuring injuries and illnesses to the

---

83 We chose to report the most current (2016) estimates of work-related injuries and illnesses to children; however, we also looked at estimates from 2003 to 2015.

84 BLS officials told us that including data on such workers in its current employer-based Survey of Occupational Injuries and Illnesses would require obtaining approval from the Office of Management and Budget and publishing a notice in the *Federal Register*. The Paperwork Reduction Act provides that agencies may not conduct or sponsor the collection of information from 10 or more non-federal persons without first taking certain required steps, including allowing an opportunity for public comment and obtaining Office of Management and Budget approval, among other things. See 44 U.S.C. § 3507.

85 BLS published some estimates for work-related injuries and illnesses to 14-year-olds in certain years, as shown in appendix IX.

86 See generally 29 U.S.C. §§ 1-8.

87 Under the OSH Act, the Secretary of Labor is required to "compile accurate statistics on work injuries and illnesses which shall include all disabling, serious, or significant injuries and illnesses, whether or not involving loss of time from work, other than minor injuries requiring only first aid treatment and which do not involve medical treatment, loss of consciousness, restriction of work or motion, or transfer to another job." 29 U.S.C. § 673(a).

88 GAO, *Standards for Internal Control in the Federal Government*, GAO-14-704G (Washington, D.C.: September 2014).

aforementioned worker populations upon the completion of its pilot, DOL is missing opportunities to more accurately quantify injuries and illnesses to children, which could better inform its compliance and enforcement efforts. Further, BLS will not know the cost of collecting this information and whether it should explore other ways to get information on work-related injuries and illnesses to vulnerable child workers. BLS officials told us in an interview that, after completing the household survey pilot at the end of fiscal year 2019, they could consider the feasibility of enhancing reporting on certain populations that are currently not measured in the pilot.

DOL Uses a Strategic Enforcement Approach to Oversee Compliance with Federal Child Labor Law, but Some Limitations Exist

DOL's Child Labor Enforcement Approach Includes Targeted Investigations and Outreach, but It Has Not Evaluated These Efforts

Investigations

DOL's Wage and Hour Division (WHD) uses a strategic enforcement approach to oversee compliance with the child labor provisions of the FLSA. This approach uses data to establish annual priorities and identify goals for investigations—agency-initiated (directed) and those initiated from complaints (complaint-based)—and compliance assistance, including outreach. Specifically, WHD uses data to create strategic initiatives, which include both enforcement and outreach activities, that focus on the working conditions of vulnerable workers, including children, and the industries that employ them.[89] Officials from WHD's national office told us they use complaint data from their internal investigation database (WHISARD) and CPS data to determine priority industries for outreach and investigations. In addition, WHD officials use federal data, such as CPS data, to assess labor market trends affecting vulnerable workers.[90]

WHD officials told us that child labor is an enforcement priority and child labor complaints from the public—particularly those involving hazardous working conditions—are assigned to a WHD investigator for immediate action. For example, one WHD investigator described going to a worksite to conduct an investigation into a child labor complaint within 2 hours of receiving the complaint. In addition, WHD officials told us that investigators look for potential child labor violations in every full investigation they conduct under the FLSA.[91]

[89] For purposes of its enforcement and compliance assistance efforts, WHD defines vulnerable worker populations as those who are at higher risk of exploitation by employers or less likely to submit complaints in response to employer violations of worker protections, such as workers with disabilities, young workers, agricultural workers, and workers with no private right to pursue remedies on their own behalf.

[90] Officials stated that priority industries are those with a high prevalence of minimum wage and overtime violations, and those in which workers experiencing violations are less likely to complain. Officials stated that WHD's priority industry list includes those industries employing children and those with historically high violations, such as retail, hospitality, and food service.

[91] WHD registers each investigation for internal WHD tracking purposes under the specific act that is the focus of the investigation, but the investigation may also cover other acts that WHD is responsible for enforcing. WHD may conduct several types of investigations including full investigations, in which investigators look for child labor violations as one part of the investigation, or limited investigations, such as one focused primarily on

For example, five of six WHD investigators we spoke with told us they include specific questions in their interviews with employers and workers, which are designed to uncover potential child labor violations during worksite visits. WHD guidance also instructs investigators to look for the presence of children and the pieces of equipment covered by hazardous occupations orders when conducting worksite visits.

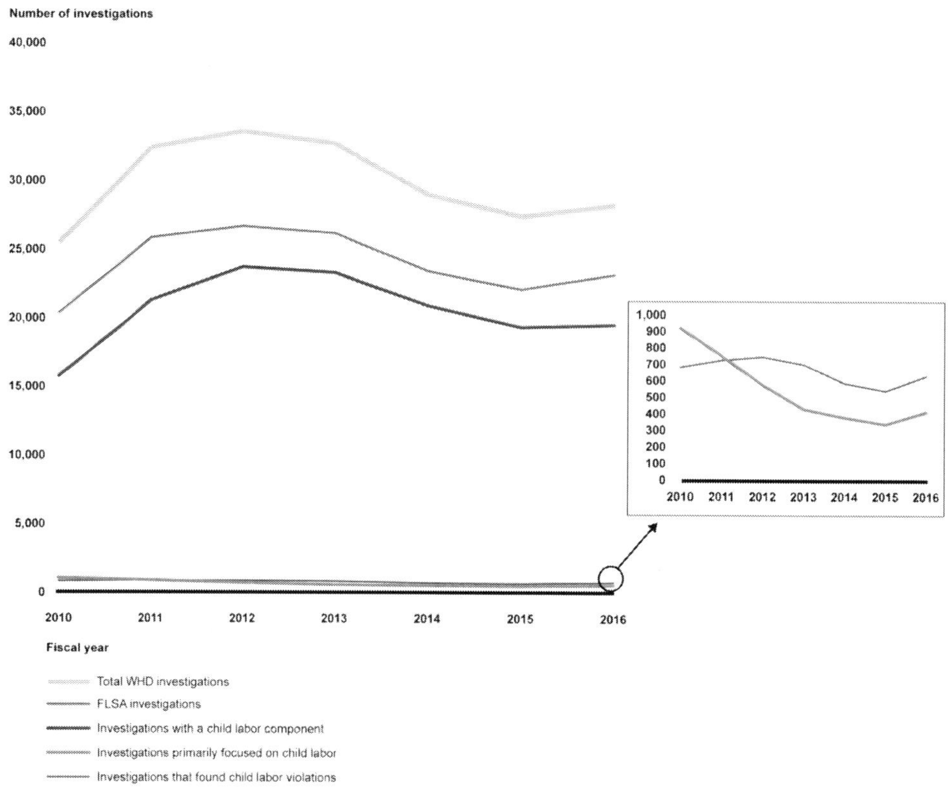

Source: GAO analysis of Wage and Hour Investigative Support and Reporting Database data. | GAO-19-26.

Notes: In addition to the Fair Labor Standards Act (FLSA), WHD enforces multiple other statutes, such as the Family and Medical Leave Act, among others. In this figure, "total WHD investigations" includes all investigations conducted under the authority of any of the laws enforced by WHD. Any WHD investigation may include a child labor component if a WHD investigator checks for potential child labor violations during the investigation, and child labor violations may be found during any WHD investigation. Not all FLSA investigations include a child labor component because some are limited investigations, which may focus on enforcing other provisions of the FLSA.

Figure 7. Wage and Hour Division (WHD) Investigation and Child Labor Violation Trends, Fiscal Years 2010 to 2016.

WHD officials we interviewed said that, as of 2010, child labor had been incorporated within the agency's broader FLSA investigatory activity, and our analysis of WHISARD data indicates that there has been a general decline in its child labor-specific investigations since

---

enforcing the child labor provisions (or other provisions) of the FLSA. WHD may find child labor violations in all types of investigations.

2010. According to our analysis of WHISARD data, the trends in the number of FLSA investigations and the number of investigations with a child labor component generally aligned from fiscal years 2010 to 2016. During the same period, our analysis shows a decline in investigations primarily focused on child labor from fiscal years 2010 to 2015, with a slight increase in 2016 (see inset of Figure 7). Further, the number of investigations that found child labor violations stayed about the same, with a slight dip in fiscal years 2014 and 2015.[92]

Child labor violations have been found across many industries, often in investigations that are not specifically focused on child labor. As previously noted, the industries in which children most commonly work are leisure and hospitality; wholesale and retail; and professional and other services, financial activities, and information. According to our analysis of WHISARD data for fiscal years 2010 to 2016, WHD found most child labor violations in the leisure and hospitality and wholesale and retail industries (see Figure 8). As illustrated in Figure 8, WHD also found violations across other industries including those that employ substantially fewer children, such as construction and mining.[93]

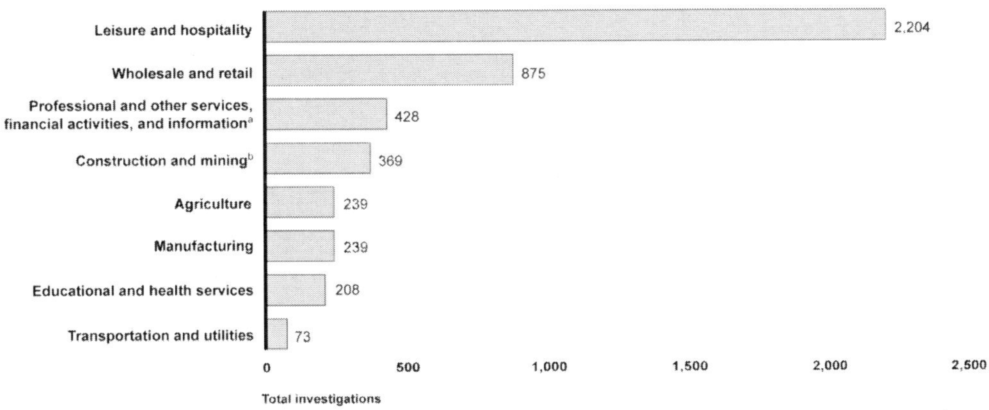

Source: GAO analysis of Wage and Hour Investigative Support and Reporting Database data. | GAO-19-26.

[a]Professional and other services, financial activities, and information includes professional, scientific, and technical services, among others, as well as finance and real estate, and information.

[b]Construction and mining also includes quarrying, and oil and gas extraction.

Figure 8. Wage and Hour Division Investigations That Found a Child Labor Violation, by Industry, Fiscal Years 2010 to 2016.

The most common child labor violations WHD found across all industries for this period were related to (1) hours standards, non-agricultural; (2) all prohibited occupations, non-

[92] WHD may assess civil monetary penalties for child labor violations. The amount of the penalty depends on various factors, such as the size of the business and the gravity of the violations. WHISARD data indicate that the total amount of child labor civil monetary penalties assessed generally decreased from a high of $2.9 million for investigations concluded in fiscal year 2010 to a low of $1.4 million in fiscal year 2015. For investigations that concluded in fiscal year 2016, WHD assessed $1.9 million in child labor civil monetary penalties.

[93] Construction and mining also includes quarrying, and oil and gas extraction.

agricultural; and (3) recordkeeping, such as employer failure to maintain records of a child worker's date of birth (see Figure 9).[94]

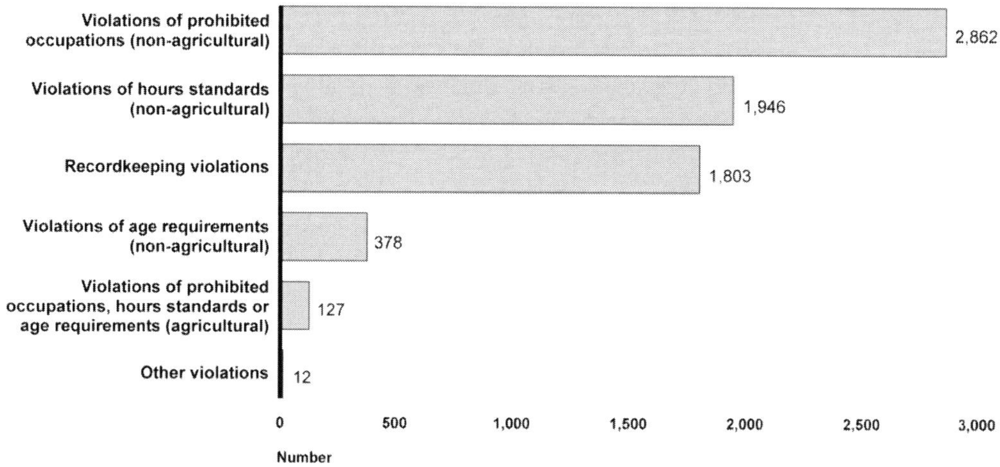

Source: GAO analysis of Wage and Hour Investigative Support and Reporting Database data. | GAO-19-26.

Notes: Categories are not mutually exclusive because an investigation may find more than one type of violation. The "other violations" category includes investigations that found violations for shipping of goods in interstate commerce that have been produced in violation of the child labor provisions, 29 U.S.C. § 212(a). "Other" and "recordkeeping" violations may be found in both agricultural and non- agricultural investigations. We also excluded 13 investigations that found a child labor violation but did not identify the type.

Figure 9. Number of Investigations That Found Child Labor Violations across All Industries, by Type, Fiscal Years 2010 to 2016.

Outreach

WHD Community Outreach and Resource Planning Specialists support WHD's strategic enforcement approach in the field offices by conducting compliance assistance outreach to stakeholder groups associated with WHD's priority industries.[95] These outreach and planning specialists aim to increase voluntary compliance with the child labor provisions of the FLSA and other worker protections. Outreach specialists shared examples of these efforts, such as providing child labor and FLSA presentations and materials to stakeholders, including associations representing employers or teachers, and disseminating information to high schools about DOL-approved apprenticeship programs and the applicable hazardous occupations orders and exemptions.

Outreach and planning specialists told us that they also stay informed about workplace conditions in the community, particularly those affecting children, through their outreach efforts. For example, one specialist told us that they contact stakeholders in a specific industry

[94] With respect to an employee subject to the FLSA's minimum wage provisions or both the minimum wage and overtime pay provisions, employers are required to maintain and preserve records containing certain information, including the employee's date of birth if the employee is under age 19. 29 C.F.R. § 516.2(a)(3).

[95] In addition to the national office, WHD operates offices at the regional, district, area, and field levels. For the purposes of this report, we generally refer to all WHD offices outside of the national office as "field offices," unless otherwise noted.

in part to gather information on potential violations and compliance issues while also raising awareness about WHD's enforcement role. Another outreach and planning specialist discusses child labor at interagency trainings held on farms, and has received some worker complaints at these events.

Over time WHD has emphasized the importance of its outreach efforts related to child labor in agriculture to varying degrees. In 2012, when DOL withdrew its proposed revisions to the agricultural child labor regulations, DOL stated that it would conduct outreach to agricultural stakeholders, such as professional farming organizations.[96] In addition, from fiscal years 2011 to 2014, WHD gave explicit guidance to field offices to incorporate child labor-related efforts in agriculture.

However, WHD has not included child labor-related outreach efforts in agriculture in its guidance to the field since fiscal year 2014, and officials could not identify other directives asking its field staff to focus more on child labor in agriculture. Further, five of the six field office outreach and planning specialists we interviewed could not identify WHD agriculture outreach conducted specifically in response to the 2012 proposed rule withdrawal.[97] While WHD established a metric for the number of outreach events involving child labor in 2018, it has not developed metrics and associated targets for a desired level of child labor outreach in agriculture, where our analysis of federal data shows a disproportionate amount of injuries to and fatalities of working children. Federal internal controls state that management should define objectives clearly to enable the identifications of risks, such as by defining objectives in specific and measurable terms to enable the design of internal control for related risks. Without establishing metrics and associated targets for child labor-related outreach in agriculture, WHD may not be effectively addressing the risk faced by children working in agriculture or helping to reduce their injuries and fatalities.

In addition, WHD has not conducted an evaluation of the effectiveness of its overall child labor enforcement approach since implementing the strategic enforcement program in 2010, which would allow WHD to draw conclusions about the impact or outcomes of outreach and enforcement activities on employers or working children. WHD officials said that they have used a variety of tools and techniques to evaluate progress and guide continuous program improvement, such as developing communities of practice across field offices. WHD has also had a performance metric for child labor in place from fiscal year 2011 to 2017, which assessed the extent to which WHD investigators checked for child labor violations during an investigation.[98] However, this metric would not allow WHD to assess whether its child labor enforcement strategies were achieving their desired outcomes, nor would it allow WHD to determine the extent to which it was investigating establishments where substantial numbers

---

[96] Child Labor Regulations, Orders and Statements of Interpretation; Child Labor Violations—Civil Money Penalties, 77 Fed. Reg. 31,549 (May 29, 2012).

[97] In July 2018, WHD officials provided us with the number of agriculture outreach events from fiscal year 2011 to fiscal year 2015. However, they were not able to identify which of these events focused on child labor. WHD officials stated that, prior to fiscal year 2017, WHD field staff may not have added a secondary "child labor" designation to agricultural outreach, because they usually cover child labor during agricultural outreach presentations. As a result, we were not able to accurately assess the relevance and the meaning of the data provided for child labor outreach in agriculture from fiscal years 2011 to 2015.

[98] In fiscal year 2011, WHD identified two primary performance metrics for child labor: (1) the number of investigations in which child labor is examined, and (2) the percent of enforcement time devoted to child labor. From fiscal years 2012 to 2017, WHD identified one primary performance metric for child labor: the percent of investigations in which child labor is examined.

of children work.[99] Under federal standards for internal control, management should design control activities to achieve objectives and respond to risks, such as by comparing actual performance to planned or expected results and analyzing significant differences.[100] Without developing additional performance metrics, or other measures specific to its child labor enforcement approach, WHD cannot determine whether its investigations are conducted at establishments where children are likely to be working, and effectively targeting its limited resources.

WHD Incorporates Data into Its Child Labor Compliance Strategies

WHD aims to supplement its internal investigation data with external data—including state, local, and other federal data sets—to identify compliance targets for its strategic enforcement approach. According to WHD officials, field offices plan initiatives at the beginning of the fiscal year to allocate resources for investigations and outreach. WHD directs field offices to use a range of evidence, including data, to develop these initiative plans, which reflect where each office expects to have the greatest impact, including finding violations.

WHD Internal Investigation Data

According to WHD officials, they have used trend data from WHISARD, based on past investigation data patterns, to determine future enforcement and compliance activity. However, WHD national office officials we interviewed said WHISARD is not suited for targeting future enforcement action because, as an administrative database, it appropriately reflects past decisions and outcomes that are not generalizable to the general population. Further, officials told us that WHISARD should not be used for predictive enforcement planning as it does not describe current labor market conditions and anticipate future labor trends. However, WHD field staff in five of the six district offices we reviewed told us that they partly rely on WHISARD data for developing enforcement and compliance targets.

State and Local Data

To supplement WHISARD data, WHD has been using external data sources to inform enforcement and compliance planning since approximately 2009. In addition, WHD national office officials reported creating a data team in 2016 to implement multiple data strategies for the agency, including the use of external data sources for enforcement planning. This data team provides data training and other support services to field staff, such as identifying data sources available to answer research questions, according to WHD officials.

WHD's outreach and planning specialists use information from other data sources—including stakeholders—to help identify enforcement and compliance targets in local field offices. For example, one specialist told us that some of the data sources they use for strategic planning and developing initiatives include (1) local economic data, (2) information from

[99] In 2017, DOL's Chief Evaluation Office contracted for an external evaluation examining the efficiency and effectiveness of WHD's overall enforcement approach and compliance assistance outcomes. DOL officials told us that this evaluation will not be examining outcomes specific to child labor, as WHD intends to apply any insights gained from the evaluation into its compliance assistance across all of its program areas.

[100] GAO-14-704G.

community stakeholders, (3) reports from industry groups and employer associations, and (4) discussions with business roundtables. Another outreach and planning specialist told us they use workplace injury data collected by a state agency to monitor trends in demographic characteristics and employing industries. The specialist said they used these data to inform the field office's decision to focus on the local restaurant and hospitality industry. In two districts, outreach and planning specialists told us they collaborate with local educational stakeholders, such as an association representing high school employment counselors, to identify where children are working and inform local strategic efforts for child labor compliance.

Other Federal Data

Some WHD planning staff also use other federal data sources, such as BLS data sets, to identify enforcement and compliance targets. One outreach and planning specialist we met with uses federally compiled county specific data from the Census Bureau to assess the local prevalence of different industries to help inform the district office's strategic enforcement. These data in conjunction with BLS data sets facilitated efforts to monitor local employment trends in traditional low- wage industries—such as retail and food service—overall as well as to track emerging trends in the local labor market. One WHD region is piloting a team of regional data experts that identifies and reviews federal data sets, among others, and helps staff incorporate useful data into their work. WHD officials also stated that they have reviewed BLS injury and illness data for general information on industries where children are being hurt, but the survey's sample size limits WHD's ability to use the data for more specific information on injuries and illnesses to working children. As noted earlier in the report, the BLS injury and illness data has some limitations regarding data on working children, including those working in agriculture, and exploring ways to more comprehensively measure injuries and illnesses to children could inform WHD's strategic approach on how to focus their compliance and enforcement efforts.

WHD has recently begun providing training to key planning staff on the use of external data sources. WHD national office officials told us that in order to encourage field staff to use external data more consistently; they intend to offer more training on available external data sources. In addition, WHD officials stated that the data resources used by each of WHD's five regions may vary based on the different competencies of field staff in terms of analyzing and using external data. As part of its planning for fiscal year 2019, WHD provided training on the use of external data in June 2018, and officials stated that training on external data sources would evolve as field office staff and WHD officials learn of promising practices with data.

WHD Does Not Consistently Collaborate with the Occupational Safety and Health Administration in Its Efforts to Ensure Compliance with Federal Child Labor Law

WHD and OSHA are each responsible for enforcing certain federal workplace protections and have an agreement to coordinate and share information. OSHA inspectors conduct worksite inspections to enforce occupational health and safety standards, but they are not responsible for enforcing potential child labor violations, which are WHD's responsibility. However, when OSHA inspectors discover information indicating potential child labor violations, they may refer the cases to WHD. WHD and OSHA currently have a memorandum of understanding, which was signed in 1990, to facilitate coordination by establishing a referral system to convey complaints and information about potential violations between the two agencies. The memorandum of understanding documents policies WHD and OSHA have agreed to implement to coordinate their enforcement and compliance efforts. These policies include, among other things, (1) providing field personnel with information and training on the types of issues that will be referred; (2) evaluating referrals on a priority basis and taking appropriate action; (3) transmitting to the other agency the results of inspections conducted in response to referrals; (4) establishing a system to monitor the progress of actions taken on referrals; and (5) conducting periodic meetings to report on the progress of actions taken on the other agency's referrals and evaluate the system.

WHD and OSHA staff told us that they exchange information with each other informally, and both agencies acknowledged the importance of collaboration in their memorandum of understanding. Some WHD field officials told us their offices maintain informal relationships with their counterparts in local OSHA field offices, which include exchanging referrals, sharing information, and, in some instances, coordinating on investigations. WHD field officials from every region we spoke with said their offices receive referrals or information from OSHA. For example, one district official told us that their office occasionally coordinates with OSHA to exchange referrals and assist with investigations. Another district official told us they meet with officials from the local OSHA office to discuss violation trends and national targeting guidance.

Although the memorandum of understanding between WHD and OSHA states that the agencies will establish a system to monitor the progress of actions taken on referrals, WHD and OSHA officials told us they do not have a systematic way to do so. Specifically, they have no formal systems or consistent processes for tracking or monitoring referrals. Further, WHD officials told us that their internal investigations system does not have a way to easily track and systematically report on the disposition of referrals from OSHA.[101] In addition, OSHA officials told us that they do not systematically track referrals made to WHD. OSHA officials told us that their field officials may periodically meet with their WHD counterparts, but there is no formal requirement to do so, nor any requirements to document such discussions. Further, WHD and OSHA officials acknowledged that they have not updated their memorandum of understanding since the original 1990 agreement. We have reported that agencies can strengthen their commitment to work collaboratively by developing ways to continually update and monitor written agreements.[102]

While the memorandum of understanding between WHD and OSHA provides a framework for sharing information, updating the memorandum of understanding and establishing procedures for WHD and OSHA when monitoring the exchange of and actions taken on referrals can help ensure agency officials better track the disposition of referrals. Without such documentation, WHD and OSHA lack the ability to ensure that they consistently take appropriate action to protect children from unsafe working conditions.

---

[101] According to WHD national officials, while a data element for OSHA referrals exists within WHISARD, this data element has not been included in WHD reports and it is not widely known or used by field staff.

[102] GAO, *Managing for Results: Key Considerations for Implementing Interagency Collaborative Mechanisms,* GAO-12-1022 (Washington, D.C.: Sept. 27, 2012).

CONCLUSION

For many children, working can result in benefits such as independence and responsibility. However, work may also interfere with their education or present a physical danger to children working in certain industries, such as agriculture. Since our 2002 report, the overall number of working children in the United States has varied and, since 2011, data indicate that the number of children working is increasing. While most children do not suffer injuries at work, our analyses of BLS data show that injuries to and fatalities among working children persist, that children in agriculture comprise more than half of work-related fatalities, and work-related fatalities among children have increased since 2013. However, BLS data on work-related injuries and illnesses do not measure certain populations—such as children working on farms with 10 or fewer workers and household workers, and its pilot household-based injury survey does not include children aged 17 and under. Without improved data regarding injuries and illnesses to working children in the United States, DOL will not have the information necessary to reliably identify types of establishments with a high number of work-related injuries to children, such as farms employing with 10 or fewer workers.

WHD officials said they have made it a priority to enforce the child labor provisions of the FLSA, and since 2010 they have been using available data to inform their strategic approach to enforcement and compliance. WHD has recently begun increasing the resources available to field staff regarding how to analyze and use external data in their enforcement and compliance planning, according to officials—and these efforts will continue to be critical to WHD's strategic approach. However, WHD has not yet taken actions to determine whether its strategic efforts are paying off. For example, WHD has not yet developed metrics and targets for outreach efforts related to children working in agriculture, nor has it developed performance metrics specific to its strategic approach on child labor. In addition, WHD and OSHA have not updated their memorandum of understanding or established current procedures for monitoring referrals exchanged between the two agencies or actions taken in response. Establishing metrics for goals within the strategic enforcement approach could help ensure that actions are yielding results and children can safely work in a variety of industries, particularly agriculture.

RECOMMENDATIONS FOR EXECUTIVE ACTION

We are making four recommendations to DOL:

The Acting Commissioner of the Bureau of Labor Statistics should, upon completion of the pilot Household Survey of Occupational Injuries and Illnesses, evaluate the feasibility of measuring injuries and illnesses to certain worker populations—specifically, children aged 17 and under, child household workers, and those employed on farms with 10 or fewer workers—in any final survey scope, or determine a way to gather information on these populations. (Recommendation 1)

The Administrator of the Wage and Hour Division should establish specific metrics and associated targets for child labor-related outreach in agriculture. (Recommendation 2)

The Administrator of the Wage and Hour Division should develop performance metrics or other measures specific to its child labor enforcement approach, such as whether WHD investigations are conducted at establishments where children are likely to be working. (Recommendation 3)

The Administrator of the Wage and Hour Division and the Assistant Secretary of the Occupational Safety and Health Administration should update and routinely monitor the 1990 WHD and OSHA memorandum of understanding and establish documented procedures for monitoring the exchange of and actions taken on referrals. (Recommendation 4)

AGENCY COMMENTS AND OUR EVALUATION

We provided a draft of this chapter to the Departments of Health and Human Services (HHS) and Labor (DOL) for review and comment. DOL's Occupational Safety and Health Administration (OSHA) provided written comments that are reproduced in appendix XI. DOL's Wage and Hour Division (WHD) provided written comments that are reproduced in appendix XII. HHS did not provide written comments on our report. HHS and DOL provided technical comments, which we incorporated in the report, as appropriate.

In its technical comments, DOL's Bureau of Labor Statistics (BLS) generally agreed with the recommendation that it evaluate the feasibility of measuring injuries and illnesses to certain worker populations— specifically, children aged 17 and under, child household workers, and those employed on farms with 10 or fewer workers—in any final survey scope, or determine a way to gather information on these populations. However, BLS stated that its ability to complete a feasibility study is subject to budget availability. We note that this recommendation also allows for alternate ways, other than a feasibility study, to determine how best to gather information on these populations of working children, and maintain that it is important to do so. Given the importance of this issue, we encourage BLS to explore cost-effective ways to implement this recommendation.

In its written comments, DOL's Wage and Hour Division stated that it agreed with our second recommendation to establish specific metrics and associated targets for child-labor related outreach in agriculture. WHD noted that it has existing performance measures that separately track the number of employer outreach events and the number of events involving child labor, and that a new, combined metric would provide an additional incentive for WHD field offices to conduct child labor-related outreach events in agriculture. WHD generally agreed with the third recommendation, which originally recommended that WHD develop a performance metric specific to its child labor enforcement approach. In its written comments, WHD agreed that it could develop either an internal performance metric or new planning guidance and reporting requirements to ensure that WHD's child labor enforcement efforts focus on industries, establishments, and time periods in which children are likely to be working or injured. Although we agree that planning guidance and reporting requirements can encourage field office staff to focus more on child labor; we continue to believe it is important to include a measurement of WHD's overall child labor enforcement approach as part of any new planning guidance and reporting requirements. We have thus broadened the recommendation to include other measures.

WHD and OSHA generally agreed with our fourth recommendation, to update the memorandum of understanding between WHD and OSHA and establish documented procedures for monitoring the exchange of and actions taken on referrals. Specifically, WHD and OSHA agreed to work together to review and update their memorandum of understanding and to evaluate the efficacy of the existing referral process, and propose actions to improve the process as appropriate. While WHD and OSHA correctly observe that we do not identify any instances where WHD or OSHA failed to take action on a referral, we also note in the report that the agencies have no formal systems or consistent processes for tracking or monitoring referrals. As we stated in our report, we believe that without establishing documented procedures for tracking the disposition of referrals, WHD and OSHA cannot ensure that they are consistently taking appropriate action to protect children from unsafe working conditions.

As agreed with your offices, unless you publicly announce the contents of this chapter earlier, we plan no further distribution until 30 days from the report date. At that time, we will send copies to the appropriate congressional committees, the Secretary of the Department of Health and Human Services, and the Secretary of the Department of Labor.

Cindy Brown Barnes
Director, Education, Workforce and Income Security

Steve D. Morris
Director, Natural Resources and Environment

APPENDIX I: OBJECTIVES, SCOPE, AND METHODOLOGY

Objective I Data Sources

To identify what is known about children working in the United States, including those working in agriculture,[103] we obtained and analyzed monthly and yearly data from two national data sets from the Department of Labor (DOL):

- Bureau of Labor Statistics' (BLS) Current Population Survey (CPS)[104] from 2003 to 2017, and
- Employment and Training Administration's National Agricultural Workers Survey (NAWS) for 2003 to 2016.[105]

We also collected information from two other sets of survey data for certain non-contiguous years:

---

[103] None of the analyses in this report are intended to assess compliance with the Fair Labor Standards Act (FLSA). Among other reasons, the definitions of terms used in these data sets may not be the same as the definitions in the FLSA and DOL's regulations.

[104] CPS is sponsored jointly by BLS and the Census Bureau.

[105] NAWS data are organized by fiscal year.

- Department of Health and Human Services' National Institute for Occupational Safety and Health's (NIOSH) Childhood Agricultural Injury Survey (CAIS), and
- U.S. Department of Agriculture's (USDA) National Agricultural Statistics Service's Census of Agriculture.

The years of data we analyzed varied by data source, based on the availability of data and the number of cases needed to develop national estimates (see Table 9).

Table 9. Data Sources Used in GAO Analyses for Objective I

Data file	Organization responsible	Type of information in file used in analyses	Population GAO examined	Time frame covered by data
Current Population Survey (CPS), including its Annual Social and Economic Supplement (ASEC)	Department of Labor (DOL)'s Bureau of Labor Statistics (BLS); Census Bureau	Hours, occupations, and industries in which children worked; and demographic characteristics of child workforce, including gender, race and ethnicity, and low-income status	Children aged 15 to 17	2003 to 2017[a]
National Agricultural Worker Survey (NAWS)	DOL's Employment and Training Administration	Age first worked in agriculture, demographic characteristics of child hired agricultural labor workforce, including gender, race and ethnicity, poverty status, experience mixing and applying pesticides	Hired farm workers in crop agriculture, aged 14 to 17	Fiscal years 2003 to 2016
Childhood Agricultural Injury Survey (CAIS)	Department of Health and Human Services' National Institute for Occupational Safety and Health (NIOSH)	Number and characteristics of children on farms who worked	Household and hired children aged 17 and under on U.S. crop or livestock farms	2004, 2006, 2009, 2012, 2014b
Census of Agriculture	U.S. Department of Agriculture's National Agricultural Statistics Service	Number of farms that employ 10 or fewer workers	All farm operations	2002, 2007, 2012

Source: GAO analysis of various data sets. | GAO-19-26.

[a]We analyzed data from the 2017 ASEC, which provides information about the industries and occupations that children reported they were working in, as well as about working children families' low-income status during the prior year (i.e., calendar year 2016).

[b]The CAIS was conducted in 2001, 2004, 2006, 2009, 2012, 2014. This chapter's scope is from 2003 onward.

The CPS is the primary source of federal government statistics on employment and unemployment in the United States. The basic monthly survey collects information on employment, such as employment status, occupation, and industry, as well as demographic characteristics, among other things. The survey is based on a sample of the civilian, non-institutionalized population of the United States. About 55,000 households are interviewed monthly based on area of residence, to represent individual states and the country as a whole.[106] In addition to the standard questions from the basic CPS monthly survey, the Annual Social and Economic Supplement (ASEC) includes additional questions of households and provides supplemental data on work experience; income components, such as earnings from employment; and noncash benefits, such as health insurance coverage, among other things. ASEC data on employment and income refer to the preceding calendar year, although demographic data refer to the time of the survey. This chapter used data from the March 2017 ASEC, which refers to employment and income during calendar year 2016.

DOL's NAWS is an employment-based, annual survey of demographic, employment, and health characteristics of hired farm workers in crop agriculture, including crop workers, workers at nurseries, workers at packing houses,[107] and includes workers brought to farms by contractors. NAWS does not include animal agricultural workers, unpaid household workers, or H-2A visa workers.[108] Each year, approximately 1,500 workers are randomly selected for an interview. Interviews are conducted three times per year to account for the seasonal and regional fluctuations of agricultural production and employment. All interviews are conducted in person and the interviewer documents respondents' answers directly on the paper questionnaire. Respondents are generally interviewed directly at their work site, and only currently employed persons are interviewed.

The CAIS farm operator survey is a NIOSH collaborative effort with the U.S. Department of Agriculture's National Agricultural Statistics Service (NASS) to produce national and regional estimates of the number of individuals under age 20 on U.S. operated farms by various demographic characteristics.[109] NIOSH has collaborated with NASS to collect injury and demographic data regarding farm workers aged 20 and under via the CAIS for certain years, including the years 2001, 2004, 2006, 2009, 2012, and 2014. From 2001 through 2012, CAIS was based on a sample of 50,000 U.S. farm operations from the Census of Agriculture, which was increased to 75,000 farming operations for the 2014 survey. For this chapter, we analyzed CAIS results for children aged 17 and under from the 2004 to 2014 surveys. Estimates include household children (a member of a farm operator's household), hired children (a paid worker hired directly by a farm operator), and visiting child (a visitor to the farm, whether a relative or not).

The Census of Agriculture is sponsored by the USDA's National Agricultural Statistics Service (NASS), and collects information about any operation from which $1,000 or more of agricultural products were produced and sold, or normally would have been sold, during the census year. To do this, NASS creates a list of agricultural operations that potentially meet the definition of a farm in order to provide information on the characteristics of farm operations and farm operators at the national, state, and county levels. The Census of Agriculture includes information regarding the number of farms by size and type, inventory and values for crops and livestock, and operator demographic characteristics. When NASS

---

[106] The total sample also includes additional households that are not interviewed for various reasons, such as not being reachable.

[107] Packing and canning operation workers are eligible to be interviewed if the operation is adjacent to or located on the contacted employer's farm and at least 50 percent of the produce being packed or canned originated from the employer's farm.

[108] An H-2A visa is a temporary work visa for foreign agricultural workers with a job offer for temporary or seasonal agricultural work in the United States. The H-2A visa program is generally open to nationals of countries that the Secretary of Homeland Security has designated as eligible to participate and that list is renewed annually.

[109] CAIS defines a farm as being any crop and/or livestock operation with $1,000 or more of gross agricultural production within a calendar year.

summarizes the Census of Agriculture, it assigns the data from an individual report to the principal county—which is the county in which the majority of the operator's agricultural products are produced.

Objective I Quantitative Methodology

To describe what is known regarding children working in the United States, including those working in agriculture, we analyzed CPS data in a variety of ways. Table 10 presents a list of the CPS variables we analyzed.

Table 10. GAO Analysis of Selected Current Population Survey (CPS) Data Variables, 2003 to 2017

	CPS variable	Use in report
CPS monthly data		
Number of working children	Pemlr	Determine number of working children in summer and non-summer months for children aged 15 to 17.
Hours usually worked	Pehruslt	Determine hours usually worked in summer and non-summermonths for children aged 15 to 17.
Self employed	Prdtcow1	Identify self-employed persons based on primary job.
Race and ethnicity	Pehspnon, Prdtrace, Ptdtrace[a]	Determine race and ethnicity information.
Gender	Pesex	Determine trends in employment by gender.
Agricultural work	Pragna, Prdtcow1	To identify those working in agricultural, or non-agricultural industries.
Non-paid working in a family business	Prdtcow1	To identify an unpaid child working in a family business or farm
CPS 2017 Annual Social And Economic Supplement (ASEC) Data[b]		
Industry	Industry	To identify the industry of the longest job in which the respondent worked.
Occupation	Wemocg, Occup	To identify the occupation of the longest job among major groups, and occupation of longest job among more detailed groups.
Low-income status	Famlis	To identify whether a respondent is from a household experiencing poverty, and to determine the ratio of the family's income to the CPS's low-income level.

Source: GAO analysis of Current Population Survey (CPS) data. | GAO-19-26.

Notes: For Annual Social and Economic Supplement (ASEC) data, we determined whether a respondent had worked the previous year by identifying those respondents who had checked yes for the WRK_CK variable, which indicates the interviewer checked yes that the respondent had worked the previous year.

[a]The prdtrace variable changed in August 2005. Accordingly, we analyzed prdtrace from 2003 to July 2005 and ptdtrace from August 2005 to 2017.

[b]2017 Annual Social and Economic Supplement data reports calendar year 2016 information.

- Number of children who worked. To estimate the extent to which children aged 15 to 17 worked during summer and non-summer months, we defined summer months as June through August, and defined non-summer months as January through May and September through December for each calendar year, and averaged estimates for summer and non-summer months.[110] We analyzed the pemlr variable, which is based

[110] Our definitions of summer and non-summer months are not intended to align with how summer is defined in the FLSA child labor regulations. We used our definition of summer and non-summer months in our analysis as

on BLS's definition of an employed person, to determine the number of children who worked. According to BLS's definition, employed people are those who, during the reference week (a) did any work at all (for at least 1 hour) as paid employees; worked in their own businesses, professions, or on their own farms; or worked 15 hours or more as unpaid workers in an enterprise operated by a family member or (b) were not working, but who had a job or business from which they were temporarily absent because of vacation, illness, bad weather, childcare problems, maternity or paternity leave, labor- management dispute, job training, or other family or personal reasons whether or not they were paid for the time off or were seeking other jobs. Each employed person is counted only once, even if he or she holds more than one job.

- Weekly hours worked. To estimate the hours worked during summer and non-summer months, we analyzed the pehruslt variable—the sum of the pehrusl1 and perhrusl2 variables indicating primary and secondary jobs—that indicates a respondent's usual weekly work hours worked. In addition, we developed categorical thresholds to describe hours worked per week in the summer and non-summer months, and we included both primary and secondary jobs in this analysis.
- Industries worked. To identify the industries in which children aged 15 to 17 worked and the occupations they held in 2016, we obtained and analyzed 2017 CPS Annual and Social Economic Supplement (ASEC) data. More specifically, we categorized the industries that children may be working in using the following crosswalk of the Census Bureau classification systems regarding industry information. See Table 11.
- Gender. To describe trends in the gender of working children, we analyzed 2003-2017 CPS basic monthly data.
- Race and ethnicity. This analysis is of the pehspnon, prdtrace and ptdtrace variables,[111] which indicate a respondent's identified race and ethnicity, and the pemlr variable, which indicates the child was employed, as defined by CPS. CPS treats ethnicity separately from race. As a result, a child can be identified in CPS as both white and Hispanic, or as both black and Hispanic, among other considerations. For the purposes of our report, we categorized any respondent identifying as Hispanic, irrespective of their reported race, as Hispanic. We further categorized respondents who identified as not being bi- or multiracial white or black as being white only and black only. We categorized respondents of two or more races, as well as Asians and other specific races such as Native American or Pacific Islander, as other races.[112]
- Low-income status. We obtained data from CPS's March 2017 ASEC to identify children aged 15 to 17 who had had worked in calendar year 2016. We analyzed their reported family income (famlis variable) as it compares to the CPS ASEC's poverty thresholds.[113] For this analysis, we defined "low-income" as any individual whose

we found this categorization to be the most workable given the arrangement and contents of the CPS data set. We did not account for the extent to which some schools may have year-round calendars, or differentiate between varying school calendars between schools.

[111] The race variable changed from prdtrace to ptdtrace in August 2005.

[112] Due to relatively small numbers of respondents identifying themselves as Asian and other races, as well as certain bi-racial and other racial categories, we are only able to report white only, black only, Hispanic, and "other races" race and ethnicity information.

[113] Poverty thresholds are set by the U.S. Census Bureau and take into account family size and composition to determine who is in poverty. Famlis is the CPS ASEC variable that describes the ratio of family income to the

family income was below 150 percent of their poverty threshold.[114] We utilized CPS ASEC data to determine the percentage of working children that were from low-income families and the percentage who were from higher income families (with income at least 150 percent of the poverty threshold), compared to non-working children. We also determined the percentage of working children from low-income families who worked 20 hours or more per week.

Table 11. Crosswalk of Census Bureau Industry Codes Used in GAO Analyses

GAO categorical variable	2012 Census industry classification code	2012 North American Industry Classification System (NAICS) code
All agriculture	0170, 0180-0290	111-115
Agriculture: crop production	0170	111
Agriculture: non-crop agriculture	0180-0290	112-115
Construction and mininga	0370-0490, 0770	21, 23
Educational and health services	7860-8470	61-62
Manufacturing	1070–3990	31-33
Wholesale and retail trade	4070–5790	42, 44 -45
Transportation and utilities	6070–6390, 0570–0690	22, 48- 49
Leisure and hospitality	8560–8690	71-72
Other	6470-6780, 6870-7190, 7270-7790, 8770-9290, 9370-9590	51, 52-53, 54-56, 81, 92

Source: GAO analysis of Census Bureau information. | GAO-19-26.

Note: "Other" includes financial activities, information, professional and business services, other services, and public administration.

[a]Construction and mining industry includes quarrying, and oil and gas extraction.

CPS estimates contained in this chapter are estimated standard errors and presented along with an approximate margin of error at the 95 percent confidence level or relative standard errors. We express our confidence in the precision of a particular sample's estimates with a confidence interval. By adding and subtracting the margin of error from the estimate, we construct a confidence interval that would contain the actual population value for 95 percent of the samples that CPS could have drawn. All margins of error for CPS estimates presented in this chapter are approximations. We calculated the approximate margins of error following CPS guidance and technical documentation. In order to estimate the margin of error for estimates of our subgroups of interest, a number of approximations were required. As a result, the margins of error provide a general order of magnitude. A relative standard error is equal to the standard error of a survey estimate divided by the survey estimate.

We conducted a data reliability assessment of the CPS variables included in our analyses. We reviewed technical documentation and related publications and websites with information about the data. We spoke with the appropriate officials at BLS to resolve any questions about the data and identify any known limitations. We also conducted electronic testing, where

poverty threshold, and is available for all individuals, regardless of family type. A person whose family income is less than 100 percent of the poverty thresholds is categorized as "in poverty." CPS ASEC documentation notes that a family is a group of two persons or more residing together and related by birth, marriage, or adoption. Any related subfamily member is counted as within a primary family. For the purposes of our analysis, the poverty status of an individual in a family is based on their family's income. The poverty status of individuals who are not in a family is based on their own income.

[114] According to a Census Bureau official, the Census Bureau does not officially define low- income.

feasible, to check for logical consistency, missing data, and consistency with data reported in technical documentation. In general, we analyzed our estimates and determined they had relative standard errors of 10 percent or less, except where noted.[115] We determined that the variables we used from the data we reviewed from the CPS were sufficiently reliable for the purposes of our reporting objectives.

Table 12. Selected National Agricultural Worker Survey (NAWS) Data Variables Used in GAO Analyses

Report topic	Variable	Use in report
Gender	Gender	Report percentage of hired crop workers aged 17 and under by gender in 2005 to 2008, fiscal years 2009 to 2012, and 2013 to 2016.
Race and ethnicity	B01 and B02	Report percentage and estimated population of hired crop workers aged 17 and under in fiscal years 2005 to 2008, 2009 to 2012, and 2013 to 2016.
Family poverty status	Fampov	Percentage of hired crop workers aged 17 and under below the poverty level in 2005 to 2008, 2009 to 2012, and 2013 to 2016.
Intensity of work: days worked	Fwrdays	Mean working days for hired crop workers aged 14 to 17 working on U.S. farms, by age in 2005 to 2008, 2009 to 2012, and 2013 to 2016.
Age first worked in agriculture	Agefrstfw	Age range that respondent reported he or she began working, for 2005 to 2008, 2009 to 2012, and 2013 to 2016.
Documentation status	Currstat	Report percentage of hired crop workers aged 17 and under by documentation status in 2013 to 2016.
Region worked	Region6	Report percentage of hired crop workers aged 17 and under by region worked in 2005 to 2016.
Mixed/applied pesticides in last year	Np01f	Report percentage of hired crop workers aged 14 to 17 working on U.S. farms, by age that loaded, mixed or applied pesticides in last 5 years.

Source: GAO analysis of Department of Labor Employment and Training Administration's National Agricultural Workers Survey (NAWS) data. | GAO-19-26.

Notes: NAWS data are organized by fiscal year. According to Employment and Training Administration officials, to determine farm workers' poverty status as reported in NAWS, a poverty threshold was calculated for each worker based on the worker's family size and the U.S. Department of Health and Human Services' poverty guidelines for the calendar year that matches the year for which the worker answered the family income question. Workers' family incomes were then compared to the poverty thresholds calculated for their family size and poverty status was assigned. Income was not adjusted for the amount of time the respondent was present in the United States in the calendar year in which income was reported.

To provide additional information regarding the agricultural child labor work force—in particular hired child crop workers—we analyzed NAWS data regarding hired farm workers in crop agriculture aged 17 and under. More specifically, to determine trend information where possible, we constructed a time variable by aggregating fiscal year 2005 to 2008, fiscal year 2009 to 2012, and fiscal year 2013 to 2016 data to develop a set of responses filtered for 17-year-olds and under that we would be able to report in a statistically reliable fashion at the 95 percent confidence level. To estimate the percentage of 14-, 15-, 16-, and 17-year-olds, we worked with ETA officials to determine a methodology to apply the NAWS population inflator to our estimated percentages and determine a population estimate for our time

[115] For our estimates of the numbers of working children, we analyzed the estimates for 15-, 16-, and 17-year-olds for all years from 2003 to 2017 and determined they have relative standard errors of 10 percent or less.

periods.[116] With respect to our analysis of NAWS data regarding identified characteristics of farm workers in crop agriculture, we analyzed the variables shown in Table 12.

Due to the relatively small samples, at least 2 years of data are to be combined for national-level analyses, according to a NAWS methodology document.[117] All mean estimates were rounded to the nearest whole number. Given the relatively small size of the data sets, to present conservative estimates, we rounded estimates' margin of errors up to the nearest whole number. We conducted a data reliability assessment of the NAWS variables included in our analyses. We reviewed technical documentation and related publications and websites with information about the data. We spoke with the appropriate officials at the Employment and Training Administration to resolve any questions about the data and identify any known limitations. We also conducted electronic testing, where feasible, to check for logical consistency, missing data, and consistency with data reported in technical documentation. We determined that the variables we used from the data we reviewed from NAWS were sufficiently reliable for the purposes of our reporting objectives.

To provide additional information regarding children working in agriculture—in particular, household children working on farms and livestock agriculture—we obtained information from the Department of Health and Human Services' National Institute for Occupational Safety and Health (NIOSH) Childhood Agricultural Injury Survey (CAIS). We reviewed agency documentation regarding its methodology for compiling the data, and interviewed agency officials regarding our results. We reviewed the agency's code used to tabulate results and reported results only within CAIS reporting parameters, with a relative standard error of 33 percent of less.

To provide information regarding the extent to which the agricultural workforce worked on farms employing 10 or fewer workers, we obtained information from the United States Department of Agriculture's Census of Agriculture. We reviewed agency documentation regarding its methodology for compiling the data, and interviewed agency officials regarding our results. We reviewed the agency's code used to tabulate results and reported results only within USDA reporting parameters.

We interviewed officials from DOL's Bureau of Labor Statistics, Employment and Training Administration, and Wage and Hour Division; the Department of Health and Human Services' NIOSH; and the Department of Agriculture regarding the data available and our analyses of the numbers and demographic characteristics of working children.

Objective II Data Sources and Methodology

To describe what is known about the work-related fatalities and injuries to working children, including those in agriculture, we primarily relied on data from two national data sets maintained by Bureau of Labor Statistics—the Census of Fatal Occupational Injuries

[116] The NAWS population inflator is derived from the USDA's Census of Agriculture, which was conducted in 2002, 2007, 2012, and 2017. Because the time frames covered by the NAWS population inflator in some cases fall in the midst of the time period variable we constructed, we worked with NAWS to determine the appropriate population inflator measure.

[117] Due to relatively small sample sizes for respondents aged 17 and under, we opted to present one aggregated estimate for fiscal years 2003 to 2016 for the region a respondent worked in and the variable indicating whether a respondent had mixed or applied pesticides in the last year.

(CFOI) and the Survey of Occupational Injuries and Illnesses (SOII). We also collected information from two other injury and illness data sets, the National Electronic Injury Surveillance System—Occupational Supplement (NEISS-Work) and the Childhood Agricultural Injury Survey (CAIS) (see Table 13). The years of data we analyzed were from 2003 to 2016 for the CFOI, SOII, and NEISS-Work, and selected years for CAIS.

Table 13. Data Sources Used in GAO Analyses of Work-Related Fatalities and Injuries and Illnesses to Children in Objective II

Data file	Organization responsible	Type of information in file used in analyses	Population GAO examined	Time frame covered by data
Census of Fatal Occupational Injuries	Department of Labor's Bureau of Labor Statistics	Ages, occupations, and industries in which children suffered work-related fatalities, including demographic characteristics of child fatalities including gender and race and ethnicity of child	Working children aged 17 and under	2003 to 2016
Survey of Occupational Injuries and Illnesses	Department of Labor's Bureau of Labor Statistics	Numbers of, ages, and industries in which children incurred work-related injuries and illnesses	Working children aged 15 to 17	2003 to 2016
National Electronic Injury Surveillance System—Occupational Supplement	Department of Health and Human Services' National Institute for Occupational Safety and Health	Numbers of and ages in which children incurred work-related injuries and illnesses	Working children aged 14 to 17	2003 to 2016
Childhood Agricultural Injury Survey	Department of Health and Human Services' National Institute for Occupational Safety and Health	Extent to which children on farms incurred work-related injuries	Household and hired children aged 17 and under on U.S. crop or livestock farms	2004, 2006, 2009, 2012, 2014[a]

Source: GAO analysis of Department of Labor and Department of Health and Human Services' National Institute for Occupational Safety and Health data. | GAO-19-26.

[a]The Childhood Agricultural Injury Survey was conducted in 2001, 2004, 2006, 2009, 2012, 2014. This chapter's scope is from 2003 onward.

The Census of Fatal Occupational Injuries (CFOI) is an annual count of fatal workplace injuries, and is a federal-state cooperative program that has been implemented in all 50 states, and the District of Columbia. BLS uses diverse state, federal, and independent data sources to identify, verify, and describe fatal work injuries to ensure counts are as complete and accurate as possible. The CFOI also covers workers on farms of any size, including those employing 10 or fewer workers, and self-employed, family, and federal government workers. We conducted a data reliability assessment of the CFOI variables included in our analyses. We reviewed technical documentation and related publications and websites with information about the data. We spoke with the appropriate officials at BLS to resolve any questions about the data and identify any known limitations. We reviewed the CFOI analyses conducted by BLS to identify any unexpected values or logical inconsistencies in the results. We determined that the summary data provided were sufficiently reliable for the purposes of our reporting objectives. The Survey of Occupational Injuries and Illnesses (SOII) is an annual estimate of workplace injuries and illnesses based on a survey of employers. The SOII is the largest occupational injury and illness surveillance system in the country, providing injury and illness counts and rates for a variety of employer, employee, and case characteristics based on a sample of approximately 230,000 establishments. According to BLS, for the purposes of the SOII an occupational injury is any injury, such as a cut, fracture, sprain, amputation, and so forth, which results from a work- related event or from a single instantaneous exposure in the work environment. Detailed case data and worker demographics, including race and ethnicity, are collected for cases that require a day away from work. SOII estimates the number and frequency (incidence rates) of workplace injuries and illnesses based on recordkeeping logs kept by employers during the year. These records reflect the employer's understanding of which cases are work-related and meet other recordkeeping requirements established by the U.S. Department of Labor's Occupational Safety and Health Administration.[118]

In addition to injury and illness counts, survey respondents are asked to provide additional information for the subset of nonfatal cases that involved at least 1 day away from work, beyond the day of injury or illness. Employers answer several questions about these cases, including the demographics of the worker, the nature of the disabling condition, the event and source producing that condition, and the part of body affected. We conducted a data reliability assessment of the SOII variables included in our analyses. We reviewed technical documentation and related publications and websites with information about the data. We spoke with the appropriate officials at BLS to resolve any questions about the data and identify any known limitations. We reviewed the SOII analyses conducted by BLS to identify any unexpected values or logical inconsistencies in the results. We determined that the summary data provided were sufficiently reliable for the purposes of our reporting objectives.

To provide additional information regarding work-related injuries incurred by children, we obtained and analyzed data from the NEISS-Work public portal. The NEISS-Work data are collected by the NIOSH Division of Safety Research in partnership with the U.S. Consumer Product Safety Commission. NIOSH collects data from a nationally representative sample of 67 U.S. hospital emergency departments. Coders at participating hospitals review all emergency department records to capture nonfatal work-related injuries and illnesses that occurred on the job to civilian workers.[119] An injury is considered work-related if the work was for pay or other compensation; doing agricultural production; or working as a volunteer for an organized group. NEISS-Work data from 2003 to 2014 include data for illnesses that began at work, such as heart attacks and strokes, and chronic conditions. According to NIOSH, illness cases comprise about 5 to 10 percent of all total annual NEISS-Work case estimates. Data from 2015 do not capture most illnesses that began at work. We conducted a data reliability assessment of the NEISS-Work variables included in our analyses. We reviewed technical documentation and related publications and websites with information about the data. We spoke with the appropriate officials at NIOSH to resolve any questions about the data and identify any known limitations. We determined that the variables we used

---

[118] See generally 29 C.F.R. pt. 1904.

[119] According to NIOSH officials, each case in NEISS-Work represents a "worker" who sought treatment in one of the NEISS-Work sampled emergency departments for an occupational injury, including occupational exposures. Hospital coders abstracting the medical records for NEISS-Work are instructed by NIOSH to identify a case as a "worker" if at least one place in his or her emergency department medical record notes that injury occurred while the patient was working.

from the data we reviewed from NEISS-Work were sufficiently reliable for the purposes of our reporting objectives. To provide additional information regarding the number of work-related injuries incurred by child workers, including household workers, on U.S. farms, we worked with NIOSH to obtain information from its Childhood Agricultural Injury Survey (CAIS). This survey is designed to produce national and regional estimates of the number of individuals under age 20 on U.S. operated farms by various injury characteristics. CAIS injury information is for all individuals under age 20 on farms for the years 2001, 2004, 2006, 2009, 2012, and 2014. This includes children aged 17 and under living on, working on, or visiting the farm. More specifically, CAIS defines a household worker as being a member of the farm operator's household (farm operator, his/her spouse, child/step child); a visitor as being a visiting relative to the farm operation or a non-relative visitor; and a hired worker as being a paid worker or laborer hired directly by the farm operator. Injury data include information on whether an injury was work- related or not, the nature of the injury, the source of injury, the type of injury event, and the body part injured. Demographic information for all injured children was also collected. CAIS defines an injury as being any nonfatal traumatic event occurring on the farm operation resulting in at least 4 hours of restricted activity, or requiring professional medical treatment. CAIS defines a work injury as being any injury that occurred while performing work or chores on the farm that was associated with the farm business, regardless of whether the work was performed for pay.

We reviewed the code NIOSH used to tabulate our requested results and only reported results within CAIS reporting parameters, i.e., those with a relative standard error of 33 percent or less. We conducted a data reliability assessment of the CAIS variables included in our analyses. We reviewed technical documentation and related publications and websites with information about the data. We spoke with the appropriate officials at NIOSH to resolve any questions about the data and identify any known limitations. We reviewed the CAIS analyses conducted by NIOSH to identify any unexpected values or logical inconsistencies in the results. We determined that the summary data provided were sufficiently reliable for the purposes of our reporting objectives.

We performed additional analyses with CPS data to support our work for this objective. To calculate total worked hours for each year, we calculated monthly hours worked from CPS basic monthly data by multiplying the pehruslt variable (usual weekly worked hours) by 52 and divided by 12. We then estimated the total hours worked by multiplying the monthly hours worked by our population estimations of the number of working children.[120] We analyzed the prdtcow1 variable to estimate the percentage of unpaid children working in a family business and self- employed children aged 15 to 17. We analyzed the CPS ASEC noemp variable to estimate the percentage of children working for employers with 9 or fewer workers, and 10 to 49 workers.

We identified limitations with the comparability of data across data sets, which results in risks in analyzing data across data sets. To minimize such risks, we reviewed documentation, and interviewed or obtained information from officials responsible for the data to ensure our characterization of the data and our results is accurate and the data are sufficiently reliable for the purposes of our reporting objectives.

---

[120] BLS officials stated the agency does not have research regarding standard errors for estimated total hours worked for 15- to 17-year-olds, and did not provide guidance on how to calculate such standard errors. GAO did not calculate the standard errors for the number of annual hours worked.

Objective III Data Sources and Methodology

To assess how DOL oversees compliance with the child labor provisions of the FLSA, we analyzed administrative data collected by DOL's Wage and Hour Division (WHD), conducted interviews with WHD and OSHA, and reviewed relevant federal laws, regulations, and guidance. To examine WHD's child labor enforcement efforts over time, we analyzed data from WHD's Wage and Hour Investigative Support and Reporting Database (WHISARD), which includes information on investigations and violations related to child labor. For our reporting period of fiscal years 2010 to 2016, we requested data on all WHD investigations and findings.[121] We analyzed total number of investigations with child labor findings and violations by fiscal year,[122] registration act,[123] and industry. Before performing our own analysis, we requested many of these numbers from WHD, which we then calculated on our own and highlighted differences for WHD to comment on. After consulting with WHD officials, we excluded certain unusual types of investigations and investigations with no violations or penalties assessed that were closed due to the employer shutting down or being unlocatable.

In addition, we interviewed officials from DOL's Wage and Hour Division and Occupational Safety and Health Administration. We also conducted interviews with WHD staff at the national office, all five regional offices, and six selected district offices. We identified and selected WHD district offices based on the concentration of investigations with at least one child labor violation and geographical diversity, including areas with representation across agricultural and non-agricultural sectors.

We measured the concentration of investigations with child labor violations, by using WHISARD summary data provided by WHD officials to calculate an average total number of these investigations for the most recent 3 fiscal years (2014 to 2016) and our total 7 fiscal year reporting period (2010 to 2016), for each district office.[124] We then categorized district offices by high, medium, and low averages for investigations with child labor violations using the 3-year average.[125] For our final selections, we primarily used the 3-year averages to ensure that the selected offices had recent experience with investigations that resulted in child labor violations. Our final selections—Austin, Des Moines, Pittsburgh, Raleigh, Sacramento, and San Francisco—represent locations with a mix of high, medium, and low average number of investigations with child labor violations, across all five WHD regions.

---

[121] WHD provided data for all investigations that were not dropped and that concluded during the time period, except for non-enforcement agency investigations under the Davis- Bacon Act and certain other investigations where complainants did not give permission to use their names. WHD identified at least one child labor violation that was not in our data because the permission to use the complainant's name was lacking.

[122] Throughout this report, investigations—and any violations found and resulting penalties—are counted in the fiscal year in which they concluded, although the investigations work may have been done in a prior fiscal year.

[123] In WHISARD, each investigation is registered under the act that was the official focus of the investigation. However, investigations registered under acts other than the FLSA can check for, identify, and result in penalties for child labor violations.

[124] WHD began a new data-driven enforcement strategy and also revised the non- agriculture child labor regulations in fiscal year 2010. As such, we reviewed DOL's actions from fiscal year 2010 to fiscal year 2016 to focus on the most current DOL enforcement practices and regulations.

[125] The 3-year averages for "total investigations with child labor violations" were categorized as follows: "low" was 0-9 investigations, "medium" was 10-19 investigations, and "high" was 20 or more investigations.

In each WHD region we conducted semi-structured interviews with the regional Child Labor Coordinator, and in each district office we interviewed a WHD investigator, Community Outreach Resource and Planning specialist, and district director. The findings from our discussions with regional and district WHD staff are not generalizable. However, the interviews provide examples of WHD's enforcement and compliance assistance efforts with regard to the child labor provisions of the FLSA.

In addition, we interviewed representatives from a range of organizations, including those focused on business and advocacy, such as the National Consumers League, National Children's Center for Rural and Agricultural Health and Safety, Farmworker Action Network, Center for Worker Health at Wake Forest School of Medicine, North Carolina Agribusiness Council, California Farm Bureau Federation, AgSafe, Labor Occupational Health Program University of California-Berkeley, Iowa Federation of Labor AFL- CIO, and Iowa Farm Bureau. We also held one group interview with the Association of Farmworker Opportunity Programs, with representatives from a variety of farm worker and labor organizations.

Finally, we reviewed relevant federal laws, regulations, and guidance pertaining to child labor. We also reviewed WHD's guidance to the field for fiscal years 2011 to 2018 and federal standards for internal control.[126]

We conducted a data reliability assessment of WHISARD variables included in our analyses. We reviewed technical documentation and spoke with officials to discuss our analysis plan, as well as to resolve any questions about the data and any known limitations. We also conducted electronic testing, where feasible, to check for logical consistency and missing data. We found some deficiencies in variables we used from the data, including that according to the integrity report, several variables we used in our analysis were less than 95 percent reliable when traced back to original investigation records. However, we determined that this was the best available data and that it was unlikely that our findings would be materially different due to the probable amount of incorrectly recorded data.

We conducted this performance audit from March 2017 through November 2018 in accordance with generally accepted government auditing standards. Those standards require that we plan and perform the audit to obtain sufficient, appropriate evidence to provide a reasonable basis for our findings and conclusions based on our audit objectives. We believe that the evidence obtained provides a reasonable basis for our findings and conclusions based on our audit objectives.

[126] WHD's fiscal year 2018 enforcement and compliance assistance plans regarding child labor were finalized during the course of our review and were incorporated into our analysis.

APPENDIX II: DETAILED INFORMATION ON CHILDREN IN THE UNITED STATES WHO WORKED IN SUMMER AND NON-SUMMER MONTHS

Table 14. Estimated Number of Children Who Worked in an Average Summer Month, by Age, 2003 to 2017 (In thousands)

Year	15-year-olds	16-year-olds	17-year-olds	Total
2003	499	1,108	1,703	3,310
2004	434	1,070	1,467	2,970
2005	486	1,125	1,618	3,228
2006	444	1,253	1,676	3,373
2007	358	1,068	1,673	3,099
2008	353	947	1,402	2,702
2009	254	787	1,257	2,297
2010	240	545	1,141	1,925
2011	243	590	1,083	1,916
2012	267	638	1,106	2,012
2013	240	641	1,111	1,993
2014	257	647	1,127	2,031
2015	283	717	1,262	2,263
2016	310	799	1,321	2,430
2017	274	857	1,353	2,485

Source: GAO analysis of Current Population Survey (CPS) monthly data. | GAO-19-26.

Notes: Numbers rounded to nearest thousands. Individual age totals may not sum to combined total due to rounding. Summer months include June, July, and August for each calendar year. These definitions are not intended to align with how summer is defined in federal child labor regulations. The estimates averaged these summer months. We analyzed the estimates for 15-, 16-, and 17-year-olds in 2003, 2011, and 2017 and determined they have relative standard errors of 10 percent or less.

Table 15. Estimated Number of Children Who Worked in an Average Non-Summer Month, by Age, 2003 to 2017 (In thousands)

Year	15-year-olds	16-year-olds	17-year-olds	Total
2003	294	807	1,376	2,476
2004	273	851	1,287	2,411
2005	281	843	1,362	2,486
2006	275	891	1,448	2,613
2007	252	802	1,401	2,455
2008	220	688	1,223	2,131
2009	189	537	1,024	1,749
2010	152	457	933	1,542
2011	142	421	849	1,412
2012	157	462	828	1,446
2013	141	493	905	1,538
2014	164	496	990	1,650
2015	186	536	1,004	1,726
2016	185	575	1,049	1,810
2017	171	668	1,099	1,938

Source: GAO analysis of Current Population Survey (CPS) monthly data. | GAO-19-26.

Notes: Numbers rounded to nearest thousands. Individual age totals may not sum to combined total due to rounding. Non-summer months include January through May and September through December for each calendar year. These definitions are not intended to align with how summer is defined in federal child labor regulations.

The estimates averaged these non-summer months. We analyzed the estimates for 15-, 16-, and 17-year-olds in 2003, 2011, and 2017 and determined they have relative standard errors of 10 percent or less.

Table 16. Estimated Number and Percentage of Children Employed during Summer Months and Non-Summer Months, by Age, 2003 and 2017 (In thousands)

	2003		2017	
	Number (percentage) during summer month	Number (percentage) during non-summer month	Number (percentage) during summer month	Number (percentage) during non-summer month
15-year-olds	499 (11.7%)a	294 (7.2%)	274 (6.7%)	171 (4.1%)
16-year-olds	1,108 (26.1%)	807 (19.0%)	857 (19.2%)	668 (14.7%)
17-year-olds	1,703 (39.8%)	1,376 (32.1%)	1,353 (31.4%)	1,099 (24.4%)

Source: GAO analysis of Current Population Survey (CPS) monthly data. | GAO-19-26.

Notes: Percentages rounded to nearest tenth of a percent. Summer months include June, July, and August for each calendar year. Non-summer months include January through May and September through December for each calendar year. These definitions are not intended to align with how summer is defined in federal child labor regulations. The estimates averaged these summer and non- summer months.

[a]The percentage estimate for 15-year-olds in 2003 non-summer months has a relative standard error that is higher than 10 percent but less than 30 percent.

Table 17. Estimated Hours Worked by Working Children Aged 15 to 17 Who Worked in Non-Agricultural Industries, 2003 to 2017 (Numbers in thousands)

	Summer months			Non-summer months		
Year	Worked 40 hours or more	Percentage worked 40 hours or more	Estimated number of working 15- to 17- year-olds that year	Worked 19 hours or more	Percentage Worked 19 hours or more	Estimated number of working 15- to 17- year-olds that year
2003	342	10.7	3,197	745	30.9	2,413
2004	329	11.5	2,852	723	30.9	2,337
2005	384	12.4	3,109	767	31.7	2,417
2006	393	12.1	3,239	850	33.4	2,544
2007	389	13.0	2,984	818	34.4	2,376
2008	317	12.4	2,553	665	32.2	2,065
2009	230	10.5	2,185	527	31.2	1,692
2010	214	11.6	1,837	415	27.9	1,487
2011	188	10.3	1,819	402	29.8	1,347
2012	202	10.5	1,919	405	29.2	1,390
2013	229	12.0	1,900	476	32.0	1,488
2014	235	12.1	1,943	540	33.7	1,603
2015	282	13.0	2,175	558	33.2	1,679
2016	349	15.0	2,323	587	33.6	1,747
2017	326	13.6	2,407	663	35.2	1,882

Source: GAO analysis of Current Population Survey (CPS) monthly data. | GAO-19-26.

Notes: For our analysis, we did not estimate the number of hours for respondents reporting their hours as "varies" based on the results of what other respondents reporting discrete numbers of hours worked. Summer months include June, July, and August for each calendar year. Non-summer months include January through May and September through December for each calendar year. These definitions are not intended to align with how summer is defined in federal child labor regulations, and this analysis is not intended to assess whether this work complied with federal child labor requirements.

Table 18. Estimated Hours Worked by Children Aged 15 Who Worked in Non-Agricultural Industries, 2003 to 2017, by Hours per Week (Numbers in thousands)

	Summer months			Non-summer months		
Year	Worked 40 hours or more	Percentage worked 40 hours or more	Total estimated number of working 15- year-olds	Worked 19 hours or more	Percentage worked 19 hours or more	Total estimated number of working 15-year-olds
2003	40	8.5[a]	465	47	16.9[a]	278
2004	31	7.6[a]	405	35	13.8[a]	254
2005	46	10.5[a]	442	40	15.4[a]	258
2006	50	12.1[a]	410	49	19.0[a]	260
2007	38	11.6[a]	325	48	20.7[a]	234
2008	38	11.6[a]	325	42	20.7[a]	203
2009	19	8.3[b]	232	41	23.2a	176
2010	27	12.5[a]	216	32	22.7[a]	141
2011	28	12.5[a]	222	33	25.5[a]	128
2012	28	11.7[a]	237	34	23.4[a]	145
2013	33	15.0[a]	217	38	30.2[a]	127
2014	44	18.6[a]	239	46	30.4[a]	152
2015	32	12.2[a]	267	53	30.5[a]	173
2016	43	15.1[a]	283	48	27.8[a]	173
2017	36	14.2[a]	257	42	26.0[a]	160

Source: GAO analysis of Current Population Survey monthly data. | GAO-19-26.

Notes: For our analysis, we did not estimate the number of hours for respondents reporting their hours as "varies" based on the results of what other respondents reporting discrete numbers of hours worked. Summer months include June, July, and August for each calendar year. Non-summer months include January through May and September through December for each calendar year. These definitions are not intended to align with how summer is defined in federal child labor regulations, and this analysis is not intended to assess whether this work complied with federal child labor requirements.

[a]Estimate has a relative standard error greater than 10 percent but less than 30 percent.

[b]Estimate should be interpreted with caution because it has a relative standard error between 31 and 50 percent.

Table 19. Estimated Number of Children Aged 15 to 17 Working in Agricultural Industries, Summer and Non-Summer Months, 2003 to 2017 (Numbers in thousands)

	Summer months	Non-summer months
Year	Estimated number	Estimated number
2003	104	59
2004	111	67
2005	113	65
2006	130	65
2007	109	74
2008	145	63
2009	109	53
2010	82	47
2011	89	59
2012	88	52
2013	83	48
2014	86	42
2015	84	43
2016	101	57
2017	71	49

Source: GAO analysis of Current Population Survey (CPS) data. | GAO-19-26.

Notes: Estimates are rounded to the nearest thousand. Summer months include June, July, and August for each calendar year. Non-summer months include January through May and September through December for each calendar year. These definitions are not intended to align with how summer is defined in federal child labor regulations, and this analysis is not intended to assess whether this work complied with federal child labor requirements. All estimates have a relative standard error of less than 30 percent.

APPENDIX III: DEMOGRAPHIC CHARACTERISTICS OF CHILDREN IN THE UNITED STATES WHO WORKED IN SUMMER AND NON-SUMMER MONTHS

Gender

Our analysis of Current Population Survey (CPS) basic monthly data found that working females aged 15 to 17 comprised about 52 percent of the working child population in 2017 summer months, and 53 percent in non-summer months. Tables 20 and 21 present detailed results of our analysis.

Table 20. Estimated Number of Children Aged 15 to 17 Who Worked in an Average Summer Month, by Gender, 2003 to 2017 (In thousands)

Year	Female	Male
2003	1,614	1,697
2004	1,525	1,446
2005	1,653	1,575
2006	1,621	1,753
2007	1,524	1,576
2008	1,357	1,346
2009	1,123	1,174
2010	945	980
2011	968	948
2012	1,054	958
2013	1,027	966
2014	1,034	997
2015	1,114	1,148
2016	1,214	1,217
2017	1,294	1,190

Source: GAO analysis of Current Population Survey (CPS) monthly data. | GAO-19-26.

Notes: Summer months include June, July, and August for each calendar year. These definitions are not intended to align with how summer is defined in federal child labor regulations. The estimates averaged these summer months.

Table 21. Estimated Number of Children Who Worked in an Average Non-Summer Month, by Gender, 2003 to 2017 (In thousands)

Year	Female	Male
2003	1,280	1,196
2004	1,267	1,144
2005	1,297	1,189
2006	1,379	1,235
2007	1,277	1,177
2008	1,148	983
2009	928	821
2010	822	720
2011	753	659
2012	753	693
2013	815	723
2014	867	782
2015	883	842
2016	986	823
2017	1,034	904

Source: GAO analysis of Current Population Survey (CPS) monthly data. | GAO-19-26.

Notes: Non-summer months include January through May and September through December for each calendar year. These definitions are not intended to align with how summer is defined in federal child labor regulations.

Race and Ethnicity

Table 22. Estimated Number of Children Aged 15 to 17 Who Worked in an Average Summer Month, by Race and Ethnicity, 2003 to 2017 (In thousands)

Year	White only	Black only	Hispanic	Other races
2003	2,544	252	351	164[a]
2004	2,314	240	270	147[a]
2005	2,503	222	351	152[a]
2006	2,598	265	349	161[a]
2007	2,334	264	349	152[a]
2008	2,002	248	322	131[a]
2009	1,730	191[a]	271	104[a]
2010	1,458	137[a]	243	87[a]
2011	1,455	168[a]	225	69[a]
2012	1,444	177[a]	272	119[a]
2013	1,405	159[a]	300	128[a]
2014	1,446	169[a]	290	126[a]
2015	1,573	212	312	166[a]
2016	1,621	232	377	200[a]
2017	1,651	240	389	205[a]

Source: GAO analysis of Current Population Survey (CPS) monthly data. | GAO-19-26.

Notes: CPS treats ethnicity separately from race. As a result, a child can be identified in CPS as both white and Hispanic, or as both black and Hispanic, among other considerations. For the purposes of our report, we categorized any respondent identifying as Hispanic, irrespective of their reported race, as Hispanic. We further categorized respondents who identified as not being bi- or multiracial white or black as being white only and black only. We counted bi- and multiracial respondents, as well as Asians, and other specific races such as Native American or Pacific Islander, as other races. Summer months include June, July, and August for each calendar year. These definitions are not intended to align with how summer is defined in federal child labor regulations.

[a]This estimate has a relative standard error greater than 10 percent and less than 30 percent.

Our analysis of CPS basic monthly data found that from 2003 to 2017 the percentage of children aged 15 to 17 who worked during summer months and identified as white only declined, and the percentage of this age group that identified as other races or ethnicities—black only, Hispanic, or other races combined—increased.[127] More specifically, the percentage of working Hispanic children was 15.7 percent in 2017; the percentage of black only children was 9.7 percent; other races was 8.3 percent; and working white only children was 66 percent in 2017.[128]

---

[127] These estimates have relative standard errors of less than 10 percent. CPS treats ethnicity separately from race. As a result, a child can be identified in CPS as both white and Hispanic, or as both black and Hispanic, among other considerations. For the purposes of our report, we categorized any respondent identifying as Hispanic, irrespective of their reported race, as Hispanic. We further categorized respondents who identified as not being bi- or multiracial white or black as being white only and black only. We counted the following respondents as other races: respondents of two or more races, Asians, and other races such as Native American or Pacific Islander.

[128] These estimates are for children working during summer months. The race and ethnic composition of working children during non-summer months was similar. More specifically, the percentage of working Hispanic children during non-summer months was 16.7 percent in 2017, the percentage of black only children was 8.9 percent, and working children of other races increased was 7.8 percent, while working white only children was 67 percent in 2017.

Table 23. Estimated Number of Children Aged 15 to 17 Who Worked in an Average Non-Summer Month, by Race and Ethnicity, 2003 to 2017 (In thousands)

Year	White only	Black only	Hispanic	Other races
2003	1,902	196	268	110a
2004	1,876	175	235	125a
2005	1,915	181	268	122a
2006	1,948	225	308	132
2007	1,816	218	296	125a
2008	1,581	177	268	105a
2009	1,340	133	204	73a
2010	1,176	125	179	61a
2011	1,082	104a	166	60a
2012	1,047	110a	200	89a
2013	1,121	106a	218	93a
2014	1,141	145	257	107a
2015	1,173	162	267	123a
2016	1,210	158	308	133
2017	1,291	172	324	152

Source: GAO analysis of Current Population Survey (CPS) monthly data. | GAO-19-26.

Notes: CPS treats ethnicity separately from race. As a result, a child can be identified in CPS as both white and Hispanic, or as both black and Hispanic, among other considerations. For the purposes of our report, we categorized any respondent identifying as Hispanic, irrespective of their reported race, as Hispanic. We further categorized respondents who identified as not being bi- or multiracial white or black as being white only and black only. We counted bi- and multiracial respondents, as well as Asians, and other specific races such as Native American or Pacific Islander, as other races. Non- summer months include January through May and September through December for each calendar year. These definitions are not intended to align with how summer is defined in federal child labor regulations.

[a]This estimate has a relative standard error greater than 10 percent and less than 30 percent.

Low-Income Status[129]

Our analysis of CPS ASEC data found that for 2016, working children aged 15 to 17 were less likely to be from low- income families than children who did not work: 15 percent and 27 percent, respectively.[130] Further, our analysis found that this trend was consistent across varying working hours; in 2016 about 16 percent of children working 20 or more hours per week and about 14 percent of children working less than 20 hours were from low-income families.

---

[129] In this report, we defined low-income as having income below 150 percent of the poverty threshold. Poverty thresholds are set by the U.S. Census Bureau and take into account family size and composition to determine who is in poverty. According to a Census Bureau official, the Census Bureau does not have an official definition of low-income.

[130] This analysis was conducted for all individuals, regardless of family type. The poverty status for persons aged 15 to 17 who are not related to anyone in a household (e.g., living alone or a foster child) is determined by their own income. CPS ASEC documentation notes that a family is a group of two persons or more residing together and related by birth, marriage, or adoption. Any related subfamily member is counted as within a primary family. For the purposes of our analysis, the poverty status or low-income status of individuals in a family is based on their family's income. The poverty/low-income status of individuals who are not in a family is based on their own income.

Appendix IV: Detailed Information on Occupations in Which Children Aged 15 to 17 Worked, 2016

Table 24. Occupations in Which Children Aged 15 to 17 Were Estimated to Have Worked, 2016 (In thousands)

Occupation title	Estimated number of working children (margin of error)
Cashiers	375 (+/-52)
Waiters and waitresses	141 (+/-36)
Athletes, coaches, umpires, and related workers	103 (+/-27)
Child care workers	90 (+/-24)
Miscellaneous agricultural workers, including animal breeders	87 (+/-23)
Cooks	86 (+/-26)
Retail salespersons	84 (+/-26)
Food preparation workers	83 (+/-22)
Lifeguards and other recreational and all other protective service workers	79 (+/-24)
Food preparation and serving related workers, all other including dining room and cafeteria attendants and bartender helpers	77 (+/-23)
Hosts and hostesses, restaurant, lounge, and coffee shop	71 (+/-22)
Counter attendants, cafeteria, food concession, and coffee shop	69 (+/-24)
Janitors and building cleaners	64 (+/-21)
Laborers and freight, stock, and material movers, hand	58 (+/-20)
Packers and packagers, hand	58 (+/-27)
Grounds maintenance workers	55 (+/-20)
Stock clerks and order fillers	54 (+/-21)
Office clerks, general	52 (+/-21)
Customer service representatives	51 (+/-21)
Dishwashers	49 (+/-22)
Recreation and fitness workers	46 (+/-19)
Other teachers and instructors	45 (+/-18)
Combined food preparation and serving workers, including fast food	42 (+/-17)
Miscellaneous entertainment attendants and related workers	37 (+/-18)
Cleaners of vehicles and equipment	33 (+/-18)
Receptionists and information clerks	25 (+/-13)
Construction laborers	22 (+/-15)[a]
Food servers, non-restaurant	21 (+/-12)[a]
Driver/sales workers and truck drivers	15 (+/-11)[a]
Nonfarm animal caretaker	14 (+/-11)[a]
Teacher assistants	11 (+/-9)[a]
Secretaries and administrative assistants	11 (+/-9)[a]
Carpenters	11 (+/-10)[a]
Maids and housekeeping cleaners	11 (+/-8)[a]
Bookkeeping,accounting, and auditing clerks	10 (+/-9)[a]
Ushers, lobby attendants, and ticket takers	10 (+/-9)[a]
Counselors	10 (+/-8)[a]
Nursing, psychiatric, and home health aides	10 (+/-7)[a]
Security guards and gaming surveillance officers	9 (+/-8)[a]
Miscellaneous healthcare support occupations, including medical equipment preparers	9 (+/-7)[a]

Source: GAO analysis of Current Population Survey (CPS) 2017 Annual Social and Economic Supplement (ASEC) data, which reports calendar year 2016 information. | GAO-19-26.

Notes: Data in parentheses represent the margin of error at the 95 percent confidence level. This analysis is not intended to assess whether this work complied with federal child labor requirements.

[a]This estimate has a relative standard error between 30 and 50 percent and should be interpreted with caution.

APPENDIX V: DETAILED INFORMATION ON HIRED CHILD CROP WORKERS IN THE UNITED STATES

Estimated Number of Hired Working Children in Crop Agriculture

Our analysis of National Agricultural Worker Survey (NAWS) data found that from fiscal years 2005 to 2008 about 43,000 children aged 17 and under on average worked on U.S. crop farms—about 3.1 percent of the total hired crop worker population. Further, from fiscal years 2009 to 2012 there were about 30,000 children aged 17 and under on average (1.8 percent), and from fiscal years 2013 to 2016 about 34,000 on average (2.1 percent).

Age First Worked in Agriculture

Table 25. Age Hired Crop Workers First Worked in U.S. Agriculture, by Estimated Percentage, Fiscal Years 2003 to 2016

Age first worked in U.S. agriculture	Estimated percentage of all hired crop workers (margin of error)
0- to 13-years-old	7 (+/-1)
14- to 18-years-old	32 (+/-2)
19- to 21-years-old	18 (+/-1)
22- to 24-years-old	11 (+/-1)
25- to 34-years-old	32 (+/-2)

Source: GAO analysis of National Agricultural Worker Survey (NAWS) data. | GAO-19-26.

Notes: Data in parentheses represent the margin of error at the 95 percent confidence level. All mean estimates are rounded to the nearest whole number, and margin of errors are rounded up to the next whole number. The National Agricultural Worker Survey (NAWS) survey does not identify the discrete age at which a respondent first worked in U.S. agriculture. Accordingly, it is not possible to identify the extent to which those reporting they first worked in U.S. agriculture between age 14 and 18 started working at age 14, 15, etc. This analysis is not intended to assess whether this work complied with federal child labor requirements.

Our analysis of NAWS data indicates that more than one-third of hired crop workers—both adults and children—began working in U.S. agriculture at age 18 or under. More specifically, in the fiscal year 2003 to 2016 reporting period, between 6 and 8 percent of hired crop workers began working at age 13 or under, and another 30 to 34 percent began working at age 14 to 18.[131] Table 25 presents specific results.

Gender

Our analysis of National Agricultural Worker Survey (NAWS) data identified no discernible trends with respect to the gender of the hired child crop workers during the time periods we reviewed. However, our analysis shows that hired crop workers aged 17 and under were more often male than female. See Table 26.

[131] These ranges are estimates at the 95 percent confidence level.

Table 26. Estimated Percentage of Hired Crop Workers Aged 17 and under by Gender, Fiscal Years 2005 to 2016

Fiscal years	Percentage of females (margin of error)	Percentage of males (margin of error)
2005 to 2008	19 (+/-18)a	81 (+/-18)
2009 to 2012	24 (+/-9)	76 (+/-9)
2013 to 2016	30 (+/-15)	70 (+/-15)

Source: GAO analysis of National Agricultural Worker Survey (NAWS) data. | GAO-19-26.

Note: Data in parentheses represent the margin of error at the 95 percent confidence level. All mean estimates are rounded to the nearest whole number, and margin of errors are rounded up to the next whole number. While the estimated percentage of female hired child crop workers appears to increase, and the percentage of males decrease, the margin of errors overlap among mean estimates. Therefore, we cannot with confidence state that the trends are statistically reliable and instead note that there are no discernible trends.

[a]Estimate has a relative standard error between 31 and 50 percent and should be interpreted with caution.

Race and Ethnicity

Table 27. Estimated Percentage of Hired Crop Workers Aged 17 and under by Race and Ethnicity, Fiscal Years 2005 to 2016

Fiscal years	Percentage Hispanic (margin of error)	Percentage white only (margin of error)
2005 to 2008	74 (+/-18)	25 (+/-18)a
2009 to 2012	50 (+/-17)	50 (+/-17)
2013 to 2016	65 (+/-17)	34 (+/-17)

Source: GAO analysis of National Agricultural Worker Survey (NAWS) data. | GAO-19-26.

Notes: Data in parentheses represent the margin of error at the 95 percent confidence level. All mean estimates are rounded to the nearest whole number, and margin of errors are rounded up to the next whole number. We separately analyzed black only and "other races"—defined as Native American, Pacific Islander, and persons of two or more races—for the time periods noted, but did not obtain statistically reportable results for respondents aged 17 and under.

[a]Estimate has a relative standard error between 31 and 50 percent and should be interpreted with caution.

Our analysis of NAWS data found no discernible trends with respect to the trends in Hispanic and white only hired child crop workers during the time periods we reviewed. Table 27 presents detailed results.

Poverty Status

Our analysis of NAWS data indicates a substantial percentage of hired child crop workers come from families experiencing poverty. More specifically, our analysis shows that between 74 and 92 percent of hired crop workers aged 17 and under in the fiscal year 2005 to 2008 review period came from families below the poverty level, as defined for purposes of NAWS,[132] whereas in the fiscal year 2013 to 2016 review period, between 42 and 76 percent

[132] According to Employment and Training Administration officials, to determine farm workers' poverty status as reported in NAWS, a poverty threshold was calculated for each worker based on the worker's family size and the U.S. Department of Health and Human Services' poverty guidelines for the calendar year that matches the year for which the worker answered the family income question. Workers' family incomes were then compared to the poverty thresholds calculated for their family size and poverty status was assigned. Income

did. Table 28 presents specific details for the fiscal year 2005 to 2008, 2009 to 2012, and 2013 to 2016 reporting periods.

Table 28. Estimated Percentage of Hired Crop Workers Aged 17 and under from Families below the Poverty Level, Fiscal Years 2005 to 2016

Fiscal years	Percentage below the poverty level (margin of error)	Percentage above the poverty level (margin of error)
2005 to 2008	83 (+/-9)	17 (+/-9)
2009 to 2012	77 (+/-13)	23 (+/-13)
2013 to 2016	59 (+/-17)	41 (+/-17)

Source: GAO analysis of National Agricultural Worker Survey (NAWS) data. | GAO-19-26.

Notes: Data in parentheses represent the margin of error at the 95 percent confidence level. Percentages may not total to 100 due to rounding. According to Employment and Training Administration officials, to determine farm workers' poverty status as reported in NAWS, a poverty threshold was calculated for each worker based on the worker's family size and the U.S. Department of Health and Human Services' poverty guidelines for the calendar year that matches the year for which the worker answered the family income question. Workers' family incomes were then compared to the poverty thresholds calculated for their family size and poverty status was assigned. Income was not adjusted for the amount of time the respondent was present in the United States in the calendar year in which income was reported.

Mean Farm Work Days per Year

Our analysis of NAWS data indicates that hired crop workers aged 17 and under worked an estimated 70 days in the fiscal year 2013 to 2016 reporting period.[133] Table 29 presents the detailed results of the mean estimated number of days worked for children aged 14 to 17.

Table 29. Trends in Estimated Mean Working Days for Hired Crop Workers Aged 14 to 17 Working on U.S. Farms, by Age and Year Grouping

	Fiscal years 2005 to 2008	Fiscal years 2009 to 2012	Fiscal years 2013 to 2016
Worker age	Mean estimated number of days (margin of error days)	Mean estimated number of days (margin of error days)	Mean estimated number of days (margin of error days)
14-years-old	126 (+/-74)	82 (+/-35)[a]	65(+/-42)[a]
15-years-old	77 (+/-13)	71 (+/-50)[a]	101 (+/-43)[a]
16-years-old	94 (+/-31)	63 (+/-14)	57 (+/-16)
17-years-old	95 (+/-42)	94 (+/-31)	74 (+/-24)
Total aged 17 years and under	93 (+/-24)[a]	78 (+/-16)	70 (+/-15)
Total aged 18 years and older	195 (+/-8)	190 (+/-8)	194 (+/-8)

Source: GAO analysis of National Agricultural Worker Survey (NAWS) data. | GAO-19-26.

Notes: Data in parentheses represent the margin of error at the 95 percent confidence level. All mean estimates are rounded to the nearest whole number, and margin of errors are rounded up to the next whole number. This analysis is not intended to assess whether this work complied with federal child labor requirements.

[a]Estimate has a relative standard error between 31 and 50 percent and should be interpreted with caution.

---

was not adjusted for the amount of time the respondent was present in the United States in the calendar year in which income was reported.

[133] At the 95 percent confidence level, the estimated number of days that crop workers on U.S. farms aged 17 or under worked were between 55 and 85 days for the fiscal year 2013 to 2016 reporting period.

Documentation Status

According to our analysis of NAWS data, which is self-reported by workers, from 2013 to 2016, the majority of hired crop workers aged 17 and under were U.S. citizens, with some participation in the hired crop work force by children holding green cards or who were unauthorized workers, as defined for purposes of NAWS. Table 30 presents details.

Table 30. Estimated Percentage of Hired Crop Workers Aged 17 and Under by Documentation Status, Fiscal Years 2013 to 2016

Fiscal years	Citizen (margin of error)	Green card (margin of error)	Unauthorized (margin of error)
2013 to 2016	73 (+/-16)	12 (+/-10)[a]	15 (+/-13)[a]

Source: GAO analysis of National Agricultural Worker Survey (NAWS) data. | GAO-19-26.

Notes: Data in parentheses represent the margin of error at the 95 percent confidence level. All mean estimates are rounded to the nearest whole number, and margin of errors are rounded up to the next whole number. Table does not include results for Other Work Authorization, the results of which were not reportable for the time periods. NAWS also does not include workers employed on H-2A visas in its survey or in the survey results.

[a]Estimate has a relative standard error between 31 and 50 percent and should be interpreted with caution.

Region Worked

Our analysis of NAWS data found a relatively even distribution of hired crop workers in the California, Midwest, and Northwest regions, with somewhat fewer workers in the Southeast and Southwest, for the time period from fiscal year 2005 to 2016. Table 31 presents the detailed results.

Table 31. Estimated Percentage of Hired Crop Workers Aged 17 and Under by Region, Fiscal Years 2005 to 2016

Region	States	Percentage of workers in region (margin of error)
California	California	21 (+/-9)
East	Connecticut, Delaware, Kentucky, Maine, Maryland, Massachusetts, New Hampshire, New Jersey, New York, North Carolina, Pennsylvania, Rhode Island, Tennessee, Vermont, Virginia, and West Virginia	15 (+/-8)
Midwest	Illinois, Indiana, Iowa, Kansas, Michigan, Minnesota, Missouri, Nebraska, North Dakota, Ohio, South Dakota, and Wisconsin	23 (+/-10)
Northwest	Colorado, Idaho, Montana, Nevada, Oregon, Utah, Washington, and Wyoming	21 (+/-8)
Southeast	Alabama, Arkansas, Florida, Georgia, Louisiana, Mississippi, and South Carolina	11 (+/-5)
Southwest	Arizona, New Mexico, Oklahoma, and Texas	10 (+/-6)

Source: GAO analysis of National Agricultural Worker Survey (NAWS) data. | GAO-19-26.

Notes: Data in parentheses represent the margin of error at the 95 percent confidence level. All mean estimates are rounded to the nearest whole number, and margin of errors are rounded up to the next whole number. The NAWS is not administered in Alaska or Hawaii.

Applied or Mixed Pesticides within the Last Year

Our analysis of NAWS data shows that from 2003 to 2016, an estimated 14 percent (+/-13 percent) of 16-year-olds and 8 percent (+/-7 percent) of 17-year-olds reported that in the past 12 months they had loaded, mixed, or applied pesticides.[134]

APPENDIX VI: DETAILED INFORMATION ON CHILDREN IN THE UNITED STATES WHO WORK ON FARMS

Table 32. National Estimates of Children Working on U.S. Farms by Type of Farm, Type of Worker and Age, 2004, 2006, 2009, 2012, 2014

Farm type	Worker type	Age	2004 (margin of error)	2006 (margin of error)	2009 (margin of error)	2012 (margin of error)	2014 (margin of error)
Crop	Working household	14 and under	158,811 (+/-10,676)	121,513 (+/-9,855)	107,097 (+/-9,259)	99,571 (+/-10,474)	100,288 (+/-8,522)
		15 to 17	87,811 (+/-6,315)	76,662 (+/-5,998)	64,350 (+/-5,894)	64,448 (+/-18,853)	52,132 (+/-4,733)
		Total under 18	246,622 (+/-13,275)	198,175 (+/-12,177)	171,447 (+/-12,038)	164,019 (+/-13,777)	152,420 (+/-10,539)
	Hired	14 and under	21,799 (+/-4,929)	15,378 (+/-3,967)	11,454 (+/-4,092)	10,059 (+/-2,656)	12,131 (+/-2,954)
		15 to 17	84,561 (+/-9,816)	75,446 (+/-9,179)	52,101 (+/-7,619)	56,194 (+/-9,243)	67,195 (+/-8,653)
		Total under 18	106,360 (+/-11,785)	90,823 (+/-10,741)	63,556 (+/-9,937)	66,253 (+/-9,967)	79,326 (+/-9,643)
Livestock	Working household	14 and under	228,838 (+/-14,388)	192,802 (+/-12,571)	171,374 (+/-12,681)	142,377 (+/-13,255)	145,549 (+/-10,108)
		15 to 17	115,245 (+/-8,110)	106,205 (+/-7,844)	94,087 (+/-7,589)	81,688 (+/-8,171)	77,866 (+/-5,892)
		Total under 18	344,083 (+/-17,587)	299,007 (+/-16,064)	265,460 (+/-15,996)	224,064 (+/-17,301)	223,415 (+/-13,073)
	Hired	14 and under	21,460 (+/-5,917)	14,036 (+/-3,169)	8,836 (+/-2,325)	12,934 (+/-3,083)	10,130 (+/-2,785)
		15 to 17	71,190 (+/-8,677)	79,360 (+/-9,424)	51,003 (+/-7,562)	51,505 (+/-7,697)	58,389 (+/-7,824)
		Total under 18	92,649 (+/-11,358)	93,396 (+/-10,635)	59,838 (+/-8,103)	64,439 (+/-8,953)	68,519 (+/-8,522)
Total crop and livestock	Working household and hired	All under 18	789,714 (+/-54,006)	681,401 (+/-49,617)	560,301 (+/-46,074)	518,775 (+/-49,998)	523,680 (+/-41,777)

Source: GAO analysis of Childhood Agricultural Injury Survey 2004, 2006, 2009, 2012, 2014 data. | GAO-19-26.

Notes: The National Institute for Occupational Safety and Health's (NIOSH) Childhood Agricultural Injury Survey defines a farm as being any crop and/or livestock operation with $1,000 or more of gross agricultural production within a calendar year. Farm type is determined by the type of production indicated for the respondent which represents the largest proportion of gross income for the farm operation. Working household children are defined as a member of the farm operator's household who performed work or chores on the farm (regardless of pay), and is a subset of household children. Hired children are defined as children hired directly by the farm operator and paid for work performed on the farm. These exclude working household children and contract laborers. Data in parentheses represent the margin of error at the 95 percent confidence level. This analysis is not intended to assess whether this work complied with federal child labor requirements.

[134] These estimates have relative standard errors of between 31 and 50 percent and should be interpreted with caution. This analysis is not intended to assess whether this work complied with any applicable federal requirements, such as federal child labor requirements or the Environmental Protection Agency's Worker Protection Standard.

NIOSH also calculated the estimated number of children aged 12 and under in 2014 that worked on a U.S. farm, and estimated there were 68,866 (+/-7,023) working household children on crop farms, and 102,260 (+/-8,328) working household children on livestock farms. Further, NIOSH calculations estimate the number of hired children aged 12 and under that worked on a U.S. farm in 2014 as being 2,693 (+/-1,186) on crop farms and 3,538 (+/-1,936) on livestock farms. Data in parentheses represent the margin of error at the 95 percent confidence level.

APPENDIX VII: INFORMATION ON WORK-RELATED CHILD FATALITIES BY INDUSTRY, 2003 TO 2016

Table 33. Number of Work-Related Child Fatalities, by Detailed Industry, 2003 to 2016

General industry	Detailed industry	Sub-industry	Number	Percentage of total
Agriculture			237	52.4
	Crop production		143	31.6
		Oilseed and grain farming	19	4.2
		Vegetable and melon farming	8	1.8
		Fruit and tree nut farming	6	1.3
		Other crop farming	24	5.3
	Animal production and aquaculture		67	14.8
		Cattle ranching and farming	56	12.4
		Other animal production	6	1.3
	Forestry and logging		5	1.1
	Fishing, hunting and trapping		9	2.0
	Support activities for agriculture and forestry		11	2.4
Construction and Mining			59	13.1
	Mining, quarrying, and oil and gas extraction		3	0.7
	Construction		56	12.4
Manufacturing			10	2.2
	Wood product manufacturing		5	1.1
Wholesale and Retail Trade			33	7.3
	Wholesale trade		14	3.1
	Retail trade		19	4.2
Transportation and Warehousing			12	2.7
	Truck transportation		9	2.0
Leisure and Hospitality			34	7.5
	Arts, entertainment, and recreation		14	3.1
	Accommodation and food services		20	4.4

General industry	Detailed industry	Sub-industry	Number	Percentage of total
Professional, business, and other services			55	12.2
	Information		3	0.7
	Professional and business services		31	6.9
		Professional, scientific, and technical services	3	0.7
		Administrative and support and waste management and remediation services	28	6.2
	Educational and health services		5	1.1
		Health care and social assistance	4	0.9
	Other services, except public administration		16	3.5
Government, including public administration			11	2.4
	Public administration		6	1.3

Source: GAO analysis of Census of Fatal Occupational Injuries (CFOI) data. | GAO-19-26.

Note: Totals for general industries may not total the sum of detailed industries and sub-industries, because some data for detailed industries or sub-industries did not meet BLS publication criteria.

Appendix VIII: Selected Demographic Characteristics of Work-Related Fatalities, Children Aged 17 and under, 2003 to 2016

With respect to gender, the data from BLS's Census of Fatal Occupational Injuries show that 87 percent of the children killed due to work-related injuries were boys,[135] and about 56 percent of the work-related fatalities were incurred by children aged 16 or older. Boys aged 17 and under suffered a work-related fatality about seven times more often than girls.

With respect to race and ethnicity, most children incurring work-related fatalities were white only (75 percent), as shown in Table 34.

Table 34. Number and Percentage of Work-Related Child Fatalities, by Race and Ethnicity, 2003 to 2016

	White only	Hispanic	Black only	Other races	Total
Number of children	340	89	11	11	451
Percentage of children	75	20	2	2	99[a]

Source: GAO analysis of Census of Fatal Occupational Injuries (CFOI) data. | GAO-19-26.

Notes: The number of work-related fatalities reported in this table is one less than reported in Table 3 because, according to BLS, the fatality in Table 3 did not meet publication criteria. Respondents who reported they were of Hispanic ethnicity and any race (for example, black and Hispanic) were counted as Hispanic; respondents who report they were of Hispanic ethnicity and two or more races were counted as Hispanic; respondents who did not report Hispanic ethnicity who also identified as two or more races were counted as "other races."

[a]Percentage does not sum to 100 percent due to rounding.

[135] BLS reported gender information for 451 of the 452 work-related fatalities to children during the time period.

With respect to the event or exposure that contributed to a child's death,[136] our analysis of BLS data indicate that, from 2012 to 2016, 61 percent of the 119 work-related fatalities incurred by children aged 17 and under were due to a work- and transportation-related accident, including roadway incidents involving motorized land vehicles. Table 35 provides details on the types of event or exposure that caused the work-related child fatalities from 2012 to 2016.

Table 35. Causes of Work-Related Child Fatalities, 2012 to 2016

Event or exposure general category	Event or exposure specific category	Number	Percentage to total for time period
Violence and other injuries by persons or animals		11	9
	Intentional injury by person	6	5
	Injury by person— unintentional or intent unknown	3	3
	Animal and insect related incidents	2	2
Transportation incidents		72	61
	Animal and other non- motorized vehicle transportation incidents	5	4
	Pedestrian vehicular incident	4	3
	Water vehicle incident	3	3
Transportation incidents	Roadway incident involving motorized land vehicle	26	22
	Non-roadway incident involving motorized land vehicle	33	28
	Fire	1	1
Fall, slip, trip		5	4
	Fall to lower level	5	4
Exposure to harmful substances or environments		5	4
	Exposure to electricity	3	3
	Exposure to other harmful substances	2	2
Contact with objects and equipment		23	19
	Struck by objects or equipment	14	12
	Caught in or compressed by equipment or objects	8	7

Source: GAO analysis of Census of Fatal Occupational Injuries (CFOI) data. | GAO-19-26.

Notes: Totals for categories may contain subcategories not shown elsewhere, which did not meet Bureau of Labor Statistics publication criteria. Accordingly, some totals do not sum to that total's specific subcategories. This analysis is not intended to assess whether this work complied with federal child labor requirements.

[136] Our analysis was of the event or exposure, but not the source for a work-related fatality.

APPENDIX IX: ESTIMATED WORK-RELATED INJURIES AND ILLNESSES TO CHILDREN AGED 17 AND UNDER, 15 AND UNDER, AND 14 AND UNDER

Table 36. Estimated Work-Related Injuries and Illnesses to Children Aged 17 and Under, Aged 15 and Under, and Aged 14 and Under, 2003 to 2016

	Bureau of Labor Statistics (BLS) Survey of Occupational Illness and Injuries (SOII)					National Institute for Occupational Safety and Health (NIOSH) National Electronic Injury Surveillance System – Occupational Supplement (NEISS-Work)			
Year	Total estimated number of work related injuries and illnesses involving days away from work in thousands	Aged 15to 17, estimated number of injuries and illnesses in thousands(margin of error)	Aged 15to 17, estimated percentage of total injuries and illnesses that involved a day away from work	Aged 15 and under, estimated number of injuries and illnesses (margin of error)[a]	Aged 15 and under, estimated percentage of total injuries and illnesses	Aged 17 and under, estimated number of injuries and illnesses in thousands (margin of error)	Aged 17 and under, estimated percentage of injuries and illnesses to total injuries and illnesses	Aged 14 and under estimated number of injuries and illnesses in thousands (margin of error)	Aged 14and under, estimated percentage of total injuries and illnesses
2003	1,316	9.0 (+/-.457)	0.68%	220 (+/-69)	.02%	54.8 (+/-11.1)	1.6%	3.8 (+/-1.6)	0.10%
2004	1,259	7.9 (+/-.431)	0.62%	200 (+/-67)	.02%	53.9 (+/-11.7)	1.6%	3.7 (+/-1.7)	0.10%
2005	1,235	7.7 (+/-.423)	0.62%	90 (+/-44)	.01%	54.7 (+/-13.7)	1.6%	3.2 (+/-1.4)	0.10%
2006	1,184	7.6 (+/-.313)	0.64%	190 (+/-47)	.02%	56.1 (+/-14.8)	1.6%	3.4 (+/-1.7)	0.10%
2007	1,159	6.2 (+/-.301)	0.53%	420 (+/-76)	.04%	53.6 (+/-13.5)	1.6%	4.8 (+/-2.3)	0.10%
2008	1,078	6.6 (+/-.325)	0.61%	130 (+/-42)	.01%	40.1 (+/-12.2)	1.3%	Not Reportable	
2009	965	4.8 (+/-.291)	0.50%	180 (+/-52)	.02%	29.4 (+/-7.5)	1.1%	2.8 (+/-1.5)	0.10%
2010	933	4.2 (+/-.245)	0.45%	280 (+/-59)	.03%	27.3 (+/-6.9)	1.0%	2.7 (+/-1.5)	0.10%
2011	918	3.3 (+/-.232)	0.36%	200 (+/-53)	.02%	28.0 (+/-7.7)	1.0%	Not Reportable	
2012	919	4.1 (+/-.250)	0.45%	110 (+/-38)	.01%	27.2 (+/-6.3)	1.0%	3.2 (+/-1.5)	0.10%
2013	917	4.1 (+/-.259)	0.45%	120 (+/-42)	.01%	30.4 (+/-8.2)	1.10%	Not Reportable	
2014	916	4.3 (+/-.268)	0.47%	140 (+/-91)[b]	.02%	25.2 (+/-5.4)	0.90%	Not Reportable	
2015	902	5.2 (+/-.294)	0.57%	140 (+/-45)	.02%	22.9 (+/-4.4)	0.90%	Not Reportable	
2016	892	5.1 (+/-.288)	0.57%	270 (+/-64)	.03%	26.3 (+/-5.8)	0.80%	3.2 (+/-1.9)b	0.10%

Source: GAO analysis of Survey of Occupational Injuries and Illnesses (SOII) and National Electronic Injury Surveillance System—Occupational Supplement (NEISS-Work) data. | GAO-19-26.

Notes: BLS published some estimates for work-related injuries and illnesses to 14-year-olds in certain years. More specifically, BLS from 2003 to 2015 estimated that there were 40 work-related injuries and illnesses to 14-year-olds in private industry in

2003; 20 in 2006; 120 in 2007; 60 in 2010; 120 in 2011; 70 in 2012; 20 in 2013; 70 in 2014; and it estimated that there were 30 work-related injuries and illnesses to 14-year-olds in local government in 2009. These estimates have relative standard errors of 30 percent or less, except for the 2003, 2009 and 2013 estimates, which have relative standard errors higher than 30 but less than 50 percent and should be interpreted with caution; and a 2005 estimate which we are not reporting because it has a relative standard error greater than 50 percent. Further, estimates for 2008 to 2013 are for workers at private and public entities, while estimates from 2003 to 2008 are for private entities only. Total days away from work in this table are for private industry only. BLS estimated that in its data about 5 percent of injuries and illnesses in private industry and federal, local, and state government were illnesses. NIOSH technical information notes that NEISS-Work data from 2003 to 2014 include illnesses such as those that began at work (heart attacks or stroke), chronic conditions, and exacerbated long-term injuries; it estimates 5 to 10 percent of all cases were such illnesses. The mean estimate for NEISS-Work may be higher than that listed because some observations were omitted to protect confidentiality related to the underlying individual data or other reasons. NEISS-Work data from 2015 onward do not capture most illnesses. Data in parentheses represent the margin of error at the 95 percent confidence level.

[a]Table shows only private sector data for BLS's SOII work-related injuries to children aged 15 and under. Number represents BLS's estimate for children 15 or under who incurred a work-related injury resulting in at least one day of missed work. Estimates ranged from 90 to 420 such children.

[b]This estimate has a relative standard error above 30 percent and less than 50 percent and should be interpreted with caution.

Appendix X: Estimated Work-Related Injuries and Illnesses to Children Aged 17 and Under, by Industry, 2003 and 2016

Table 37. Estimated Number of Work-Related Injuries and Illnesses to Children Aged 17 and Under, 2003 and 2016

		2003			2016		
Industry	Sub-industry	Weighted estimate (margin of error)	Number of working children aged 15 to 17 in industry	Median days away from work	Weighted estimate (margin of error)	Number of working children aged 15 to 17 in industry (margin of error)	Median days away from work
Construction		500 (+/-133)	99,938	44	80 (+/-58)[a]	64,939 (+/-24,587)	4
Educational and health services		560 (+/-101)	292,337	4	290 (+/-54)	259,092 (+/-41,430)	4
	Educational services[c]		136,596		60 (+/-25)	131,098 (+/-30,663)	6
	Health care and social assistance	550 (+/-102)	155,741	4	230 (+/-49)	127,994 (+/-29,966)	4
Financial Activities		130 (+/-52)	59,770	2		35,304 (+/-16,933)	
	Finance and insurance	20 (+/-19)[a]	31,877	25		24,231 (+/-15,462)[a]	
	Real estate and rental and leasing[c]	120 (+/-62)	27,893	2		11,072 (+/-7,632)[a]	
Information		100 (+/-40)	81,240	2	30 (+/-23)[a]	28,425 (+/-15,947)	2
Leisure and hospitality		3,940 (+/-448)	1,352,958	3	2,900 (+/-284)	1,150,060 (+/-95,973)	3
	Accommodation and food services	3,560 (+/-502)	1,031,256	3	2,500 (+/-284)	879,821 (+/-85,907)	3
	Arts entertainment and recreation	380 (+/-73)	321,702	3	400 (+/-82)	270,239 (+/-39,682)	5

Table 37. (Continued)

		2003			2016		
Industry	Sub-industry	Weighted estimate (margin of error)	Number of working children aged 15 to 17 in industry	Median days away from work	Weighted estimate (margin of error)	Number of working children aged 15 to 17 in industry (margin of error)	Median days away from work
Manufacturing		280 (+/-61)	52,923	5	80 (+/-28)	48,977 (+/-19,248)	3
Natural resources and mining		100 (+/-31)	138,563	2	110 (+/-35)	109,900 (+/-28,488)	38
	Agriculture forestry fishing and hunting	100 (+/-51)	138,080	2	50 (+/-30)[a]	109,900 (+/-28,488)	7
Other services except public administration		290 (+/-85)	234,527	2	80 (+/-63)[a]	130,511 (+/-31,631)	10
Professional and business services	Administrative and waste services	190 (+/-92)	135,612	23	30 (+/-28)[a]	72,773 (+/-23,535)	3
	Professional and technical services[c]		53,307		110 (+/-65)[a]	38,727 (+/-20,008)	2
Trade transportation and utilities		2,830 (+/-283)	718,283	6	1,040 (+/-122)	468,038 (+/-65,025)	3
	Retail trade	2,250 (+/-273)	665,917	5	960 (+/-124)	431,141 (+/-63,186)	3
	Transportation and warehousing	440 (+/-97)	18,537	8	60 (+/-25)	27,168 (+/-15,908)[a]	6
	Wholesale trade	130 (+/-63)	33,829	2	Not reportable[b]	9,728 (+/-7,366)[a]	Not reportable[b]
Total		8,970 (+/-457)	3,234,645	4	4,760 (+/-271)	2,433,501	3

Source: GAO analysis of Survey of Occupational Injuries and Illnesses and Current Population Survey March 2017 ASEC data. | GAO-19-26.

Notes: Annual Social and Economic Supplement (ASEC) data report information for the previous calendar year. Subcategories will not always add to totals because some data do not meet publication criteria. Industries combine into two domains: goods producing and service producing. Goods producing—with a weighted estimate of 270 (+/-62) and median days away from work of 7 in 2016—includes construction, manufacturing, and natural resources and mining. Service providing— with a weighted estimate of 4,490 (+/- 273) and median days away from work of 3 in 2016—includes educational and health services, information, leisure and hospitality, other services except public administration, professional and business services, and trade transportation and utilities.

[a]Relative standard error greater than 30 and less than 50, and should be interpreted with caution.

[b]Estimate is not reportable as relative standard error is 50 or higher.

[c]Educational services, as well as professional and technical services subcategories do not have data for 2003. Real estate and rental and leasing subcategory does not have estimate for 2016.

Appendix XI: Comments from the Department of Labor's Occupational Safety and Health Administration

U.S. Department of Labor

Occupational Safety and Health Administration
Washington, D.C. 20210

OCT 19 2018

Ms. Cindy Brown Barnes, Director
Education, Workforce and Income Security Issues
U.S. Government Accountability Office
441 G Street, NW
Washington, DC 20548

Dear Ms. Brown Barnes:

Thank you for the opportunity to comment on the Government Accountability Office's (GAO) draft report, *Working Children: Federal Injury Data and Compliance Strategies Could be Strengthened.* The following comments are submitted on behalf of the Department of Labor's Occupational Safety and Health Administration (OSHA) and relate only to those sections of the report that address OSHA directly.

The report notes that field staff from both the Wage and Hour Division (WHD) and OSHA stated there is a regular exchange of information, and officials from every WHD region acknowledge receipt of "referrals or information" from OSHA. While we concede that the 1990 Memorandum of Understanding between the two agencies is dated, the report recognized that this has no impact on the cooperation between OSHA and WHD and the effective sharing of information. Further, as OSHA and WHD are agencies within the same department, there is no barrier to interagency communication and cooperation.

The report recommends OSHA should update the MOU and establish procedures for monitoring the actions taken on referrals. To be clear, there was no indication in the report that OSHA failed to take appropriate action following a referral from WHD, and there is no indication from WHD that there is dissatisfaction on their part with the current process. However, OSHA will coordinate with WHD on updating the MOU, including discussing whether any referral issues exist and how to work together to share referral data, as appropriate.

OSHA welcomes this process review, and appreciates the opportunity to respond to GAO's draft report.

Sincerely,

Loren Sweatt
Deputy Assistant Secretary

APPENDIX XII: COMMENTS FROM THE DEPARTMENT OF LABOR'S WAGE AND HOUR DIVISION

U.S. Department of Labor Wage and Hour Division
Washington, D.C. 20210

October 19, 2018

Ms. Cindy Brown Barnes
Director
Education, Workforce and
Income Security
U.S. Government Accountability Office
Washington, D.C. 20548

Dear Ms. Brown Barnes,

The Department of Labor's Wage and Hour Division (WHD) appreciates the opportunity to respond to the Government Accountability Office (GAO) Draft Report (Report) entitled "*Working Children: Federal Injury Data and Compliance Strategies Could be Strengthened*" (GAO-19-26).

GAO's objectives in conducting this study, as outlined to then Acting Secretary of Labor Edward Hugler on April 17, 2017, were to examine: (1) the trends, since 2002, in the number of children working in the United States in agricultural and non-agricultural occupations, (2) the trends, since 2002, in the characteristics of these children, including their safety, health, and educational attainment, particularly for those employed in work deemed hazardous, and the extent to which these children may be employed in a manner not consistent with FLSA provisions, (3) what, if any, gaps exist in data on children working in U.S. agricultural and nonagricultural occupations, and (4) the federal role in enforcing Fair Labor Standards Act restrictions on child labor and reducing the risks.

The report contains four recommendations for the Department, two specific to WHD and a joint recommendation for both WHD and OSHA. WHD plans to take the following actions to address GAO's recommendations.

Recommendation 2

> *The Administrator of the Wage and Hour Division should establish specific metrics and associated targets for child-labor related outreach in agriculture.*

WHD Response:
WHD agrees that it can develop a more specific internal performance measure and associated target for child labor outreach in agriculture. In 2018, WHD introduced performance measures to track the number of outreach events to employers and the number of hours associated with those events. WHD also introduced an internal program-specific measure to track the number of events involving child labor. WHD already conducts the vast majority of child labor investigations and outreach in the industries GAO identifies because they are WHD priority industries. A new, combined metric would provide an additional incentive for WHD field offices to conduct outreach events in the agriculture industry that address child labor issues.

Recommendation 3

> *The Administrator of the Wage and Hour Division should develop performance metrics specific to its child labor enforcement approach, such as whether their investigations are conducted at establishments where children are likely to be working.*

WHD Response:
Data sources to identify establishments where children are likely to be working are limited. WHD agrees it can develop either an internal performance metric or new planning guidance and reporting requirements for the FY 2020 planning cycle to ensure that adequate resources are dedicated to child labor enforcement and that child labor enforcement efforts focus on industries, establishments, and time periods in which children are likely to be working or injured. In FY 2019, WHD's Division of Strategic Planning and Performance and FLSA Branch will work with Planning and Review Officers (PROs) and Community Outreach Resource and Planning Specialists (CORPS) in the field to identify ongoing initiatives that could be expanded or refined to include a more targeted child labor focus.

Recommendation 4

> *The Administrator of the Wage and Hour Division and the Assistant Secretary of the Occupational Safety and Health Administration should update and routinely monitor the 1990 WHD and OSHA memorandum of understanding and establish documented procedures for monitoring the exchange of and actions taken on referrals.*

WHD/OSHA Response:

WHD agrees to work with OSHA to review and update the existing memorandum of understanding (MOU). GAO's report also recommends that WHD and OSHA establish documented procedures for monitoring the exchange of and actions taken on referrals, but does not identify any instances in which either OSHA or WHD failed to take appropriate action on a referral. WHD agrees to explore the efficacy of the existing referral process with OSHA, identify any weaknesses, and propose actions to improve the efficacy of the referral process, as appropriate.

Again, thank you for the opportunity to comment on the report. If you have any questions, please do not hesitate to contact us.

Sincerely,

Bryan Jarrett
Acting Administrator

INDEX

#

2018 Census Test, vii, 49, 50, 51, 52, 54, 55, 61, 66, 67, 68, 69, 71
9/11, 88, 171

A

access, 29, 42, 57, 58, 60, 61, 68, 84, 85, 95, 153, 186, 189, 190, 196, 198, 199, 200, 201, 212, 213, 225, 226, 260, 282, 304, 335, 342
accountability, viii, 128, 137, 138, 140, 144, 146, 152, 154, 155, 156, 157, 159, 160, 162, 168, 171, 188, 227
accountability report, viii, 137, 138, 144, 157, 168, 171
accounting, 84, 107, 130, 267, 273, 321, 368, 408
administrative support, 368
advance contracts, v, vii, 1, 2, 3, 4, 5, 6, 8, 9, 12, 14, 15, 16, 17, 18, 19, 21, 23, 24, 25, 26, 27, 28, 29, 30, 31, 32, 33, 34, 36, 37, 38, 39, 40, 45
age, 43, 129, 241, 268, 314, 354, 356, 357, 358, 359, 360, 361, 363, 368, 369, 376, 382, 391, 395, 399, 402, 406, 409, 411
agencies, viii, ix, xi, 5, 7, 9, 10, 11, 12, 14, 22, 27, 39, 56, 59, 64, 79, 82, 85, 86, 88, 91, 92, 93, 94, 95, 97, 105, 108, 111, 112, 114, 117, 125, 138, 139, 140, 141, 142, 143, 144, 145, 146, 147, 148, 149, 150, 151, 152, 153, 154, 155, 156, 157, 158, 159, 160, 161, 162, 163, 164, 168, 171, 172, 178, 179, 180, 181, 182, 183, 184, 185, 186, 187, 188, 189, 190, 191, 192, 193, 194, 195, 196, 197, 198, 199, 200, 201, 202, 203, 205, 206, 207, 208, 209, 210, 211, 212, 213, 214, 215, 216, 217, 218, 219, 220, 221, 222, 223, 224, 227, 228, 229, 238, 239, 249, 292, 332, 336, 340, 341, 344, 352, 354, 376, 378, 386, 387, 389
agriculture, x, 12, 86, 138, 139, 150, 152, 153, 164, 169, 171, 172, 182, 199, 202, 219, 221, 223, 228, 351, 352, 353, 354, 355, 356, 358, 359, 360, 361, 362, 363, 364, 369, 370, 371, 372, 373, 376, 377, 383, 385, 387, 388, 389, 390, 391, 392, 394, 395, 396, 400, 409, 414, 419
airports, 41, 82, 99, 104, 108, 130
armed forces, 11, 259
assessment, 60, 66, 76, 80, 93, 95, 96, 101, 102, 105, 106, 107, 108, 109, 110, 119, 121, 124, 125, 126, 128, 130, 131, 168, 169, 170, 186, 187, 194, 198, 202, 203, 205, 210, 211, 218, 219, 222, 223, 266, 273, 275, 278, 281, 284, 326, 365, 394, 396, 397, 398, 399, 401
assets, 43, 78, 83, 84, 86, 91, 92, 93, 96, 102, 108, 109, 110, 113, 125, 130, 181, 185, 186, 187, 200, 204, 212, 213, 218, 219, 220, 224, 225, 226, 227, 271, 284, 285, 291, 296, 300, 302, 305, 308, 309, 310, 311, 312, 313, 315, 316, 317, 318, 319, 320, 321, 322, 324, 327, 328
audit, 6, 39, 52, 72, 81, 142, 143, 145, 146, 162, 179, 183, 194, 196, 222, 223, 240, 253, 258, 277, 333, 355, 356, 401, 408
awareness, x, 4, 90, 92, 93, 94, 111, 113, 179, 193, 198, 205, 213, 216, 225, 227, 282, 329, 330, 331, 336, 341, 342, 343, 344, 345, 383

B

balanced budget, 292
barriers, 63, 212, 335
benefits, 209, 211, 212, 218, 220, 261, 273, 278, 285, 291, 292, 294, 297, 298, 299, 300, 304, 312, 313, 315, 316, 319, 320, 387, 391
bilateral, 240, 241

budget surplus, 321
Bureau of Labor Statistics, 290, 293, 294, 296, 297, 298, 299, 301, 302, 306, 307, 308, 309, 351, 354, 369, 372, 375, 387, 388, 389, 390, 396, 397, 416, 417
business partners, 204, 206
businesses, 16, 17, 77, 299, 310, 317, 318, 319, 361, 363, 393

C

cable television, 19, 38
California wildfires, vii, 2, 3, 4, 5, 6, 12, 13, 18, 27, 28, 29, 36, 37, 45
capacity building, 243
capital consumption, 313, 319, 320
capital expenditure, 312
capital goods, 312
capital investment, x, 255, 257, 276, 313
Census, v, vii, 49, 50, 51, 52, 53, 54, 55, 56, 57, 59, 60, 61, 63, 64, 65, 66, 67, 68, 69, 70, 71, 290, 293, 294, 296, 297, 298, 299, 301, 302, 306, 307, 308, 309, 351, 354, 355, 363, 364, 367, 369, 370, 371, 372, 373, 377, 385, 389, 390, 391, 393, 394, 396, 397, 407, 415, 416
challenges, vii, viii, ix, x, 2, 4, 5, 16, 17, 18, 22, 24, 27, 28, 32, 36, 37, 38, 39, 50, 51, 59, 65, 69, 78, 79, 91, 128, 140, 152, 154, 156, 159, 178, 182, 206, 212, 218, 241, 255, 256, 257, 258, 259, 260, 261, 264, 265, 267, 268, 269, 270, 271, 272, 274, 277, 286, 292, 295
child labor, x, xi, 352, 353, 354, 355, 356, 357, 358, 360, 361, 362, 365, 366, 368, 379, 380, 381, 382, 383, 384, 385, 387, 388, 392, 395, 400, 401, 402, 403, 404, 405, 406, 407, 408, 409, 411, 413, 416
childcare, 393
childhood, 374
children, x, 41, 43, 352, 353, 354, 355, 356, 357, 358, 359, 360, 361, 362, 363, 364, 365, 366, 367, 368, 369, 370, 371, 372, 373, 374, 375, 376, 377, 378, 379, 380, 381, 382, 383, 385, 386, 387, 388, 389, 390, 391, 392, 393, 395, 396, 397, 398, 399, 406, 407, 408, 409, 411, 412, 413, 414, 415, 416, 418, 419
citizens, 77, 204, 291, 363, 412
citizenship, 51
clarity, 77, 100, 112, 114, 120, 122, 154
climate, 107, 129, 238, 242, 246
climate change, 107, 129, 238, 242, 246
commerce, 83, 99, 361, 382
commercial, 9, 10, 44, 85, 117, 180, 211, 212, 218, 220, 269, 284, 294, 312
communication, 8, 30, 41, 42, 85, 94, 111, 190, 224, 283, 285, 335
compensation, 294, 296, 299, 310, 312, 319, 322, 364, 398
competition, 5, 8, 10, 15, 16, 18, 25, 37, 240, 269
competitive advantage, 243
compliance, viii, xi, 88, 97, 110, 111, 113, 114, 138, 139, 140, 142, 143, 144, 145, 146, 147, 148, 151, 152, 153, 154, 155, 156, 157, 158, 159, 161, 162, 163, 164, 168, 171, 172, 185, 186, 195, 223, 303, 352, 353, 354, 355, 361, 362, 365, 379, 382, 383, 384, 385, 386, 387, 389, 400, 401
computer, 81, 84, 85, 93, 180, 181, 182, 184, 190, 196, 204, 208
computer systems, 84, 85, 181
configuration, 84, 191, 196, 197, 198, 216, 226, 277
conflict, 238, 239, 240, 241, 242, 243, 252, 258, 272
Congress, vii, viii, ix, 1, 8, 11, 15, 26, 32, 37, 77, 83, 109, 115, 123, 138, 139, 140, 142, 143, 144, 145, 146, 151, 152, 153, 154, 155, 156, 159, 160, 161, 162, 178, 180, 184, 189, 191, 198, 201, 202, 203, 205, 207, 208, 209, 210, 211, 218, 219, 257, 264, 266, 276, 277, 278, 284, 289, 291
congressional budget, 110, 112, 114, 115
construction, 7, 8, 25, 44, 84, 129, 273, 277, 278, 367, 368, 373, 381, 419
consumption, 312, 314, 318, 319, 320, 321, 322, 324
coordination, 2, 5, 7, 27, 29, 30, 31, 39, 88, 92, 94, 115, 153, 179, 201, 203, 226, 273, 275, 282, 283, 386
corruption, 239, 242, 252
cost, vii, x, 8, 10, 14, 15, 17, 20, 22, 25, 26, 28, 32, 49, 51, 84, 112, 180, 188, 189, 264, 266, 267, 277, 278, 282, 283, 286, 287, 297, 298, 304, 305, 306, 307, 312, 314, 315, 316, 318, 320, 327, 328, 330, 336, 337, 341, 376, 379, 388
criminal activity, 86, 111, 127
critical infrastructure, vii, 74, 77, 78, 79, 84, 85, 86, 87, 88, 90, 91, 92, 93, 94, 96, 105, 106, 108, 109, 111, 120, 121, 125, 127, 128, 129, 130, 182, 185, 187, 188, 205, 224, 225, 242, 243
crop, 359, 364, 369, 373, 390, 391, 394, 395, 397, 409, 410, 411, 412, 413, 414
crop production, 394
cybersecurity, viii, ix, 73, 74, 75, 76, 77, 78, 79, 84, 85, 88, 90, 91, 92, 93, 94, 95, 96, 97, 98, 99, 103, 104, 105, 106, 107, 111, 115, 118, 119, 121, 122, 123, 124, 125, 126, 127, 128, 130, 177, 178, 179, 180, 181, 182, 183, 184, 185, 186, 187, 188, 189, 190, 191,192, 194, 198, 199, 200, 201, 203, 206, 207, 208, 210, 212, 213, 217, 219, 220, 221, 222, 223, 224, 225, 226, 227, 228, 229, 230
cyberspace, 182

D

data collection, 5, 25, 38, 39, 42, 50, 54, 55, 56, 67, 69, 71, 81, 162, 279, 354, 365
data set, 354, 355, 356, 366, 369, 374, 375, 378, 384, 385, 389, 390, 393, 396, 399
database, 80, 110, 111, 112, 113, 114, 115, 116, 117, 216, 365, 379, 384
decennial census, vii, 49, 51, 59
decision makers, 86, 188, 277, 284, 286
decision-making process, 109
defense mechanisms, 191
deficiencies, 128, 179, 194, 196, 197, 217, 222, 277, 278, 281, 401
deficits, x, 289, 295, 310
defined benefit pension, 294, 313, 315, 317, 320
demographic change, ix, 235, 238, 246
demographic characteristics, 52, 66, 354, 367, 374, 385, 390, 391, 396, 397
demographic data, 376, 391
Department of Agriculture, 228, 396
Department of Commerce, 50, 68, 69, 70, 72, 169, 219, 220, 228, 232, 291
Department of Defense (DOD), ix, 1, 3, 4, 10, 11, 12, 33, 37, 80, 109, 112, 137, 150, 152, 154, 155, 156, 157, 158, 165, 168, 169, 171, 172, 183, 188, 212, 221, 235, 236, 237, 238, 239, 240, 241, 243, 244, 245, 246, 247, 248, 249, 250, 251, 252, 253, 256, 257, 258, 259, 261, 264, 267, 269, 270, 271, 272, 273, 274, 275, 277, 278, 279, 280, 281, 282, 283, 284, 285, 286, 287
Department of Education, 137, 155, 157, 165, 169, 172, 228
Department of Energy, 73, 79, 84, 90, 93, 124, 228
Department of Health and Human Services, 137, 139, 149, 150, 155, 157, 165, 168, 169, 228, 353, 354, 364, 375, 389, 390, 395, 396, 397, 410, 411
Department of Homeland Security (DHS), vii, ix, 1, 3, 4, 5, 7, 8, 9, 10, 12, 15, 22, 23, 24, 25, 29, 33, 37, 39, 73, 74, 75, 80, 85, 86, 87, 88, 90, 91, 92, 97, 103, 105, 106, 107, 108, 109, 110, 111, 112, 114, 117, 118, 120, 121, 122, 124, 125, 127, 128, 129, 130, 131, 137, 148, 150, 152, 154, 155, 156, 160, 166, 169, 172, 177, 178, 179, 180, 182, 183, 184, 185, 186, 187, 188, 189, 190, 191, 194, 198, 201, 202, 203, 204, 205, 206, 207, 208, 209, 210, 211, 212, 213, 214, 216, 217, 218, 219, 220, 221, 222, 223, 228, 235, 236, 237, 238, 239, 243, 244, 245, 246, 247, 248, 249, 250, 251, 252
Department of Justice, 83, 93, 184, 228
Department of Labor, 137, 150, 152, 167, 170, 172, 228, 352, 354, 357, 358, 359, 360, 369, 389, 390, 395, 397, 420, 421
Department of State, ix, 228, 235, 236, 238, 249, 251
Department of the Interior, 228
Department of the Treasury, 138, 139, 149, 150, 167, 170, 172, 228
Department of Transportation, 73, 79, 82, 92, 124, 167, 170, 228
Departments of Agriculture, 182, 199, 202, 219, 221, 223
depreciation, 293, 306, 307, 308, 311, 312, 313, 319, 320
detection, viii, ix, 178, 180, 182, 183, 185, 186, 187, 190, 191, 192, 201, 202, 203, 204, 205, 206, 209, 210, 211, 212, 213, 214, 216, 218, 219, 220, 221, 222, 223, 227
disaster, v, vii, 1, 2, 3, 4, 5, 7, 8, 9, 10, 12, 14, 15, 16, 17, 19, 23, 25, 26, 27, 28, 29, 30, 31, 32, 33, 36, 37, 38, 39, 40, 41, 42, 44, 45, 143, 164, 166, 167, 169, 170, 171, 226, 243, 312
disaster area, 41
disaster assistance, 7, 41
disaster relief, 7, 10, 12
distribution, 16, 43, 44, 81, 85, 88, 94, 111, 122, 285, 286, 346, 389, 412

E

economic consequences, 131
economic growth, 241, 242, 291, 302, 305, 326
economic indicator, 326
economic well-being, 84
education, 104, 225, 294, 301, 312, 326, 357, 387
educational programs, 362
emergency, 3, 4, 7, 8, 10, 16, 19, 31, 37, 42, 44, 45, 93, 99, 364, 374, 375, 376, 398
Emergency Assistance, 7
Emergency Relief Program, 170
emergency response, 16, 93, 99
employee compensation, 294, 295, 298, 299, 300, 319, 320
employee labor groups, xi, 352, 355
employees, 19, 38, 50, 52, 60, 62, 84, 94, 103, 111, 113, 117, 167, 185, 196, 291, 292, 294, 297, 298, 299, 300, 309, 310, 312, 313, 315, 316, 319, 320, 322, 358, 359, 360, 361, 393
employer, xi, 352, 355, 360, 362, 371, 374, 376, 378, 379, 382, 385, 388, 391, 398, 400
employment, 62, 181, 314, 315, 316, 320, 354, 356, 357, 359, 360, 364, 385, 390, 391, 392
employment status, 62, 390
energy, vii, 7, 74, 77, 82, 84, 85, 89, 90, 108, 111, 129, 130, 185
energy sector, vii, 74, 77, 84, 85, 90

enforcement, 88, 304, 353, 354, 355, 361, 362, 379, 382, 383, 384, 385, 386, 387, 388, 400, 401
enumerators, vii, 49, 50, 51, 52, 53, 54, 55, 56, 57, 58, 59, 60, 61, 62, 63, 64, 65, 66, 67, 68, 69, 70, 71, 72
environment, viii, ix, 52, 59, 65, 74, 75, 77, 78, 79, 85, 97, 99, 104, 106, 118, 126, 127, 155, 198, 225, 226, 241, 242, 255, 257, 258, 261, 333, 340, 341
environmental conditions, 81, 204
environmental issues, 238
equipment, 8, 42, 44, 45, 62, 84, 184, 263, 264, 276, 277, 294, 300, 312, 359, 380, 408, 416
equity, 326
ethnicity, 354, 363, 367, 374, 390, 392, 393, 395, 397, 398, 406, 407, 415
evidence, 6, 39, 52, 64, 72, 81, 143, 162, 183, 223, 240, 253, 258, 293, 300, 333, 346, 356, 362, 384, 401
execution, 111, 192, 215, 262
executive branch, viii, 90, 138, 143, 186, 187, 188, 201, 203, 212, 238, 249
Executive Order, ix, 79, 85, 87, 88, 96, 178, 179, 182, 185, 187, 188, 189, 201, 212, 221, 228, 285
exercises, 111, 113, 116, 214, 275
expenditures, x, 290, 291, 292, 293, 294, 295, 297, 298, 300, 302, 304, 305, 306, 307, 308, 309, 310, 311, 312, 313, 314, 318, 319, 320, 321, 322, 324, 325, 326, 327, 328
expertise, 50, 76, 94, 103, 104, 109
exploitation, 84, 86, 107, 129, 379
exposure, 57, 86, 127, 354, 398, 415, 416
extraction, 368, 372, 373, 381, 394, 414

F

Fair Labor Standards Act, xi, 351, 352, 353, 354, 356, 357, 358, 360, 361, 366, 368, 380, 389
families, 335, 336, 342, 367, 390, 394, 407, 410
family income, 363, 393, 395, 410, 411
family members, 371, 373
farms, 363, 364, 369, 376, 377, 378, 383, 387, 388, 390, 391, 393, 395, 396, 397, 399, 409, 411, 414
fatalities, x, 258, 352, 353, 354, 355, 364, 370, 371, 372, 373, 374, 376, 377, 378, 383, 387, 396, 397, 414, 415, 416
federal agency, 77, 180, 182, 190, 221, 222, 229, 354, 361, 378
federal assistance, 7, 19, 38
federal authorities, 83
Federal Cybersecurity Enhancement Act, ix, 178, 182, 183, 185, 186, 203, 207, 209, 210, 211, 212, 219, 220, 221, 222
Federal Emergency Management Agency, 1, 2, 3, 6, 8, 13, 14, 15, 26, 28, 34, 36, 38, 40, 107, 127, 166, 170, 172, 251
federal government, vii, viii, 2, 4, 7, 10, 32, 36, 87, 88, 91, 94, 141, 150, 178, 179, 181, 182, 183, 184, 188, 189, 191, 193, 200, 204, 212, 218, 219, 221, 222, 229, 249, 257, 291, 304, 305, 310, 314, 317, 318, 319, 320, 321, 322, 323, 324, 372, 390, 397
federal information security, viii, 78, 177, 178, 179, 180, 181, 182, 184, 185, 191, 193, 194, 195, 196, 198, 201, 202, 205, 207, 208, 210, 221, 228, 229
Federal Information Security Modernization Act, ix, 177, 178, 179, 180, 181, 185, 191, 193, 194, 195, 196, 198, 201, 202, 205, 207, 208, 210, 221, 228, 229
federal law, xi, 7, 185, 228, 352, 354, 355, 356, 361, 400, 401
Federal Procurement Data System-Next Generation, vii, 1, 2, 3, 4, 13, 14, 36
Federal Register, 378
Federal Reserve, 290, 292, 293, 294, 296, 297, 298, 299, 301, 302, 306, 307, 308, 309
field supervisors, vii, 49, 50, 53, 56, 57, 58, 61, 64, 67, 69, 71
fighter pilot workforce, x, 255, 257, 270, 272, 274
financial, viii, x, 10, 18, 38, 137, 138, 142, 144, 156, 157, 160, 168, 171, 177, 179, 181, 183, 193, 194, 196, 197, 217, 222, 229, 238, 241, 296, 310, 313, 315, 317, 318, 321, 322, 324, 326, 352, 353, 368, 381, 394
financial report, viii, 137, 138, 144, 157, 168, 171, 179, 193, 194, 196, 197, 217, 228, 229
financial resources, 238
financial system, 222
fire fighting, 358
first responders, 111
fiscal pressures, x, 289, 290, 291, 292, 304
fiscal sustainability, x, 289, 291
fiscal year, viii, ix, x, 5, 20, 21, 25, 45, 51, 76, 80, 102, 103, 110, 111, 112, 113, 114, 115, 116, 117, 138, 139, 140, 141, 142, 143, 144, 145, 146, 147, 148, 149, 150, 151, 152, 153, 154, 155, 156, 157, 158, 159, 160, 161, 162, 163, 164, 168, 171, 172, 178, 179, 183, 184, 189, 191, 193, 194, 195, 196, 197, 198, 199, 200, 201, 207, 208, 214, 219, 220, 221, 222, 223, 229, 256, 261, 262, 265, 266, 267, 268, 269, 270, 276, 283, 303, 305, 330, 332, 333, 334, 336, 338, 339, 340, 341, 342, 345, 354, 355, 362, 378, 379, 381, 383, 384, 385, 389, 395, 396, 400, 401, 409, 410, 411, 412
foreign affairs, 243
foreign language, 30

funding, viii, 138, 140, 142, 143, 145, 146, 156, 157, 158, 159, 161, 162, 264, 266, 269, 271, 282, 299, 304
funds, 25, 26, 144, 294, 295, 305, 311, 312, 313, 315, 317, 320, 339, 340

G

GDP per capita, 298, 307, 320
global economy, 241
globalization, 241
goods and services, vii, 1, 2, 3, 8, 9, 12, 14, 15, 16, 17, 23, 27, 28, 29, 32, 37, 38, 303, 305, 310, 312, 319, 325, 326
government spending, 314
governments, 4, 27, 29, 30, 31, 238, 241, 242, 245, 291, 292, 295, 297, 298, 299, 300, 302, 305, 307, 309, 313, 315, 316, 319, 321, 326
grant programs, 165
gross domestic product, 289, 291, 295, 314, 318, 320, 321, 325, 327, 328
gross investment, 312, 320, 321, 322, 323, 324
growth, 204, 246, 256, 266, 279, 291, 292, 297, 298, 300, 301, 304, 305, 306, 307, 314, 315, 316, 318, 320, 325, 327, 328
growth rate, 314, 315, 316, 327, 328
guidance, viii, 2, 4, 11, 12, 14, 15, 16, 17, 18, 21, 22, 23, 29, 31, 32, 33, 34, 37, 38, 50, 57, 58, 59, 64, 67, 68, 69, 70, 74, 78, 79, 80, 94, 95, 97, 98, 100, 101, 118, 123, 127, 138, 139, 140, 141, 144, 145, 146, 152, 153, 154, 156, 158, 159, 160, 161, 162, 178, 180, 186, 187, 188, 192, 203, 205, 208, 209, 213, 215, 218, 222, 223, 265, 274, 276, 277, 278, 279, 355, 357, 358, 360, 362, 363, 365, 372, 380, 383, 386, 388, 394, 399, 400, 401
guidelines, viii, 74, 75, 78, 79, 88, 95, 96, 97, 98, 100, 107, 110, 111, 113, 114, 118, 126, 129, 185, 186, 192, 208, 276, 395, 410, 411

H

hazardous materials, 90
hazardous waste, 45
health, 99, 100, 242, 285, 291, 292, 294, 297, 298, 299, 302, 304, 305, 307, 313, 314, 316, 319, 320, 326, 327, 328, 331, 335, 336, 340, 341, 356, 357, 358, 361, 362, 364, 378, 391, 394, 408, 415, 418, 419
health care, 291, 292, 297, 298, 302, 304, 305, 307, 313, 316, 319, 320, 326, 327, 331, 335
health effects, 99
health expenditure, 298, 299, 307, 308, 314, 320, 327, 328
health insurance, 299, 391
health services, 394, 415, 418, 419
historical data, 106, 107, 127, 302, 313, 316
history, 5, 23, 24, 39, 335, 362
homeland security, 87, 92, 94
hospitality, 352, 367, 376, 379, 381, 385, 394, 418, 419
House of Representatives, 35, 36, 70, 71, 123, 141, 181, 249, 329, 331, 353
Housing and Urban Development, 12, 150, 160, 168, 169, 172, 182, 199, 202, 219, 221, 223, 228
human, 104, 190, 226, 238
Hurricane Katrina, vii, 1, 8, 14
hurricanes, vii, 2, 3, 4, 5, 6, 10, 12, 14, 15, 16, 18, 27, 29, 36, 37, 45, 130

I

identification, 62, 79, 80, 100, 353
improper payment, v, viii, 137, 138, 139, 140, 141, 142, 143, 144, 145, 146, 147, 149, 150, 151, 153, 154, 155, 156, 157, 158, 159, 160, 161, 162, 163, 164, 168, 171, 172
improper payment rate, viii, 138, 143, 144, 149
improper payment reduction targets, viii, 138
improvements, 93, 115, 128, 188, 194, 203, 220, 305, 346
income, 291, 296, 301, 303, 304, 310, 311, 314, 317, 318, 319, 322, 323, 324, 325, 326, 363, 367, 390, 391, 392, 393, 394, 395, 407, 411, 413
income tax, 291, 296, 301, 303, 310, 317, 318, 319, 323, 324
independent variable, 323, 324, 325
individual taxpayers, 303
inflation, 300, 309, 314, 318, 319, 320
information exchange, 215
information processing, 186
information sharing, 27, 88, 91, 93, 94, 183, 212, 224, 227, 244
information systems, viii, 90, 98, 124, 130, 178, 179, 181, 182, 185, 186, 189, 190, 192, 193, 194, 203, 205, 210, 211, 214, 217, 220, 221, 222, 224, 225, 226, 228
information technology, 8, 64, 85, 90, 93, 192, 198, 212, 223, 226, 229
infrastructure, 27, 51, 78, 82, 84, 85, 86, 87, 88, 90, 92, 93, 99, 106, 107, 109, 121, 127, 128, 129, 130, 131, 188, 189, 191, 192, 216, 242, 243, 264, 291, 296, 300, 301, 326
infrastructure cyber incidents, vii, 74

inspectors, 139, 142, 150, 160, 163, 164, 171, 177, 179, 181, 193, 194, 195, 196, 197, 201, 217, 220, 221, 385
integration, 109, 191, 245, 276, 323, 324, 325
integrity, 129, 181, 182, 191, 216, 225, 401
intellectual property, 240, 294, 312
intelligence, 87, 92, 94, 111, 113, 224, 238, 243, 244, 250
interstate pipelines, vii, 74
intrusion, vii, viii, 74, 77, 85, 92, 178, 180, 182, 183, 185, 186, 187, 190, 191, 192, 193, 201, 202, 203, 204, 205, 206, 209, 210, 211, 212, 213, 214, 215, 216, 218, 219, 220, 221, 222, 223
intrusion detection, viii, 178, 180, 182, 183, 187, 190, 191, 192, 201, 202, 203, 204, 205, 206, 209, 210, 211, 212, 213, 214, 216, 218, 219, 220, 221, 222, 223
investment, x, 255, 257, 264, 276, 296, 300, 301, 310, 311, 312, 313, 317, 318, 319, 320, 321, 322, 323, 324
IPERA, viii, 137, 138, 139, 140, 142, 143, 144, 145, 146, 147, 148, 149, 150, 151, 152, 153, 154, 155, 156, 157, 158, 159, 160, 161, 162, 163, 164, 168, 169, 171, 172
issues, vii, 4, 7, 28, 31, 49, 50, 51, 52, 57, 58, 59, 62, 63, 64, 69, 70, 71, 86, 91, 92, 108, 110, 111, 138, 140, 142, 143, 150, 152, 154, 155, 156, 159, 162, 200, 242, 243, 249, 257, 258, 259, 269, 271, 279, 280, 284, 286, 287, 292, 383, 386

J

jurisdiction, 53, 142
justification, 10, 11, 38, 110, 112, 114, 115

L

labor force, 363
labor market, 379, 384, 385
language barrier, 51, 57, 59, 63, 66
law enforcement, 84, 92, 115, 185, 227
laws and regulations, 354
legislation, 143, 153, 159, 292, 303, 304
livestock, 358, 364, 373, 390, 391, 396, 397, 413, 414
loans, 317, 320, 321, 322, 324
local government, x, 4, 5, 7, 8, 9, 19, 27, 29, 30, 31, 33, 38, 39, 99, 289, 290, 291, 292, 293, 294, 295, 296, 297, 298, 299, 300, 301, 302, 303, 304, 305, 306, 307, 308, 309, 310, 311, 312, 313, 314, 315, 316, 317, 318, 319, 320, 321, 322, 323, 324, 325, 326, 327, 328, 372, 418
logging, 358, 373, 414
logistics, 27, 266, 271, 285, 286
long-term debt, 293, 296, 306, 307, 308, 312, 317, 320, 321, 322, 323, 324
long-term fiscal trends, x, 289

M

magnitude, 7, 28, 77, 87, 186, 260, 261, 270, 295, 303, 363, 374, 394
majority, 7, 10, 214, 331, 343, 345, 352, 362, 363, 367, 392, 412
malware, 85, 179, 192, 198, 199, 200, 207
management, 4, 5, 17, 23, 25, 31, 33, 36, 37, 39, 42, 43, 56, 57, 58, 59, 60, 62, 63, 69, 71, 74, 79, 80, 85, 86, 96, 100, 104, 106, 109, 110, 113, 114, 117, 118, 128, 131, 142, 143, 160, 161, 177, 187, 191, 193, 196, 197, 198, 199, 200, 201, 206, 214, 216, 224, 225, 226, 227, 258, 263, 269, 272, 276, 285, 333, 341, 353, 383, 384, 393
manufactured housing, 14, 19, 30, 38
manufacturing, 82, 85, 98, 185, 268, 269, 356, 357, 358, 414, 419
Marine Corps, v, ix, x, 251, 255, 256, 257, 259, 260, 267, 268, 269, 270, 271, 272, 273, 274, 275, 276, 281, 282, 285, 286, 287
Maritime Transportation Security Act, 97, 124
media, x, 226, 329, 330, 331, 332, 333, 335, 336, 337, 338, 339, 340, 341, 342, 343, 344, 345, 346
Medicaid, 139, 150, 151, 155, 165, 169, 172, 289, 290, 291, 293, 294, 296, 297, 298, 299, 300, 301, 302, 304, 305, 306, 307, 308, 309, 312, 314, 317, 318, 319, 320, 327, 328
medical, 43, 44, 181, 294, 312, 376, 377, 378, 398, 399, 408
medical assistance, 294
Medicare, 149, 166, 172, 289, 290, 293, 294, 296, 297, 298, 299, 301, 302, 306, 307, 308, 309, 314, 317, 318, 319, 327, 328
mental health, 332, 336, 339, 340, 341
mental illness, 335
methodology, 2, 5, 6, 25, 26, 33, 39, 74, 75, 76, 86, 101, 105, 106, 109, 112, 113, 115, 125, 126, 127, 128, 143, 183, 196, 222, 238, 240, 249, 250, 258, 292, 356, 395, 396
military, ix, 82, 85, 108, 130, 235, 237, 238, 240, 242, 243, 244, 245, 246, 253, 258, 259, 260, 271, 279, 280, 281, 282, 284, 285, 286, 331, 335, 338
minimum wage, 354, 356, 357, 360, 379, 382
mission, 7, 21, 26, 90, 92, 94, 104, 106, 112, 114, 127, 187, 196, 200, 224, 229, 257, 267, 269, 270, 271, 277, 282, 284, 285, 344, 378
modernization, 212, 229, 268, 277

modifications, 5, 11, 24, 25, 26, 39, 55, 67, 69
modules, 58, 59

N

National Academy of Sciences, 252
National Aeronautics and Space Administration, 12, 183, 199, 202, 219, 221, 229
National Defense Authorization Act, ix, 4, 10, 11, 37, 235, 238, 259, 263, 277, 284
National Institute for Occupational Safety and Health, 351, 353, 354, 375, 390, 396, 397, 413
National Research Council, 108, 109
National Response Framework, 7, 8
National School Lunch Program, 150, 152, 164, 169, 172
national security, v, ix, 34, 83, 84, 88, 90, 185, 188, 235, 236, 237, 238, 239, 240, 243, 244, 245, 246, 247, 249, 251, 252, 257
National Security Agency, 238, 251
National Security Council, 243
National Strategy, 73, 77, 83, 110, 111, 188, 335, 341, 344
natural disaster, 8, 15, 16, 29, 84, 85, 86, 106, 127, 155, 243
natural gas, vii, 73, 74, 77, 78, 79, 81, 82, 83, 84, 85, 86, 87, 88, 89, 90, 91, 92, 93, 94, 96, 101, 120, 124, 126, 127
natural gas pipeline, 78, 81, 83, 84, 85, 91, 92, 93, 101
natural hazards, 105, 106, 107, 120, 121, 125, 126, 127, 129
natural resources, 419
Navy, v, ix, 157, 165, 169, 172, 251, 255, 256, 257, 258, 260, 261, 262, 263, 264, 265, 266, 267, 268, 269, 270, 271, 272, 273, 274, 275, 276, 277, 278, 279, 280, 281, 282, 285, 286, 287
Navy ship, ix, 255, 257, 258, 266, 273, 277, 285, 286
networks, viii, 42, 77, 78, 83, 85, 88, 90, 93, 178, 180, 181, 182, 185, 186, 187, 189, 190, 191, 192, 200, 203, 204, 206, 207, 210, 216, 220, 221, 226, 228, 336
Nuclear Regulatory Commission, 183, 199, 202, 219, 221, 229

O

Occupational Safety and Health Act, 351, 361
Office of Management and Budget, 137, 140, 141, 142, 144, 145, 146, 150, 157, 159, 160, 161, 162, 177, 179, 180, 182, 184, 191, 192, 198, 201, 202, 205, 207, 208, 210, 220, 221, 229, 378
Office of the Director of National Intelligence (ODNI), ix, 235, 236, 237, 238, 239, 240, 241, 243, 244, 245, 246, 247, 248, 249, 250, 251, 252
Office of the Inspector General, 24
oil, vii, 74, 77, 79, 81, 83, 90, 94, 126, 127, 130, 294, 312, 357, 368, 372, 373, 381, 394, 414
online learning, 59
operating revenues, 295, 296
operating system, 118, 192, 216
operations, vii, viii, 7, 16, 27, 32, 42, 43, 44, 45, 49, 50, 51, 52, 53, 54, 57, 63, 64, 69, 71, 72, 84, 86, 91, 92, 93, 95, 96, 99, 100, 106, 111, 118, 123, 127, 130, 151, 178, 181, 185, 186, 187, 196, 215, 224, 226, 227, 243, 244, 245, 256, 258, 259, 260, 261, 264, 266, 268, 271, 275, 276, 281, 286, 287, 313, 358, 363, 364, 368, 390, 391
opportunities, 94, 111, 125, 242, 260, 270, 275, 276, 277, 353, 361, 379
outreach, x, 4, 27, 29, 32, 33, 91, 92, 115, 329, 330, 331, 332, 333, 335, 336, 337, 338, 339, 340, 341, 342, 343, 344, 345, 346, 352, 353, 362, 379, 382, 383, 384, 385, 387, 388
oversight, vii, 42, 74, 77, 88, 142, 144, 155, 162, 182, 185, 210, 212, 214, 238, 249, 277, 278, 332, 333, 342, 345, 346

P

Pacific, x, 41, 127, 240, 251, 255, 258, 271, 272, 274, 275, 281, 367, 393, 406, 407, 410
Pacific fleet, x, 255, 258
payment risk assessments, viii, 138
payroll, vii, 49, 53, 58, 62, 72, 166
peer review, 75, 76, 101, 108, 109, 119, 120, 121
performance indicator, 53, 198, 200, 201, 229, 335
performance measurement, 112
personally identifiable information, viii, 78, 178, 181, 182
pipeline, v, vii, viii, 73, 74, 75, 76, 77, 78, 79, 80, 81, 82, 83, 84, 85, 86, 87, 88, 89, 90, 91, 92, 93, 94, 95, 96, 97, 98, 99, 100, 101, 102, 103, 104, 105, 106, 107, 108, 109, 110, 111, 112, 113, 114, 115, 116, 117, 118, 119, 120, 121, 122, 123, 124, 125, 126, 127, 128, 129, 130, 131
pipeline security, vii, 73, 74, 75, 76, 77, 78, 79, 80, 84, 88, 89, 90, 91, 93, 95, 96, 97, 98, 99, 100, 101, 102, 103, 104, 105, 106, 107, 108, 109, 110, 111, 112, 113, 114, 115, 116, 117, 118, 119, 120, 121, 122, 124, 125, 126, 127, 128, 129, 130, 131
policy, x, 25, 26, 85, 86, 87, 94, 104, 182, 185, 187, 202, 205, 209, 212, 213, 214, 218, 224, 226, 228, 277, 278, 285, 290, 291, 292, 295, 302, 305, 309, 325, 326

population, x, 7, 42, 51, 53, 54, 55, 56, 65, 66, 82, 238, 241, 304, 314, 315, 316, 318, 319, 320, 327, 328, 329, 331, 352, 363, 367, 369, 371, 373, 384, 390, 394, 395, 396, 399, 405, 409
population growth, 319, 328
poverty, 294, 304, 312, 354, 367, 390, 392, 393, 395, 407, 410, 411
preparation, 8, 43, 50, 59, 159, 275, 358, 408
preparedness, 3, 4, 7, 8, 32, 36, 42, 90, 108, 111, 113, 125, 130
prescription drugs, 299
present value, 316, 325
prevention, viii, ix, x, 178, 180, 182, 183, 185, 186, 187, 190, 192, 201, 202, 203, 204, 205, 206, 209, 210, 211, 212, 213, 214, 215, 216, 218, 219, 220, 221, 222, 223, 329, 330, 331, 332, 333, 334, 335, 336, 337, 338, 339, 340, 341, 342, 343, 344, 345, 346, 358
price competition, 16
price index, 314, 318, 320
primary data, x, 290, 291
principles, 75, 79, 80, 96, 97, 104, 118, 185, 208, 225, 226
private sector, 7, 86, 88, 91, 92, 94, 188, 223, 245, 310, 314, 315, 320, 418
protection, 78, 84, 85, 86, 87, 91, 92, 93, 94, 109, 111, 180, 192, 201, 205, 214, 215, 226, 291, 292
protective factors, 335
protective mechanisms, 192
public administration, 372, 394, 415, 419
public assistance, 38, 41, 312
public awareness, 115
public goods, 319, 325, 326
public health, 79, 83, 84, 85, 88, 118, 331, 341

Q

quality assurance, 28, 335
quality of service, 326
questionnaire, ix, 236, 237, 239, 244, 245, 246, 247, 250, 251, 252, 391

R

race, 354, 363, 367, 374, 376, 390, 392, 393, 397, 398, 406, 407, 415
rate of return, 305, 308, 309, 315, 327, 328
real estate, 314, 318, 322, 324, 381
real time, 52, 59, 93
recommendations, x, 2, 4, 5, 11, 27, 31, 32, 33, 39, 50, 69, 70, 74, 75, 77, 78, 80, 88, 93, 95, 109, 110, 111, 113, 115, 116, 117, 118, 119, 120, 122, 125, 140, 153, 155, 158, 178, 180, 181, 183, 188, 190, 204, 205, 218, 219, 220, 222, 255, 256, 257, 258, 259, 269, 271, 272, 273, 275, 278, 282, 330, 335, 345, 346, 352, 362, 365, 387
recovery, ix, 3, 4, 9, 10, 12, 28, 36, 41, 90, 113, 224, 225, 226, 227, 243, 255, 259, 261, 267, 280
regulations, xi, 39, 88, 96, 129, 226, 352, 354, 355, 356, 357, 358, 360, 361, 362, 366, 368, 383, 389, 392, 400, 401, 402, 403, 404, 405, 406, 407
regulatory requirements, 97, 224
reliability, 4, 37, 80, 110, 112, 115, 139, 223, 271, 281, 356, 394, 396, 397, 398, 399, 401
remediation, 222, 264, 415
repair, 19, 43, 226, 264, 266, 271, 274, 282, 358
requirements, viii, x, 4, 5, 8, 9, 10, 11, 15, 16, 17, 18, 19, 20, 21, 25, 28, 29, 31, 33, 36, 37, 39, 58, 64, 91, 101, 138, 140, 141, 142, 143, 145, 146, 152, 153, 154, 155, 156, 160, 161, 183, 185, 186, 190, 194, 195, 204, 206, 211, 212, 213, 214, 222, 224, 226, 227, 261, 264, 265, 270, 271, 273, 274, 275, 276, 279, 281, 282, 285, 289, 292, 295, 304, 305, 333, 346, 354, 356, 357, 358, 359, 360, 361, 366, 368, 386, 388, 398, 403, 404, 408, 409, 411, 413, 416
residuals, 323, 324, 325
resilience, 79, 86, 90, 96, 106, 108, 127, 128, 130, 187, 226
resource allocation, 86, 101
resources, vii, x, 1, 7, 8, 12, 15, 17, 28, 30, 31, 32, 53, 66, 84, 92, 94, 104, 106, 127, 128, 158, 181, 185, 188, 191, 192, 196, 198, 203, 208, 212, 213, 219, 220, 238, 244, 250, 262, 267, 275, 276, 279, 280, 282, 329, 330, 332, 336, 341, 342, 343, 344, 345, 384,385, 387, 419
response, vii, ix, 2, 3, 4, 5, 7, 8, 9, 12, 14, 15, 16, 17, 18, 25, 26, 27, 28, 30, 32, 34, 36, 37, 38, 39, 41, 42, 44, 45, 49, 51, 52, 56, 62, 71, 79, 90, 92, 96, 97, 98, 101, 109, 113, 116, 128, 139, 180, 212, 219, 220, 227, 236, 239, 243, 250, 251, 258, 263, 273, 275, 280, 283, 304, 334, 338, 346, 379, 383, 386, 387
restrictions, 102, 354, 357, 358, 360, 361, 366, 368
revenue, x, 290, 291, 294, 295, 296, 302, 303, 310, 317, 318, 319, 322, 323, 324, 326
risk assessment, viii, 74, 75, 76, 80, 86, 101, 105, 106, 107, 108, 109, 118, 120, 121, 124, 125, 126, 127, 128, 129, 130, 131, 138, 143, 144, 157, 164, 165, 166, 167, 168, 187, 225, 252
risk factors, 155, 276, 334
risk management, 79, 80, 86, 87, 96, 98, 101, 107, 108, 128, 129, 131, 201, 202, 222, 224, 225
root, 138, 140, 154, 155, 156, 159, 323
routes, 99

S

safety, 45, 77, 79, 84, 85, 88, 90, 92, 96, 118, 129, 181, 258, 265, 355, 361, 362, 378, 385
schedule delays, 261
school, 310, 335, 356, 357, 360, 366, 367, 393
schooling, 356, 357, 361
Secretary of Commerce, 69, 70
Secretary of Defense, 11, 34, 251, 257, 259, 269, 271, 272, 273, 274, 280, 282, 283, 284, 285, 286, 287
Secretary of Homeland Security, 7, 34, 88, 391
security, vii, viii, ix, 29, 74, 75, 76, 77, 78, 79, 80, 82, 84, 86, 88, 89, 90, 91, 92, 93, 94, 95, 96, 97, 98, 99, 100, 101, 102, 103, 104, 105, 106, 107, 108, 110, 111, 113, 114, 115, 116, 117, 118, 119, 120, 122, 123, 125, 126, 127, 128, 129, 130, 177, 178, 179, 180, 181, 182, 183, 184, 185, 186, 187, 188, 190, 193, 194, 195, 196, 197, 198, 199, 200, 201, 204, 205, 206, 207, 208, 209, 210, 212, 213, 214, 215, 216, 217, 218, 220, 221, 222, 223, 225, 226, 227, 228, 229, 235, 236, 238, 240, 241, 242, 243, 249, 255, 258, 282
security practices, ix, 91, 95, 178, 193, 194, 197
security risks, viii, 74, 77, 78, 79, 80, 81, 87, 96, 101, 105, 118, 119, 185
security threats, viii, 92, 178, 181, 183
self-employed, 371, 373, 392, 397
self-response rates, vii, 49
semi-structured interviews, 183, 214, 222, 223, 401
service provider, 190, 192, 204, 205, 206, 207, 215, 226
services, ix, x, 3, 7, 8, 9, 10, 11, 14, 15, 18, 20, 28, 30, 32, 38, 40, 41, 42, 43, 44, 45, 53, 98, 180, 183, 187, 189, 190, 191, 192, 202, 206, 207, 209, 213, 214, 223, 224, 225, 238, 255, 259, 260, 267, 268, 270, 272, 275, 279, 280, 281, 282, 283, 284, 286,290, 291, 292, 295, 299, 304, 305, 310, 312, 314, 318, 319, 322, 324, 325, 326, 331, 332, 335, 336, 342, 345, 368, 372, 381, 394, 415, 419
ship crewing, x, 255, 257
shipyard workforce, x, 255, 257, 264
simulation, 291, 292, 295, 297, 298, 300, 301, 306, 307, 308, 309, 313, 315, 327, 328
social benefits, 310, 312, 319
social institutions, 335
social programs, 291
Social Security, 12, 54, 137, 138, 140, 149, 150, 155, 168, 171, 172, 181, 183, 199, 202, 219, 220, 221, 229, 233, 305
Social Security Administration, 12, 137, 138, 140, 149, 150, 155, 168, 171, 183, 199, 202, 219, 220, 221, 229, 233
software, 78, 84, 85, 191, 192, 196, 200, 216, 224, 225, 227
spending, x, 2, 32, 223, 257, 290, 291, 292, 294, 295, 296, 297, 298, 299, 300, 304, 305, 307, 310, 312, 313, 314, 315, 318, 320, 321, 322, 327, 328
staffing, 18, 27, 65, 66, 69, 76, 80, 96, 101, 103, 104, 116, 118
stakeholders, xi, 10, 78, 79, 90, 92, 93, 97, 113, 115, 122, 127, 210, 211, 212, 219, 224, 225, 227, 274, 276, 277, 279, 283, 352, 355, 382, 383, 384
standard error, 355, 363, 366, 367, 368, 369, 370, 371, 372, 373, 376, 377, 394, 395, 396, 399, 402, 403, 404, 406, 407, 408, 410, 411, 412, 413, 418, 419
storage, 24, 45, 81, 83, 96, 192, 285, 286, 358, 359
structure, x, 7, 62, 71, 86, 109, 110, 255, 257, 258, 266, 272, 279, 283, 341, 346
subgroups, 363, 394
submarine fleet, ix, 255, 257, 261, 272, 273
submarines, 261, 262, 263, 264, 266, 267, 273
Subsidies, 311, 312
subsidy, 294, 319, 320, 322
substance abuse, 335
suicide, v, x, 329, 330, 331, 332, 333, 334, 335, 336, 337, 338, 339, 340, 341, 342, 343, 344, 345, 346
suicide prevention, v, x, 329, 330, 331, 332, 333, 334, 335, 336, 337, 338, 339, 340, 341, 342, 343, 344, 345, 346
supply chain, 98, 127, 130, 224, 225, 271, 274, 283, 285
support services, 41, 42, 43, 45, 335, 344, 384
surplus, 293, 306, 307, 308, 310, 311, 312, 313, 319, 322

T

target, 92, 102, 103, 112, 114, 115, 155, 157, 164, 165, 166, 167, 168, 169, 170, 198, 200, 229, 242, 270, 276, 331, 340, 343, 344, 365
target number, 114
tax base, 291, 301
tax collection, 303
tax increase, 292, 296
tax rates, 303
tax system, 303
taxes, 291, 295, 296, 301, 302, 303, 310, 311, 317, 318, 319
technical assistance, 45, 208
technical comments, 33, 50, 70, 120, 139, 160, 220, 248, 346, 388
techniques, 85, 92, 124, 126, 334, 338, 383
technological advancement, 242

technologies, 84, 107, 130, 179, 180, 187, 198, 203, 211, 212, 218, 220, 226, 239, 242, 245, 252
technology, ix, 57, 93, 124, 181, 196, 229, 235, 238, 242, 276
telecommunications, 18, 28, 30, 42
terrorism, 85, 86, 90, 92, 111, 127, 243
terrorist attack, 77, 97, 101, 109, 111, 113, 243
test planning, vii, 49, 71
test procedure, 50, 56, 68
test scores, 59
testing, 4, 24, 37, 52, 54, 55, 56, 58, 59, 61, 62, 64, 65, 67, 68, 69, 71, 80, 91, 201, 225, 227, 394, 396, 401
threat assessment, 79, 92, 97, 101, 126
threats, ix, 74, 76, 77, 84, 86, 87, 88, 91, 92, 93, 101, 105, 106, 125, 126, 128, 129, 178, 179, 180, 181, 187, 188, 189, 190, 198, 204, 206, 207, 208, 211, 212, 216, 218, 219, 235, 236, 237, 238, 239, 241, 242, 243, 244, 245, 246, 249, 250, 251, 252, 257, 259, 260, 271
time frame, 16, 51, 53, 103, 188, 213, 218, 219, 220, 238, 239, 249, 250, 275, 280, 313, 315, 333, 335, 396
training, vii, 5, 15, 17, 23, 30, 31, 32, 33, 34, 39, 41, 49, 50, 57, 58, 59, 60, 64, 65, 66, 67, 69, 70, 71, 104, 111, 113, 115, 178, 180, 192, 198, 203, 208, 209, 213, 214, 218, 220, 222, 256, 257, 258, 260, 261, 262, 264, 270, 275, 276, 280, 281, 360, 361, 362,365, 384, 385, 386
transfer payments, 311, 312, 313, 320, 322
transportation, 7, 8, 28, 29, 42, 44, 77, 86, 88, 90, 92, 93, 94, 99, 101, 102, 105, 107, 110, 111, 127, 129, 130, 243, 300, 310, 357, 358, 374, 414, 416, 419
transportation infrastructure, 107, 110, 129
transportation security, 90, 130, 243
Treasury, 12, 138, 139, 149, 150, 151, 152, 153, 154, 155, 160, 183, 199, 202, 219, 221, 314, 317, 318, 322, 325
treatment, 310, 335, 375, 376, 377, 378, 398, 399
Trust Fund, 170, 289, 290, 293, 294, 296, 297, 298, 299, 301, 302, 305, 306, 307, 308, 309, 314, 327, 328
turnover, 20, 24, 330, 340, 342, 345, 346

U

U.S. Army Corps of Engineers, 1, 2, 3, 13, 14, 28, 34, 36, 38, 40, 45, 157, 165, 169, 172
U.S. Department of Agriculture, 138, 139, 150, 152, 153, 164, 169, 351, 355, 363, 364, 369, 377, 390, 391
U.S. Department of Commerce, 88, 310, 352
U.S. Department of Labor, 351, 398
U.S. economy, 118
U.S. history, 8
U.S. policy, 88
United States, v, vi, vii, ix, x, xi, 1, 3, 6, 7, 28, 34, 35, 49, 68, 73, 74, 79, 81, 82, 84, 90, 123, 127, 137, 141, 142, 160, 174, 177, 178, 181, 184, 186, 235, 236, 237, 238, 239, 240, 241, 243, 244, 245, 246, 248, 249, 255, 257, 289, 299, 329, 331, 339, 340, 351, 352, 353, 354, 363, 364, 366, 378, 387, 389, 390, 391, 392, 395, 396, 402, 405, 409, 411, 413

V

veterans, x, 12, 112, 150, 157, 160, 167, 170, 172, 183, 199, 202, 219, 221, 223, 228, 263, 329, 330, 331, 332, 334, 335, 336, 337, 338, 339, 341, 342, 343, 344, 345, 346, 347
vulnerability, 76, 78, 80, 86, 92, 96, 97, 101, 105, 106, 107, 109, 110, 114, 115, 118, 120, 121, 124, 125, 126, 128, 129, 130, 190, 191, 204, 206, 216, 226, 243

W

wages, 294, 300, 309, 313, 314, 315, 316, 318, 319, 320
weapon system sustainment, x, 255, 257, 267, 272, 274
weapons, ix, 83, 235, 236, 238, 242, 243, 244, 246, 247, 251, 252
weapons of mass destruction, 242, 243
work activities, 358, 368
workers, 242, 262, 264, 269, 294, 296, 299, 312, 353, 354, 356, 358, 361, 363, 364, 369, 370, 371, 373, 374, 375, 376, 377, 378, 379, 380, 387, 388, 390, 391, 393, 395, 396, 397, 398, 399, 408, 409, 410, 411, 412, 418
workforce, x, 7, 42, 50, 52, 65, 71, 74, 76, 80, 101, 104, 118, 119, 121, 224, 255, 257, 264, 300, 316, 355, 371, 373, 390, 396
working children, vi, x, 351, 352, 353, 354, 355, 356, 363, 364, 365, 366, 367, 368, 369, 370, 371, 372, 373, 374, 378, 383, 385, 387, 388, 390, 392, 393, 394, 395, 396, 397, 399, 403, 406, 407, 408, 409, 418, 419
working conditions, 379, 386, 389
workplace, 361, 374, 377, 382, 385, 397, 398
work-related injuries, x, 352, 353, 355, 364, 370, 374, 375, 376, 377, 378, 387, 397, 398, 415, 417, 418